D1590179

Tissue Engineering

Tissue Engineering

*Engineering Principles for the Design of
Replacement Organs and Tissues*

W. MARK SALTZMAN

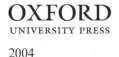

UNIVERSITY PRESS

2004

OXFORD
UNIVERSITY PRESS

Oxford   New York
Auckland   Bangkok   Buenos Aires   Cape Town   Chennai
Dar es Salaam   Delhi   Hong Kong   Istanbul   Karachi   Kolkata
Kuala Lumpur   Madrid   Melbourne   Mexico City   Mumbai   Nairobi
São Paulo   Shanghai   Taipei   Tokyo   Toronto

Published by Oxford University Press, Inc.,
198 Madison Avenue, New York, New York, 10016

www.oup.com

Oxford is a registered trademark of Oxford University Press

Library of Congress Cataloging-in-Publication Data
Saltzman, W. Mark.
Tissue engineering: engineering principles for the design of replacement organs and
tissues / W. Mark Saltzman
p. cm.
Includes bibliographical references and index.
ISBN 0-19-514130-X
1. Tissue engineering.   I. Title.

R857.T55S358 2004
617.9'5—dc21   2003049865

9 8 7 6 5 4 3 2 1
Printed in the United States of America
on acid-free paper

To Melissa,
my best friend during the years that fell into this text

Preface

What It Means to Me

It is awkward to admit that, although I have now written a book on the subject, I am reluctant to tell people that tissue engineering is one of my primary academic interests. It is a reluctance of the heart, not the head, although several practical reasons for this aversion have occurred to me. Tissue engineering is difficult to define. There are few examples of successful tissue engineering that one can use to illustrate a definition; therefore, telling someone that you are a tissue engineer can lead to a long and unsatisfying conversation. Sometimes, in the right company, I feel like a lengthy conversation; now, on those other occasions, I can recommend this book. There is another emotional barrier: the concept of making replacement tissues sounds so fantastic, insinuating science fiction more than actual engineering practice, that I find it difficult to stake so bold a claim.

In spite of these reservations, I am certain that tissue engineering is a concept whose time has arrived. Within its embrace is the real possibility of new tools for plastic surgery, for treatment of diabetes, for repair of spinal cord injuries; these new discoveries will change the length and quality of life of many individuals in the coming decades. In breaking the subject down into chapters and headings, I hope that tissue engineering will become accessible to anyone interested in engineering and modern medicine. The goals of tissue engineering are grand and important and increasingly achievable; even a modest step toward progress in the area is worthy of effort and sacrifice.

Tissue Engineering is my second book; my first, *Drug Delivery*, was published in 2001. These two books were born conjoined, in the early 1990s, as a single project with the working title "Biomaterials for Drug Delivery and Tissue Engineering" (affectionately, BDDTE). Five years of work on this initial project earned me two bulging notebooks of chapter drafts and little hope that they could be corralled to even a tentative conclusion. I was fortunate to have two advisors at that time, Doug Lauffenburger of MIT and Bob Rogers, then of Oxford University Press, who, at a breakfast meeting on a mid-November Chicago day, confirmed my suspicion that my ambition for BDDTE was running far ahead of my accomplishment. One possible solution was to split the project, publish *Drug Delivery* first (since it was the more manageable of the two subjects), and leave *Tissue Engineering* to ripen and (hopefully) find its own path to harvest.

That *Tissue Engineering* survived, and even prospered, is due largely to the generosity of the Whitaker Foundation, which provided a grant that permitted me to take a two-semester sabbatical during the 2000–2001 academic year. The most important elements of this book—the themes that toil to hold it together—were developed during that period. I am grateful to members of the Whitaker Foundation for their enthusiasm and support for this project. I especially thank John Linehan, who supplied vital encouragement at several key points and enthusiasm continuously.

My own interest in tissue engineering was born in 1986, when I was fortunate to work with two irreplaceable mentors, Joseph Vacanti and Robert Langer. Bob is a force of nature, and it is impossible to move within his field of action without absorbing some of his enthusiasm. For the subject of tissue engineering, as in drug delivery, Bob is my first and best teacher. Jay is a scientist-surgeon and extraordinary person. He showed me the connection between transplant surgeons and biomedical engineers. He taught me that even busy people can find the time to be kind.

Here is another good reason to be a tissue engineer: you get to have terrific colleagues. Many of them proofread chapters and provided homework problems. Each homework problem has an acknowledgement to indicate the donor (where no one is indicated, I am the donor). I thank Keith Gooch, Linda Griffith, Erin Lavik, Song Li, Christine Schmidt, Michael Sefton, Rebecca Kuntz Willits, and Peter Zandstra for contributing problems from their courses. I owe a special thanks to Linda, who provided some spectacular exercises and also encouraged me to add a section on mass transfer fundamentals. I thank Malcolm Steinberg and Martin Kluger for their critical reviews of Chapters 3 and 10, respectively. I thank Christine Schmidt and her students for their helpful and thorough review of the entire book, which led to several changes that improved the quality of the text. I thank Greg Rutkowski, Robert Sah, William Olbricht, William Miller and Elizabeth Geller for their comments. Every picture saved me a thousand words (this is most acutely true for the pictures that I got from friends): I appreciate the generosity of Guenter Albrecht-Buehler, Kristi Anseth, Peter Fong, Steven Goldstein, Erin Lavik, Peter Ma, and Andrew Zydney who provided photographs. I thank Sylvia Yoo, Chris Anker, Chun Kuo, and Michael McWay for helping with figure preparation. I thank Sara Royce for help with organization and preparation of solutions to the exercises. I thank Kirk Jenson of Oxford University Press for his patient and thoughtful guidance throughout this period. And, with a special enthusiasm, I thank Malgorzata Cartiera, who helped me in too many different ways to enumerate (from proofreading to copying), always with a smile, always perfect and prompt, and always wonderful.

Lastly, I thank Alison Wittenberg for her encouragement, her enthusiasm, and her voice—patient, wise, and soothing—which leads me when I lose my own.

How To Use This Book

This book was prepared from lecture notes that I have used over the past 10 years to teach senior undergraduate and graduate students at Johns Hopkins, Cornell, and Yale. The course issued in different disguises, but always with an accompanying numerical code (to certify and legitimize); it was Biomaterials for Drug Delivery and Tissue Engineering (540.641) at Hopkins from 1993 to 1995, Artificial Organs and Tissue Engineering (ENGRG 606.2) at Cornell, 1997–2002, and Senior Seminar in Biomedical Engineering (BENG 480) at Yale in 2002. I thank my colleagues for allowing me to teach these courses (all but one were done voluntarily as an overload on my regular teaching schedule).

The book is, as the courses were, intended for engineering students. I have found some non-engineering students who enjoyed and profited from the material, although, in all of these cases, these students had strong mathematics backgrounds. Some background in biology, particularly cell and molecular biology, is useful but not necessary. Most students find that they profit from extra reading on biology topics that are unfamiliar or difficult; the latest editions of the Molecular Cell Biology books by Lodisch et al.—or Alberts et al.—and some aptitude with use of an index—are highly recommended for that purpose. I have included background information on two subjects that are particularly important for tissue engineering—polymers and mass transfer—in the appendix. I realize that these tutorials will be unnecessary for many readers, particularly those who are studying chemical engineering, but by adding this background I hope to make the textbook accessible to biomedical engineering, electrical engineering and mechanical engineering, and other students who do not usually take separate courses in these areas.

One of the most influential early papers in tissue engineering was a review, published in 1993, that defined the field by breaking it down according to tissue types and approaches [1]. An encyclopedic and important book, *Textbook of Tissue Engineering*, follows a similar outline, but adds flesh to it by also incorporating chapters on materials science and biological science in areas of importance [2]. Both of these works are valuable and serve their purposes, for introduction and explication, admirably.

This textbook explores the same wooded region, but encourages you to wander along a different path by first presenting developmental biology as a foundational science and then exploring certain areas of biology (adhesion, growth, and motility of cells) that are presumed fundamental to the practice of tissue engineering. It is now possible to write about these fundamentals in quantitative terms, to think about rates of cell movement, to define rate constants for cell growth processes, and to develop models of the physics cell adhesion. Only in the third section of the book are the core elements of tissue engineering—based on the use of synthetic materials—presented. With a quantitative background in the fundamentals behind them, a few readers will be able to distinguish something bright and alluring between the lines in the third section—some rays of sunlight between the neatly planted trees. Write to me: I am eager to hear about what you see in these places.

The final edits on this preface were typed in my most familiar office: the waiting area at a U.S. airport, which is currently undergoing the renovation that seems to be chronic in these places. Within my view are the faces (and too often the voices) of the American traveling public. Rushing, shuffling papers, re-checking boarding passes, eager to get somewhere, many of these people will spend some fraction of their future life in surgical suites, in hospital rooms, or in the receding familiarity of their own bedrooms wishing for better treatments for heart disease, diabetes, or Alzheimer s disease. I am ready to sign off on this project during a strange period for Americans, in which we wait (with increasing skepticism and vocalization) while our political leaders muster support to bloody, and then heal, a foreign nation that might someday threaten our national security (and certainly imperils our foreign oil supply). There are many areas of life in which you can invest your effort; a few of them will make things better for all of us.

References

1. Langer, R. and J.P. Vacanti, Tissue engineering. *Science*, 1993, **260**, 920–932.
2. Lanza, R., R. Langer, and J. Vacanti, eds., *Textbook of Tissue Engineering*, 2nd ed. New York: Academic Press, 2000.

Contents

Tissue Engineering

Part 1

TISSUE EXCHANGE AND
TISSUE DEVELOPMENT

1

The State-of-the-Art in
Tissue Exchange

tissue n [L, *texere*, to weave.]...an aggregate of cells usu. of a particular kind together with their intercellular substance.

Webster's Ninth New Collegiate Dictionary, 1984.

On Arachne, the weaver:

"Oft, to admire, the niceness of her skill,
The Nymphs would quit their fountain, shade, or hill:
...
Nor would the work, when finish'd please so much,
As, while she wrought, to view each graceful touch."

Ovid, *Book the Sixth*, in *Metamorphoses*, translated under direction of Sir Samuel Garth by Dryden, Pope, Addison, Congreve et al. (1717).

It is an impressive spectacle. Multicellular organisms—from fruitflies to humans—emerge from a single cell through a coordinated sequence of cell division, movement, and specialization. Many of the fundamental mechanisms of animal development are known: differentiated cells arise from less specialized precursor or stem cells, cells organize into functional units by migration and selective adhesion, and cell-secreted growth factors stimulate growth or differentiation in other cells. Despite extensive progress in acquiring basic knowledge, however, therapeutic opportunities for patients with tissue loss due to trauma or disease remain extremely limited. Degeneration within the nervous system can reduce the quality and length of life for individuals with Parkinson's disease. Inadequate healing can cause various problems, including liver failure after hepatitis infections, as well as chronic pain from venous leg ulcers and severe infections in burn victims. The symphony of development is difficult to conduct in adults.

Tissue or whole-organ transplantation is one of the few options currently available for patients with many common ailments including excessive skin loss and artery occlusion. During the past century, many of the obstacles to transplantation were cleared: immunosuppressive drugs and advanced surgical techniques make liver, heart, kidney, blood vessel, and other major organ transplantations a daily reality. But transplantation technology has encountered another severe limitation. The number of patients requiring a transplant far exceeds the available supply of donor tissues. New technology is needed to reduce this deficit. Some advances will come from individuals trained to synthesize basic scientific discoveries (for example, in developmental biology) with modern bioengineering principles.

Tissue engineering grew from the challenge presented by tissue shortage. Tissue engineers are working to develop new approaches for encouraging tissue growth and repair; these approaches are founded on basic science of organ development and wound healing. A few pioneering efforts are already being tested in patients; these include engineered skin equivalents for wound repair, transplanted cells that are isolated from the immune system by encapsulation in polymer membranes for treatment of diabetes, and chondrocyte implantation for repair of articular cartilage defects. It is clear from these studies that novel tissue replacement strategies will work in certain cases, but success does not come easily and hybrid approaches involving cultured cells, manufactured matrices, and advanced materials are required.

1.1 History

While the study of tissue engineering is new, it has antecedents that stretch to the distant past. Perhaps a more appropriate title for this introductory chapter is "How have we been engineering tissue?" One answer is presented in the sections that follow.

1.1.1 Tissue Exchange Between Individuals

The idea of replacing organs or tissues is as old as the human imagination. In Egypt, it was commonly believed that this exchange could occur by supernatural forces, even between species, as in the Sphinx [1]. Greek mythology presented the feared and dangerous Chimera, a hybrid creature that inspired modern use of the term "chimera" for an organism containing cells from another animal. Ancient folklore refers to the transplantation of certain body parts, particularly the nose, which was frequently destroyed by uncontrolled syphilis or lost in battle. Indians, including the surgeon Sushruta, performed successful nose transplants as early as 1000 B.C. The Italian surgeon Tagliacozzi performed many successful autografts to the nose during the Renaissance [1]. Skin grafts to other sites, even transplants between donors, became common by the 1800s; for example, Sir Winston Churchill donated skin to a fellow soldier in 1898 [2]. Corneal transplants were developed in the 1800s, when a captive surgeon named Bigger transplanted a cornea into a gazelle favored by his captors [3]. Transplantation of teeth was common in Britain in the mid-1700s and briefly popular in colonial America until it was discovered that the transplanted tooth could possibly carry syphilis and tuberculosis [1].

The "modern" age of organ and tissue transplantation is now many decades old [1]. Kidney transplants were attempted during the 1940s and 1950s, but usually failed due to rejection. John Merrill and his transplant team successfully transplanted a kidney between identical twin boys on December 23, 1954; the recipient, Richard Merrick, lived for 8 years following the operation. Chimpanzee- and baboon-to-human kidney transplants were tested during the early 1960s, but without much long-term success. A cadaver kidney was successfully transplanted into a human in 1962. Liver transplants, performed in animals starting from the mid-1950s, were first attempted in humans in 1963. Pioneers such as Thomas Starzl and Roy Calne developed many of the surgical techniques required for this difficult procedure. The first human lung transplant was performed by James Hardy in 1963. Bone marrow transplants, since they were introduced by Georges Mathe in France in the 1960s, have been used to treat leukemia and other disorders.

Heart transplantation is arguably the most impressive of the organ replacements. Although accomplished relatively recently, there is evidence that the concept of heart transplants existed in China during the third century A.D., in which the surgeon Huo T'o routinely used a self-made anesthetic to permit a variety of surgeries [1]. Alexis Carrel developed the technique for suturing blood vessels and performed the first experimental heart transplant in 1905, when he connected the heart of a small dog to vessels of another dog. Several groups, including Mann's at the Mayo Clinic, worked with this technique. It was eventually perfected, thus allowing complete replacement of a dog's heart by Norman Shumway at Stanford in 1961. A chimpanzee heart was transplanted into a human patient by James Hardy in 1964. The first human-to-human heart transplant—perhaps the most dramatic surgical procedure in medical history—was performed December 3, 1967, in Capetown, South Africa. In this operation, Christiaan Barnard replaced the heart of Louis Washkansky with the heart of a young accident victim [4]; Mr. Washkansky lived for 18 days with the woman's heart.

Plastic surgery, or reconstructive surgery, also has a long and distinguished history, which intersects with the history of transplantation at several key points. Plastic surgery has its ancient origins in reconstructive procedures that were performed in India as early as 800 B.C. The field was established in the United States in the early 1800s, when the innovator and Virginian doctor John Peter Mettauer performed reconstructive surgery for cleft palate, using instruments that he designed. Reconstructive surgery gained importance through the horror of war, particularly World War I, which was a rich source of devastating head and facial injuries. Although plastic surgeons now rely heavily on synthetic materials, the descriptor "plastic" actually derives from the Greek word "plastikos," meaning to mold or give form.

1.1.2 Origins of Tissue Engineering

As in almost every field of biomedical research, research in organ transplantation has been facilitated by the use of cell and tissue culture techniques. The first tissue culture was performed at Johns Hopkins in 1907, when Ross Harrison demonstrated that frog neural tissue could be maintained in a dish outside the organism [5]. Methods for collection, purification, storage, characterization, and use of donor blood have improved continuously over the last century, particularly after the discovery of blood typing by Landsteiner. Genetically engineered cells were first introduced into patients in the late 1980s; in these patients, cells were engineered to express marker genes that permitted their identification in the body [6]. The first use of therapeutic gene transfer occurred several years later, when cells containing an inserted adenosine deaminase gene were introduced into children with severe immunodeficiency [7].

The past decade has brought tremendous progress in transplantation, primarily because of improved surgical techniques and immunosuppressive agents. Unfortunately, all transplantation procedures suffer from a common problem: the demand for viable tissues or organs from donors far exceeds the supply. This problem will become more pronounced with time, as population growth and better treatments for other diseases produce more candidates for organ transplantation or tissue repair. In fact, a staggering number of patients presently suffer from organ and tissue deficiencies in this country (Table 1.1); transplantation, transfusions, and grafts are the only hope for survival in many cases. The ethical dilemmas surrounding the availability of human organ transplantation were recognized early [8], and are still frequently debated. Moral and legal problems will increase in the future as technology advances. Consider, for example, the ongoing debate regarding the use of human fetal tissue in experimental therapies.

One possible solution for many of the tissue and organ deficiencies is the development of better methods for tissue engineering. In tissue engineering, organ or tissue substitutes are constructed in the laboratory—for example, by combining living cells with artificial components—for subsequent introduction into a patient. Tissue engineering is an evolving discipline; a precise definition is difficult, but it has been described as [9]: "the application of principles and methods of engineering and life sciences toward fundamental understanding of structure–function relationships in normal and pathological mammalian tissues and the development of biological substitutes to restore, maintain, or improve tissue function." Alternatively, biologically active molecules or synthetic constructs may be placed into a diseased tissue to stimulate tissue repair or regeneration.

1.1.3 Materials in Tissue Engineering

As in the development of new drug delivery systems and artificial organs, the design of novel methods for tissue engineering will be improved by the use of synthetic materials that are integrated with biological components in a rational manner. Frequently, these materials are polymers (see Table 1.2). For example, polymers are already routinely used in vascular grafts, and better materials—particularly materials that provide key biological signals [10]—should lead to

Table 1.1
Incidence of Organ and Tissue Deficiencies, or the Number of Surgical
Procedures Related to These Deficiencies, in the United States

Indication	Procedures or Patients per Year
Skin	
Burns[a]	2,150,000
Pressure sores	1,500,000
Venous stasis ulcers	500,000
Diabetic ulcers	600,000
Neuromuscular disorders	200,000
Spinal cord and nerves	40,000
Bone	
Joint replacement	558,200
Bone graft	275,000
Internal fixation	480,000
Facial reconstruction	30,000
Cartilage	
Patella resurfacing	216,000
Chondromalacia patellae	103,400
Meniscal repair	250,000
Arthritis (knee)	149,900
Arthritis (hip)	219,300
Fingers and small joints	179,000
Osteochondritis dissecans	14,500
Tendon repair	33,000
Ligament repair	90,000
Blood vessels	
Heart	754,000
Large and small vessels	606,000
Liver	
Metabolic disorders	5,000
Liver cirrhosis	175,000
Liver cancer	25,000
Pancreas (diabetes)	728,000
Intestine	100,000
Kidney	600,000
Bladder	57,200
Ureter	30,000
Hernia	290,000
Breast	261,000
Blood transfusions	18,000,000
Dental	10,000,000

Source: [24]. [a]Approximately 150,000 of these individuals are hospitalized
and 10,000 die annually.

improved performance. Combinations of synthetic polymers and living cells
may someday lead to implantable replacement cartilage, liver, or nervous tissue
[11].

Much of the initial progress in biomaterials was related to repair in the
vascular system, primarily in an effort to reapproximate severed vessels. From
ancient times until the early 1970s, only collagenous materials like catgut found

Table 1.2
Some of the Polymers that Might be Useful in Tissue Engineering, Based on Past
Use in Biomedical Devices

Materials	Typical Applications
Polydimethylsiloxane, silicone elastomers (PDMS)	Breast, penile, and testicular prostheses Catheters Drug delivery devices Heart valves Hydrocephalus shunts Membrane oxygenators
Polyurethanes (PEU)	Artificial hearts and ventricular assist devices Catheters Pacemaker leads
Poly(tetrafluoroethylene) (PTFE)	Heart valves Vascular grafts Facial prostheses Hydrocephalus shunts Membrane oxygenators Catheters and sutures
Polyethylene (PE)	Hip prostheses Catheters
Polysulphone (PSu)	Heart valves Penile prostheses
Poly(methyl methacrylate) (pMMA)	Bone cement for fracture fixation Intraocular lenses Dentures
Poly(2-hydroxyethylmethacrylate) (pHEMA)	Contact lenses Catheters
Polyacrylonitrile (PAN)	Dialysis membranes
Polyamides	Dialysis membranes Sutures
Polypropylene (PP)	Plasmapheresis membranes Sutures
Poly(vinyl chloride) (PVC)	Plasmapheresis membranes Blood bags
Poly(ethylene-co-vinyl acetate)	Drug delivery devices
Poly(L-lactic acid), Poly(glycolic acid), and Poly(lactide-co-glycolide) (PLA, PGA, and PLGA)	Drug delivery devices Sutures
Polystyrene (PS)	Tissue culture flasks
Poly(vinyl pyrrolidone) (PVP)	Blood substitutes
Poly(ethylene terephthalate) (PET)	Artificial hearts Vascular grafts
Hydroxyapatite	Bone repair
Collagen	Artificial skin

Sources: [25–27] [a]Trade name Dacron.
[b]Trade names Teflon, Goretex.

general acceptance as absorbable sutures, although a variety of innovative approaches were used. Absorbable sutures derived from animal sinews were described by Sushruta, an Indian surgeon, in 600 B.C. [12]. Hallowell used a wooden peg and thread to repair a brachial artery in 1759; Gluck used ivory clamps and Jassinowsky used silk and needles to repair vessels in the 1880s [13]. The first absorbable synthetic material, poly(glycolic acid), was developed by American Cyanamid in the 1960s (see [14] for a historical review of this development).

Polymers have been used as biomaterials in dental applications since the last century (see [15] for a review): gutta-percha was used for dental impressions beginning in 1848, vulcanized caoutchouc was used in 1854 for dental bases, and celluloid was used in 1868 for dental prostheses. In 1909, bakelite was first used, and poly(methyl methacrylate) (PMMA) has been used since 1930 for denture bases, artificial teeth, removable orthodontics, surgical splinting, and fillings. Many new polymers appeared during the 1930s, including polyamides, polyesters, and polyethylene. The use of polymers as biomedical materials has expanded enormously in recent years, as described in the following paragraphs.

Catheters are an important tool in diagnosis and disease management. Fritz Bleichroeder was the first individual to perform catheterization when he inserted a catheter into his own femoral artery. The first cardiac catheterization was performed by another brave individual, Werner Forssman, in 1929. Forssman, a 23-year-old urology student, inserted a urethral catheter via the antecubital vein into his heart. With the catheter in place, Forssman reportedly ascended a flight of stairs to the X-ray room where he documented this experiment. This risky but prescient decision eventually earned him a Nobel Prize.

Synthetic materials are critical components in extracorporeal systems for blood purification or treatment. Willem Kolff, a Dutch physician, developed the first successful kidney dialysis unit in 1943, using cellophane to remove urea from the blood of diabetics [1]. The first implanted synthetic polymeric biomaterial appears to be poly(methyl methacrylate), which was used as a hip prosthesis in 1947 [16]. Polyethylene, and then other polymers, were used as implants in the middle ear in the early 1950s. Although they yielded good initial results, local inflammation limited the use of these materials.

An artificial heart valve composed of a plastic ball in a metal socket was implanted by Charles A. Hufnagel in 1952. Implantable cardiac pacemakers were also developed in the 1950s. Research on artificial hearts began during this same period. An artificial ventricle, the Liotta–DeBakey tube pump composed of PET-reinforced silicone, was implanted into a patient in 1963 [17]. A large, bedside artificial heart machine was first used on a human in Houston in 1969 [18]. This device, designed by Domingo Liotta and Michael DeBakey, was used to keep Haskell Karp alive and awaiting a donor for 63 hours. The first permanent total artificial heart (the Jarvik 7-100, composed of PET with a polyurethane diaphragm) was implanted into a human in 1982 by DeVries [19]; the longest duration of survival to date has been 620 days.

Vascular surgeons have been traumatizing arteries for wound treatment since this was first demonstrated by Sushruta in India and Galien in Rome (see historical review in [20]). Hufnagel used smooth, poly(methyl methacrylate) tubes as vascular grafts in the late 1940s [21]. In the early 1950s textile grafts were first introduced, initially primarily composed of silk fibers and then of poly(vinyl chloride-co-acrylonitrile). Currently, PET and PTFE grafts are the most widely used.

Biomaterials have been used frequently in the nervous system, particularly as shunts to divert excess cerebrospinal fluid from the ventricular system in patients with hydrocephalus (see [22] for a review of early work). Miculicz reported the use of a glass wool "nail" for this purpose in 1890. Autologous vessels and rubber tubes were used in the period from 1900 to 1930 with some success (see [23]). Poly(vinyl chloride) and silicone tubing were first employed in the 1950s, yielding better results. Implanted polymeric materials are now being used in a variety of neurological settings, including regeneration of damaged peripheral nerves and drug delivery to the brain.

Today, many medical devices involve polymeric biomaterials (see Table 1.2). Polymers of a variety of chemistries, in many shapes and forms, are introduced into patients around the world each day. Many of these materials are now common: catheters, coatings for pacemaker leads, and contact lenses. In some cases, appropriate synthetic polymer materials have enabled dramatic and heroic technologies, like the artificial hip and total artificial heart. Still, there is considerable work remaining: even the most modern artificial hips are a pale replacement of the natural material, and no patient has survived for long on a totally artificial heart.

The development of improved materials and smarter ways of using existing materials will improve human health care. Our understanding of the molecular mechanisms of cell interaction with synthetic materials has advanced rapidly in the last decade. This knowledge has led to a more rational thinking about the design of materials and the role of materials in tissue replacement and regeneration. One can consider cell interactions with polymers at several levels of complexity (Figure 1.1). Within one dimension, features such as cell adhesion and cell spreading can be examined. In two dimensions, the shape and orientation of cells can now be considered, as well as patterns of cell migration and growth and the response of cells to surface gradients. Expanding to three dimensions additionally makes structural anisotropy available for observation. Three dimensional structures provide opportunities for cell interaction unavailable in experimental systems (such as traditional cell culture) that confine cells to a two-dimensional surface.

1.2 Prospects for the Future

Organ transplantation has increased human longevity and changed our understanding of individuality. "I could live with the beating heart of another." It is an accepted miracle that people of the 21st century can outlive a vital organ, an

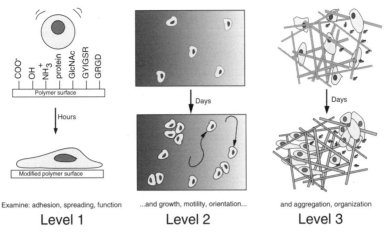

Figure 1.1. Development of polymeric biomaterials for tissue engineering. Biomaterials for tissue engineering are characterized by evaluating (Level 1) cell adhesion and spreading, (Level 2) cell migration and growth, and (Level 3) cell aggregation and tissue organization.

organ suffused with our parents' genes and born in parallel with our own minds; our bodies can accommodate the genes, cells, and organs of another.

Tissue engineering pushes hard on the edge of this reality, asking if new tissues and organs can be regenerated from components, some natural and some synthetic. "Can I live with a beating heart that came from no one?" A positive answer to this question depends on unveiling the mysterious forces at play during development. Tissue engineering can take its cues from the biophysical processes that control development (Figure 1.2). For that reason, this book on tissue engineering begins with a modest review of development (Chapter 3).

Engineers have a unique role in the development of new strategies to regenerate and regrow tissues. Chemical and biomedical engineers are trained to integrate basic biological science (for example, quantitative physiology and pathophysiology, cell and molecular biology), advanced engineering technology (for example, polymer engineering or microfabrication technology), and complex mathematical analysis (for example, pharmacokinetics and transport phenomena). Understanding and manipulating the fate of proteins or cells in humans is a classical engineering endeavor, where basic science and mathematical analysis can be used to achieve an important practical end. Tissue engineers must begin to ask the same questions already asked by engineers of bridges and aircraft: how can this be accomplished efficiently and safely?

This text is concerned with the engineering of tissues for treating human disease, particularly tissue replacements that use polymers as biomaterials. While the development of new chemical entities is clearly important, our approach is biophysical. We will emphasize approaches—which are based on the physiology of drug distribution, cell migration, and tissue organization— for using materials in the most effective way or for designing new materials that are motivated by biochemical or biophysical findings.

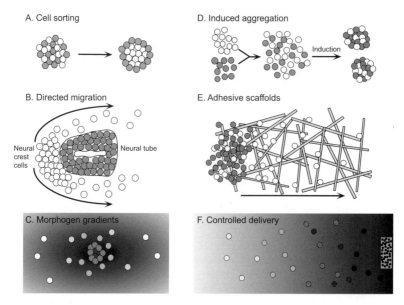

Figure 1.2. Analogies between developmental processes and tissue engineering. During histogenesis, cells (indicated by open and filled spheres) assemble into a functional tissue. Cell assembly and differentiation occurs by a number of mechanisms during embryogenesis including (A) cell sorting into layers, which is guided by cell–cell adhesion molecules, (B) directed migration along adhesive pathways, which requires interactions with extracellular matrix, cell surfaces, and diffusible substances, and (C) differentiation in gradients of morphogens, which provide positional information in the developing tissue. In B, cells from the neural crest migrate around the neural tube and aggregate to form ganglia at distal tissue sites. In C, the white cells acquire positional information by the local concentration of a factor released by the darker cells. In tissue engineering, these natural processes are mimicked using cells and synthetic approaches such as (D) induction of aggregation, which can occur by addition of polymers that stimulate cell adhesion, (E) provision of scaffolds, which control microarchitecture and adhesion for invasion by specific cells, and (F) sustained release of bioactive agents from localized sources. In D, assembly of a suspension of cultured cells, mixed to form the correct proportions, is induced by addition of a soluble cell–cell adhesion promoter; in E, the matrix of polymer fibers supports the adhesion and migration of the white cells, but not the grey; and in F, the gradient of morphogen, which gives positional information only to the light-colored cells, is provided by a controlled release implant. (B adapted from [28], Figures 19–21.)

References

1. Deaton, J.G., *New Parts for Old: the age of organ transplants*. Palisades, NJ: Franklin Publishing Company, 1974.
2. Churchill, W.L.S., *My Early Life, a Roving Commission*. London: Butterworth, 1930.
3. Bigger, S. L., An enquiry into the possibility of transplanting the cornea with the view of relieving blindness (hitherto deemed impossible) caused by several diseases of that structure. *Dublin Q. J. Med. Sci.*, 1837, **11**, 1.

4. Barnard, C. N. and C. B. Pepper, *One Life*. London: George G. Harrap, 1969.
5. Harrison, R. G., *Observations on the living developing nerve fiber. Proc. Soc. Exp. Biol. Med.*, 1907, **4**, 140–143.
6. Rosenberg, S. A., et al., Gene transfer into humans: immunotherapy of patients with advanced melanoma, using tumor-infiltrating lymphocytes modified by retroviral gene transduction. *New England Journal of Medicine*, 1990, **323**(9), 570–578.
7. Blaese, R. M., et al., T Lymphocyte-directed gene therapy for ADA-SCID: initial trial results after 4 years. *Science*, 1995, **270**, 474–480.
8. Porzio, R., *The Transplant Age: reflections on the legal and moral aspects of organ transplants*. New York: Vantage Press, 1969.
9. Skalak, R. and C. F. Fox, eds., *Tissue Engineering*. New York: Alan R. Liss, 1988.
10. Hubbell, J. A., et al., Endothelial cell-selective materials for tissue engineering in the vascular graft via a new receptor. *Bio/Technology*, 1991, **9**, 568–572.
11. Vacanti, J. P., et al., Selective cell transplantation using bioabsorbable artificial polymers as matrices. *Journal of Pediatric Surgery*, 1988, **23**, 3–9.
12. Goldenberg, I. S., *Surgery*, 1959, **46**, 908.
13. Greco, R. S., ed., *Implantation Biology: The Host Response and Biomedical Devices*. Boca Raton, FL: CRC Press, 1994.
14. Frazza, E. J. and E. E. Schmitt, A new absorbable suture. *Journal of Biomedical Materials Research Symposium*, 1971, **1**, 43–58.
15. Bascones, A., et al., Polymers for dental and maxillofacial surgery, in S. Dimitriu, ed., *Polymeric Biomaterials*. New York: Marcel Dekker, 1994, 277–311.
16. USP XVIII. *The Pharmacopia of the USA* (18th revision). Rockville, MD: US Pharmacopoeial Convention, 1980.
17. Liotta, D., et al., Prolonged assisted circulation during and after cardiac or aortic surgery. *American Journal of Cardiology*, 1963, **18**, 399.
18. Cooley, D., et al., *American Journal of Cardiology*, 1969, **24**, 723.
19. DeVries, W., et al., *New England Journal of Medicine*, 1984, **310**, 273.
20. Paris, E., et al., Innovations and deviations in therapeutic vascular devices, in S. Dimitriu, ed., *Polymeric Biomaterials*. New York: Marcel Dekker, 1994, 245–275.
21. Hufnagel, C.A., Permanent intubation of the thoracic aorta. *Archives of Surgery*, 1947, **54**, 382.
22. Davidoff, L. M., Treatment of hydrocephalus. Historical review and description of a new method. *Archives of Surgery*, 1927, **18**, 1737.
23. Nosko, M. G. and L. D. Frenkel, Biomaterials used in neurosurgery, in R. S. Greco, ed., *Implantation Biology*. Boca Raton, FL: CRC Press, 1994.
24. Langer, R. and J. P. Vacanti, Tissue engineering. *Science*, 1993, **260**, 920–932.
25. Peppas, N. A. and R. Langer, New challenges in biomaterials. *Science*, 1994, **263**, 1715–1720.
26. Ratner, B., et al., eds., *Biomaterials Science: an Introduction to Materials in Medicine*. San Diego, CA: Academic Press, 1996.
27. Marchant, R. E. and I. Wang, Physical and chemical aspects of biomaterials used in humans, in R. S. Greco, ed., *Implantation Biology*. Boca Raton, FL: CRC Press, 1994, 13–53.
28. Alberts, B., et al., *Molecular Biology of the Cell*, 3rd ed. New York: Garland Publishing, 1994.

2

Objectives of Tissue Engineering

OUT-WORN heart, in a time out-worn

William Butler Yeats, *Into the Twilight*

Tissue exchange is an ancient art, but tissue engineering is a new concept. The new thinking about tissue engineering is supported by technologies that were developed during the twentieth century, including advanced cell culture, gene transfer, and materials synthesis. Tissue engineering arose from a diverse group of historical precedents that included pharmacology, surgery, and materials science; each historical line of inquiry engaged different motivations and diverse tools. Therefore, as a substitute for a single definition, this chapter observes tissue engineering from several different angles and attempts to illustrate the field by practical example.

The field of tissue engineering can be subdivided in various ways; usually it is organized by organ system, as in hepatic tissue engineering or bone tissue engineering, which are concerned with engineering replacements for liver and bone function, respectively. A coarse subdivision can also be made according to the general objective; most tissue engineering strategies involve replacement of a tissue's metabolic function, structural function, or both (Figure 2.1). Here, several overlapping views of tissue engineering are presented: tissue engineering as a logical extension of contemporary medical and surgical therapies; tissue engineering as a method for controlling the normal healing response of tissues; tissue engineering as an effort to repopulate the cellular component of tissues without replacement of the whole organ; tissue engineering as a variety of controlled drug delivery; and tissue engineering as a new method for developing models of human physiology.

2.1 Tissue Engineering Is an Alternative to Drug Therapy, Gene Therapy, and Whole-Organ Transplantation

Metabolism is a coordinated ensemble of chemical transformations that are individually regulated by the action of enzymes. Many metabolic disorders are caused by the defective production of a single enzyme. It is sometimes possible to identify, produce, and use enzymes to reconstitute missing elements of

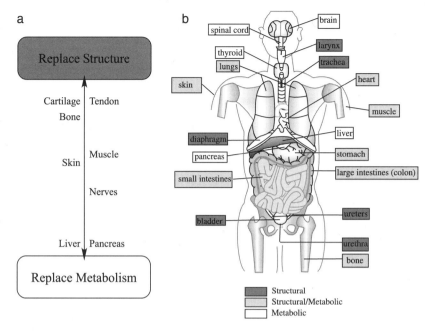

Figure 2.1. Tissue engineering approaches can be subdivided by organ system or by strategy. Here are some examples of tissue engineering approaches, which emphasize the replacement of either tissue structure or metabolism.

metabolism. For example, the enzyme adenosine deaminase (ADA) is involved in the degradation of purine nucleosides; individuals who lack the gene for ADA cannot produce the enzyme in their bodies. As a result, high concentrations of certain purine nucleoside metabolites accumulate within cells; toxicity due to these metabolites is particularly harmful to B and T lymphocytes. Although the mechanisms of disease progress are not completely understood, this genetic defect produces a severe form of immunodeficiency, which results in early death for most patients. Biotechnological processes can be used to produce the protein ADA in recombinant cells; injection of the purified enzyme is one of the best current therapies for ADA-deficient patients.

Replacement of a single enzyme is a useful therapy for ADA deficiency and other diseases including Gaucher's disease and Lesch-Nyhan disease, which is due to an almost complete deficiency of the enzyme hypoxanthine-guanine phosphoribosyltransferase. Gene therapy—in which a functional copy of the gene encoding the missing enzyme is permanently inserted into cells of the patient—is a potentially curative therapy for these patients. In fact, gene therapy is being vigorously pursued for many of the illnesses caused by a single defective gene (Table 2.1).

In other diseases, the defect cannot be localized to a single molecule. For example, liver failure involves the large-scale loss of hepatocytes, the primary functional cells of the liver. Hepatocytes, which comprise 80% of the liver

Table 2.1
Incidence of Single Gene Metabolic Deficiencies

Disease	Enzyme Involved	Incidence	Treatment	Reference
Lesch-Nyhan syndrome	hypoxanthine-guanine phosphoribosyltransferase	1 in 100,000–380,000 (males only)		[4]
ADA deficiency	adenosine deaminase		enzyme infusion; gene therapy	
Gaucher's disease	lysosomal glucocerebrosidase		enzyme infusion	[5]
Phenylketonuria	phenylalanine hydroxylase		diet	
Sickle cell anemia	hemoglobin	0.4% of African-American males		[5], p. 42
Hemophilia	factor VIII	1 in 10,000 males	blood transfusion; protein infusion	
Membrane Protein Involved				
Cystic fibrosis	cystic fibrosis transmembrane conductance receptor (CFTR)	1 in 2,000 live births in Caucasians	gene therapy not yet successful	[5], p. 202
Disaccharidase deficiency (lactose intolerance)	lactase	frequent	diet	[5], p. 1075
Duchenne's muscular dystrophy	dystrophin gene product	1 in 3,500 males	none	[5], p. 822
Protein Involved				
Huntington's disease	huntingtin		none	[5], p. 823

Information derived from a number of sources, as indicated. These diseases are cased by a defect in a single gene, which results in the deficiency of an enzyme, membrane proteins, or other gene product.

mass, are usually lost because of an underlying disease process, such as biliary atresia in children or cirrhosis secondary to toxins or viral infection in adults. When a cell—such as a hepatocyte within the liver—dies, the patient loses all of the metabolic functions that were provided by that cell. Since hepatocytes are responsible for thousands of metabolic reactions (see a condensed summary of functions in Table 2.2), patients in liver failure experience a diverse set of symptoms including jaundice (due to accumulation of unexcreted bile pigments), clotting disorders, and edema (due to loss of protein synthesis). Gene therapy and drug therapy may be an option for treating the underlying disease (if the molecular basis of the underlying disease is understood), but

Table 2.2
Partial List of Functions of Hepatocytes in the Liver

Function	Description
Endocrine	• secretion of IGF-I, which stimulates cell division in other tissues and promotes growth • activation of vitamin D • production of thyroid hormones • secretion of angiotensin, a key hormone in regulation of blood pressure • metabolism of hormones
Clotting	• production of many protein clotting factors • production of bile salts, which are essential for vitamin K absorption
Plasma protein	• synthesis of albumin, lipoproteins, and many others
Exocrine	• synthesis and secretion of bile acids, which regulate fat absorption • secretion of inorganic ions, including bicarbonate, which neutralize acid
Organic metabolism	• conversion of glucose to glycogen and triacylglycerols • conversion of amino acids to fatty acids • synthesis and secretion of triacylglycerols • production of glucose from glycogen and other sources • conversion of fats into ketones • production of urea, the major end product of amino acid breakdown
Cholesterol metabolism	• synthesis and release of cholesterol • secretion of cholesterol into bile • conversion of cholesterol into bile salts
Excretory	• secretion of bilirubin and other pigments into bile • excretion of endogenous and foreign organics via the bile • biotransformation of many endogenous and foreign organic molecules • destruction of aged red blood cells

these approaches are less suitable for replacing the multifarious function of a hepatocyte.

Early technological approaches for managing patients with liver failure were patterned after the success of hemodialysis in treating renal failure. Blood treatments—including dialysis, plasmapheresis, and charcoal hemoperfusion—can remove toxic metabolic wastes from the blood. But even aggressive blood purification coupled with infusion of liver proteins and other supportive procedures cannot support patients in end-stage liver disease for very long. Experience with blood treatments in patients with liver failure suggests that replacement of the excretory function of the liver is not sufficient to increase survival. However, patients with end-stage liver failure do respond well to liver transplantation or perfusion of their blood through living liver tissue. Therefore, replacement of the metabolic function of liver cells is essential for prolonging survival. An analogous situation exists for type I diabetics;

some of the function of the pancreas can be replaced by insulin injection, but the long-term health and survival of patients is improved with interventions (such as pancreas transplantation) that replace the dynamic metabolic function of the diseased organ.

For certain diseases, cell-based therapy is a logical alternative to drug therapy, gene therapy, or whole organ transplantation. Transplanted liver or pancreatic cells provide a readily available source of integrated metabolic activity. For example, each hepatocyte is capable of performing thousands of metabolic reactions that are fundamental to normal liver function. In addition, viable cells can often be isolated from donor tissue and reproduced outside of the body. Recently, direct transplantation of human pancreatic islet cells has been used to replace daily insulin injections in some patients [1].

From this perspective, tissue engineering encompasses the diverse ways that cells and materials can be used to extend modern pharmacological and surgical therapy.

2.2 Tissue Engineering Attempts to Inspire or Control the Normal Processes of Tissue Repair and Healing

The body is remarkably efficient at self-repair. Even the most careful among us acquire cuts, scrapes, and other trauma during the routine activities of life. In most of these cases, the body initiates a process that leads to rapid, and usually complete, repair of the wounded tissue (Figure 2.2). In some cases, such as the

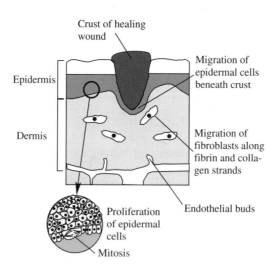

Figure 2.2. Tissue engineering involves control of healing. Sometimes the body can repair itself, but the control mechanisms are inadequate. When the tissue response is overly aggressive, as in the healing of minor skin wounds, a scar is formed. When the tissue response is inadequate, as in the cases of excessive skin loss, the normal process of regeneration cannot replace tissue function quickly enough.

excessive loss of tissue that occurs with severe burns, the repair mechanisms are not sufficient. Without intensive care, burn patients will die from infection or fluid loss before an adequate repair has occurred. In other cases, wound healing can be overly aggressive, resulting in scars or residual wound repair tissue that can impair the aesthetics and function of the repaired tissue.

An important aspect of tissue engineering is the search for methods to control the normal processes of wound healing and repair. Tissue engineers are exploring a number of strategies for control of healing; some of these strategies involve cell replacement, some involve synthetic materials, and some involve a combination (Figure 2.3). When only cells are employed, the cells must produce their own supportive matrix and must integrate with the existing tissue. When only materials are used, migration of cells into the desired area is often essential for repair. When materials and cells are applied simultaneously, there may by an evolution of the tissue construct in culture or an evolution of the tissue structure in situ. A basic tenet of tissue engineering is

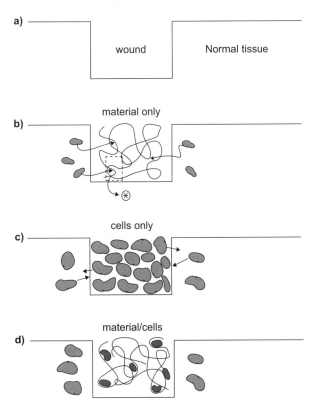

Figure 2.3. Materials and cells for repair of a tissue defect. Schematic of a wound site (a), showing tissue engineering by the use of cells only (b), material only (c), or material and cell combinations (d). (*) See the detail of the inset region provided in Figure 2.10.

that the material can provide signals or cues which guide the development of this normal tissue structure. But, in all of these cases, natural wound healing processes are essential for the formation of correct tissue structure.

Manipulation of wound healing is also an ancient practice. The long history of tissue autografts for repair was outlined in Chapter 1. More recently, physicians have begun to experiment with the use of cellular autografts: chondrocytes for cartilage defects (Genzyme Tissue Repair, $> 1,000$ patients); adrenal medullary cells and fetal neurons for Parkinson's disease; stem cells for corneal reconstruction [2, 3]; and pancreatic islets for diabetes [1].

Cell/polymer constructs are also being explored for the creation of replacement tissue; in some cases this may lead to approaches for adding mixtures of cells and synthetic components to a site of tissue damage in an effort to facilitate regeneration. An example of this approach includes the development of polymeric guides to aid in nerve repair (Figure 2.4). Here, the materials serve to isolate a "tissue compartment," defining the region of the body in which repair should occur. This approach can be supplemented by adding chemical factors or cells into the isolated chamber; components are added as needed to encourage or support the healing response. Alternately, materials may be used as physical supports for transplanted cells, providing a physical substrate that localizes and facilitates cell function. Microcarriers have been used to aid in the transplantation of hepatocytes, for example (Figure 2.5).

Another possible result of this exploration could be the production of functional tissues in the laboratory. Is it possible to assemble, outside of a living organism, all of the materials and conditions that are necessary for the formation of a functional tissue? These approaches will be discussed in more detail in Chapter 13, but already there is evidence that cartilage, bone, and liver tissue can be produced and maintained outside the body. None of these approaches is perfect, and many fundamental issues remain to be understood

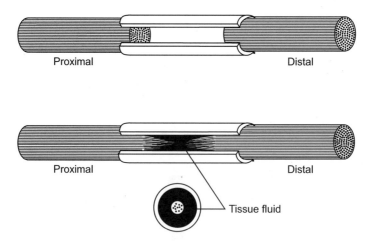

Figure 2.4. A schematic of a nerve guide. This isolates the region of the tissue in which regeneration is desired (adapted from [6]).

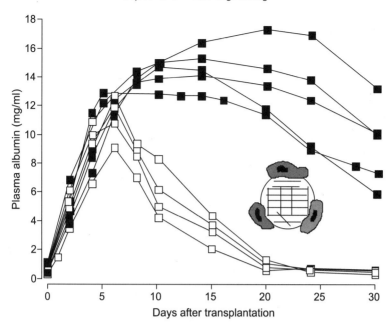

Figure 2.5. Albumin production after transplantation of hepatocytes on microspheres. Adapted from Figure 1 of [7], the graph shows albumin production by transplanted cells (into rats that are naturally deficient in albumin). The open symbols represent animals that did not receive immunosuppression; the closed symbols represent animals that did receive immunosuppression, which prolonged the life of the transplanted cells.

including the choice of materials, control of the culture conditions, timing of implantation, immunosuppression, and the source of the living cells.

Therefore, tissue engineering involves the design of new methods to control the normal processes of healing and tissue repair.

2.3 Tissue Engineering Attempts to Replace Cells that are Missing Within an Otherwise Functional Tissue or Organ

Sometimes, cells can be introduced into the body by injection or infusion. We have long experience with transfusion of blood and the cellular components of blood (see Chapter 10). Cell injection into the circulation is an obvious approach for replacement of cells that operate in the bloodstream, including red blood cells and platelets. In addition, some cells that are introduced into the circulation will crawl into tissues at certain sites of the body, through natural processes of cellular homing. For example, bone marrow precursor cells can be injected into the bloodstream of patients with depleted marrow; the injected cells will find their way to appropriate sites and reconstitute the marrow.

In other cases, it may be useful to inject cells directly into a tissue site where they are needed. For example, neurosurgeons have been injecting dopaminergic cells into the brain to replace the cells lost during Parkinson's disease. Some of the biological signals that ordinarily prohibit exchange of tissues are understood; many of these signals can be overcome by tissue matching or immunosuppression. Tissue engineering may play an important role in these new therapies by identifying new ways to grow cells—perhaps cells collected from a healthy tissue of the person needing treatment—for use in subsequent cellular therapies. An important aspect of tissue engineering is the development of engineering methods for growing specialized cells and tissues outside of the body. Much progress has already been made in this area, particularly for hematopoeitic and connective tissue cells.

Injection of cells into a tissue site does not guarantee production of a functional tissue. We know very little about the process of cellular integration into tissues. Consider, for example, the different outcomes that one would like to achieve in supplementing the tissues of the heart. The injection of cardiac muscle cells into a region of damaged heart tissue is conceptually simple and appealing (Figure 2.6), but functioning myocardium contains not only healthy cells but also a specialized tissue architecture that is critical for its function. Imagine the practical problems that an individual cell must overcome in order to mingle and cooperate within this complex fabric. Current cardiac therapies involve the replacement of assembled tissue segments; cardiac bypass operations using scavenged vessels are prolonging life for millions of patients with heart disease. But will it someday be possible to inject new blood vessel cells into the proper region of the heart? What if these cells have been pre-trained to form new functional vessels? Although these questions cannot currently be answered, they are no longer found only in remote speculations and science fiction. Fortunately, we are beginning to understand the underlying cellular processes that lead to an integrated tissue, processes that occur during development and adulthood such as cell adhesion, cell migration, and cell differentiation. These subjects are explored in the chapters of Part 2 of this book.

An important aspect of tissue engineering is the production of large numbers of healthy tissue cells and the use of these cells to repopulate damaged tissues.

2.4 Tissue Engineering Uses Cellular Control Mechanisms to Enhance Drug Delivery

The development of efficient methods for producing drugs, such as antibiotics and insulin, has greatly prolonged life around the world. Life expectancy for diabetics increased dramatically after the introduction of insulin in the 1920s (Table 2.3). Life expectancy continues to rise as a result of better methods for insulin production, formulation, and delivery. But insulin-dependent diabetics must still inject insulin every day in order to receive its benefits.

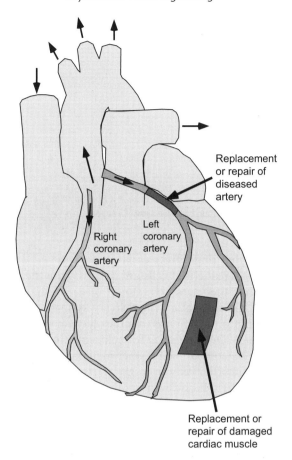

Replacement
or repair of
diseased
artery

Left
coronary
artery

Right
coronary
artery

Replacement or
repair of damaged
cardiac muscle

Figure 2.6. Tissue engineering for a damaged heart. As an alternative to whole heart transplant, or the replacement of heart components with appropriated or synthetic substitutes, tissue engineers hope to produce new, functional blood vessels and to develop methods for supplementing the cellular components of living cardiac muscle.

Cells of the pancreas respond automatically to changes in blood glucose level by changing their rate of insulin secretion. In normal patients, the cells of the pancreas produce insulin periodically throughout the day as a direct response to the amount of glucose that is ingested and accumulated in the blood. Diabetics must adjust their intake of carbohydrates, and their dose of insulin, in order to maintain blood glucose levels that are near normal. The balancing of insulin dose, diet, and level of activity is difficult; most diabetics must check their blood glucose level regularly in order to insure that they are taking the proper dose of insulin to match their daily need. The long-term health consequences of diabetes—including blindness, heart disease, and kidney disease—appear to be related to the degree of control that the diabetic can maintain over his or her glucose level.

Table 2.3
Life Expectancy for Patients Diagnosed with Diabetes Has Greatly Increased during the Last Century

Time Period	Ten Years Old	Thirty Years Old	Fifty Years Old
1897–1913*	1.3	4.1	8.0
1914–1922*	2.6	6.3	9.5
1922–1925	14.3	16.8	12.3
1926–1928	31.7	22.7	13.2
1929–1938	39.8	27.6	14.4
1939–1947	44.2	29.5	16.0

Life expectancy after initial diagnosis, in years. Symbol (*) indicates pre-insulin era. This is a cohort age chart, source George F. Baker Clinic. Analysis by Metropolitan Life Insurance Company.

Many tissue engineering efforts could impact the care and treatment of diabetes. Healthy pancreatic islet cells are able to sense the local glucose concentration and secrete the necessary amount of insulin in response. Islet cells can therefore form the basis of a drug delivery system for diabetics, in which cells are introduced into the body so that they have contact with the blood (or other interstitial fluid). One approach for achieving this contact is by encapsulating cells within a biocompatible polymer material (Figure 2.7). The polymer encapsulation separates the cells from the patient's immune system, so that cells from another individual or even another species can be used. This same concept can be used to deliver other agents to a patient by transplantation of cells that secrete that agent; this idea has been used with neurotransmitters, proteins, and anti-cancer drugs. For the tissue engineer, an important element of this system is the ability to coordinate the need for drug with the delivery of drug by exploiting the metabolic machinery of the cell.

In pursuing this approach, tissue engineering attempts to use cellular mechanisms to control the rate, location, or duration of drug delivery.

2.5 Tissue Engineering Leads to New Models of Human Physiology

Our ability to treat human disease is directly related to our understanding of the operation of the human system. Human physiology has progressed tremendously throughout the last century, to the point where we have uncovered the genetic blueprint that directs all of the processes of human metabolism and behavior. But we do not yet understand how the components specified by that blueprint are assembled into a healthy human. The mapping of human genes, proteins, and other components into the operation of cells and the function of a human organism is the subject of human physiology.

Human physiology is often studied by means of experiments on people, although this approach has important limitations. For example, carefully conducted experiments involving human volunteers can teach us about the relationship between the composition of inhaled gas and the rate of breathing or

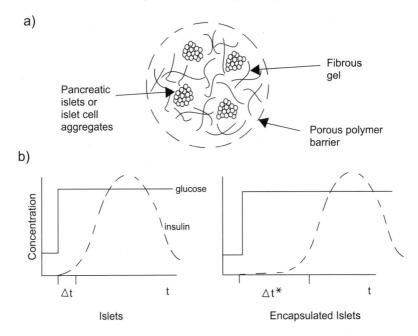

a)

Pancreatic islets or islet cell aggregates

Fibrous gel

Porous polymer barrier

b)

Concentration

glucose

insulin

Δt   t

Islets

Δt*   t

Encapsulated Islets

Figure 2.7. Insulin release from encapsulated islets. (a) Schematic of islet cells encapsulated within a gel that is surrounded by a porous polymer membrane barrier. (b) Islets respond to an increase in glucose concentration by secreting insulin. When they are surrounded by a polymer barrier the lag time for the islet response is increased, due to the extra time it takes for glucose to diffuse across the membrane.

the relationship between gene structure and the incidence of disease in families. But most of the detailed information that we have on human physiology is obtained by study of other animal species, or cells derived from animals, or even reconstituted systems that are built from purified components. Tissue engineering represents a logical progression of this line of study; one of the main thrusts of tissue engineering has been the development of reconstituted systems of cells and synthetic components. For example, microfabricated systems are permitting study of the relationship between extracellular environment and cell migration (Figure 2.8), and microparticulate aggregated cell systems are permitting the study of drug delivery and metabolism under conditions that closely mimic tissue architecture (Figure 2.9). As we learn more about rebuilding tissues in the laboratory, we are also learning more about the role of tissue structure and assembly in physiology.

In this manner, tissue engineering is leading to the development of new model systems that illuminate previously unknown aspects of human physiology.

2.6 Tissue Engineering

Advances in one aspect of tissue engineering provide new opportunities in other areas. Synthetic materials are being used to define the relationship

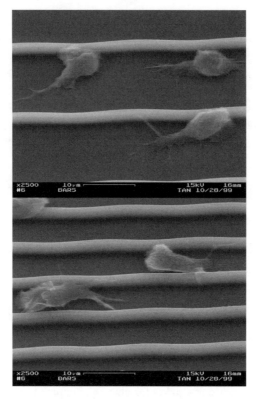

Figure 2.8. Human neutrophils migrate along synthetic microfabricated barriers. Human leukocytes orient with respect to physical features that were produced by microfabrication techniques (photo courtesy of Jian Tan [8]).

between cell behavior and properties of the extracellular environment (as illustrated in Figure 2.8). For example, as described in more detail in Chapter 7, synthetic materials are valuable tools in defining the relationship between extracellular matrix structure/chemistry and rates of cell migration. These relationships can now form the basis for predicting the properties of materials that will be useful in a tissue engineering application (Figures 2.3 and 2.10). As we use tissue engineering approaches to learn more about cell behavior and physiology, we are also increasing the set of tools that are available to improve medical and surgical practice.

Summary

Tissue engineering is difficult to define, but approaches to tissue engineering can be organized around several general principles:

- Tissue engineering is a logical extension of conventional medical and surgical practices.

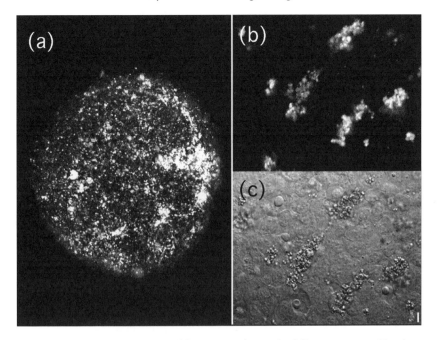

Figure 2.9. Brain cell aggregates with entrapped protein delivery systems. Neotissues can be formed by assembly of cells and synthetic particles [9]. Images of neotissue obtained with fluorescence microscopy (panel a, low magnification; panel b, high magnification) or DIC optics (c). Microparticles contained FITC-BSA; note that regions of fluorescence co-localize with the presence of microparticles on the neotissue surface.

- Tissue engineering involves control or regulation of the normal healing process.
- Tissue engineering attempts to replace or supplement the cellular component of diseased tissues.
- Tissue engineering uses cellular processes to control drug delivery.
- Tissue engineering produces new models for the study of human physiology.

Exercises

Exercise 2.1 (provided by Keith Gooch)

a) Briefly describe the three general strategies for creating new tissues mentioned in the article: Langer, R. and J.P. Vacanti, Tissue engineering. *Science*, 1993, **260**, 920–932.

b) From the applications discussed in the review article, give one example of each general strategy.

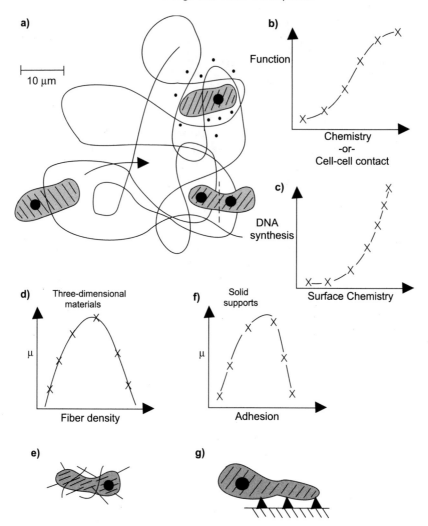

Figure 2.10. Materials properties influence cell behavior and function. Tissue engineering relies on synthetic materials; these can be used to define mechanisms of cell behavior. Assume, for example, that you are interested in using a synthetic material at a wound site to influence the behavior of migrating cells (see * in Figure 2.3). (a) Close-up view of cells crawling into the synthetic material of Figure 2.3. Function (b) and growth potential (c) for attached cells are known to depend on properties of the material. Rates of cell migration also depend on the chemistry and geometry of the three-dimensional material (d and e) or chemistry of the solid surface (f and g). The properties of the material can therefore be used to manipulate the behavior of associated cells.

Exercise 2.2 (provided by Song Li)

Artificial skin may or may not contain living cells. What are the advantages and disadvantages of having cells in the artificial skin? Are keratinocytes immunogenic? Why? If you are going to make artificial skin with cells, where are you going to get the cells?

References

1. Shapiro, A.M.J., et al., Islet transplantation in seven patients with type 1 diabetes mellitus using a glucocorticoid-free immunosupressive regimen. *The New England Journal of Medicine*, 2000, **343**, 230–238.
2. Tsubota, K., et al., Treatment of sever ocular-surface disorders with corneal epithelial stem-cell transplantation. *The New England Journal of Medicine*, 1999, **340**, 1697–1703.
3. Tsai, R.J., L. Li, and J. Chen, Reconstruction of damaged corneas by transplantation of autologous limbal epithelial cells. *The New England Journal of Medicine*, 2000, **343**, 86–93.
4. Sege-Peterson, K., W.L. Nyhan, and T. Page, Lesch-Nyhan disease and HPRT deficiency, in R.N. Rosenberg, et al., eds., *The Molecular and Genetic Basis of Neurological Disease*. Boston: Butterworth-Heinemann, 1993, 241–259.
5. Devlin, T.M., ed. *Textbook of Biochemistry with Clinical Correlations*. New York: Wiley-Liss, 1997.
6. Lundborg, G., et al., In vivo regeneration of cut nerves encased in silicone tubes. *Journal of Neuropathology and Experimental Neurology*, 1982, **41**(4), 412–422.
7. Demetriou, A., et al., Replacement of liver function in rats by transplantation of microcarrier-attached hepatocytes. *Science*, 1986. **23**, 1190–1192.
8. Tan, J. and W.M. Saltzman, Topographical control of human neutrophil motility on micropatterned materials with various surface chemistry. *Biomaterials*, 2002, **23**, 3215–3225.
9. Mahoney, M.J. and W.M. Saltzman, Transplantation of brain cells assembled around a programmable synthetic microenvironment. *Nature Biotechnology*, 2001, **19**, 934–939.

3

Elements of Tissue Development

> Lord, thou hast given me a cell,
> Wherein to dwell;
>
> Robert Herrick, *A thanksgiving to God, for his house*

This book began with a reflection on the miracle of development, wherein a single cell transforms into a human. The transformation from fertilized egg to adult results from a complex tapestry of events, which scientists are only beginning to dissect and unravel. Certain processes occur frequently during development; that is, the tapestry is woven from threads of elemental colors and textures.

A central assumption of subsequent chapters is that key concepts underlying tissue regeneration first appear during fetal development (recall Figure 1.2). The elements of developmental biology are presented in this chapter; more complete descriptions are available in any of several excellent textbooks [1, 2]. The relevance of developmental processes in the study of tissue engineering is detailed in subsequent chapters. One of the most intimidating aspects of developmental biology is the vocabulary; therefore, important words are indicated in small capitals on first occurrence and collected in a glossary at the end of the chapter.

Developmental biology is an ancient science. One of the central concepts in developmental biology, EPIGENESIS, came from Aristotle in the fourth century B.C. Epigenesis is a continuous, stepwise process in which a simple initial structure becomes complex. Through much of history between Aristotle and the present, epigenesis was not widely accepted as operating in development; many scientists, particularly during the 17th and 18th centuries, were preformationists who believed that the structure of animals was preformed at conception. To the preformationist, the embryo begins as a small replica of an individual which changes only in size during the course of development. Preformationists differed as to whether the preformed individual resided in the ovum or the sperm, but they agreed that all of the attributes of an adult were present from the outset of development. Epigenesis is now well established and many of the steps underlying epigenesis are understood.

Human development is part of a larger cyclic process; fertilized eggs develop into newborns who grow to adults and produce new eggs and sperm

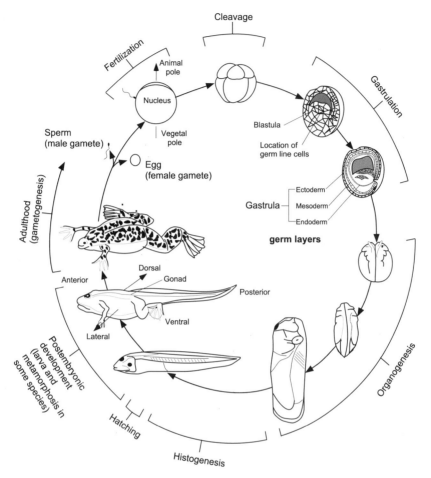

Figure 3.1. Life cycle, including the period of development, illustrated for an amphibian. Schematic diagram illustrating the steps in the life cycle of an amphibian. Human development is different from amphibian development in several important ways, but the basic elements of the life cycle are similar. Cleavage, a period of development characterized by rapid cell division, follows fertilization of the egg. The blastula, which is now separated into a region that develops into the embryo (the inner cell mass) and extra-embryonic tissues, forms by processes that depend on cell adhesion and polarization. Gastrulation comprises a series of coordinated cellular movements, which results in the formation of the three germ layers. Organogenesis and histogenesis are developmental periods in which the specialized organs and tissues are formed.

(Figure 3.1). This chapter will introduce some of the mechanisms underlying human development from egg to newborn. These mechanisms are introduced primarily through examples of development in other species, such as the frog *Xenopus* and the fruitfly *Drosophila melanogaster*, which are more easily studied in the laboratory. As tissue engineers, we are primarily concerned with understanding the events of development for clues that will lead to new methods for regenerating or repairing tissue in adult mammals, particularly humans.

3.1 Early Transformations in the Embryo

The union of sperm and egg creates a single hybrid cell, called a ZYGOTE, that develops into a complete human infant. The zygote is a large cell, but it is not physiologically symmetrical. Most zygotes have at least one axis of polarity: the ANIMAL POLE and VEGETAL POLE correspond to the regions closest to and farthest from the egg nucleus. Zygotes differ among species in size, shape, and distribution of cytoplasmic contents. Human eggs are nearly symmetrical, with a relatively small volume of yolk that is distributed evenly throughout the egg; zygotes with this characteristic are called isolecithal (from the Greek for "equal yolk"). The yolk volume is split among new cells, called BLASTOMERES, during early cell divisions; this type of division is called holoblastic cleavage (from the Greek for "whole germ").

3.1.1 Before Implantation

The signature event in early development is cell division, the coordinated process by which a single cell produces two daughter cells. Cell division persists in some tissues throughout the human life span: for example, cells on epithelial surfaces such as skin are continuously replicated and replaced. Cell division during early embryogenesis differs from cell division during adulthood; the early developmental process is called CLEAVAGE. Divisions are usually more rapid during cleavage (cleavage cell cycles are about 12 hours in mammalian embryos, very slow compared to cleavage times in other species, but rapid when compared to cell division in adults; see Chapter 4). In addition, cells do not increase in volume between cleavage divisions; blastomeres therefore become progressively smaller during each round of cleavage.

Early cleavage occurs in the human embryo during its movement along the oviduct (Figure 3.2), from the distal portion of the oviduct where fertilization occurs, to the uterus. During this journey, which takes about 4 days, the embryo undergoes dramatic changes. Cleavage divisions produce an 8-cell embryo, which is about the same size as the zygote. The embryo becomes more compact during the transition from 8-cell to 16-cell; the more compact 16-cell embryo has polarized cells with organized junctional contacts between cells. Tight junctions link cells on the outside of the embryo and gap junctions link cells within the interior (see Chapter 6 for additional information on junctional complexes); consequently, junctional complexes create a functional distinction between cell populations. The presence of tight junctions produces a permeability barrier at the outer cell layer; molecules must pass through the outer cells to enter the embryo. Polarized cells, with a distinguishable outside (or apical) face and inside (or basal) surface, can participate in directional

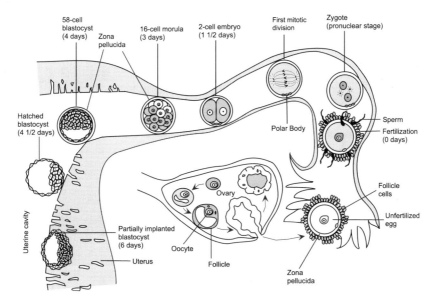

Figure 3.2. Changes that occur during the cleavage divisions of a human embryo. In mammals, fertilization of the egg occurs after its release from the ovary. The first cell divisions, known as cleavage, and the formation of the blastula occur prior to implantation of the embryo into the uterine wall. Figure adapted from Figures 5.8 and 5.10 of [1].

transport of nutrients. For example, cells at the surface of the MORULA, the 16- to 32-cell embryo, collect uterine fluid and transport it into the center of the embryo; this fluid eventually accumulates to produce an internal cavity called the blastocoel. Just prior to implantation in the uterine wall, the embryo, now called a BLASTOCYST, consists of two distinguishable populations of cells: TROPHOBLAST surrounding the blastocoel, and INNER CELL MASS. After implantation, the trophoblast participates in formation of the placenta, the anatomical structure that allows communication between the growing fetus and the mother. The inner cell mass—now assured of a stable, protective environment with a steady source of nutrition—becomes the developing fetus.

3.1.2 Development of Germ Layers

The inner cell mass of the implanted blastocyst develops a new level of complexity by a process called GASTRULATION. In the first step of gastrulation, a layer of cells peels away from the inner cell mass and spreads to surround the blastocoel (the "peeling away" process is called DELAMINATION). This cell layer, the HYPOBLAST, encloses the blastocoel, which is now called the yolk sac. The residual cells of the inner cell mass are called the epiblast; another delamination from the epiblast produces the AMNIOTIC ECTODERM, leaving the EMBRYONIC EPIBLAST (Figure 3.3). In addition to the formation of new cell layers, these

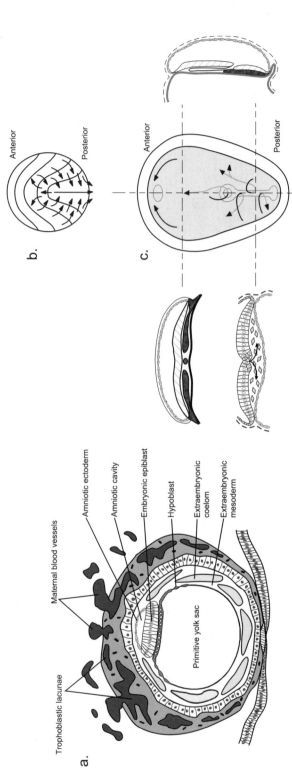

Figure 3.3. Schematic diagram of changes that occur during gastrulation in the human embryo. Dramatic changes in the organization of the embryo occur during gastrulation, a developmental process that is characterized by the coordinated movements of cell populations. The inner cell mass of the implanted blastula develops into the two cell layers, the hypoblast and the epiblast. These layers develop into the gastrula (a), which possesses cylindrical body form and three germ layers. The embryo proper is viewed from the top (i.e. from the perspective of looking down onto the surface cells from the yolk sac) in (b) and (c). Arrows in (b) indicate the direction of cell migration, which causes the embryo to elongate in the anterior–posterior direction, as shown in (c). Also in (c), several cross-sections are shown to illustrate the role of cell migration in the rearrangement of cells during gastrulation. Figure adapted from Figures 10.33 and 10.34 of [1].

delaminations result in the formation of two fluid-filled spaces, the yolk sac and the amniotic cavity.

As described earlier, cell multiplication is central to development of the blastocyst from the zygote. In addition to cell division, movements of individual cells and coordinated movements of cell groups are essential for gastrulation. Delamination to form the yolk sac is an example of a coordinated change that occurs during gastrulation; others are illustrated in Figure 3.4. This type of coordinated activity requires specialized abilities of cells (for example, the ability to move or to generate force; see Section 3.3.5). Directed cell movements transform the epiblast (Figure 3.3a), creating axial elongation and the formation of a central valley and ridges (the primitive streak, Figure 3.3c). Involution and ingression through the primitive streak produce embryonic endoderm and mesoderm. The end result of this complex morphological rearrangement is the development of the three germ layers: the hypoblast is covered by embryonic endoderm; epiblast cells that invaded through the primitive streak become mesoderm; and the residual epiblast cells form the embryonic ectoderm (Figure 3.5). These three layers eventually transform into all of the specialized cells and tissues of the adult.

3.2 Control of Development

The first cleavage divisions produce blastomeres that are similar in size, shape, and composition. But adult organisms possess cells of many different sizes, shapes, and properties. Between zygote and adult, processes of diversification and differentiation accompany cell division to generate cells with distinct and mature characteristics. DIFFERENTIATION refers to later processes by which a cell attains its specialized, mature characteristic form; for example, blood precursor cells differentiate into B and T lymphocytes. DETERMINATION is an earlier event, as when blastomeres become committed to different fates.

3.2.1 Regulative Development or Stepwise Approximation

Some species exhibit invariant cleavage, in which every new individual develops by an identical set of cleavage divisions. In these species, there are no significant differences between two individuals at the same stage of development. In embryos from these organisms, such as roundworms and snails, the distribution of cytoplasm among blastomeres is a major determinant of diversification. In contrast, vertebrates exhibit variant cleavage, which is more relaxed and allows for variation in outcome among individuals. The 16-cell mouse morula, for example, varies in the number of cells within the inner and outer regions (Figure 3.6a). Therefore, control of mouse development requires a second process to correct for the deviations that occur during variant cleavage; this process is called REGULATIVE DEVELOPMENT or, sometimes, STEPWISE APPROXIMATION [1].

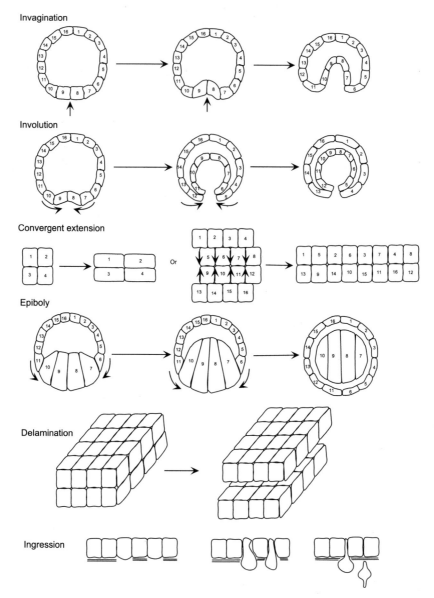

Figure 3.4. Characteristic movements and transformations that occur during development. The types of coordinated cell movements that occur in gastrulation and later stages of development can be classified into generalized types: invagination, involution, convergent extension, epiboly, delamination, and ingression are shown here. Adapted from Figure 10.3 of [1].

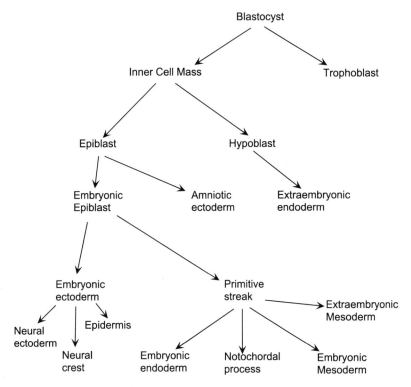

Figure 3.5. Flowchart showing the origins of tissues in the adult from the early embryo. The two layers of the inner cell mass develop into the three germ layers of the embryo (embryonic ectoderm, mesoderm, and endoderm). Adapted from Figure 10.32 of [1].

Control of diversification in embryos with variant cleavage depends on communication between cells; cell interactions modulate cell diversification and development. This form of diversification requires that cells have more choices in development than they are able to exercise. A 16-cell mouse morula has inner cells and outer cells; these cells differ with respect to junctional contacts, ability to endocytose, and other properties. The transformation from morula to blastocyst could occur by a simple process; for example, proliferation of the inner cells of the morula to produce the inner cell mass and the outer cells to produce the trophoblast. But not all 16-cell mouse morulas are identical; variant cleavage produces morulas with between two and seven inner cells. If the simple proliferation process was invoked, the morula possessing only two inner cells might have a problem generating a sufficient cell number for a viable inner cell mass.

Stepwise approximation solves this problem by allowing morula outer cells to join the inner cell mass (Figure 3.6); the number of cells converting from the outer to the inner cell mass varies inversely with the number of inner cells in the

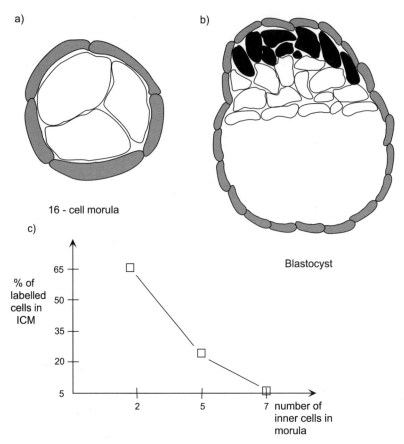

a)

b)

16 - cell morula

c)

% of labelled cells in ICM

65
50
35
20
5

2   5   7 number of inner cells in morula

Blastocyst

Figure 3.6. Stepwise approximation illustrated in early mouse development. Variant cleavage leads to different morphologies at the morula stage, which results in a variable number of inner cells for the developing inner cell mass. (a) The outer cells of the morula are labeled (grey) to allow tracking of their progeny as the inner cell mass develops. (b) The colored cells (both black and grey) are progeny of the outer cells from (a). (c) Morulas that have fewer inner cells develop into blastocysts in which a greater fraction of the inner mass cells derive from outer cells of the morula. Adapted from Figure 5.19 of [1].

morula. In this more complicated process, the fate of each morula outer cell is determined by its position after cleavage and by its ability to interact with other cells, such as the inner cells with inadequate numbers of neighbors. Interactions with the local environment provide information to an individual cell; this information influences cell choice. Stepwise approximation allows for variation in any particular stage of development by providing a subsequent correction mechanism to insure balanced development of the whole organism. But this process can only work if cells, such as the morula outer cells, have the potential to develop into both inner cells and trophoblast cells.

3.2.2 Fate, Potency, Determination, and Regulation

The FATE of an embryonic cell is equivalent to the structure that it becomes. Fate can be illustrated by FATE MAPS, which are depictions of an embryo with the fate of each cell identified. Experimentally, such maps are constructed by labeling cells in an early embryo and observing the location of labeled progeny at a later stage (Figure 3.7). Labeling can be achieved by using dyes or genetic markers; in either case, the label must be passed to all of the cell's progeny, but not to other cells.

Although cells within an embryo are destined, as illustrated in the fate map, most cells are capable of participating in more than one outcome. For example, if a collection of cells taken from any two positions (call them X and Y) (Figure 3.7) are exchanged and the embryo still develops normally, these cells have the POTENCY to achieve either fate X or fate Y. Such a cell is PLURIPOTENT and, in different environments, can achieve more than one fate. A cell that can produce a whole organism is TOTIPOTENT. Experimentally, potency is determined either by removing a cell or a group of cells from an embryo and observing its development under controlled conditions (isolation) or by transplanting a cell or group of cells from a donor to a different location in a host (heterotopic transplantation). With either technique, the observed potency depends on the actual potency of the cell, but it can also be influenced by the experimental procedure. During the period of development in which a cell is pluripotent (that is, still capable of more than one fate), the cell is capable of REGULATION. Signals from the environment influence cell development; external information guides the cell in selection of its fate.

As development progresses, each cell moves closer to its ultimate fate or mature position and function within the organism. At some stage during this

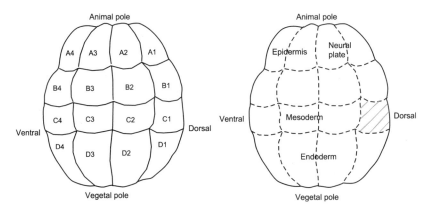

Figure 3.7. Fate map of a *Xenopus* embryo. A fate map illustrates the outcome of normal development. In this frog embryo, the cells of an early embryo are labeled to show the tissue that they become if development proceeds normally. Adapted from Figure 6.2 of [1].

sequential process, the fate of the cell becomes "determined"; the cell is destined to one fate. (Although it was once believed that a determined cell was no longer capable of other fates, it is now believed that many cells remain pluripotent throughout development.) Determination is also a gradual process, part of the overall diversification that occurs during development, in which negative and positive signals from the environment suppress and encourage the pluripotent cell to adopt different fates. Mammalian cells appear to become determined late in the blastocyst stage (Figure 3.2); at the morula and early blastocyst stages, inner and outer cells are biased toward inner cell mass and trophoblast fates, respectively, but heterotransplanted cells are still capable of both fates. Cells, or groups of cells, are SPECIFIED if they will develop normally (that is, according to their normal fate) when isolated from the embryo and cultured in a neutral environment.

3.2.3 Genomic Equivalence and Cytoplasmic Variation

The process of development leads to a complex, multicellular organism in which diverse cell types cooperate to function as a community. But every cell in the adult body, even cells that differ dramatically in function and appearance (Table 3.1), is a descendent of the single fertilized egg. How do cells diversify to accomplish these different fates? Shape and size differences are obvious, but cell types also differ in the molecular content of their cytoplasm. What is different about a neuron and a pancreatic islet cell and how are these

Table 3.1
Examples of Characteristics of Differentiated Cells

Cell Type	Function in Organism	Example Biochemical Produced by This Differentiated Cell
Keratinocyte	Mechanical barrier	Keratin
Red blood cell	Oxygen transport	Hemoglobin
Lens cell	Transmission of light	Crystallins
B lymphocyte	Antibody synthesis	Immunoglobulins
T lymphocyte	Regulation of the immune response	Cytokines and cell surface antigens
Chondrocyte	Physical support	Type II collagen
Pancreatic islet cell	Sugar metabolism	Insulin
Myocyte	Contraction and force generation	Acin and myosin
Hepatocyte	See Table 2.2	Albumin
Neuron	Transmission of electrical impulses	Neurotransmitter (e.g. dopamine, acetylcholine)

A few examples of differentiated cells from the adults are listed, with a brief description of their function and an example of a specialized biochemical that is produced in the cell. The protein or biochemical contributes to the specialized function of each cell. Adapted from Table 13.1 of [2].

differences generated? More specifically, why do some cells produce insulin, while others do not?

Cells can become specialized in two different ways. In *autonomous specification*, the cell is internally endowed with the capacity to achieve its fate; that is, the mixture of biochemicals that are needed for development is contained within the cell's cytoplasm. For example, segregation of cytoplasmic contents during division can lead to daughter cells with different compositions of cytoplasm (see subsequent section on spatial segregation of the egg). In *conditional specification*, the cell depends on an interaction with other cells or materials in its environment to achieve its fate. These conditions can be achieved by a variety of mechanisms, as elaborated in the following paragraphs.

A key question of development involves the role of genes in specification. When cells become more specialized, do they lose some of the genes that are no longer required? Have neurons lost their ability to produce insulin because the gene for insulin is no longer present in their nucleus? The search for answers to these questions has formed an important linkage between the scientific disciplines of genetics (which is usually concerned with the transmission of traits through generations) and development (which is focused on the expression of traits in individuals).

There is now substantial evidence that genes are not lost from cells during development, but that individual cells regulate the expression of genes within their nucleus. This concept, called *genomic equivalence* because every cell in an organism is equipped with the same nuclear genes, is logical, on the basis of the observation that chromosomes are duplicated and passed unchanged from the fertilized egg to all daughter cells. Experiments with heterotopic transplantation, an experimental technique in which cells are moved from one part of the developing organism to another, demonstrate that many cells are able to recover traits that appear to be lost during specification. For example, fully differentiated cells from the salamander eye can produce other cell types upon transplantation into a different tissue environment, thus demonstrating that the unused genes are still present within the differentiated cell. Other examples of cell de-differentiation or re-differentation will be discussed throughout this text. In fact, the concept of encouraging cells to express old, other, or previously unused traits is essential to many practical approaches in tissue engineering.

3.2.4 Pattern Formation and Fields

If all cells have the same genetic information, how do cells within a developing organism know that they are destined to become brain or muscle or bone? The concepts of embryonic fields and inductive interactions are critical for understanding the mechanisms of differentiation and formation of specialized features. In tissue engineering, cells are moved from one organism to another, or from one region of an individual to another. Therefore, the concept of tissue-specific fields may be a useful way for thinking about the changes that occur during tissue engineering as well (how does the local field influence cell development after transplantation? what is the mechanism for generating a field in a tissue?). The concepts of embryonic fields, patterns, and inductive interactions are presented in this section.

Embryonic Fields.   The vertebrate limb is a common experimental system for studying development. In amphibians, the limb and supporting structures arise from a cell region called the limb disc (Figure 3.8), which includes the cells that are fated to form the limb, the peribrachial flank, and the shoulder girdle. If the limb region is removed from the embryo, cells from the surrounding shoulder girdle and flank area will change their fate and become the limb proper. Further, if the entire limb disc is removed, cells from the region immediately surrounding the disc will accept the fate of the limb, shoulder, and flank; an entire limb structure will still be produced. If a sufficiently large region of embryonic cells is removed, however, no limb will develop. The region that is *capable* of forming a limb is called the limb FIELD. In general, embryonic fields are regions of tissue that are capable of producing a particular feature, even though they might not form this feature if development proceeds normally.

Pattern Formation.   Features, such as the limb, are recognizable because matter is arranged into detectable patterns. During development, characteristic patterns emerge from an unpatterned cell mass. PATTERN FORMATION in the limb, for example, occurs as the amorphous limb disc develops into a recognizable pattern of bones and muscles with a prescribed arrangement of digits and other definable characteristics. Some patterns are spectacular, as in the plumage of a peacock; other patterns are subtle. In all cases, patterns form by exchange of signals between cells that are capable of participating in the pattern. To create a pattern, cells must differ in some noticeable way. But if all cells arise from sequential division of a single fertilized egg, how are differences between cells generated?

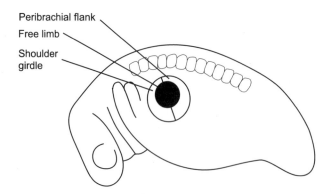

Figure 3.8. Cell regions associated with limb formation in an amphibian. Adapted from Figure 20.3 of [1].

Polarity in the Embryo from Localization of Components in the Egg.   The creation of differences between cells as a function of spatial location is a defining event in development. This process of "difference-making" begins very early in development. The fertilized egg of most species has an identifiable animal pole and a vegetal pole, as illustrated in Figure 3.9. In many species, the first cleavage bisects the animal and vegetal poles, yielding two cells that are equal, or nearly so. Blastomere separation in the sea urchin, for example, leads to two complete embryos. But the egg cytoplasm also contains localized components, which can become segregated into different cells during cleavage. This segregation of components in cleavage division can create differences between adjacent blastomeres that are the precursors to polarity (for example, head-to-tail or anterior–posterior polarity) in the embryo.

Polarity can form in the absence of cellularization. In early development—after fertilization and for the first nine divisions—the *Drosophila* embryo is a syncytium in which all of the cell nuclei are contained within a common cytoplasm. During the syncytial phase, there are no "cells" within the embryo; the entire embryo is a large, multinucleated, single cell in which proteins and other signaling molecules can diffuse freely throughout the blastoderm. In *Drosophila*, localized components are provided by the mother and placed at spatial locations in the egg during development in the ovary. These

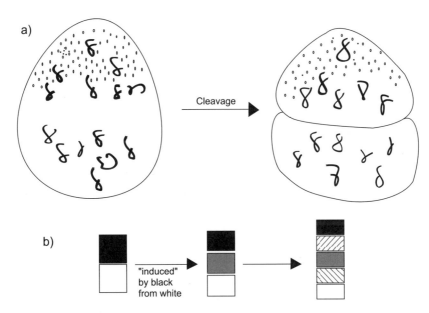

Figure 3.9. Differences arise from spatial segregation of the egg. (a) Differences in the cytoplasm of blastomeres can be generated during cleavage. (b) Inductive interactions generate detail in the pattern produced on the first division. For example, the grey region is induced by contact with both the black region and the white region. Similarly, the hatched regions are induced by contact with unique combinations of black, grey, and white.

components, produced by maternal effect genes, are produced by the ovary during oogenesis and localized within the embryo after fertilization. The influence of one of the maternal effect genes—the gene encoding bicoid proteins—is discussed later in this chapter, but introduced briefly here. Bicoid mRNA, which is provided by the mother and concentrated at the anterior end of the egg, binds to fixed components of the egg cytoskeleton and is not translated until after fertilization. The translated protein is present in the highest concentration at the anterior end of the embryo, nearest the site of translation. The protein is freely soluble in the embryo, so that it diffuses toward the posterior end, but it is also degraded during diffusion (with a half-life of ~30 min); these factors act together to create an anterior–posterior concentration gradient of protein.

In the *Drosophila* embryo, bicoid gradient formation occurs within the syncytial blastoderm. The bicoid protein is a transcription factor that regulates the level of expression of other genes within the many nuclei of the embryo (see more detail in Section 3.3.4). In this situation, the localized production of protein provides polarity to the embryo in the form of a bicoid protein gradient; this transcription factor gradient leads to spatial gradients in the expression of other genes; this polarity determines the anterior–posterior axis of the full-grown organism. Other genes and their proteins act—in ways that are similar to bicoid and in ways that are different—to form the posterior pattern (*nanos* and *caudal*, for example) or the dorsoventral pattern (*toll* and *dorsal*, for example).

Inductive Interactions.   The concept of molecular gradients providing patterning signals in *Drosophila* is simplified by the syncytial structure of the embryo; since all of the blastoderm is connected (without any cellular membranes or boundaries), a diffusible molecule can act in a simple manner. In other species, cleavage produces thousands of distinct cells during early development. Patterning can occur because of molecular gradients in the fluid surrounding the cells, but it can also occur because of interactions between cells. The development of an individual cell depends on its environment; that is, on the types of cells that surround it.

Consider the process of development in an embryo that first forms cells with different cytoplasmic contents in the first cleavage division. Once the initial difference between two blastomeres is established, further refinement can occur by inductive interactions between adjacent cells. To illustrate this process, consider a population of cells expressing different properties, which is symbolized by color in Figure 3.9b. The first cleavage results in one "black" and one "white" cell and, importantly, one cell–cell interface with the property "black/white." The region of contact provides another source of information that can be used on the next cleavage; new cells created in the "black/white" region are induced—because of their spatial relationship to both "black" and "white"—to produce a new cell with property "grey." The development of "grey" cells creates even more potential for pattern formation because the "grey/black" and "grey/white" interfaces also provide specific spatial information, which may induce the generation of cells with new properties. This simple inductive process, originating from the polarized two-cell embryo and repeated through a sequence of cleavages, can yield a multicellular embryo with complex and detailed patterns of a cell property. In the example illustrated here, induction leads to the generation of segments, which occur in a specific order along the anterior–posterior axis.

INDUCTIVE signaling is a means for creating embryonic fields in which one cell region induces another group of cells to follow a particular developmental path. The most famous example of induction involves Spemann's organizer, which is located within the dorsal lip of the amphibian blastopore. (The dorsal lip of the amphibian blastopore is analogous to Hensen's node in mammalian embryos (Figure 3.3).) When the dorsal blastopore lip of a donor embryo is implanted into a recipient, but at a location on the recipient's ventral surface, the transplanted tissue causes the development of a second neural plate. The transplanted tissue follows its normal fate, becoming the notochord and somites. In addition, the presence of this developing transplant tissue induces the surrounding host tissue to form structures associated with the neural axis. The tissue transplant not only follows a developmental pathway that is programmed within itself, but causes cells of the host to change their fate and participate in the formation of an integrated embryonic structure.

The fate of cells within the blastopore lip is determined early in development; these cells will mature according to their fate even when moved to a new position in the embryo. In addition, these cells induce the formation of appropriate embryonic fields at a secondary location. Other cells develop according to their position within an embryonic field, rather than their history. When these cells are transplanted into another embryonic location, they participate in the formation of the tissues associated with their new neighborhood. Rather than inducing a change in their surroundings, these cells are regulated by interactions with the surroundings; their fate and mature function depend on their location within an embryonic field.

Transplantation experiments demonstrate that cell responses during development depend on the genetic information in the cell as well as the experience, or history, of that cell during development. Many experimental observations can be explained by the concept of a POSITIONAL VALUE within an embryonic field; cell fate, in vertebrate embryos, depends on location within the embryo. Pattern formation, then, occurs in two steps: cells receive information from their environment and interpret that information to determine their fate. This two-step process is illustrated famously by French and US flags, in which the two-dimensional flag is analogous to an embryonic field (Figure 3.10a). If regions from the French and U.S. flags are exchanged, then the transplanted regions will develop according to their new positions, but only within the context of their history (that is, they can only express fates that are possible for the flag of origin). In the flag analogy, the transplanted cells will develop as cells do in that particular position, but they will develop according to their native pattern (Figure 3.10b). This analogy is

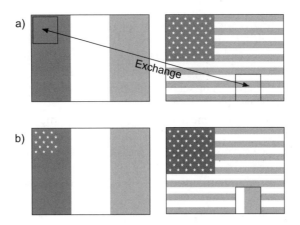

Figure 3.10. French and U.S. flag model of positional value. (a) French and U.S. flags are used to illustrate the pattern within a two-dimensional embryonic field. Colors or shapes within the flag may correspond to expression of certain genes or acquisition of certain characteristics. (b) Heterotransplantation experiments reveal that the fate of transplanted regions depends on both information intrinsic to the transplant and information contained within the field.

consistent with experimental data; when cell regions are excised from the future brain region of a frog embryo and transplanted into the future epidermal region of a newt embryo, a region of frog epidermis is produced within the newt. This example illustrates a critical principle: both genetic information within the cell and the position of the cell contribute to the final form of the tissue.

3.2.5 Example of Limb Regeneration

To further illustrate the relationship between positional value and cell fate, consider again the development of the limb, which grows from a small bud to form a fully developed arm or leg. In adult salamanders, an amputated limb will completely regenerate from cells that dedifferentiate at the site of amputation (the clump of dedifferentiated cells is called the regeneration blastema); this regeneration is an excellent model for studying embryonic limb development. The salamander limb can be amputated at any position—arm, elbow, or wrist—and only the lost parts of the limb (that is those elements that are distal to the amputation site) will re-develop (compare Figure 3.11a and 3.11b).

But how do the dedifferentiated cells in the regeneration blastema know how much of the limb to reconstruct? When a blastema that is formed at a distal site is transplanted onto a recipient with a proximal amputation, the cells in the blastema produce only the distal tissues; the intervening elements are produced from host tissue (Figure 3.11c). How do the cells within the blastema remember their position? Experimental studies of amputation and transplanta-

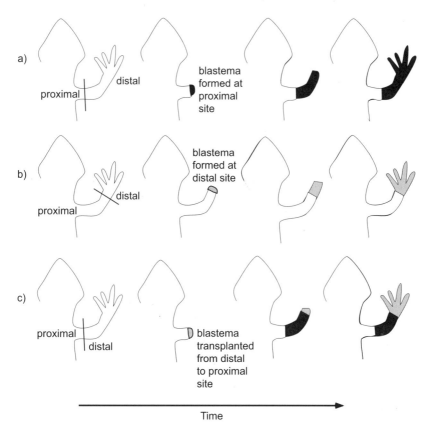

Figure 3.11. Limb regeneration in the salamander. The limbs of amphibians, such as the salamander, can regenerate completely after amputation; this regeneration in an adult serves as a convenient model for limb formation during development. (a) When the amputation is produced at a proximal site, the regeneration blastema is formed at that site (black region in 2nd panel) and cells from the blastema regenerate the lost portions of the limb. (b) When the amputation is produced at a distal site, the blastema is formed at that site (grey region in 2nd panel) and cells from the distal blastema regenerate the lost portions of the limb. (c) When a distal blastema (formed as in 2nd panel of b) is transplanted onto an amputation stump in a proximal location (produced as in 1st panel of a), the blastema cells reform only the parts that they would have formed by following the natural outcome (grey region, analogous to 4th panel of b). The intervening portions of the limb are regenerated correctly, but from cells of the recepient animal (black region, analogous to 3rd panel of a).

tion suggest that cells within the developing (or regenerating) limb experience a gradient of adhesion—extending from the proximal to the distal—that provides information to cells regarding their location on the limb. Limb regeneration in the amphibian has been used to test hypotheses regarding the molecular mechanisms for determination of positional value within the developing organism.

3.3 Mechanisms of Development

The preceding section of this chapter outlined some of the events that act to control and direct development. These events depend on mechanisms, such as cell division and differentiation, for generation of complexity within the embryo. In this final section, some additional mechanisms that operate during development are presented. These basic mechanisms are described in more detail in subsequent chapters, since they provide a conceptual framework for new approaches to tissue engineering. For example, cell mechanics is discussed in Chapter 5, cell adhesion in Chapter 6, and cell migration in Chapter 7. The purpose of this section is to illustrate the profound influence of cellular behaviors (that is growth, adhesion, migration) on development. Later chapters, which dissect each of these attributes individually, focus on understanding each element in order to control properties of engineered tissues.

3.3.1 Cell Shape Change

Cells of an adult appear in an astonishing variety of shapes and sizes (Figure 3.12a). But each cell has the same essential components. What is the machinery that permits this spectrum of morphologies within units of the same basic composition?

The outer surface of the cell, the plasma membrane, is a deformable fluid sheet that completely surrounds the internal contents of the cell, or cytoplasm. If the cell contents were completely homogeneous and liquid—that is, if the cell was a bag full of water—and if the membrane was under tension—that is, the bag was elastic like a balloon—then the overall cell shape would be spherical. On the other hand, if this same membrane-bound liquid bag enclosed a number of incompressible sticks, then its overall shape would depend on both the tension in the membrane and the stiffness of the sticks (Figure 3.12b). For this imaginary cell, morphology depends on the properties of the membrane (for example, tension and deformability) and the characteristics of the internal sticks (for example, their size, number, position, and mechanical properties).

Cells are considerably more complicated than balloons filled with sticks, but they appear to share some common characteristics. The elastic and fluid properties of the membrane have already been mentioned. The cytoplasm also contains a wide spectrum of molecules that probably serve as molecular struts (Figure 3.12c). Microfilaments, microtubules, and intermediate filaments are nanometer-scale fibers that extend throughout the cytoplasm, creating interconnected and entangled networks. The influence of these systems on the mechanical properties of cytoplasm and, therefore, the whole cell are discussed in Chapter 5.

3.3.2 Cell Adhesion

Cells adhere to their surroundings through specialized membrane proteins called adhesion molecules. Several families of adhesion molecules have been

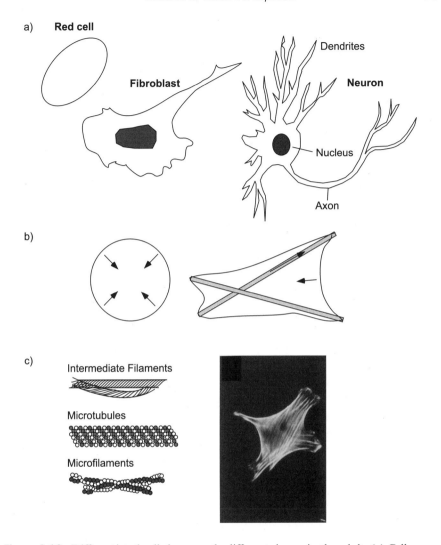

Figure 3.12. Differentiated cells have vastly different shapes in the adult. (a) Cells can have diverse shapes, which are illustrated here by a red cell, fibroblast, and neuron. (b) The cytoskeleton underlies cell shape and morphology. (c) The cytoskeleton consists of a variety of filamentous components including microfilaments, microtubules, and intermediate filaments; the photograph shows a cultured fibroblast in which microfilaments have been fluorescently labelled. These components are integrated within the cell to form a continuous network-like structure [10].

identified including integrins, which are primarily involved in cell adhesion to the extracellular matrix, and cadherins, which are primarily involved in cell–cell adhesion. Cadherins are particularly important during development. The properties of integrins, cadherins, selectins, and Ig-like adhesion molecules are described in Chapter 6. For the present discussion, it is sufficient to know that these molecules enable specific binding between the surface of a cell and a neighboring cell or extracellular matrix. Since there are different kinds of adhesion molecules, and each kind of molecule interacts or adheres only to certain types of counter-adhesion ligands, the overall "adhesiveness" of a cell is determined by the number and type of receptors that are expressed on its surface.

The influence of cell adhesion on morphology of the developing embryo is illustrated by rearrangement of embryonic cells dissociated from different embryonic tissues [3]. Dissociated epidermal cells and neural plate cells are dispersed and then reaggregated to form an initial aggregate in which epidermal and neural plate cells are intermixed. Over time, cells within the aggregate rearrange to produce a final structure in which the epidermal cells surround a core of neural plate cells (Figure 3.13).

Rearrangement is driven by cell adhesion; cells differing in their adhesive properties rearrange to diminish the aggregate's adhesive free energy. The importance of cell adhesion in rearrangement has been best documented for cadherin-dependent cell adhesion. Two cell lines with different amounts of P-cadherin on the surface were produced. Aggregates composed of mixtures of these two cell populations rearrange so that cells are sorted according to the density of cadherin on the surface; cells with more cadherin are in the interior of the aggregate and cells with less are at the periphery (Figure 3.14).

What forces drive this spontaneous rearrangement to a stable, sorted state? Cells within the initial aggregate migrate randomly. Random migration provides a mechanism for cells to leave regions of poor adhesion and find regions of strong adhesion. As cells randomly migrate, they enter regions of the aggregate in which they experience poor adhesion and other regions in which they experience strong adhesion. Once in the strong adhesion zone, the cell is less likely to migrate away from this region. The physical process that accounts for cell sorting appears to be analogous to the property of surface tension in fluids; when two immiscible liquid phases are placed in contact, the liquid with the lower surface tension (that is, with the lower cohesive forces between the fluid molecules) surrounds the liquid with the higher surface tension.

The physical process of cell aggregation into tissue-like units is described in Chapter 8.

3.3.3 Cell Migration

The astonishing transformations that occur during gastrulation (Figure 3.3) involve the coordinated movements of populations of cells (Figure 3.15). The ability of individual units to migrate with respect to the whole organism can have a profound impact on tissue structure, in the same way that the individuals in a marching band can move (either singly or as small groups in coordination) to form patterns on a football field. From the perspective of an individual cell, movement has at least two requirements: generation of mechanical force, and traction with another surface.

Because of the requirement for cell traction, cell migration is intimately related to cell adhesion. For example, the molecular linkages that cells use to

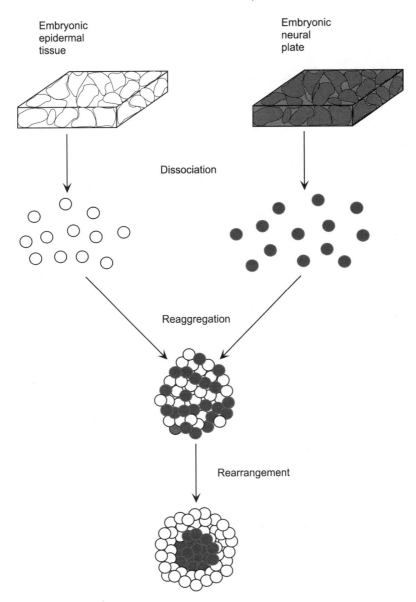

Figure 3.13. Spontaneous rearrangement of reaggregated embryonic cells. Cells that are derived from different tissues of the embryo will rearrange into aggregates of predictable form.

hold themselves to surfaces or to other cells must be able to withstand the forces that are generated during migration. In addition, changes in cell adhesion can sometimes provide a mechanism for directed cell migration. Consider the adhesive situation experienced by cells in the sea urchin blastula (Figure 3.16). Some of the blastocyst cells leave the outer cell layer, crawling into the blastocoel to

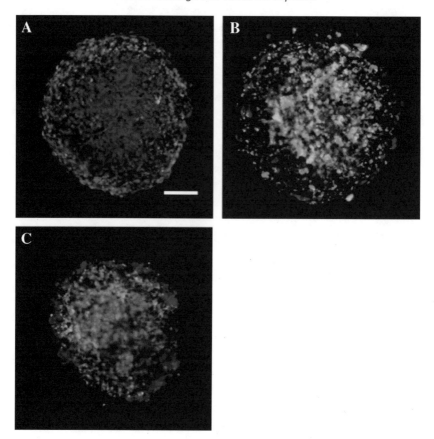

Figure 3.14. Spontaneous rearrangement of cells expressing different quantities of the P-cadherin adhesion molecule. Steinberg and coworkers produced and co-aggregated cell lines expressing different E- and P-cadherins in the same or different amounts [11]. If the cadherin expression levels differed (a, c), then the cells expressing the lower amount enveloped those expressing the higher amount, regardless of cadherin subtype. However, when the cadherin expression levels were equal, no sorting-out occurred despite the difference in cadherin subtypes (b). Bar = 100 μm.

form the mesenchyme (Figure 3.16a). This process of ingression (recall Figure 3.4) involves migration of the cells from their initial position within the outer cell layer radially inward to the blastocoel. Cell migration appears to be driven by changes in the adhesive properties of the cells: the cells that will become mesenchyme become less adhesive to both hyalin (on the outer surface of the blastocyst) and adjacent blastocysts while at the same time becoming more adhesive to the proteins found in the blastocoel (Figure 3.16b) [4].

The ability of cells to move within an organism enables the formation of complex structures during embryogenesis and organogenesis. Cell migration is also a fundamental operation of tissue engineering. In many cases, the engineering of tissue will not be possible unless the migration of individual

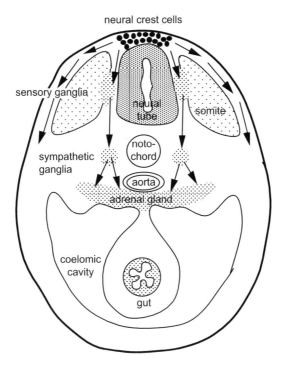

neural crest cells

sensory ganglia

neural tube

somite

sympathetic ganglia

noto-chord

aorta

adrenal gland

coelomic cavity

gut

Figure 3.15. Migration of neural crest cells during development. Cells from the neural crest migrate to a variety of positions in the developing embryo. Redrawn from Figure 16-84 of [9].

cells and/or cell populations can be controlled. Cell migration is considered more completely in Chapter 7.

Diffusion of Soluble Signals

How do cells know about their location within an embryonic field? In the example of limb regeneration, cell adhesion differences appear to provide locational information during development. Soluble, diffusible agents can also provide spatial information. A common model for positional information involves gradients of signaling molecules called MORPHOGENS. If cells in one region of an embryo are producing a signaling molecule, and cells in another region are consuming that molecule, a gradient of concentration is developed (Figure 3.17). A simple diffusion–elimination model is useful for studying mechanisms of gradient formation. Local concentration of the diffusible morphogen, c, depends on its rate of diffusion and its local rate of disappearance within the embryo:

$$\frac{\partial c}{\partial t} = D^* \frac{\partial^2 c}{\partial x^2} - k^* c \qquad (3\text{-}1)$$

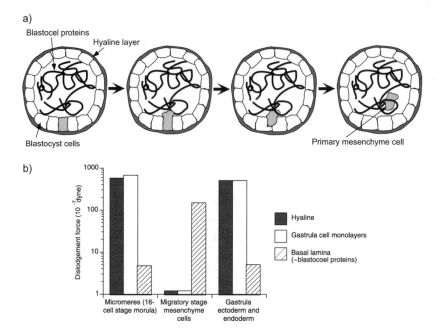

Figure 3.16. Migration of primary mesenchyme cells in the sea urchin blastula. The sea urchin blastocyst consists of a continuous cell monolayer enclosing the blastocoel. The outer surface of the blastula is covered by a hyaline layer. (a) Certain blastocyst cells migrate, through a process of ingression, from the monolayer into the blastocoel. (b) Cells that migrate have characteristic adhesion properties: the migrating cells exhibit a loss of adhesion for the hyaline layer and adjacent cells, and an increase in adhesion for the blastocoel extracellular proteins.

where D^* is the diffusion coefficient and k^* is a constant characterizing the first-order elimination reaction. For simplicity, assume that the morphogen is produced at one end of the embryo at a constant rate and eliminated uniformly throughout the embryo. Morphogen concentration will vary with time and position according to Equation 3-1. This equation can be solved subject to the initial and boundary conditions:

$$c(x, t) = 0 \quad \text{for } x > 0 \quad\quad t = 0$$
$$c(x, t) = c_0 \quad \text{for } x = 0 \quad\quad t > 0$$
$$c(x, t) = 0; \quad \text{for } x \to \infty \quad t > 0$$

to yield:

$$\frac{c}{c_0} = \frac{1}{2}\exp\left\{-x\sqrt{k/D_A}\right\}\text{erfc}\left\{\frac{x}{2\sqrt{D_A t}} - \sqrt{kt}\right\}$$
$$+ \frac{1}{2}\exp\left\{x\sqrt{k/D_A}\right\}\text{erfc}\left\{\frac{x}{2\sqrt{D_A t}} + \sqrt{kt}\right\}$$

(3-2)

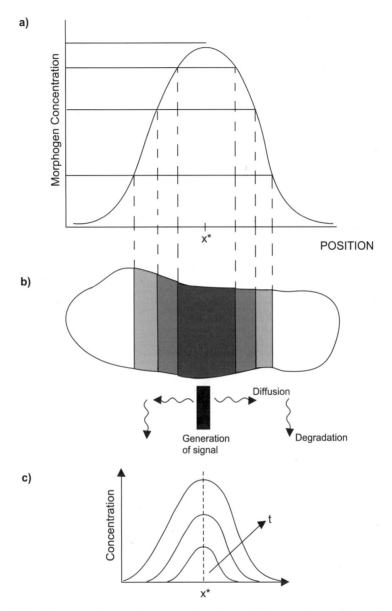

Figure 3.17. Creation of a morphogen gradient by spatial separation of sites of synthesis and consumption. (a) Morphogen concentration profiles for diffusion and first-order consumption. (b) Schematic model illustrating the physical factors (generation of signal, diffusion, and degradation) that lead to formation a gradient of a soluble signal. (c) The concentration and concentration gradient may change with time.

where c_0 is the concentration at the site of morphogen production, which is assumed constant. The corresponding steady-state solution to Equation 3-1 can be found:

$$\frac{c_A}{c_0} = \exp\left(-x\sqrt{\frac{k}{D_A}}\right) \tag{3-3}$$

Concentration profiles predicted by these simple calculations are shown in Figure 3.18. In panel a, the approach to steady state is shown for the situation where D^* is 1×10^{-7} cm^2/s and k^* is 1×10^{-4} s^{-1}. After sufficient time, the transient equations are identical to the steady-state solution. In panel b, steady-state solutions are shown for the same D, with k varying between 1×10^{-2} and

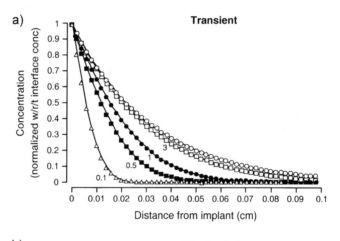

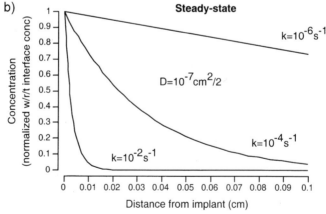

Figure 3.18. Morphogen gradients depend on time, rate of diffusion, and rate of degradation. (a) The approach to steady state is illustrated from concentration gradients formed by a morphogen with diffusion coefficient D equal to 10^{-7} cm^2/s and degradation rate k equal to 10^{-4} s^{-1}. (b) The steepness of the gradient depends on k, which is varied here between 10^{-2} and 10^{-6} s^{-1} for a fixed D of 10^{-7} cm^2/s.

1×10^{-6} s^{-1}. This range of degradation constants corresponds to a range of half-lives from 0.02 to 200 h. Clearly, the rate of degradation of a morphogen within the embryo has a profound influence on the gradient of morphogen concentration and, therefore, its effectiveness in providing positional information.

A well-studied example of gradient formation involves expression of the protein Bicoid in *Drosophila* embryos. Embryos that arise from mothers lacking the *bicoid+* gene do not develop normally; they possess an extended abdomen, but no head or thorax. Bicoid is produced by a maternal effect gene; mRNA from the maternal gene is segregated to the anterior pole of the developing egg, resulting in localized synthesis of bicoid protein (Figure 3.19). Because insects undergo superficial cleavage—and cellularization of the embryo has not yet occurred at this point in development—bicoid protein diffuses freely within the cytoplasm. As it diffuses it is also degraded, producing a gradient of bicoid concentration. Bicoid protein is a transcription factor (Figure 3.19); when present at sufficient concentration, bicoid regulates the expression of other genes such as *hunchback*. Bicoid regulates hunchback expression by binding to sites in the promoter region of *hunchback*; the promoter region has both high- and low-affinity sites for bicoid binding. The affinity of the binding site is related to the threshold concentration required to enhance expression.

This simple model assumed that a single diffusible agent is responsible for providing positional information. More complex patterns can be formed by assuming that multiple factors influence the differentiation of a cell, and that each of these factors is potentially present in gradients. Some analyses of the influence of multiple diffusible factors on pattern formation are available; for example, a model for the outgrowth and patterning of the limb which involves multiple interacting morphogens has been studied [5].

3.3.5 Tissue Mechanics and Morphogenesis

Earlier in this chapter, the process of gastrulation was described as a series of morphological changes, in which each change can be classified as one of several basic types (Figure 3.4). These changes involve coordination between populations of cells. But how are these coordinated movements of groups of cells accomplished? Communication between cells is essential if each cell is to know when to enact its special role in the community event. In addition, cells must be capable of exerting forces that are sufficient to create the mechanical deformations that are required for the change. Little is known about the detailed mechanisms underlying any of the specialized transformations shown in Figure 3.4, but it may be possible to learn about mechanisms by comparing the physical changes that occur with known mechanical properties of the cells and tissues. Chapter 5 will consider this aspect of tissue engineering in more detail, but one example is provided here.

Invagination is one of the fundamental categories of morphological change; it requires the bending of an epithelial sheet (Figure 3.4).

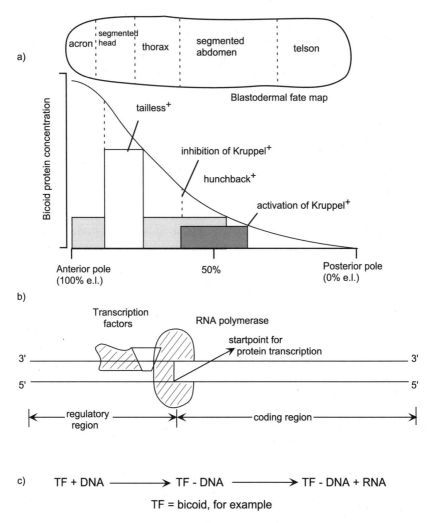

Figure 3.19. Mechanism of gene regulation by transcription factors. (a) Gradients of a transcription factor can lead to spatial localization of gene expression. In this case, the anterior–posterior gradient of bicoid protein leads to differential expression of the genes for tailless, Kruppel, and hunchback. When present at high levels, bicoid activates the gene tailless; at intermediate levels, it inhibits the gene Kruppel and activates hunchback. (b) Transcription factor proteins bind to the regulatory region and facilitate or inhibit the binding of RNA transcriptase and therefore transcription of the protein-coding region. (c) Transcription factor proteins have characteristic DNA-binding domains such as zinc fingers and homeodomains.

Invagination (and epithelial bending in general) occurs during development of all animals, but is most easily studied in some species such as the sea urchin. What are the mechanisms that cause sheets of cells to bend in controlled and predictable fashion?

The answer to this question is not known and, in fact, it is probable that different mechanisms operate in different circumstances. A common model for epithelial bending is the primary invagination of the sea urchin blastula (Figure 3.20). The characteristic change of shape in the blastula is well documented: the flattened ventral plate bends inward and intrudes on the blastocoel. What physical factors lead to coordination between the movement of this population of cells? Over the past 100 years, at least seven distinct mechanisms for invagination in the sea urchin have been proposed; a few of the mechanisms can be ruled out, because they depend on events that are

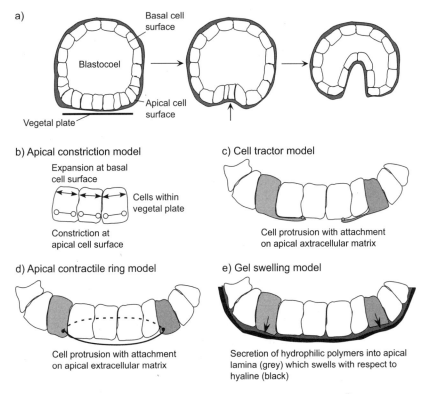

Figure 3.20. Postulated mechanisms for invagination in the sea urchin. (a) The morphology of the blastula during invagination. Invagination occurs on the flattened vegetal plate. Several mechanical models have been proposed to account for invagination in the blastula including: (b) the apical constriction model, in which individual cells constrict at the apical end, causing expansion at the basal end (to maintain constant cell volume) and shifting of the cytoplasmic contents; (c) the cell tractor model, in which cells send thin contractile protrusions towards the center of the vegetal plate that adhere to the apical ECM; (d) the apical contractile ring model, in which a continuous ring of contractile fibers closes, like a purse string, to create the invagination, and (e) the gel swelling model, in which hydrophilic polysaccharides are secreted by cells into the apical lamina, causing swelling of the lamina with respect to the outer hyaline layer, which leads to bending of the sheet.

known not to occur during invagination (such as cell division and generation of hydrostatic pressure in the blastocoel) [6]. Using finite element methods to model deformations in the blastula system, Davidson et al. examined the mechanical consequences of the remaining proposed mechanisms (some are shown in Figure 3.20). They found that all of the mechanisms are capable of achieving the deformations that are known to occur during invagination, but each of the mechanisms could function only under certain conditions. For example, cell tractoring and gel swelling mechanisms only work if the apical ECM is stiff compared to the cell layer; on the other hand, apical constriction or apical contractile ring mechanisms only work if the apical ECM is of similar or lower stiffness than the cell layer. This detailed analysis of the mechanical properties therefore suggests new approaches for evaluating the likelihood of each mechanism. In subsequent experiments, Davidson and colleagues found that the apical ECM is stiffer than the cell layer, indicating that the apical constriction and apical contractile ring models are inadequate to explain invagination [7].

Summary

- The biological process of development has been studied for centuries, most extensively in insects, amphibians, and birds; many of the basic features of development are similar among species.
- Cell division occurs throughout development, but it is the most important event of early development.
- Gastrulation occurs in a sequence involving cell division, cell migration, and the coordinated movement of groups of cells (for example, folding and bending of cell sheets). These transformations produce the three germ layers (ectoderm, mesoderm, and endoderm) that give rise to the differentiated tissues of adults.
- Cells of the early embryo are totipotent, that is, capable of becoming any of the specialized cells of the adult. As the embryo develops, individual cells lose their potency and become restricted in the fates that they can achieve. Some cells reach a stage at which they are "determined" and destined to only one fate; other cells are pluripotent, even in adults.
- All cells of an organism have the same genetic composition, but differ in the composition of their cytoplasm. The specialized fates of cells are determined by their cytoplasmic contents and by their interactions with the environment.
- The characteristic patterns of animal form arise from inductive interactions between cells and from the presence of gradient fields, which provide cells with information regarding their spatial location in the organism.
- The broad changes that occur during development are increasingly explainable in terms of molecular and cellular events, such as cell-

sorting (which is driven by adhesive differences at the cell surface) and diffusion/reaction patterns of biochemicals.

Glossary

Glossary definitions are obtained from various sources, including [1] and [8].

ANIMAL POLE   the point on the surface of an egg that is diametrically opposite to the vegetal pole and usually marks the most active part of the protoplasm or the part containing least yolk

BLASTOCYST   the modified blastula of a placental mammal

BLASTOMERE   any of the cells resulting from cleavage of a fertilized egg during early development

CLEAVAGE   the series of cell divisions that produces a blastula from a fertilized egg; can also refer to any one of those divisions

DELAMINATION   separation into constituent layers

DIFFERENTIATION   the sum of the developmental processes whereby apparently unspecialized cells, tissues, and structures attain their adult form and function.

DIVERSIFICATION   early process in development, in which daughter cells attain different properties.

EMBRYONIC EPIBLAST   the outer layer of the blastoderm

EPIGENESIS   the theory that an individual is developed by sequential differentiation of an unstructured egg

FATE   the expected result of normal development

FATE MAP   an anatomical map showing the fate of cells from every region of a developing embryo.

FIELD   a region of embryonic tissue potentially capable of a particular type of differentiation.

GASTRULA   an early metazoan embryo in which the ectoderm, mesoderm, and endoderm are established either by invagination of the blastula (as in fish and amphibians) to form a multilayered cellular cup with a blastopore opening into the archenteron or (as in reptiles, birds, and mammals) by differentiation of the upper layer of the blastodisc into the ectoderm and the lower layer into the endoderm and by the inward migration of cells through the primitive streak to form the mesoderm

GASTRULATION   the process of becoming or of forming a gastrula

HYPOBLAST   the endoderm of an embryo

INDUCTION   sum of the processes by which the fate of embryonic cells is determined and morphogenetic differentiation brought about

INNER CELL MASS   the portion of the blastocyst of a mammalian embryo that is destined to become the embryo proper

MORULA   embryo in the 16- to 32-cell stage; cells are polarized and connected by junctional complexes

PLURIPOTENT   not fixed as to developmental potential; having developmental plasticity

POTENCY   initial inherent capacity for development of a particular kind

REGULATION   the process of redistributing material to restore a damaged or lost part independent of new tissue growth

TOTIPOTENT   capable of developing into a complete organism or differentiating into any of its cells or tissues

TROPHOBLAST   the outer layer of the mammalian blastocyst that supplies nutrition to the embryo, facilitates implantation by eroding away the tissues of the uterus with which it comes in contact, allowing the blastocyst to sink into the cavity formed in the uterine wall, and differentiates into the extraembryonic membranes surrounding the embryo

VEGETAL POLE   the point on the surface of an egg that is diametrically opposite to the animal pole and usually marks the center of the protoplasm containing more yolk, dividing more slowly and into larger blastomeres than that about the animal pole, and giving rise to the hypoblast of the embryo

ZYGOTE   fertilized egg

Exercises

Exercise 3.1 (provided by Keith Gooch)

a) What are the three germ layers? Where do they reside in the embryo following gastrulation? What are two tissue types that result from each?

	Layer	Location	2 tissues	
A.	_____	_____	_____ and _____
B.	_____	_____	_____ and _____
C.	_____	_____	_____ and _____

b) Though all of a tissue type often derives from a given germ layer, what are two counter examples to this generalization? (You may need to look to an outside resource to answer this question.)

Exercise 3.2 (provided by Keith Gooch)

Prior to the cloning of Dolly, researchers were relatively success at cloning frogs but had been relatively unsuccessful at cloning mammals (for example, mice). What was a major factor contributing to previous researchers' inability to clone mammals, and how was this overcome with Dolly?

Exercise 3.3 (provided by Song Li)

Define cell determination and cell differentiation. Explain with examples.

Exercise 3.4 (provided by Keith Gooch)

Mesodermal tissue from the developing leg bud normally gives rise to the thigh but is transplanted to the tip of the wing bud.

a) Make your best prediction: what does the transplanted tissue form?
b) Relate your answer to the concept of positional values.

Exercise 3.5 (provided by Michael Sefton)

A spherical cell with the diameter of $10\,\mu m$ has a protein concentration of $20\,mg/ml$. Determine the number of protein molecules within the cell if the molecular weight of an average protein is 50,000 dalton (g/mol).

Exercise 3.6 (provided by Michael Sefton)

The sphere, cylinder, and rectangular parallelepiped are common shapes that could be used to model different living cells. Assume that you have three cells; a sphere, a cylinder, and a rectangular parallelepiped. Each cell has the same volume ($1\,\mu m^3$), and the radius of the sphere and the cylinder are equal to the width of the two sides of the rectangular cell.

a) What are the surface / volume ratios for these shapes?
b) Which shape is better? Why?
c) Why might a given weight of small cells be more metabolically active than the same weight of large cells? (Assume the density is constant.)
d) Does the answer in (c) change if you compare an equal number of cells (rather than an equal weight)?

Exercise 3.7

Consider the model for gradient development shown in Figure 3.16.

a) Show that this model can predict linear and exponential concentration gradients. Your solution should start with Equation 3-1 and involve boundary and initial conditions that you specify.
b) How long will it take to achieve a steady-state gradient within a 1 mm embryo, if the diffusion coefficient is 10^{-6} cm^2/s and the half-life for the elimination reaction is 15 min?

References

1. Kalthoff, K., *Analysis of Biological Development*. New York: McGraw Hill, 1998.
2. Gilbert, S.F., *Developmental Biology*, 5th ed. Sunderland, MA: Sinauer Associates, 1997.
3. Steinberg, M.S., Does differential adhesion govern self-assembly processes in histogenesis? Equilibrium configurations and the emergence of a hierarchy among populations of embryonic cells. *Journal of Experimental Zoology*, 1970, **173**, 395–434.
4. Fink, R.D. and D.R. McClay, Three cell recognition changes accompany the ingression of sea urchin primary mesenchyme cells. *Developmental Biology*, 1985, **107**, 66–74.
5. Dillon, R. and H.G. Othmer, A mathematical model for outgrowth and spatial patterning of the vertebrate limb bud. *Journal of Theoretical Biology*, 1999, **197**, 295–330.
6. Davidson, L.A., et al., How do sea urchins invaginate? Using biomechanics to distinguish between mechanisms of primary invagination. *Development*, 1995, **121**, 2005–2018.
7. Davidson, L.A., et al., Measurements of mechanical properties of the blastula wall reveal which hypothesized mechanisms of primary invagination are physically plausible in the sea urchin *Strongylocentrotus purpuratus*. *Developmental Biology*, 1999, **209**, 221–238.

8. Soukhanov, A., ed., *The American Heritage Dictionary of the English Language*, 3rd ed. 1992. Boston, MA: Houghton Mifflin, 1992.
9. Alberts, B., et al., *Molecular Biology of the Cell*, 2nd ed. New York: Garland Publishing, 1989, p. 1218.
10. Ingber, D.E., The architecture of life. *Scientific American*, 1998, **278**, 48–57.
11. Dugay, D., R.A. Foty and M.S. Steinberg, Cadherin-mediated cell adhesion and tissue segregation: qualitative and quantitative determinants. *Developmental Biology*, 2003, **253**, 309–323.

Part 2

TISSUE ENGINEERING FUNDAMENTALS

4

Cell Growth and Differentiation

Till in the midst of play,
transfiguring and preparing for the future,
the first white veil descended . . .

                    Rainer Maria Rilke, *The Grown-up*

The expansion in size of a region of tissue, often called growth, is critical to embryonic development and tissue repair. Growth of a tissue most often occurs by an increase in cell number. In fact, sequential cell division—and a resulting increase in total cell number—is the most important change of early development (Figure 4.1). As development proceeds, however, the rate of increase in cell number slows (Figure 4.1b) but the overall size of the organism continues to increase steadily (Figure 4.1c).

Growth throughout life can occur by a variety of mechanisms in addition to increased cell number; for example, increases in cell volume or extracellular volume also produce growth. The overall growth of an organ or tissue can involve multiple mechanisms. For example, in the nervous system, neurons increase in size, but not number, as a juvenile grows to adulthood. By contrast, glial cells within the nervous system divide and proliferate throughout life. Overall, however, cell proliferation (which occurs by the process of sequential cell division) is the most important feature of tissue growth.

Growth is only one of the changes that occurs with development. As a child grows to adulthood, her increase in size is probably less astonishing than her overall change in behavior and ability. Underlying this overall change are dramatic alterations in function and operation of individual cells; this observation is related to the discussion in Chapter 3, in which the processes of cellular differentiation and specialization were introduced. The child develops by reference to a fixed instructional program, the genome, which somehow encodes all of the molecular signals that lead to increases in size, changes in shape, and inexorable dynamics of aging. But the child is also influenced by her environment and the opportunities for change that her environment presents. One child becomes a doctor and another a cellist; the factors and forces that nudge each down her path are not programmed by the genes alone. Similarly, differentiation of a cell is influenced by its genetic composition and the environment that surrounds it.

69

Tissue Engineering Fundamentals

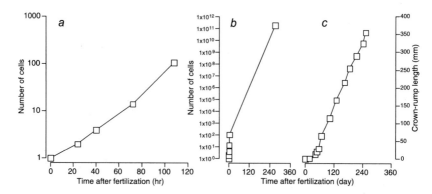

Figure 4.1. Growth of the developing human. The rate of growth is indicated by the increase in cell number during early development (panels a and b) and the increase in linear length (panel c) throughout the gestational period.

This chapter begins with a discussion of mechanisms and kinetics of cell division. Later parts of the chapter consider some of the factors that influence cell differentiation. The relationship of cell growth during development of a normal organism and cell growth in culture is introduced in the final sections.

4.1 The Cell Cycle

Cell division in animal cells occurs in an orderly sequence of steps, although the rate of progression through this sequence varies considerably among cell types. The cell cycle (Figure 4.2a) is continuously repeated as new daughter cells develop and divide. Consider the progression of a newly-formed cell, which begins in a phase called G_1 because it represents the gap between mitosis (M phase) and DNA synthesis (S phase). Cells can exit the cell cycle and remain in an indefinite period of rest called G_0; some cells (such as neurons) are suspended in G_0 for the lifetime of an individual. Re-entry into G_1 from G_0 is usually stimulated by interactions of the cell with the environment or through the action of growth factors, which are discussed in the sections that follow.

G_1 ends as the period of DNA replication, called S phase, begins. During S phase, the cell produces an exact copy of its genetic material so that equivalent genetic information is available for transmission to each daughter cell. Because DNA replication precedes the physical division of the cell, there is a period during which the cellular material has twice the normal amount of DNA. In most cells, the G_2 phase is associated with a substantial increase in cell volume; the cell prepares for division by making sufficient cytoplasm for each new cell. The collective period between mitosis events is called interphase. The kinetics of interphase—that is, the period of time a cell spends in each of the phases G_1, S, and G_2—is highly variable among different cell types. During cleavage in the early embryo, for example, the G phases are essentially absent; blastomeres

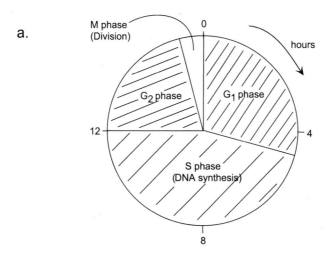

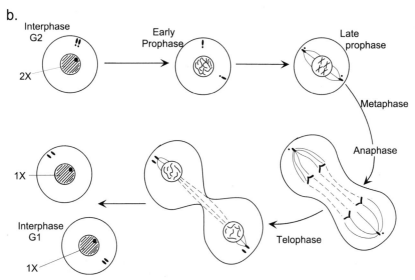

Figure 4.2. Phases of cell division and physical transformations in eukaryotic cells. (a) Phases of the cell cycle in eukaryotic cells. (b) Interphase is the stage between mitotic events. Mitosis, or M phase, is separated into identifiable stages.

synthesize DNA and divide without any substantial delay or increase in cell volume.

The most dramatic changes in cell shape and structure occur during mitosis, or M phase, as the cell undergoes the physical transformations that are necessary to divide (Figure 4.2b). At the end of interphase, the mother cell has replicated its DNA and is ready for division. Mitosis is usually divided into stages—prophase, metaphase, anaphase, telophase, and cytokinesis—which have been thoroughly described [1, 2]. The first stage, called prophase, involves the movement of cytoskeletal elements to form the mitotic spindle and the condensation of nuclear DNA into organized chromosomes (Figure 4.2b). Prometaphase begins with dissolution of the nuclear membrane. Spindle fibers assemble through the nuclear region and associate with chromosomes via protein complexes called kinetochores at a chromosome region (with a specific DNA sequence) called the centromere. During metaphase, the chromosomes become aligned along a plane that is midway between the two poles of the mitotic spindle. At this point, each of the chromosome/kinetochore complexes connects two chromatids, which are the replicated DNA complements destined for each daughter cell. Anaphase begins with the separation of each chromosome complex into two chromatids (which will become the chromosome of the daughter cell). Each member of the "chromatid:chromatid" pair is translated toward its corresponding spindle pole at a speed of ~ 1 μm/min. When the new chromosomes reach the pole, the nuclear envelope begins to reform in each emerging daughter cell. The period of envelope formation and spindle dissolution is called telophase. Finally, the plasma membrane at the midplane between the cell poles begins to constrict, causing dramatic narrowing along the equator. This narrowing, called the cleavage furrow, continues until the constriction reaches the middle of the cell at the site of the disappearing mitotic spindle. Eventually, constriction at this location is completed by breakage and resealing of the membrane to form two individual and separate cells. Each daughter cell, now in G_1 phase, contains a complete set of chromosomes and nearly equal volume of cytoplasm. The chromosomes decondense to re-establish the architecture of an interphase nucleus (Figure 4.3).

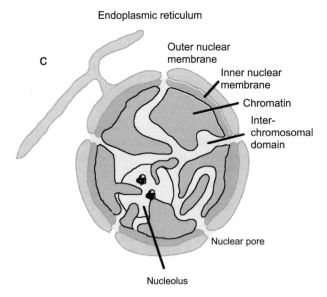

Figure 4.3. Structure of the cell nucleus. Structure of a typical interphase nucleus. (Adapted from [2, 20].)

4.2 Stem Cells and Cell Differentiation

During development, as cell division proceeds from the fertilized egg to the multicellular gastrula, several changes occur in cells. Cell division leads to an increase in the total number of cells (as in Figure 4.1). Directed cell movements cause certain populations of cells to aggregate in regions of the developing embryo. And cells begin to specialize in function, through a process called differentiation. Mammals begin as a single fertilized cell, which transmits copies of its DNA to all subsequent cell generations. Although all cells in our bodies were derived from this single cell, cells in different organs vary considerably in shape, size, and function. Differentiation is the complex process that leads to diversity in cell properties (that is, what the cell actually is and does, the cell's *phenotype*, which is often characterized by the physical appearance of the cell and the contents of its cytoplasm) from a population of cells with the same *genotype* (that is, the same genetic material).

Stem cells are precursor cells that are capable of both self-renewal and differentiation into more specialized cells. These two defining characteristics— limitless self-renewal and multilineage differentiation—were first identified in precursor cells of the hematopoietic system [3]. A third defining characteristic of stem cells is their capacity to populate tissues as functional cells after transplantation into a recipient. Putative stem cells have been isolated from the adult peripheral blood, marrow, nervous system, muscle, liver, intestine, skin, and other tissues; the classification of these cells as "stem cells" is achieved by testing their capacity for self-renewal, multilineage differentiation, and repopulation of tissues in recipients. In addition to their potential for use in repopulation and tissue regeneration, it is speculated that stem cells have an important role in normal physiology; they may exist in small amounts within the tissues of all adult organs, serving as a perennial source of differentiated tissue cells.

A stem cell that differentiates into one type of progenitor is called unipotent (Figure 4.4). Unipotent stem cells display an asymmetrical division; the stem cell divides to produce a new stem cell (for renewal) and a progenitor cell that is committed to differentiation along a certain pathway. Although successive rounds of division and differentiation may follow this initial asymmetric division, the progenitor is irreversibly committed to formation of differentiated cells.

The cell division depicted at the top of Figure 4.4 has what is termed invariant asymmetry; each division produces an identical pair of cells, one stem cell and one progenitor. Invariant asymmetrical division provides a simple mechanism for division that results in a differentiated progenitor while maintaining a constant number of stem cells. Other mechanisms for producing progenitors are possible; populational asymmetry provides additional versatility in the overall outcome. In populational asymmetry, divisions of the stem cell population result in a larger population of cells. These cells now proceed down several possible fate paths; if half of the newly formed cells become stem cells, then the total population of stem cells remains constant. Stem cell division also produces a population of cells that are capable of differentiating into cells of various lineages. The choice of each cell depends on a variety of factors,

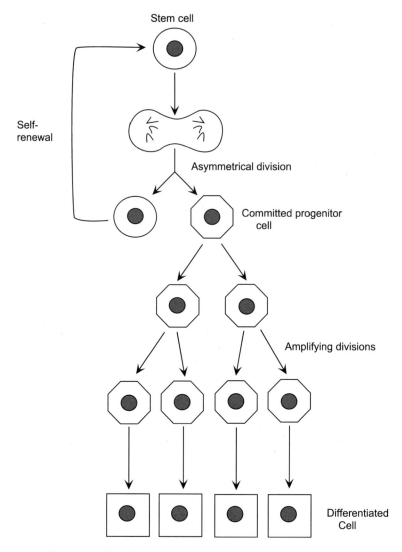

Figure 4.4. Characteristics of stem cells. This schematic diagram shows a typical pattern for differentiation of unipotent stem cells.

including asymmetry in the distribution of intracellular contents to daughter cells, and interactions with soluble and insoluble signaling molecules in the environment, which will be discussed below.

Hematopoiesis is an example of pluripotent stem cell differentiation (Figure 4.5), in which a single stem cell can produce multiple cell lineages. Progression from a stem cell to a fully differentiated cell occurs in a series of steps of successively greater commitment. At each step, cell proliferation provides for renewal of the stem cell population. Some of these new cells differentiate into progenitor cells that choose one of the fates possible for

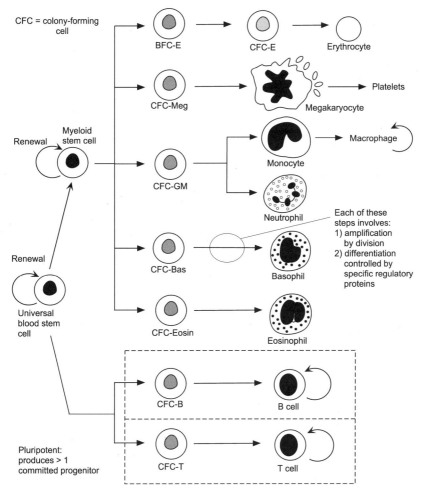

Figure 4.5. Schematic diagram of hematopoiesis, indicating a hypothesized pattern of stem cell differentiation during hematopoiesis. Notice that, in contrast to the unipotent stem cell shown in Figure 4.4, the universal stem cell can differentiate down more than one path.

this stem cell. Further proliferation and differentiation lead some of the cells down alternate pathways of differentiation, to form separate cell lineages. Each of these steps involves amplification by division and differentiation. These processes are controlled by specific regulatory proteins.

4.2.1 Hematopoietic Stem Cells

Many stem cell populations have now been discovered in tissues throughout the body, but hematopoietic stem cells (HSCs) are the most completely studied stem cell system. Isolation and identification of HSCs within the population of developing cells has been difficult; cells are most commonly identified by their surface proteins, which are uncovered by interaction with labeled monoclonal antibodies. Both human and mouse HSCs can now be isolated from donor tissue using antibody markers (Table 4.1); when transplanted into patients whose bone marrow has been ablated by radiation and chemotherapy, these cells will repopulate the marrow and initiate production of neutrophils, platelets, and other blood cells. HSCs can also be maintained in culture and expanded to form new HSC (self-renewal) or differentiated into mature, functional cells. The control of hematopoiesis outside of the body is an important example of tissue engineering, in which the function of a human tissue (in this case, bone marrow) is replicated through cell culture technologies.

HSCs within the body undergo continuous division to provide for self-renewal, differentiation, and cell migration to other sites (some fraction of the new cells may also undergo programmed cell death). The potential for migration is important throughout life, as it provides a natural mechanism for development and re-population of hematopoietic loci throughout the body. Emigration from tissue sites can be induced by signaling proteins, such as granulocyte colony-stimulating factor (G-CSF); for example, administration of a substantial dose of a G-CSF causes mobilization of stem cells to the blood where they can be more easily collected. One can envision strategies in which autologous (that is, obtained from the same patient who is to be treated) bone marrow cells are enriched, propagated, or differentiated *in vitro*; these cultured cells could be injected back into the bloodstream of the patient and then lead to engraftment and function at appropriate tissue sites.

4.2.2 Mesenchymal Stem Cells

Another class of stem cells has been found in the bone marrow. These cells, called mesenchymal stem cells (MSCs), were first isolated from marrow aspirates by their ability to adhere to surfaces during culture (HSCs do not adhere). The cultured cells, which appear similar to fibroblasts in culture, can be induced to differentiate into mature adipocytes, chondrocytes, and bone cells. There are some reports that the developmental potential of these cells is even greater, and that neurons, myocytes, and other cells can be obtained under the appropriate induction conditions.

Table 4.1
Cell surface markers for mouse and human HSCs

Species	Specific Markers	Negative for:
Mouse	Thy-1^{lo} Sca-1$^+$	B220, Mac-1, Gr-1, CD3, CD4, CD8, Ter119
Human	Thy-1$^+$ CD34$^+$	CD10, CD14, CD15, CD16, CD19, CD20

Information taken from [6].

4.2.3 Embryonic Stem Cells

Cells within the embryo have enormous potential for differentiation; therefore, the early embryo is a natural source to explore for stem cell populations. Because of their unique role in development, embryonic stem cells are the most versatile—as well as controversial—stem cells. Cells cultured from the inner cell mass (recall the discussion referring to Figure 3.6) are totipotent when transplanted into a host blastocyst, but it is not yet possible to control the differentiation of these early cells into tissue-specific stem cells. Some of the molecular characteristics of embryonic stem cells have been identified, such as the presence of transcription factors (such as oct-4, Rex-1, sox-2, and LIF-R) and enzymes (such as telomerase); the role of these molecules is described in the next section.

It is possible that all tissues are derived from tissue-specific stem cells that are differentiated descendents of an earlier, less-differentiated stem cell (Figure 4.6); these tissue stem cells may persist at scattered locations throughout adult life where they are available for activation and regeneration of damaged tissue as necessary. Likewise, the creation of specific progenitor cells within a specific tissue during development may occur in a hierarchical pattern, providing a population of ever more restricted stem cells in tissues as they develop (Figure 4.7 illustrates this concept for cells of the nervous system).

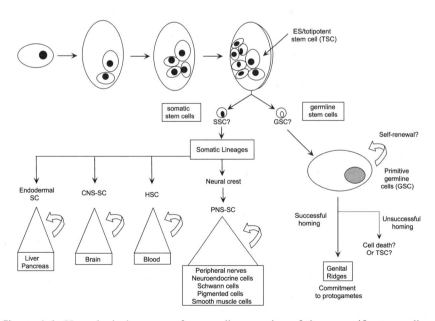

Figure 4.6. Hypothetical process of stem cell generation of tissue-specific stem cells (redrawn from [6]). Schematic model of the differentiation of a totipotent stem cell into germ and somatic cell lineages. Totipotent stem cells can differentiate into tissue- and organ-specific stem cells that have more restricted fates.

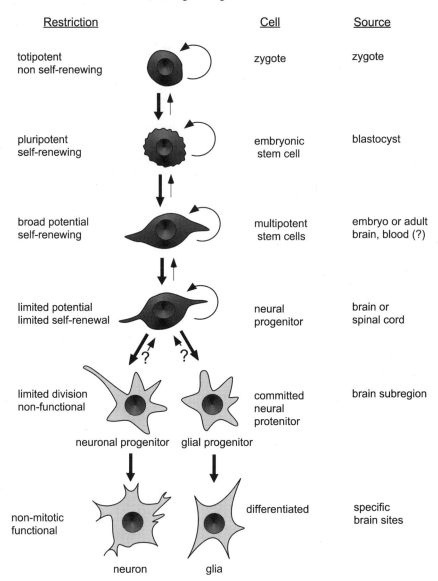

Restriction	Cell	Source
totipotent non self-renewing	zygote	zygote
pluripotent self-renewing	embryonic stem cell	blastocyst
broad potential self-renewing	multipotent stem cells	embryo or adult brain, blood (?)
limited potential limited self-renewal	neural progenitor	brain or spinal cord
limited division non-functional	committed neural protenitor	brain subregion
	neuronal progenitor glial progenitor	
non-mitotic functional	differentiated	specific brain sites
	neuron glia	

Figure 4.7. Hypothetical hierarchy of stem cell development in the nervous system (redrawn from [7]). Tissue-specific stem cells, such as those in the nervous system, differentiate by a sequential process of increasing commitment to nervous system fates. As the cells become more differentiated, they lose potency.

4.2.4 Neural Stem Cells

Neural stem cells (NSCs), stem cells with the capacity to form cells that can function as neurons and glia after transplantation, have been studied in some detail. Stem cells, which are defined by the characteristics of self-renewal and differentiation, have been isolated from the rat neural crest [4], adult rodent brain [5], and human fetal brain [6]. Like other stem cells, transplanted brain stem cells differentiate under the direction of the host microenvironment (Figure 4.8) and, therefore, can be used to repopulate lost tissue in specific regions of the brain. This capacity is consistent with the recent hypothesis that neurogenesis occurs at some sites, most notably the dentate gyrus and subventricular zone, throughout adult life (see [7] for a review, although this hypothesis remains controversial, particularly in primates [8]). Some stem cell populations appear to use unique mechanisms of cell migration in order to supply functional cells to appropriate anatomical areas. These findings have generated substantial excitement because isolation, expansion and transplantation of tissue-specific stem cells could be a powerful, generic strategy for induction of tissue repair in the nervous system.

4.2.5 Plasticity of Stem Cells

The abundance, capacity for self-renewal, developmental potential, and capacity for engraftment of adult stem cells is not clear at this time. There is still much to be learned about all stems, including HSCs, which have been studied the most extensively. For example, the developmental plasticity of HSCs is controversial. Some studies show that single mouse stem HSCs—isolated from marrow, injected back into lethally irradiated recipients, and then functionally isolated by recovery from the bone marrow of this first recipient—can engraft in secondary recipients and then develop into hematopoietic and non-hematopoietic cells within the marrow, peripheral blood, and a variety of other tissues (lung, liver, intestine, and skin) [9]. Other studies indicate that the developmental plasticity of HSCs is much more limited and confined primarily to cells of the hematopoietic system [10].

4.3 Agents that Regulate Cell Growth and Differentiation

Stem cells have the potential to differentiate along a variety of pathways. The fate of a particular stem cell depends on its source and its immediate environment, either in culture or after transplantation. What are the factors that influence a stem cell in its choice of fate?

Some decision-making factors are present within the cell. For example, certain cell proteins appear to function as biological clocks that encode an internal program for timed cell fate. Interestingly, the number of doublings that can be achieved by fibroblasts in culture correlates with the lifespan of the organism donating the cells (Figure 4.9), suggesting a linkage between cell life span and aging of the animal. Proteins can act to promote or inhibit the cell cycle; therefore, accumulation or disappearance of these proteins would affect the ability of the cell to divide. For example, telomeres are repetitive DNA sequences that appear at the end of chromosomes and function to insure accurate replication of the DNA sequences near the end. Telomere shortening

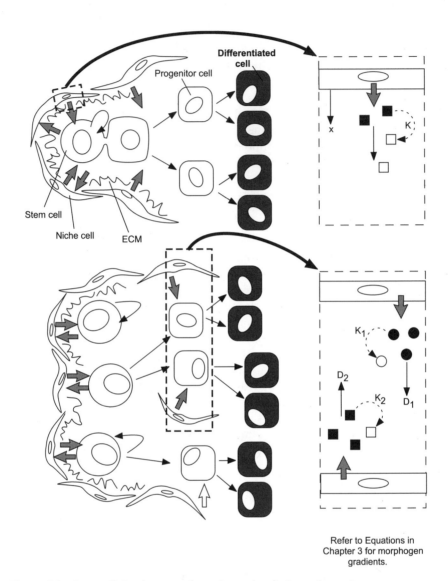

Refer to Equations in
Chapter 3 for morphogen
gradients.

Figure 4.8. Stem cell development depends on signals from the environment (redrawn from [21]). (a) The differentiation and proliferation of stem cells is influenced by the presence of soluble and insoluble factors in the local environment or stem cell niche. For example, a gradient of factor produced by cells in the periphery of the niche can signal differentiation of cells at specific spatial locations within the niche. (b) Multiple signaling molecules can be produced within a niche in order to create complex patterns of differentiation cues. In this example, two factors are released by cells on opposing sides of the niche, creating an internal environment with a wide spectrum of signaling capabilities.

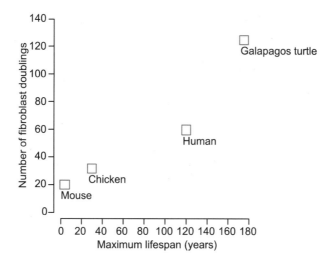

Figure 4.9. Fibroblast doublings in culture correlates with life span of animal. Most cultured cells experience a limited number of population doublings in culture before they experience a crisis that leads to senescence. For cells from different species, the number of doublings to crisis correlates well with the lifespan of the animal.

is frequently observed in cultured cells; the repetitive sequence is reduced in length by ~ 50 base pairs with each division. Telomere shortening may represent a biological mechanism for programmed cell death or senescence in culture. If this speculation about the role of telomeres in overall life span is correct, then telomerase—an enzyme that preserves telomere length and is found in stem cells—may endow cells with an extended capacity to divide.

External signals from the microenvironment are also known to be critical in the decision-making process (Figure 4.8). Secreted factors are essential for control of development in hematopoiesis; fate-specific proteins appear to enhance the survival of certain cells. These factors—such as G-CSF, interleukin 2, and erythropoietin (EPO)—appear to act by selection; presence of the factor prevents the death of certain cells, which are generated randomly from a pool of precursor cells. Secreted factors in other tissues may act by instructive mechanisms, in which the presence of the factor initiates differentiation along a specific lineage. Certain families of proteins, including TGF-β and Wnt, have been implicated in regulation of stem cell differentiation in a variety of species.

Signals for cell growth or differentiation include multiple steps and can therefore be regulated or manipulated by a variety of mechanisms. Diffusible protein growth factors, such as epidermal growth factor (EGF), bind to transmembrane receptor proteins (Figure 4.10). Binding of the growth factor ligand to its receptor initiates intracellular signals, which are transmitted through protein–tyrosine kinases and/or intracellular signal transducers such as G proteins. Action within the nucleus is mediated by proteins that are involved in control of the cell cycle, such as p53 (which regulates a tumor suppressor gene that produces a protein capable of blocking a cyclin-related signal for DNA

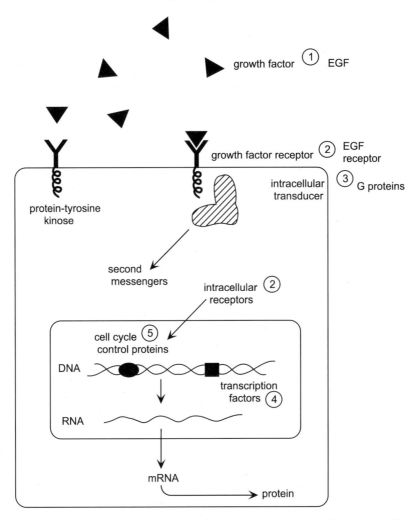

Figure 4.10. Schematic diagram showing the influence of growth factors on cell growth: (1) growth factor (e.g., epidermal growth factor, EGF); (2) extracellular or intracellular growth factor receptor (EGFR); (3) intracellular transducer (G proteins); (4) transcription factors (e.g. *jun* oncogene, which causes activation of growth-promoting genes); (5) cell cycle control proteins (e.g. cyclin p53, which is a tumor suppression gene).

synthesis), or transcription factors, such as *jun* (which activates growth promoting genes).

A wide variety of chemical agents can influence the growth and differentiation of cells in the body and in culture. Many of these molecules have been classified into groups or families, in which the members share either common functional properties (for example, *mitogens* are agents that all act to induce mitosis in a cell population) or common structural characteristics (for example, *cytokines* are small proteins, in the range 5 to 20 kilodalton, that influence cell–cell interactions and cell behavior). Some of these classifications are general and can be interchangeable: *cytokine* and *hormone* are terms that mean roughly the same thing, although the term cytokine is usually restricted to the group of molecules with well-known effects on the immune system, including interleukins, lymphokines, tumor necrosis factor (TNF), and interferons. Other groups are defined rather specifically. For example, *chemokines* are a group of inflammatory cytokines that activate and recruit leukocytes and that have common structural characteristics involving variations in a shared cysteine motif.

Some of the classifications have become inadequate, as new functions or more specific functions of their members are defined. For example, *growth factor* is used to indicate any of the proteins that are involved in cell differentiation and growth; this usage is consistent with the common practice in endocrinology of labeling substances as "factors" when their chemical composition or mechanism of action are unknown and labeling them "hormones" when they are known. As the chemical structure and biological function of "growth factors" are uncovered, the old label is less appropriate. In many cases, we now know that most "growth factors" have specific effects on specific cells, and often different effects on different cells. In addition, not all of these effects are related to "growth." For that reason, the term "growth factor" should probably be used with care, and only when a more specific term is not applicable.

4.3.1 Growth Factor and Receptor Binding Kinetics

Many aspects of action of diffusible growth factors can be understood through mathematical analysis (see [11]). Consider a single cell suspended in a solution containing a ligand L that binds to a receptor R on the cell surface (Figure 4.11). The overall binding kinetics are defined as

$$L + R \underset{k_r}{\overset{k_f}{\rightleftharpoons}} L - R \tag{4-1}$$

$$K_d = \frac{1}{K_a} = \frac{c_L c_R}{c_{L-R}} = \frac{k_r}{k_f} \tag{4-2}$$

where k_f and k_r are the overall forward and reverse rate constants, respectively, K_d is an equilibrium constant for the dissociation reaction, and K_a is an equilibrium constant for the association reaction. Concentrations of ligand, receptor, and receptor–ligand complex are indicated by c_L, c_R, and c_{L-R}, respectively. The equilibrium dissociation constant K_d is an indicator of the affinity of the interaction between the receptor and the ligand; smaller values of K_d indicate a shift in the equilibrium to the right (in Equation 4.1), such that more of the receptor molecules are in the bound state (L–R).

The dynamics of binding can be described in terms of these overall reaction rate constants. For example, the overall rate of binding can be determined from the rate of formation of new ligand receptor complexes (L–R):

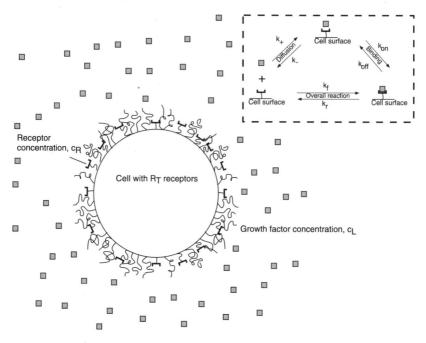

Figure 4.11. Binding of growth factor molecules to cell surface receptors. The growth factor or ligand, L indicated by grey squares, must diffuse to the cell surface prior to binding. The inset panel shows a schematic model for incorporating rates of binding and diffusion into an overall rate of ligand–receptor binding.

$$\frac{dc_{L-R}}{dt} = k_f(c_R)c_L - k_r c_{L-R} \qquad (4\text{-}3)$$

In many situations, the total number of receptors on the cell surface will be constant. If the total number of receptors is called R_T in this situation, then a balance on receptor number suggests that

$$R_T = c_R + c_{L-R} \qquad (4\text{-}4)$$

Assuming further that the concentration of ligand is sufficiently high, so that the binding reactions do not significantly change the overall concentration (that is, $c_L \sim c_{L,0}$), the differential equation 4-3 can be rewritten as

$$\frac{dc_{L-R}}{dt} = k_f(R_T - c_{L-R})c_{L,0} - k_r c_{L-R} \qquad (4\text{-}5)$$

which can be solved in the case where all of the receptors are initially unoccupied by ligand (that is, $c_{L-R} = 0$ at $t = 0$):

$$c_{L-R}(t) = \frac{k_f c_{L,0} R_T}{k_f c_{L,0} + k_r}(1 - \exp[-(k_f c_{L,0} + k_r)t]) \qquad (4\text{-}6)$$

Figure 4.12a shows the kinetics of binding for an example case. After a sufficiently long time, the rate of the forward reaction (binding) will balance the

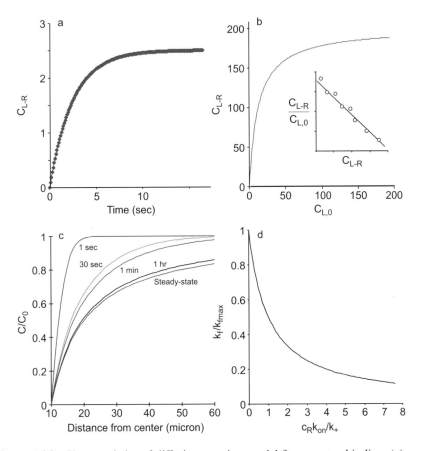

Figure 4.12. Characteristics of diffusion-reaction model for receptor binding. (a) Kinetics of ligand binding, assuming constant ligand concentration and constant receptor number. The concentration of receptors was calculated from Equation 4-6 assuming the following values, which are from Table 2-1 of [11]: $k_f = 2 \times 10^7 \, M^{-1} \, min^{-1}$, $k_r = 0.4 \, min^{-1}$, $R_T = 50,000/cell$. (b) The change in complex concentration with ligand concentration at equilibrium, from Equation 4-7. The inset shows an example of Scatchard analysis, in which a linear relation is obtained by plotting bound/free vs. free ligand concentrations (Equation 4-8). (c) Diffusion-limited concentration profiles in the vicinity of a cell with a radius of $10 \, \mu m$. The approach to steady state is shown, as well as the steady-state solution (which is indicated in Equation 4-12'). The diffusion coefficient in the liquid is $10^{-7} \, cm^2/s$. (d) In the situation where both diffusion and binding rates are important, the rate constant varies with receptor number (from Equation 4-16). The value of the forward rate constant k_f depends on the number of receptors per cell, which is indicated here by c_R in the text.

rate of the reverse reaction (unbinding) such that the total number of occupied receptors remains constant. In this limit ($t \to \infty$), the number of bound or occupied receptors is given by:

$$c_{L-R}\big|_{\text{EQUILIBRIUM}} = \frac{c_{L,0}R_T}{c_{L,0} + K_d} \tag{4-7}$$

The characteristics of receptor–ligand pairs at equilibrium are sometimes determined by reference to a linearized version of this equation:

$$\frac{c_{L-R}|_{\text{EQ}}}{c_{L,0}} = -\frac{1}{K_d}c_{L-R}|_{\text{EQ}} + \frac{R_T}{K_d} \tag{4-8}$$

This procedure is illustrated in the inset panel of Figure 4.12b.

4.3.2 Ligand Diffusion and Binding

Several different physical phenomena can contribute to the overall rates of binding that are illustrated in Equation 4-1. As shown in the inset panel of Figure 4.11, the binding event can be broken down into two steps in which the growth factor, or ligand L, must (1) diffuse to the cell surface from the bulk and (2) chemically associate (bind) to the receptor molecules R. In this formulation, the intrinsic binding kinetics are represented by rate constants k_{on} and k_{off}.

The concentration gradient in the vicinity of a spherical cell can be determined by analysis of growth factor diffusion in the vicinity of the cell. In the present situation, the rate of diffusion at the cell surface must be balanced by the rate of ligand disappearance due to the binding reaction:

$$r\pi A^2 D\frac{dc_L}{dr}\bigg|_{r=A} = k_{\text{on}}c_R c_L \qquad \text{at} \qquad r = A \tag{4-9}$$

where c_R is the number of receptors on the cell surface (molecules per cell). The differential equation governing ligand transport is, in spherical coordinates,

$$D\frac{1}{r^2}\frac{d}{dr}\left(r^2\frac{dc_L}{dr}\right) = 0 \tag{4-10}$$

and the second boundary condition is

$$c_L - c_{L,0} \qquad \text{at} \qquad r = \infty \tag{4-11}$$

The solution to Equation 4-10 subject to the two boundary conditions (Equations 4-9 and 4-11) is

$$c_L(r) = -\frac{k_{\text{on}}c_R A c_{L,0}}{4\pi DA + k_{\text{on}}c_R}\frac{1}{r} + c_{L,0} \tag{4-12}$$

The overall rate of binding at the cell surface—which accounts for a balance between diffusion of ligand to the surface and a finite rate of association with receptors at the surface—can be calculated from the flux at the cell surface:

$$\text{Rate} = -D\frac{dc_L}{dr}\bigg|_{r=A}(4\pi A^2) = \frac{k_{on}c_R Ac_{L,0}}{4\pi DA + k_{on}c_R}\frac{4\pi DA^2}{A^2} \tag{4-13}$$

The overall rate of binding is also represented by an overall forward rate constant k_f (see Figure 4.11), which is evaluated from Equation 4-13:

$$k_f = \frac{\text{Rate}}{c_{L,0}} = \frac{(4\pi DA)c_R k_{on}}{4\pi DA + c_{on}} \tag{4-14}$$

In the special case of rapid binding at the cell surface, so that ligand molecules become bound to receptors as soon as they arrive by diffusion at the surface, Equation 4-9 is replaced with $c_L = 0$ at $r = A$. Under these conditions, the rate of diffusion determines the overall rate of binding at the surface (since the surface reaction occurs instantaneously with respect to the rate of diffusion of molecules to the cell surface). The solution to Equation 4-10 with this simplified boundary condition is:

$$c_L(r) = -\frac{Ac_{L,0}}{r} + c_{L,0} \tag{4-12'}$$

The steady-state solution (Equation 4-12′) as well as the approach to steady state is shown in Figure 4.12c. The corresponding rate expression is

$$\text{Rate (rapid reaction)} = -D\frac{dc_A}{dr}\bigg|_{r=A}(4\pi A^2) = 4\pi DAc_{L,0} \tag{4-13'}$$

Therefore, the rate constant for the diffusion-limited (that is, rapid binding) reaction is

$$k_+ = 4\pi DA \tag{4-15}$$

The overall forward rate constant can therefore be written in terms of the rate constant for the diffusion-limited reaction (k_+) and the rate constant for the intrinsic binding reaction:

$$k_f = \frac{k_+ c_R k_{on}}{k_+ + c_R k_{on}}; \quad \text{or} \quad \frac{k_f}{k_{f,max}} = \frac{1}{1 + k_{f,max}}/k_+ \tag{4-16}$$

The maximum rate of the overall reaction occurs when the diffusion-limited rate constant is very large ($k_+ \gg c_R k_{on}$); $k_{f,max} = c_R k_{on}$). (Note that the rate constants k_f and k_r are defined on a per cell basis, not a per receptor molecule basis. A more detailed description of alternate conventions is available [11].) The overall rate constant k_f depends on the number of receptors per cell, c_R, as shown in Figure 4.12d. A similar analysis yields the overall reverse rate constant k_r, which describes the dissociation of growth factor molecules from the cell:

$$k_r = \frac{k_+ c_{off}}{k_+ + c_R k_{on}} \tag{4-17}$$

4.3.3 Factor Degradation and the Formation of Local Gradients

Growth factors and their receptors are often internalized and metabolized during cellular activity. The effect of internalization and intracellular trafficking has been most completely studied for EGF. Figure 4.13 shows the effectiveness of EGF at stimulating the proliferation of human fibroblasts when present in two different volumes of cell culture medium. At low medium volumes, higher concentrations of EGF are required to achieve the same level of proliferation. This difference in concentration represents the number of EGF molecules that are degraded, and therefore depleted, which in turn represents a significant fraction of the overall number of EGF molecules when a low medium volume is used.

Figure 4.13 illustrates an important feature of growth factor action: growth factor molecules are often consumed during their normal course of action. Growth factors and cytokines that are injected into the body have a finite lifetime; the overall rate of disappearance can be estimated by measuring the rate of disappearance after intravenous injection (Table 4.2). But, for some agents, the source of the molecule and the desired site of action are physically separated (Figure 4.8 illustrates one example of this). Therefore, the number of growth factor molecules that reach the target depend on both the rate of production (at the cell source) and the rate of degradation of the molecules in the diffusion pathway (usually extracellular fluid). This continuous degradation of the biologically active agent serves to limit the spatial and temporal range of action for the agent; secreted signals can operate at a distance, or over long periods of time, although activity is usually confined to a relatively small volume of tissue

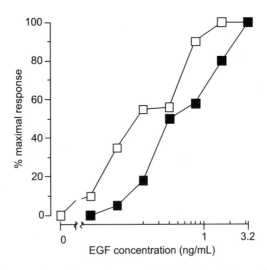

Figure 4.13. Influence of medium volume on EGF activity. The proliferation response of human fibroblasts is shown as a function of initial concentration of EGF. The EGF was provided to cells in high (80 mL, open symbols) or low (2 mL, closed symbols) volume of medium. Redrawn from [34].

Table 4.2
Half-Lives for Some Protein Therapeutic Agents

Protein	Molecular Weight	Plasma Half-life ($t_{1/2}$, min)	Source of Material and Species
Basic fibroblast growth factor (bFGF)	18,000	1.5	Recombinant bFGF in rats [27]
γ interferon	24,000	11 to 32	Partially purified protein in humans [28]
Nerve growth factor (NGF)	28,000	2.4	Purified mouse NGF in rats [29]
Interleukin-2 (IL-2)	17,000	30	Recombinant human IL-2 in humans [30]
Erythropoietin (EPO)	51,000	300	Recombinant human EPO in humans [31]
Ciliary neurotrophic factor (CNTF)	23,000	3	Recombinant human CNTF in humans [32]
Insulin	6,000	4	

The references given in the rightmost column provide more information on the specific experimental systems that were used to measure these half-lives.

surrounding the signal source, or a short period of time after release. These features of growth factor dynamics are illustrated in the next subsections.

The diffusion equation can be used to develop a simple, quantitative method for predicting the extent of growth factor penetration in a local environment, such as a stem cell niche. Consider the characteristic geometry shown in Figure 4.8, in which growth factor is secreted by the niche cells at a sufficient rate to maintain a constant value c_0 at a point just outside of the niche cell surface. After release from the niche cell, the growth factor will diffuse through the tissue space. The diffusing growth factor is also eliminated from the tissue—for example, through the binding and internal consumption processes illustrated in Figure 4.13—such that the volumetric rate of elimination is first order, with a characteristic rate constant k. The simultaneous diffusion and elimination process can be described by

$$D_A \frac{\partial^2 c_A}{\partial x^2} - k c_A = \frac{\partial c_A}{\partial t} \tag{4-18}$$

This equation is identical to that used to describe the spatial distribution of morphogens in Chapter 3. If the boundary conditions are also the same—which is a reasonable assumption for most situations—the steady-state solution for Equation 4-18 is identical to the equation found for morphogen gradients:

$$\frac{c_A}{c_0} = \exp\left(-x\sqrt{\frac{k}{D_A}}\right) \tag{4-19}$$

Concentration profiles predicted by Equation 4-19 are shown in Figure 4.14. The spatial range of distribution of the growth factor is determined by its rate of elimination within the local tissue space. To reach a progenitor cell that is 600 μm from the source, the growth factor must have a half-life of 1 hour or longer if its diffusion coefficient is $\sim 10^{-7}$ cm^2/s (Figure 4.14).

The range of signal distribution for a growth factor can be estimated from its physical and biological characteristics. For example, if we assume that the growth factor is active at all concentrations greater than 1% of the secreted concentration—and that the diffusion coefficient for the growth factor is 10^{-7} cm^2/s—the range of signal distribution is given by

$$X^* = \sqrt{k/D}\,\ln(100) \tag{4-20}$$

Complexity within the stem cell niche can create versatility in the selection of characteristics of progenitor cells. Consider, for example, a niche that is bordered by cells that secrete two different growth factors (Figure 4.8b). A progenitor cell within this niche is exposed to different concentrations of two growth factors; each growth factor will distribute throughout the niche in accord with its physical properties and half-life (Figure 4.14b). One can then

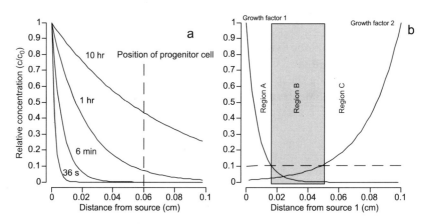

Figure 4.14. Gradients of growth factors in a stem cell niche. (a) Variation in concentration for a growth factor secreted from a single site within the stem cell niche, as shown in Figure 4.8. Equation 4-19 is plotted for a diffusion coefficient of 10^{-7} cm^2/s and an elimination rate k, where k is specified as a tissue half-life $t_{1/2} = \ln 2/k$. The range of distribution for the growth factor signal is approximately 10 μm for a growth factor with a 30 s half-life and approximately 1000 μm for a growth factor with a 10 hr half-life. (b) Variation in concentration of two growth factors that are separately secreted from two different positions within the stem cell niche. In this example, the 1 mm wide region between the growth factor sources contains a continuum of differentiation environments ranging from high 1, low 2 (at $x = 0$) to low 1, high 2 (at $x = 1$ mm). Cells that are sensitive to both factors can differentiate down a spectrum of pathways that are signaled by different concentration ranges. Here, the niche is divided into three regions that have different characteristics: region A (high 1, low 2), region B (medium 1, medium 2), and region C (low 1, high 2).

imagine a population of progenitor cells that are sensitive to both growth factors; the differentiation of each susceptible cell within the niche depends on the relative concentrations of both factors at its location.

4.3.4 Chemical Agents and Communication Distances

Some secreted factors act over long physical distances in the body. For example, the protein insulin is secreted by cells in the pancreas and circulates in the blood, eventually reaching cells at every location in the body. These *endocrine* factors, or *hormones*, are usually characterized by their long half-lives in the extracellular fluids and blood. Because they are long-lived, they can diffuse considerable distances away from the cell in which they are produced, survive transit through the extracellular space, penetrate a capillary wall, and accumulate in the blood. Other secreted signals operate over shorter distance ranges. The activity of *paracrine* factors usually is confined to a small volume of tissue surrounding the cell that secretes the molecule. *Autocrine* factors are released into the extracellular fluid, but stimulate the same cell that secreted them. The previous section described a physical mechanism for the spatial localization of paracrine factors: if the agent is degraded rapidly—compared to its rate of local diffusion—the spatial range of the factor is naturally limited.

Even in the absence of a local mechanism for degradation of the growth factor signal, the spatial range of action of an agent can be defined by analysis of its transport characteristics [12]. In this case, consider the suspended cell, such as the one illustrated in Figure 4.11, which is producing and secreting a chemical agent (rather than binding an agent which is present in the extracellular fluid). After secretion from the cell, the agent diffuses away into the extracellular space:

$$D \frac{1}{r^2} \frac{\partial}{\partial r} \left(r^2 \frac{\partial c_A}{\partial r} \right) = \frac{\partial c_A}{\partial t} \tag{4-21}$$

where c_A is the concentration of secreted agent in the extracellular space. At the cell surface, the rate of secretion is equal to the rate of diffusion into the surrounding fluid. At the time secretion begins, the concentration of the agent outside the cell is zero and, far from the cell surface, the concentration of agent is always zero:

$$\left.\begin{array}{ll} S = -D \dfrac{\partial c_A}{\partial r} \bigg|_{r=A} & ; r = A \\[2mm] c_A = -; & r \to \infty \\[2mm] c_A = 0; & t = 0, \quad r \geq A \end{array}\right\} \tag{4-22}$$

The solution to Equation 4-21, subject to the boundary conditions listed in Equation 4-22, is [12, 13]:

$$c_A(r, t) = \frac{SA}{2Dr}\sqrt{\frac{4Dt}{\pi}}\left\{\exp\left(\frac{-(r - A)^2}{4Dt}\right) - \exp\left(\frac{-(r + A)^2}{4Dt}\right)\right.$$

$$\left. -\frac{|r - A|}{\sqrt{4Dt/\pi}}\,\mathrm{erfc}\left(\frac{|r - A|}{\sqrt{4Dt}}\right) + \frac{(r + A)}{\sqrt{4Dt/\pi}}\,\mathrm{erfc}\left(\frac{r + A}{\sqrt{4Dt}}\right)\right\}$$

(4-23)

Figure 4.15 shows the changes in concentration of the agent with time and distance from the center of the suspended cell. For a spherical cell secreting into an unbounded medium, the agent concentration will eventually reach a steady-state profile. For the situation illustrated in Figure 4.15a, it takes between 3 and 24 hours to reach the steady-state value. As is typical for processes that depend on molecular diffusion (see Chapter 3 and [14]), the time constant for chemical penetration depends on the distance from the secreting cell:

$$\tau \sim \frac{1}{D}r^2$$

(4-24)

For a distance of 100 μm (0.01 cm), this approximation suggests that a large protein ($D = 10^{-7}$ cm^2/s) requires ~ 1000 s (17 min) to penetrate, which is consistent with the curves in Figure 4.15a. Some of the important consequences

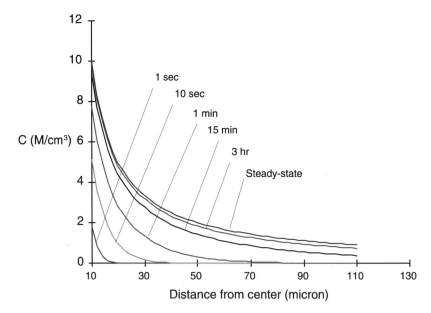

Figure 4-15. Time-dependent changes in agent concentration after secretion from a suspended cell. The concentration as a function of time and position is shown for a cell with a radius of 10 μm. The diffusion coefficient of the agent is 10^{-7} cm^2/s and the secretion rate S was set to 105 mol/cm^2/s. The result can be adjusted to another desired secretion rate (S') by multiplying the C value by the ratio S'/S.

of the relationship between cell secretion rate and local diffusion have been described in a recent analysis [12].

4.3.5 Influence of Growth Factor Binding to Insoluble Components of Tissue

Spatial localization of signaling can be even more precise through the use of cell–cell or cell–matrix interactions, which require direct contact of the signal-recipient with the cell or matrix element relaying the signal. The Notch and Delta proteins of *Drosophila* are transmembrane proteins that act as receptor and ligand, respectively, for the control of differentiation of sensory cells; Notch signaling is also important in the development of blood, retina, and muscle cells in vertebrates. Integrin–extracellular matrix interactions—which are discussed in Chapter 6—are also implicated in the differentiation of epidermal stem cells.

Soluble growth factors often bind to extracellular matrix proteins. Binding to the matrix provides a mechanism for local concentration of the growth factor. In addition, by adding a binding function to the extracellular matrix in the vicinity of a cell, the matrix can serve as a mediator for presenting the ligand to the cell; this may facilitate binding to cells with low receptor number or receptors of low affinity.

4.4 Trafficking and Signal Transduction

Binding of some ligands to membrane receptor proteins can lead to rapid internalization of both receptor and ligand by a process called endocytosis (Figure 4.16). This process has been studied extensively for a variety of ligand–receptor systems including low-density lipoprotein (LDL), transferrin, and epidermal growth factor (EGF). Endocytosis frequently leads to accumulation of ligand in intracellular vesicles, including lysosomes, in which degradation of the ligand can occur. Ligand–receptor complexes have different fates after endocytosis. In the case of LDL and LDL receptor, the LDL dissociates from the LDL receptor within the endosome and the LDL receptor is recycled to the cell surface. LDL receptors are conserved in this process and an essential nutrient is brought into the cell without sacrificing the carrier protein. Transferrin, an iron-carrying serum protein, releases bound iron in the endosome (becoming apotransferrin, the iron-free form of the protein); the transferrin–receptor complex is recycled to the cell surface, after which transferrin is released into the extracellular environment. Both protein and receptor are conserved in this process. EGF and EGF receptor are both degraded within the lysosomes. Since the receptor is degraded, EGF binding eventually leads to a decrease in the number of EGF receptors at the surface, a process called receptor down-regulation.

The versatility of receptor–ligand interactions in signal activation is illustrated in Figure 4.17 by two common biochemical pathways. In Figure 4.17a,

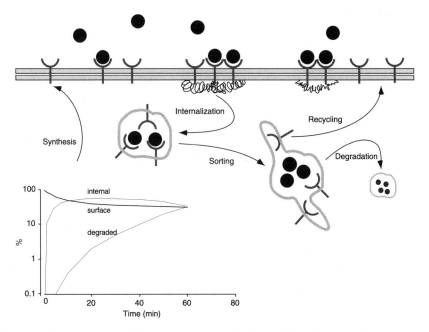

Figure 4.16. Receptor-mediated endocytosis. Binding of ligands to certain receptors leads to rapid internalization of the receptor–ligand complex in endosomes.

this concept is illustrated with the specific case of integrin binding to extracellular matrix ligands [2, 11, 15, 16]. Binding of ligand to integrin receptors at the cell surfaces causes association of cytoplasmic proteins (tensin, talin, vinculin, a-actinin, and F-actin) with the cytoplasmic domains of a transmembrane integrin receptor. The inset in Figure 4.17a shows a hypothetical model for signal transduction, based on focal adhesion kinase (FAK). The model includes tyrosine kinases (Src and Csk), adapter proteins (Grb2 and Crk), and guanine nucleotide exchange factors (SOS and C3G). Binding occurs through SH2 (Src homology 2) domains, which bind to proteins containing a phosphotyrosine (dark circles), and SH3 (Src homology 3) domains, which bind to proteins containing a proline-rich peptide motif (dark rectangles). A second example is shown in Figure 4.17b. When opioid peptides bind to opioid receptors, the receptor is internalized and signal transduction is initiated. Opioid receptor signaling occurs through the action of trimeric GTP-binding regulatory proteins; agonist binding activates a G protein, which subsequently inhibits the activity of adenylyl cyclase, a membrane-associated enzyme. G protein coupled receptors are ubiquitous; these receptors act through G-protein-mediated activation or inhibition of a second membrane protein.

Changes in receptor activation result from changes in ligand concentration in the extracellular environment. Consider the situation in which a cell is initially surrounded by a uniform concentration of ligand, which is produced in the extracellular environment at some steady rate R. Although the ligand is

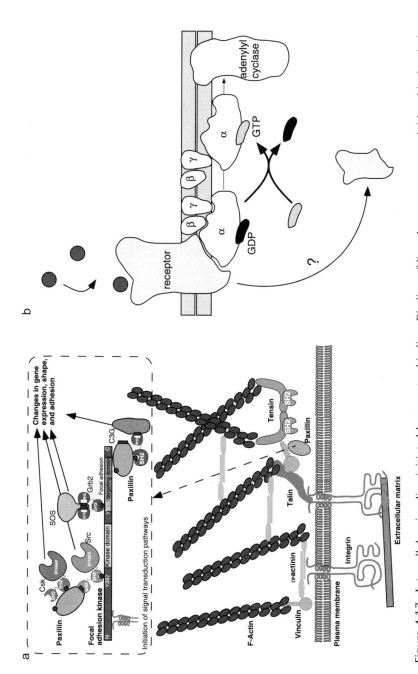

Figure 4.17. Intracellular signaling initiated by receptor binding. Binding of ligands to receptors can initiate biochemical signals within the cell. This is shown for two different, but common, biochemical pathways: (a) binding to a membrane protein with tyrosine kinase activity; and (b) binding to a G protein coupled receptor.

continuously produced, the concentration of ligand remains constant because the ligand is also degraded by some natural processes (recall the previous discussion of diffusion and degradation). For the signal to change, that is, for the concentration of the signaling agent to change, the rate of ligand generation must either increase or decrease. Modification of the rate of ligand production will eventually lead to a change in ligand concentration; change in ligand concentration will alter receptor–ligand binding and, therefore, signal activation. The ligand concentration at the cell surface will change according to the differential equation (ligand accumulation = ligand production − ligand consumption):

$$\frac{dc}{dt} = R - kc \tag{4-25}$$

At steady state, dc/dt is equal to zero, so the ligand concentration is equal to the ratio of R/k, where R is the rate of ligand production and k is the first-order rate constant for ligand degradation. If the rate of ligand production is suddenly increased to 10 times its previous level ($R = 10R_0$), then the concentration of ligand in the extracellular fluid will increase. The kinetics of ligand concentration change depend on the degradation rate (which can also be designated by the half-life for degradation, $t_{1/2} = \ln(2)/k$):

$$\frac{c}{c_0} = \frac{R}{R_0} + \left(1 - \frac{R}{R_0}\right)e^{-kt} \tag{4-26}$$

as illustrated in Figure 4.18. Rapid changes in ligand concentration, that is, rapid changes in signal activation, can only occur for compounds that are

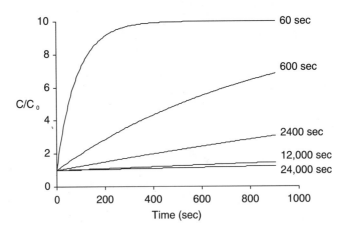

Figure 4.18. Influence of degradation on the kinetics of ligand change. Signaling molecules must have a rapid turnover in order to produce rapid changes in signal strength (i.e., the fraction of receptors bound). Each curve in this figure illustrates the influence of a ligand with a different turnover rate, which varies between 60 s and 24,000 s (or 6.7 hr).

rapidly degraded. For this reason, most naturally occurring signaling molecules often have short half-lives in the body. Rapid degradation allows cells to rapidly regulate signal activation by increasing or decreasing the ligand production rate.

4.5 Kinetics of Cell Proliferation

The fertilized egg develops into a newborn human with $\sim 200 \times 10^9$ cells. This phenomenal increase in cell number is the result of continuous cell proliferation during the period of gestation. Cell growth occurs continuously throughout adult life in some tissues such as the bone marrow, skin, and intestine. Other tissues have the capacity to regenerate lost cell mass by cell proliferation. The liver is the most famous of these tissues; all but 1/8th of the mass of a liver can be removed surgically, but proliferation of the remaining cells will eventually return the liver mass to near normal. The signals that control rates of cell proliferation in the body are incompletely understood, although regulation of proliferation by growth factors is certainly important. Other mechanisms for the control of cell growth (such as contact inhibition and nutrient limitation) have been suggested by experiments on cells that are removed from tissues and maintained in culture.

Cells that are cultured outside of the body will divide and proliferate, but only under the right conditions. Oddly, the ease with which cells can be grown *in vitro* does not always correlate with their proliferative potential in tissue; isolated liver cells are notoriously difficult to grow in culture, for example. Our ability to control cell replication and proliferation is essential for developing our abilities in tissue engineering and, therefore, as in other areas of biotechnology, progress in tissue engineering depends strongly on cell culture science.

As an example of *in vitro* cell culture, Figure 4.19 shows the growth of hybridoma cells and the associated production of monoclonal antibody. This characteristic of cultured cells may make them useful in tissue engineering; cell populations that are engineered and expanded *in vitro* can potentially be transplanted to produce a protein that is continuously released into the body. Figure 4.19 shows some of the characteristics of cell growth and protein production during continuous *in vitro* culture; cell number increases to some maximal density and decreases with depletion of a limiting nutrient (such as glucose). In general, protein production lags behind the increase in cell number, as is illustrated in Figure 4.19.

The next two sections describe some of the basic features of cell growth and analysis of the kinetics of cell growth, which is first illustrated for cells in culture.

4.5.1 Outside of the Body (*in vitro*)

Mammalian cell cultures are obtained from the tissues of an animal, usually by one of two general methods (Figure 4.20): (i) explantation or (ii) enzymatic

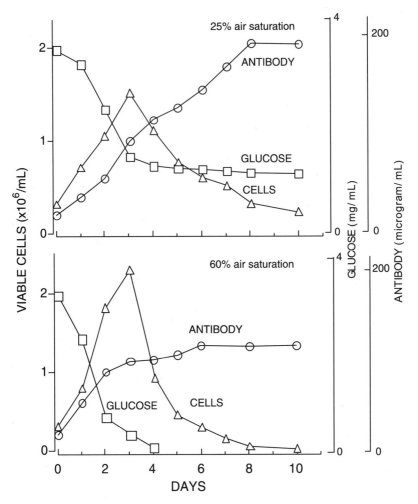

Figure 4.19. Kinetics of cell growth and antibody production by a hybridoma cell line. (redrawn from [18]). In the top panel, cell growth, glucose depletion, and antibody formation are shown for hybridoma cells growing with 25% air saturation. The bottom panel shows the same characteristics for cells grown at a higher air saturation. In these examples, the rate of antibody production lags behind the rate of cell growth.

degradation. These techniques are usually used to isolate and grow cells from rodents (embryos or adults) or from human biopsy materials. The culture that contains cells first isolated from the tissue of origin is called a primary culture. In general, these cells grow following attachment to a solid surface, usually glass or specially modified poly(styrene). In many cases, the cells will grow to form a monolayer on the surface; the cells will stop growing once a critical surface density is achieved. This inhibition of growth at a critical density is a defining feature of mammalian cell culture; it has been studied extensively,

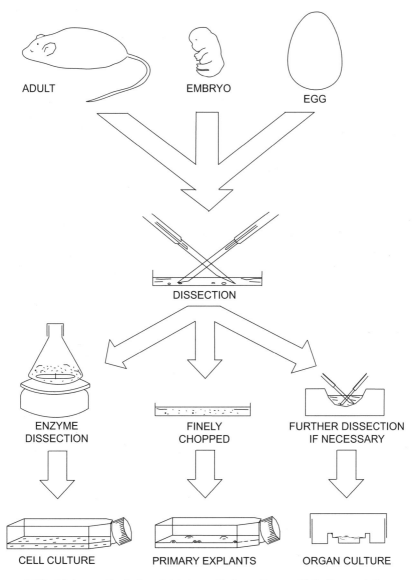

Figure 4.20. Major methods for obtaining cells from tissues. Cells from adult organs, embryos, or biopsy samples can be used as sources for cultured cells. Cells are dissociated from tissue by using enzymes or mechanical forces to disrupt the extracellular matrix and cell–cell adhesion. Cells in culture can be maintained as single cells, as small explants of intact tissue, or as whole segments of organs.

because it probably involves the mechanisms for growth control which constrain cell number within organs and tissues. To further propagate these cells beyond this point of density-dependent growth inhibition, they must be subcultured by detaching the cells with either enzymatic or chemical treatments.

Most mammalian cells have complex medium requirements: a variety of different vitamins, essential amino acids, glucose, and salts must be present in the liquid culture medium in order for cells to survive and proliferate. In most cases, the minimum essential nutrients for the cells are not known; serum from an animal (which contains hormones and growth factors such as insulin, transferrin, EPO, IL-2, etc.) is frequently added to the medium as a supplement to facilitate cell survival and growth. As mentioned previously, a solid surface is usually required for cell proliferation. Therefore, passaging or subculturing of cells is necessary to insure propagation beyond the monolayer stage. During subculture, a fraction of the cells from an adherent culture is detached from the culture dish and resuspended for propagation in a new vessel.

With repeated subculture and growth, a large number of animal cells can be produced from a single tissue source (Figure 4.21). The properties of the cells in culture frequently change as the process of subculturing and propagation is continued. Cells with characteristics that are best suited to the particular culture environment will dominate. Among the important factors that contribute to selection are: sensitivity to trypsin (or other detachment agent); nutrient, hormone, or substrate limitation; relative growth rates; and influence of cell density on individual cells. At a certain point in its history, the cell line may undergo a "crisis." At "crisis," the cells will either completely "transform," which means adapt to the culture environment (becoming a permanent cell line), or die. Transformed cells have a number of distinguishing characteristics (immortality, anchorage independence, loss of contact inhibition, loss of serum dependence, faster growth, tumorgenicity) not found in untransformed cell lines.

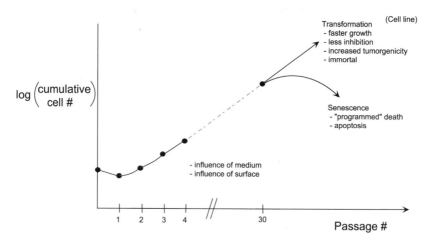

Figure 4.21. Increase of cell number with sequential culture (redrawn from Freshney and Liss [22]). Sequential passaging of cells leads to an increase in the cumulative cell number (i.e., the total number of cell progeny produced from the initial starting material). As the length of time in culture increases, the properties of the cells change.

If actively dividing cells are maintained in a uniform environment, with no constraints to their growth, the rate of growth is proportional to the number of cells:

$$\frac{dN}{dt} = k_P N \tag{4-27}$$

where N is the total number of cells and k_P is the rate constant for cell proliferation. Equation 4-27 is easily solved to reveal that the number of cells increases exponentially with time:

$$N = N_0 e^{k_P t} \tag{4-28}$$

where N_0 is the initial cell number (that is, the number of cells at $t = 0$). The rate constant is related to the doubling time for the cell population t_D:

$$t_D = \frac{\ln 2}{k_P} \tag{4-29}$$

Figure 4.22 shows the typical increase in cell number that occurs during culture of fibroblasts on a conventional tissue culture plastic surface and some other polymeric surfaces; the doubling time is approximately 1 day.

Most cells that are derived from animals are anchorage dependent; cell adhesion and spreading on a solid surface is required for proliferation and function. In addition, as the surface becomes crowded with cells, the rate of

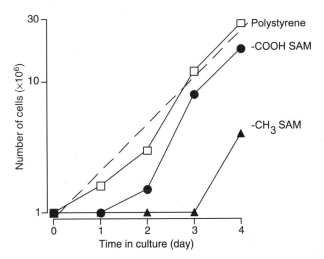

Figure 4.22. Increase in cell number of fibroblasts in culture. The rate of growth is exponential with time, as suggested by Equation 4-21. The doubling time, or the time required for the cell number to increase by a factor of 2, for many mammalian cells is ~ 24 hr. In this figure, the number of fibroblasts is shown as a function of time for three different surface treatments, indicating the influence of the surface chemistry on cell growth. (Figure redrawn from [23].)

cell growth decreases. The rate of cell division is, therefore, dependent on cell density; this phenomenon is called density-dependent cell growth.

In practice, cell proliferation will be constrained by a variety of environmental factors: cell density, nutrient availability, and waste product accumulation all contribute to the overall rate of growth. For anchorage-dependent cells, the overall rate of cell growth and death is related to cell spreading on the surface. Although it is difficult to separate the influence of cell spreading from the influence of chemical interactions between the cell and the surface, cell spreading alone can account for the variation in apoptosis and DNA synthesis that is observed in endothelial cells (Figure 4.23).

A common phenomenological model, called the Monod model, is used to describe the influence of a substrate or nutrient of limited availability that limits growth:

$$k_P = \frac{1}{N}\frac{dN}{dt} = \frac{k_{P,\max}S}{K_M + S} \tag{4-30}$$

where S is the substrate concentration and the constants $k_{P\max}$ and K_M characterize the influence of the substrate on the growth rate. The rate of substrate consumption is related to the rate of cell growth by a yield coefficient, $Y_{N/S}$, which is equal to the ratio of substrate consumption rate r_S to cell growth rate

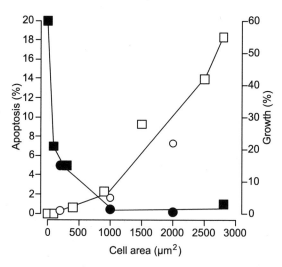

Figure 4.23. Apoptosis and DNA synthesis depend on cell spreading (redrawn from [24]). The filled symbols indicate apoptosis and the open symbols indicate DNA synthesis, both expressed as percentage of cells, for endothelial cells. The cell spreading was controlled by microfabrication of extracellular matrix patterns on a flat substrate. The square symbols are for cells in which the ECM pattern covers the entire area of cell attachment; the circle symbols are for cells in which the ECM pattern covers only a small fraction of the surface. This correlation suggests that cell spreading over a surface, but not the extent of ECM interaction, is most important in regulating cell growth and apoptotic death.

r_N (or $k_P N$): that is, $Y_{N/S} = -r_S/r_N$. Other models of growth are also available; see the chapters on modeling of cell growth kinetics in [17, 18]. The presence of growth factors also has a profound influence on rates of cell growth (Figure 4.10); perhaps the best-studied example is the influence of EGF on fibroblast growth (this work is reviewed in the text by Lauffenburger and Linderman [11]).

4.5.2 Inside the Body (*in vivo*)

The growth of individual organs and tissues within an individual is regulated. Despite individual differences in appearance, our relative body and organ proportions are roughly equivalent. Not all organs and tissues grow at the same rate, and rates of growth vary throughout life. For example, the brain increases in mass and volume early in life, while other organs lag (Figure 4.24). The overall height of an individual depends primarily on growth of the long bones, which is influenced by the environment, nutrient supply, and hormone production. Some of these factors have been quantified, but the mechanisms underlying regulation are not completely understood.

A simple description of individual growth is analogous to the expression used to characterize the increase in cell number:

$$\frac{dM}{dt} = k_{growth} M \qquad (4\text{-}31)$$

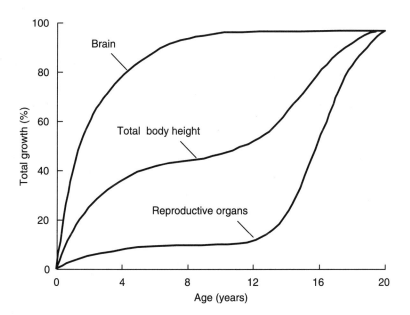

Figure 4.24. Rates of growth vary with time and differ in different organs (after [25]). The rate of growth varies with time, and can be estimated as the slope of the curves of total growth vs. age, as shown here.

where the total body mass M is assumed to increase in proportion to the mass present. The rate of growth varies with age, as is indicated by the changing slope of the curves in Figure 4.24. When different regions of the body grow at different rates, the process is called allometric growth and is characterized by

$$Y = BX^k \qquad \qquad (4\text{-}32)$$

where Y is the mass of a region of interest (for example, the brain), X is the mass of another region (or the total body mass M), and B and k are constants that characterize the differences in growth. The growth ratio k indicates the relative rate of growth of the region of interest (Y) with respect to the reference region (X); when $k > 1$, the region of interest grows more quickly than the reference region. When $k = 1$, the regions grow isometrically: that is, at the same relative rate.

During evolution, regions of the brain developed at different rates, perhaps corresponding to behavioral capabilities that enhanced survival of a particular species. For example, the relative volume of the neocortex scales allometrically within groups of primates or insectivores. There are important differences in the relative brain size between primates and insectivores. For animals of a fixed brain volume, the neocortex is substantially larger in primates than in insectivores (Figure 4.25). One can imagine that similar levels of control must be available during development of an individual; regions of a tissue grow at different rates.

It is difficult to measure the relative rates of growth for different cell populations within the body. Sometimes, cell growth and death can be studied

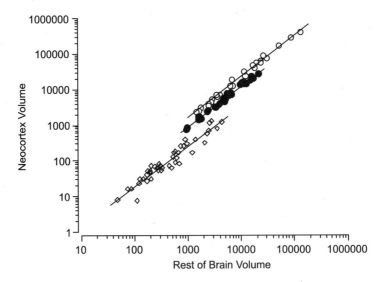

Figure 4.25. The ratio of neocortex volume to brain volume varies with species: differences between relative brain sizes in primates (circles) and insectivores (diamonds). (Redrawn from [26].)

by labeling a certain fraction of cells and observing the change in the percentage of labeled cells that occurs with time. This approach has been used to estimate growth and death rates for subpopulations of T lymphocytes [19]. In the analysis performed in [19], the proliferating T cells of monkeys were labeled by continuous administration of BrdU in the drinking water. Consider a population of cells within the circulating blood; the total number of cells N is determined by balancing the rates of proliferation, addition, and death:

$$\frac{dN}{dt} = S + pN - dN = S + (p - d)N \tag{4-33}$$

where S is the rate of cell addition (cells/min), p is a rate constant for cell growth (simplified from k_P in Equation 4-27), and d is a rate constant for cell death. If the initial cell number (at $t = 0$) is N_0, the number of cells varies with time:

$$N = \left[N_0 + \frac{S}{p - d}\right]e^{(p-d)t} - \frac{S}{p - d} \tag{4-34}$$

which reduces to Equation 4-28 (with k_P in Equation 4-28 replaced by $p - d$) in the case where $S = 0$. Equations 4-33 and 4-34 correspond to the situation illustrated in Figure 4.26a. If an agent that labels dividing cells is provided to the animal, as in [19], and it behaves as illustrated in Figure 4.26b, the overall cell balance equations during the labeling period can be written for unlabeled cells (U) and labeled cells (L):

$$\left.\begin{aligned}
\frac{dU}{dt} &= S_U - pU - dU \\[6pt]
\frac{dL}{dt} &= S_L + 2pU + pL - dL \\[6pt]
\frac{d(U + L)}{dt} &= S_U + S_L + p(U + L) - d(U + L)
\end{aligned}\right\} \tag{4-35}$$

In this set of equations, it is assumed that proliferation of an unlabeled cell produces two labeled cells and the loss of one unlabeled cell. Notice that the overall cell balance remains unchanged, since the total cell number N is equal to $L + U$ and the total rate of addition S is equal to $S_L + S_U$. After the labeling period is complete, cells continue to grow and die, as illustrated in 4.26c, but the balance equations are different:

$$\left.\begin{aligned}
\frac{dU}{dt} &= S_U' + pU - dU \\[6pt]
\frac{dL}{dt} &= S_L' + pL - dL \\[6pt]
\frac{d(U + L)}{dt} &= S_U' + S_L' + p(U + L) - d(U + L)
\end{aligned}\right\} \tag{4-36}$$

Mohri et al. [19] found an approximate solution to the set of Equations 4-35 and 4-36:

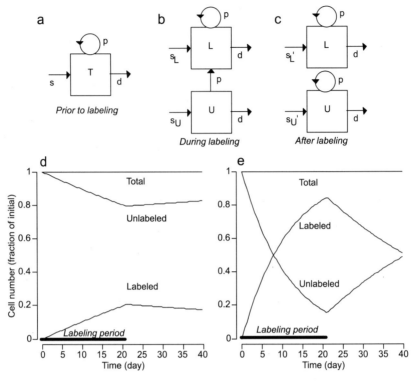

Figure 4.26. Models for determining rates of T cell growth and death in a living animal. (a) In the simplest state, the number of T cells in the blood depends on rates of growth, death, and addition from an external source. (b) During the process of labeling, there are source terms for labeled (S_L) and unlabeled (S_U) cells; the numbers of labeled and unlabeled cells are indicated as L and U, respectively. (c) After the labeling is completed, the source terms are changed to S_L' and S_U'. (d) An approximate solution to the differential cell balance equations is illustrated in the situation where no SIV infection is present: $p = 0.001$/day; $d = 0.01$/day; and cell replacement rate, $S/N_0 = 0.9\%$/day. (e) An approximate solution to the differential cell balance equations in the situation where SIV infection is present: $p = 0.031$/day; $d = 0.058$/day; and cell replacement rate, $S/N_0 = 2.7\%$/day. (Panels redrawn from [19].)

$$\left.\begin{array}{ll} f_L = C(1 - e^{-(p+d)t}), & \text{for} \quad t \le T \\[2mm] f_L = C(1 - e^{(p+d)T})e^{-(d-p)(t-T)}, & \text{for} \quad t \ge T \end{array}\right\} \quad (4\text{-}37)$$

where f_L is the fraction of labeled cells in the blood, T is the duration of the labeling period, and C is a constant equal to $1 - S_U/U(0)(p + d)$. Figure 4.26 shows this solution for two different situations; these solutions were intended to correspond to an animal that is not infected with a T cell virus (simian immunodeficiency virus, SIV, which is analogous to HIV in humans) in panel d and infected with SIV in panel e. These solutions agree with experimental data obtained by labeling cells in infected and non-infected animals and permit the estimation of cell growth and death rates in each separate situation. For this set of experiments, the mathematical model outlined in Equation 4-30 allowed the authors to conclude that T cell growth and death are accelerated in animals infected with SIV [19].

Summary

- Cell division—and the proliferation of the cell population that this produces—is an important determinant of tissue growth. As cell division proceeds, whether in development or in organ repair, cells differentiate into phenotypes that are essential for the function of the mature tissue.
- Stem cells are primitive, undifferentiated cells that are capable of giving rise to multiple cell lineages or phenotypes. Stem cells exhibit three essential properties: self-renewal, differentiation into multiple lineages, and ability to repopulate a tissue after transplantation. Stem cells can be found in both embryonic and adult tissues; embryonic stem cells, hematopoietic stem cells, and mesenchymal stem cells have been the most extensively studied and characterized.
- Soluble agents (cytokines, growth factors, hormones, etc.) influence the rate of growth and pattern of differentiation in cells. Receptor–ligand interactions are essential in the regulation of cell division and differentiation. Mathematical models, based on diffusion and chemical interactions, offer a powerful approach for understanding the mechanisms of action of soluble agents on cell growth and differentation.
- Cell culture outside of a living organism (*in vitro*) is one of the most powerful tools of modern biology. In many cases, *in vitro* cell growth and differentiation can be controlled and subsequently analyzed to determine the factors limiting growth. This analysis is more difficult to perform for cell growth *in vivo*, since many of the environmental cues are unknown or unpredictable.

Exercises

Exercise 4.1 (provided by Christine Schmidt)

For many tissue engineering applications mature differentiated cells (for example, chondrocytes, fibroblasts, osteoblasts) will be used. However, mesenchymal stem cells (MSCs) from the bone marrow are precursor cells that can differentiate into these mature connective tissue cells if they are provided with the appropriate environment. Thus, one cell would provide the source for several differentiated tissue cells. Another key advantage of using MSCs is the ease with which these cells can be cultured and expanded *in vitro*.

a) Unfortunately, MSCs only account for about 1 in every 10,000 cells in the bone marrow. Will this pose a problem with using these cells for tissue engineering applications? Why or why not?

b) Regardless of whether this will or will not pose a problem, please describe what type of procedure you could use to purify MSCs from a solution of all bone marrow cells. Be as specific as possible.

Exercise 4.2 (provided by Peter Zandstra)

Cells take up EGF from the extracellular medium by receptor-mediated endocytosis and horseradish peroxidase (HRP) by fluid-phase endocytosis. An example of the cell uptake of EGF and HRP as a function of the concentration in the medium is shown in Figure 4.27.

a) Explain why the uptake of HRP is linear whereas the EGF uptake is hyperbolic.

b) Explain why the rate of uptake of EGF is much faster than that for HRP.

Exercise 4.3 (provided by Peter Zandstra)

You have isolated a smooth muscle cell preparation that contracts when a drug (ligand) is applied. The muscle is connected to a force transducer that allows you to measure the force of contraction (cell response). The maximum force of contraction that the preparation is capable of is 1 N. A drug concentration of 1×10^{-8} M produces a contraction force of 0.75 N.

a) Determine the K_d of the drug.

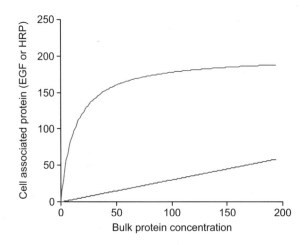

Figure 4.27. Uptake kinetics for EGF and horseradish peroxidase (HRP).

b) You add a ligand that competitively inhibits muscle contraction. When the ligand is added at a concentration of 5×10^{-7} M the contraction force is reduced to 0.25 N. Determine the K_d value for the inhibitor.
c) What concentration of the drug is necessary to achieve the original contraction force of 0.75 N in the presence of 5×10^{-7} M of the inhibitor?

Exercise 4.4 (provided by Michael Sefton)

The bigger the molecule, the slower it diffuses for the same difference in concentration; that is, bigger molecules have a smaller diffusion coefficient.

a) For a 10 μm diameter cell, calculate the difference between cell surface concentration and the concentration at the center for the following molecules if diffusion is the only means of transport. Assume a constant consumption rate.

Molecule	MW (daltons)	D (m^2/s)
Urea	60	1.20×10^{-9}
Sucrose	342	0.697×10^{-9}
Lipoxidase	97,440	5.59×10^{-11}
Albumin	67,500	6.81×10^{-11}
Urease	482,700	4.01×10^{-11}

b) Comment on the implications of these calculations on cell structure and function.

Exercise 4.5 (provided by Michael Sefton)

The "Thiele modulus" (ϕ) is a parameter that compares the rate of reaction to the rate of diffusion (actually the square root of these two). The modulus has no dimensions and hence is termed a dimensionless number.

$$\phi = R\sqrt{k/D}$$

where $R =$ sphere radius (or other characteristic dimension) (cm), $k =$ reaction rate constant (s^{-1}), and $D =$ diffusion coefficient (cm^2/s).

a) Show how this modulus can be introduced to simplify Equation 4-19.

For diffusion effects to be negligible, ϕ must be much less than 1 ($\phi \ll 1$). For most purposes, $\phi < 0.1$ is usually sufficient, so that an order-of-magnitude calculation is appropriate. Estimate the maximum or minimum order of magnitude of the other parameter if diffusion effects are to be negligible for the following situation. Specify whether it is a maximum or a minimum.

b) $D = 10^{-6}$ cm^2/s; $k = 10^{-2}$ s^{-1}
c) $D = 10^{-6}$ cm^2/s; $k = 1$ s^{-1}

d) $D = 10^{-5}$ cm^2/s; $k = 10$ s^{-1}
e) $D = 10^{-6}$ cm^2/s; $k = 10^2$ s^{-1}
f) $D = 10^{-6}$ cm^2/s; $R = 10^{-7}$ m

Comment on the significance of your calculations. *Note*: Diffusion coefficients are typically in the range from 10^{-5} to 10^{-6} cm^2/s for small molecules in liquids and 10^{-10} cm^2/s or smaller in solids. A rate constant can be converted into a characteristic time using the half-life, $t_{1/2}$, the time for half of the molecules to be consumed: $t_{1/2} = \ln 2/k$.

Exercise 4.6

For a cell of radius a, the maximum rate that the cell could absorb ligand molecules from its environment is $I_{max} = 4\pi a D L_\infty$, where D is the ligand diffusion coefficient and L_∞ is the concentration of ligand far from the cell.

a) Assume that the same cell attaches to a flat surface and takes the shape of a pancake with radius r_s. What is the maximum rate that this attached cell can absorb ligand molecules?
b) Assume that the attached pancake cell has on its surface N receptors of radius $s \ll r_s$. Find an expression for the rate of ligand absorption, assuming that the ligand molecules do not adsorb to the cell surface.

Exercise 4.7 (provided by Rebecca Kuntz Willits)

Determine both the maximum dilution rate and the dilution rate for maximum output for a CSTR with sterile feed and cells with growth kinetics according to the following equation (where C_s is the concentration of the limiting solute and μ has units of s^{-1}):

$$\mu = k_{growth} C_s$$

Be sure to define all variables used.

Exercise 4.8 (provided by Michael Sefton)

A cell culture is initially composed of 100 cells. After 12 hours the number of cells is 1.5 times the number in the initial population.

a) If the rate of growth is proportional to the number of cells present, determine the time necessary for the number of cells to triple.
b) What is the time required for a culture with 1×10^6 of the same cells to triple? Explain your results.
c) Under what conditions would the answers obtained in part b) be invalid?

Exercise 4.9 (provided by Michael Sefton)

For a specific type of cell after 3 hours, the concentration of cells per milliliter of solution is about 400/mL. After 10 hours the concentration has gone up to 2000/mL. Determine the initial concentration of cells.

Exercise 4.10 (provided by Michael Sefton)

A suspension cell culture has a maximum specific growth rate $k_{p,\max}$ of $0.2\,\text{hr}^{-1}$ when grown in the presence of glucose. The Monod constant on glucose, K_M, is $1\,\text{g/L}$ and the cell yield on glucose ($Y_{N/S}$) is 0.40 g cell/g glucose. For this example, assume steady-state operation and that all nutrients are in excess except glucose.

a) We grow this cell in a 10 L continuous reactor (CSTR) using a sterile feed stream containing 10 g/L glucose and flowing at 1 L/hr. What is the glucose concentration exiting from the CSTR?

b) If the "cell formula" is $C_{4.4}H_{7.3}N_{0.86}O_{1.2}$, estimate the rate of CO_2 production (L/hr at STP) from the CSTR in part a). State any assumptions.

Exercise 4.11 (provided by Michael Sefton)

It is expected that stem cells provide a renewable tissue-culture source of cells that can be used to regrow whole organs such as hearts and livers. The cells will then be harvested for applications in basic research or transplantation therapies. It is hypothesized that the undifferentiated proliferation of these cells follows a Monod growth model. Assume that the maximum growth rate ($k_{p,\max}$) of these cells is $0.3\,\text{hr}^{-1}$ when in presence of a specific differentiation-inhibiting factor (DIF). The Monod constant, K_M, is assumed to be $1.3\,\text{g/L}$ and the cell yields in the presence of this factor ($Y_{x/\text{DIF}}$) is 0.46 g cell/g of DIF. Assume steady-state operation for this question.

An attempt is being made to use a 10 L continuous reactor aerated with oxygen, using a sterile feed stream containing 5 g/L of DIF. What is the outlet concentration of the factor for a feed flow rate of 1 L/hr?

Exercise 4.12 (provided by Keith Gooch)

Equal numbers of fibroblasts and endothelial cells are present initially in a culture.

a) If endothelial cells double every 40 hours and fibroblasts double every 20 hours, draw a graph showing the percentage of cells in the culture that are fibroblasts as a function of time.

b) What is the time required for the culture to contain 90% fibroblasts? Write an equation that describes this situation and, when solved for time, will provide the correct answer.

Exercise 4.13 (provided by Peter Zandstra)

Your laboratory decides to test the hypothesis that the degree of cell confluence (that is, the numbers of cells per given surface area) affects equilibrium binding of epidermal growth factor (EGF) to the EGFR (epidermal growth factor receptors) on fibroblasts. On January 12, a binding experiment was done with cells ($\sim 10\,\mu m$ radius) plated at confluence in 35 mm diameter culture dishes, incubated for 6 hours at 4°C with 5 mL of media at a series of concentrations of I^{125}-labeled EGF. (The labeling was done on December 20, obtaining a specific activity of 85,000 cpm/ng.) A control for nonspecific binding was also performed, using unlabeled EGF at a concentration of 1 mg/mL. On February 3, a second experiment was done for comparison, now with cells plated at 10% confluence. But, since your stock of EGF was running low (and it is not cheap), these experiments were performed with 2 mL of medium and the nonspecific binding controls used 0.1 mg/mL. Given the data shown in Tables 4.3 and 4.4, determine the values of R_T and K_d for these cells under the two cell density conditions. Would you conclude that the degree of confluence affects intrinsic binding parameters?

Exercise 4.14 (provided by Peter Zandstra)

The binding of fibroblast growth factor (FGF) to its receptor is thought to require the presence of proteoglycans (PGs) (proteins that are a major component of the extracellular matrix) in order to elicit a biological response. Consider the model illustrated in Figure 4.28 for the binding of FGF to its cell surface receptor (FGFR) and PGs. Parameter values are enumerated

Table 4.3
January 12 Results (3 trails w/o "cold" EGF, mean ± s.e; one trail w. "cold" EGF)

EGF Concentration (ng/mL)	Binding w/o "cold" EGF (cpm)	Binding w/"cold" EGF (cpm)
0.1	1260 ± 220	15
1.0	14,810 ± 2,670	162
10	93,350 ± 19,210	1,258
100	174,800 ± 36,940	14,870

Table 4.4
February 3 Results (3 trails w/o "cold" EGF, mean ± s.e; one trail w. "cold" EGF)

EGF Concentration (ng/mL)	Binding w/o "cold" EGF (cpm)	Binding w/"cold" EGF (cpm)
0.1	76 ± 32	13
1.0	895 ± 174	86
10	6,270 ± 1,009	431
100	12,180 ± 2,314	2,876

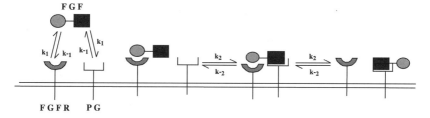

Figure 4.28. Model for binding of FGF to its cell receptor.

below. Assume that you are operating under conditions with negligible endocytic trafficking and minimal ligand depletion.

a) Generate an equilibrium Scatchard plot for total cell surface binding, and determine an effective K_d, for the following cases of cell surface PG number: 0, 10^4, 10^5, and 10^6 per cell.

b) Calculate the number of FGF/FGFR complexes as a function of FGF concentration (summing FGF/FGFR and PG/FGF/FGFR types) for the same cases.

c) Interpret your response on the basis of what you know about the biological properties of FGF.

$$k_1 = 1.5 \times 10^8 \ \text{M}^{-1} \ \text{min}^{-1}$$
$$k_{-1} = 0.05 \ \text{min}^{-1}$$
$$k_2 = 10^{-4} \ (\text{\#/cell})^{-1} \ \text{min}^{-1}$$
$$k_{-2} = 10^{-3} \ \text{min}^{-1}$$
$$\text{FGFR} = 3 \times 10^4 \ \text{\#/cell}$$

Exercise 4.15 (provided by Song Li)

How would you analyze the proliferation rate of cells in three-dimensional polymer scaffolds? Describe your experimental procedure.

Exercise 4.16 (provided by Song Li)

The cell growth in a bioreactor may be limited by the bioreactor capacity, available nutrients, and cell contact inhibition. If we assume that cell proliferation rate dX/dt is proportional to $(X_M - X)$, that is, $dX/dt = C \ (X_M - X)$, where X_M is the maximum number of cells in the bioreactor, calculate the constant C if we know the cell numbers at two time points $X(t = 0) = X_0$ and $X(t = t_1) = X_1$.

Exercise 4.17 (provided by Linda G. Griffith)

NR6 fibroblasts lack endogenous EGF receptors. Dr W has transfected a mutant internalization-deficient EGFR into NR6 cells, "c'973"; the mutant is a deletion of a large portion of the cytoplasmic domain, leaving the extra-cellular domain intact. All other properties of the receptor (for example, affi-nity for EGF and other EGFR ligands) remain the same. The steady-state receptor number obtained in the transfected cells is 60,000 EGFR/cell. In culture medium containing 5,000 cells per ml, estimate the fraction of total receptors occupied when the EGF concentration in the medium is: (a) 0.1 nM; (b) 1 nM; (c) 10 nM. Clearly state any assumptions or equations employed.

Exercise 4.18 (provided by Linda G. Griffith)

Combined effects of soluble and insoluble ligands can often be synergistic in complicated ways. Consider a soluble growth factor "A" that binds to its cell surface receptor with equilibrium dissociation constant K_{DA}, and an insoluble matrix factor "B" which mediates adhesion of the cells to the substrate and which binds to its cell surface receptor with equilibrium dissociation constant K_{DB}. It is observed that, under some conditions, A stimulates cell proliferation, whereas under other conditions A promotes cell death.

The following conceptual model can be posed to account for this observa-tion. Cells will proliferate when they are sufficiently adherent, but die when they are insufficiently adherent. When they are sufficiently adherent, their pro-liferation rate constant can be enhanced by growth factor, but growth factor also reduces cell adhesion, possibly leading to cell death. Testable predictions from this conceptual model can be made by casting it into a mathematical framework.

Let C_A be the number of steady-state complexes of growth factor with its receptor, and C_B be the number of steady-state complexes of matrix factor B with its cell receptor.

a) Assuming negligible endocytic trafficking of either factor, and constant concentrations L_A and L_B, write the expression for C_A and C_B in terms of the total receptor number of each type ($R_{T,A}$, $R_{T,B}$) and their respective equilibrium dissociation constants $K_{D,A}$ and $K_{D,B}$. Let $\mu = (1/N)dN/dt$, the net cell growth rate constant (N = cell number density), be given by

$$\mu = \begin{cases} k_{p\,max} C_A/(K_{D,A} + C_A) & \text{for} \quad C_B \geq C_B^* \\ -k_d & \text{for} \quad C_B \leq C_B^* \end{cases}$$

where C_B^* is the critical minimum number of adhesion complexes required to support cell survival proliferation. Let $K_{D,B} = \phi K_{D,B}^0 C_A/R_{T,A}$, where $K_{D,B}^0$ is the value of $K_{D,B}$ in the absence of growth factor.

b) If A decreases cell adhesion, what do you know about the value of ϕ?

c) Determine the dependence of μ on L_A.

d) Show from c) that the model does or doesn't account for the observation mentioned in the first paragraph.

e) Suggest experiments that could be done to further test this model.

Exercise 4.19 (provided by Linda G. Griffith)

Consider the ATS skin product Dermagraft^{TM} and assume that this can be modeled as a thin slab of dermis (thickness $= 2L$) containing $\sim 10\%$ cells by volume, with the remainder of the volume occupied by extracellular matrix. It has been hypothesized that the effectiveness of Dermagraft in treating dermal wounds is related to the amount of a particular growth factor—vascular endothelial cell growth factor (VEGF)—secreted by the fibroblasts in Dermagraft. VEGF produced by the fibroblasts diffuses into the surrounding tissue and induces the growth of blood vessels. For parts a)–e) below, perform the analysis for the situation where the Dermagraft is at the final stage of growing in the bioreactor—that is, it is a fully formed tissue with culture medium on both sides.

a) Assume that the production rate of VEGF by fibroblasts in Dermagraft is zero-order. For some arbitrary fixed concentration of VEGF at the surface of Dermagraft, sketch the general shape of the concentration profile of VEGF in Dermagraft at steady state.

b) Derive a differential equation governing the production and diffusion of VEGF in Dermagraft. Use the following notation: $C_v =$ molar concentration of VEGF; $x =$ distance from the surface ($x = L$ is the center of the slab); $D_{AB} =$ diffusion coefficient of VEGF in Dermagraft; $Q_{VEGF} =$ volumetric production rate of VEGF (*Hint*: pay careful attention to the sign of Q_{VEGF}).

c) Solve the equation you derived in b) to obtain an expression for the concentration of VEGF as a function of x, for a designated surface concentration C_0.

d) If $C_0 = 5$ nM and it is determined that the concentration of VEGF at the center of the Dermagraft is 100 nM, what is the cellular production rate of VEGF for a piece of Dermagraft of *total* thickness 300 µm (300×10^{-4} cm)? The diffusion coefficient of VEGF in Dermagraft is $\sim 5 \times 10^{-6}$ cm^2/s and the average diameter of a fibroblast is 12 µm. Give your answer in terms of molecules per cell per second. (Reminder: Avagadro's number $= 6.0220 \times 10^{23}$ molecules per mole.)

e) Using the production rate of VEGF you derive in part d), calculate the flux of VEGF across the outer surfaces of the graft (that is, flux at $x = 0$). Please show all calculations clearly for full credit.

f) Estimate how long it takes for VEGF to diffuse a distance of 500 µm into the local wound tissue after a piece of fresh Dermagraft is placed on the wound.

Exercise 4.20 (provided by Linda G. Griffith)

Receptor tyrosine kinases can activate a variety of pathways. Refer to a current textbook on molecular cell biology (such as [1] or [2]) and compare a few of these pathways in terms of how the signal is transmitted and what end result is achieved. How do these signal-processing pathways compare to those of G-protein-coupled receptors? How might each of these receptor types be useful to a tissue engineer?

Exercise 4.21 (provided by Linda G. Griffith)

EPO is a growth hormone secreted by the pancreas that influences red blood cell (RBC) development. The number of RBCs secreted roughly corresponds to the equilibrium number of signaling complexes. For this reason, Amgen sells a recombinant form of EPO for administration to patients who are anemic or suffering extreme blood loss.

a) In order to supply an appropriate amount of the drug, the equilibrium-binding behavior needed to be established. So a cell biology researcher measured equilibrium binding versus ligand concentration. Using the given data, calculate K_d and R_T.

Data: equilibrium binding of Epo to 110^5 cells in culture [33].

L_0 (nM)	0.025	0.05	0.075	0.15	0.25	0.33	0.66	0.75	1.25	1.75	3	10	12	16	33
C (pM)	1.05	2.2	3	5.5	8	10.5	14	16	20	22	26	35	30	32	33

b) Plot C_{eq} versus $\log(L_0)$ using the equilibrium binding equation:

$$K_d = \left(\frac{RL}{C}\right)_{eq} \approx \frac{(R_T - C_{eq})L_0}{C_{eq}}$$

In what range of ligand concentrations is the response curve linear? Where does the curve start to plateau?

c) For both cost and safety purposes, hormones are usually administered at the lowest effective concentration. Does it make sense that a "unit/ml" of EPO is defined as 0.2 nM?

References

1. Lodish, H., et al., *Molecular Cell Biology*. New York: W.H. Freeman, 1995.
2. Alberts, B., et al., *Molecular Biology of the Cell*, 3rd ed. New York: Garland Publishing, 1994.
3. Till, X. and X. McColloch, *Radiation Research*, 1961, **14**, 1419.
4. Morrison, S.J., et al., Prospective identification, isolation by flow cytometry, and in vivo self-renewal of multipotent neural crest stem cells. *Cell*, 1999, **96**, 737–749.
5. Reynolds, B.A. and S. Weiss, Generation of neurons and astrocytes from isolated cells of the adult mammalian central nervous system. *Science*, 1992, **255**, 1707–1710.
6. Weissmann, I.L., Translating stem and progenitor cell biology to the clinic: barriers and opportunities. *Science*, 2000, **287**, 1442–1446.
7. Gage, F.H., Mammalian Neural Stem Cells. *Science*, 2000, **287**, 1433–1438.
8. Kornack, D.R. and P. Racik, Cell proliferation without neurogenesis in adult primate neocortex. *Science*, 2001, **294**, 2127–2130.

9. Krause, D.S., et al., Multi-organ, multi-lineage engraftment by a single bone marrow-derived stem cell. *Cell*, 2001, **105**, 369–377.

10. Wagers, A.J., et al., Little evidence for developmental plasticity of adult hematopoietic stem cells. *Science*, 2002, **297**, 2256–2259.

11. Lauffenburger, D.A. and J.J. Linderman, *Receptors: Models for Binding, Trafficking, and Signaling.* New York: Oxford University Press, 1993, 365 pp.

12. Francis, K. and B.O. Palsson, Effective intercellular communication distances are determined by the relative time constants for cyto/chemokine secretion and diffusion. *Proc. Natl. Acad. Sci.*, 1997, **94**, 12258–12262.

13. Carslaw, H.S. and J.C. Jaeger, *Conduction of Heat in Solids*, 2nd ed. Oxford: Oxford University Press, 1959, 510 pp.

14. Saltzman, W.M., *Drug Delivery: Engineering Principles for Drug Therapy.* New York: Oxford University Press, 2001.

15. Clark, E.A. and J.S. Brugge, Integrins and signal transduction pathways: the road taken. *Science*, 1995, **268**, 233–239.

16. Longhurst, C.M. and L.K. Jennings, Integrin-mediated signal transduction. *Cellular and Molecular Life Sciences*, 1998, **54**, 514–526.

17. Bailey, J.E. and D.F. Ollis, *Biochemical Engineering Fundamentals.* New York: McGraw-Hill, 1986, 928 pp.

18. Shuler, M.L. and F. Kargi, *Bioprocess Engineering: Basic Concepts*, 2nd ed. New York: Prentice Hall, 2002.

19. Mohri, H., et al., Rapid turnover of T lymphocytes in SIV-infected rhesus macaques. *Science*, 1998, **279**, 1223–1227.

20. Lamond, A.I. and W.C. Earnshaw, Structure and function in the nucleus. *Science*, 1998, **280**, 547–553.

21. Watt, F.M. and B.L.M. Hogan, Out of Eden: stem cells and their niches. *Science*, 2000, **287**, 1427–1430.

22. Freshney, R. and A. Liss, *Culture of Animal Cells: A Manual of Basic Techniques.* New York: Alan R. Liss, 1987.

23. McClary, K.B., T. Ugarov, and D.W. Grainger, Modulating fibroblast adhesion, spreading, and proliferation using self-assembled monolayer films of alkylthiolates on gold. *Journal of Biomedical Materials Research*, 2000, **50**(3), 428–439.

24. Chen, C., et al., Geometric control of cell life and death. *Science*, 1997, **276**, 1425–1428.

25. Vander, A., J. Sherman, and D. Luciano, *Human Physiology: the Mechanisms of Body Function.* Boston: WCB McGraw-Hill, 1998.

26. Barton, R.A. and P.H. Harvey, Mosaic evolution of brain structure in mammals. *Nature*, 2000, **405**, 1055–1057.

27. Whalen, G.F., Y. Shing, and J. Folkman, The fate of intravenously administered bFGF and the effect of heparin. *Growth Factors*, 1989, **1**, 157–164.

28. Gutterman, J.U., et al., *Cancer Research*, 1984, **44**, 4164–4171.

29. Poduslo, J.F., G.L. Curran, and C.T. Berg, Macromolecular permeability across the blood–nerve and blood–brain barriers. *Proc. Natl. Acad. Sci. USA*, 1994, **91**, 5705–5709.

30. Konrad, M.W., et al., *Cancer Research*, 1990, **50**, 2009–2017.

31. Cohen, A.M., Erythropoietin and G-CSF, in A. H. C. Kung, R. A. Baughman, and J. W. Larrick, eds., *Therapeutic Proteins: Pharmacokinetics and Pharmacodynamics.* New York: W.H. Freeman, 1983, pp. 165–186.

32. Dittrich, F., H. Thoenen, and M. Sendtner, Ciliary neurotrophic factor: pharma-cokinetics and acute-phase response in rats. *Annals of Neurology*, 1994. **35**(2), 151–163.
33. Hilton, D.J., et al., *Proceedings of the National Academy of Sciences USA*, 1995, **92**, 190–194.
34. Knauer, D.J., H.S. Wiley, and D.D. Cunningham, Relationship between epidermal growth factor receptor occupancy and mitogenic response. *Journal of Biological Chemistry*, 1984, **259**, 5623–5631.

5

Cell and Tissue Mechanics

Since things in motion sooner catch the eye
Than what not stirs.

William Shakespeare, *Troilus and Cressida*

Mechanics is the branch of physics that is concerned with the action of forces on matter. Tissue engineers can encounter mechanics in various settings. Often, the mechanical properties of replacement biological materials must replicate the normal tissue: for example, there is limited use for a tissue-engineered bone that cannot support the load encountered by its natural counterpart. In addition, the mechanical properties of cells and cell–cell adhesions can determine the architecture of a tissue during development. This phenomenon can sometimes be exploited, since the final form of engineered tissues depends on the forces encountered during assembly and maturation. Finally, the mechanics of individual cells—and the molecular interactions that restrain cells—are important determinants of cell growth, movement, and function within an organism.

This chapter introduces the basic elements of mechanics applied to biological systems. Some examples of biomechanical principles that appear to be important for tissue engineering are also provided. For further reading, comprehensive treatments of various aspects of biomechanics are also available [1–3].

5.1 Elementary Solid Mechanics

5.1.1 Elastic Deformation and Young's Modulus

Consider an elongated object—for example, a segment of a biological tissue or a synthetic biomaterial—that is fixed at one end and suddenly exposed to a constant applied load (Figure 5.1). The material will change or deform in response to the load. For some materials, the deformation is instantaneous and, under conditions of low loading, deformation varies linearly with the magnitude of the applied force:

$$\sigma \left[\equiv \frac{F}{A} \right] = E\varepsilon \tag{5-1}$$

119

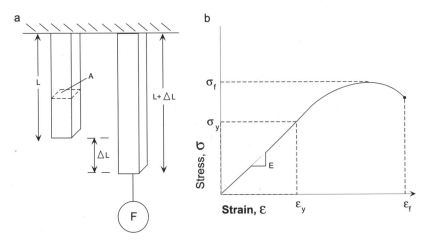

Figure 5.1. Typical characteristics of an elastic material. (a) A uniform material is subjected to an applied load. (b) Typical response of the material to tensile loads of increasing magnitude.

where σ is the applied stress and ε is the resulting strain. This relationship is called Hooke's law, after the British physicist Robert Hooke, and it describes the behavior of many elastic materials, such as springs, which deform linearly upon loading and recover their original shape upon removal of the load. The Young's modulus or tensile elastic modulus, E, is a property of the material; some typical values are provided in Table 5.1. Not all elastic materials obey Hooke's law (for example, rubber does not); some materials will recover their original shape, but strain is not linearly related to stress. Fortunately, many interesting materials do follow Equation 5-1, particularly if the deformations are small.

Materials become irreversibly altered if they are deformed beyond a critical yield strain, or elastic limit, ε_y. (Many materials obey Hooke's law for all strains less than the elastic limit; other materials obey Hooke's law over a more limited range, called the proportional limit, and continue to deform elastically, but not linearly, up to the yield stress.) This state occurs at a characteristic yield stress σ_y. Further strain of the material results in plastic (rather than elastic) deformation; an irreversible change in the material prevents it from recovering its original state after removal of the applied load. The largest stress that a material can endure without failing (that is, breaking or fracturing) is called the ultimate or failure stress, σ_f.

It is convenient to analyze deformations with respect to excursions on the stress–strain plane (Figure 5.2). If an elastic material is subjected to a load producing strain ε_A, which is less than the yield strain ε_y, it will return to its original shape (after removal of the load) by following the same locus of stress–strain coordinates that characterized its deformation. If, however, the material is deformed beyond the elastic limit, to strain ε_B for example, the material will not recover completely. Generally, the relaxation of the material occurs along a

Table 5.1
Mechanical Properties of Commonly Encountered Biological Materials

Materials	E (MPa)	Strength, Ultimate Stress (MPa)	Poisson's Ratio
Biological Materials			
Bone—long bone	15,000 to 30,000	130 to 220 in compression 80 to 150 in tension 70 in shear	
Bone—cancellous	90 to 500	2 to 5	
Bone—vertebrae	100 to 300		
Bone—skull	6,500		0.22
Cartilage		5	
Articular cartilage	1 to 10 in tension 1 in compression	9 to 40	
Human knee menisci	70 to 150		
Brain	0.067		0.48
Brain tissue—gray matter	0.005		
Brain tissue—white matter	0.014		
Tendon	1,000 to 2,000	50 to 100	
Tendon—Tendo achillis	375		
Ligament		50 to 100	
Aorta		0.3 to 0.8	
Human small artery	0.1 to 4		
Elastin	0.6		
Isolated collagen fibers	1,000	50	
Formalin-fixed myocardium	101		
Skin	0.1 to 2 (phase I)	1 to 20	
Fibroblast-populated matrix	0.08 to 0.8		
Collagen sponge	0.017 to 0.028		
Polymers			
Polyimides	3,000 to 5,000		
Polyester	1,000 to 5,000		
Polystyrene	2,300 to 3,300		
Poly(methyl methacrylate)	2,000 to 3,000		
Polyethylene—high density	1,100		
Polytetrafluoroethylene	400 to 600		
Polyethylene—low density	200 to 500		
Metals			
Stainless steel (316)	210,000	450 in tension	
Titanium	107,000		
Aluminum	69,000		
Others			
Silicon	150,000		
Aluminum oxide (Al_2O_3)	393,000		
Magnesium oxide (MgO)	225,000		
Fused silica (SiO_2)	73,000		
Concrete	2,800	4.5 in compression	
Wood	140	3.6	

Compiled from [21, 24, 29].

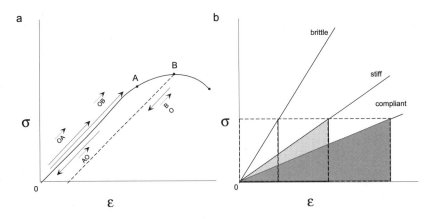

Figure 5.2. Typical characteristics of an elastic material. (a) Deformation in response to applied load for an elastic and a non-elastic material. (b) The energy stored in a material during deformation can be determined by integrating under the stress–strain curve.

line that is parallel to the initial deformation (that is, with slope equal to E, if it is a linear elastic solid).

Energy is added to a material when it is stressed; this mechanical energy, called strain energy, is stored in the material. For an elastic material, the strain energy U_0, is determined from

$$U_0 = \frac{1}{2}\sigma\varepsilon \tag{5-2}$$

which can be determined graphically from the area under the stress–strain curve. Elastic elongation and relaxation has no net energy cost; all of the energy stored in the material during elongation is returned during relaxation. But energy is lost when deformation goes beyond the elastic limit. The net loss of energy can be calculated from the difference between the strain energy required to accomplish the elongation and the energy recovered after removal of the load (net energy loss can be determined graphically, as well). The ability to store energy can be an important material property. The potential of a material for energy storage can be represented by the strain energy at failure. Brittle materials have a low U_0 at fracture, whereas compliant materials, which deform readily, can store substantial amounts of strain energy.

5.1.2 Poisson's Ratio

In the examples developed in the previous section, a stress was applied in a single direction and the response (or strain) in that same direction was observed and analyzed. Most materials will elongate when stress is applied in the axial direction, but the cross-sectional area will also decrease (Figure 5.3). The rela-

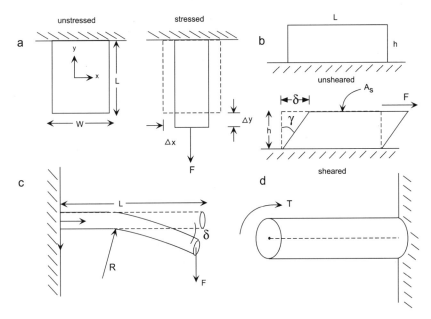

Figure 5.3. Deformation of materials under stress. (a) The extent of deformation of a material in directions other than the direction of force application is determined by Poisson's ratio. (b) Materials also deform when exposed to a shearing stress. (c) Bending deformation occurs for elongated or slender bodies. (d) Materials can deform when subjected to torsional forces.

tive magnitude of strains experienced in two dimensions is given by Poisson's ratio, ν_{xy}, which is also a property of the material:

$$\nu_{xy} = -\frac{\varepsilon_y}{\varepsilon_x} \tag{5-3}$$

In the simple example shown in Figure 5.1, the cross-sectional area decreases continuously with loading. Stresses are usually defined on the basis of the unstressed area and therefore underestimate the actual stress in the material. This discrepancy between "stress" (which is defined for convenience) and the true stress in the material accounts for the decrease in "stress" near the fracture point. The true stress is increasing up to the point of fracture but the rapid decrease in cross-sectional area that precedes failure leads to the apparent decrease in "stress".

5.1.3 Quantifying Deformations in Other Geometries

Stress that is applied to a material tangentially causes shear deformation (Figure 5.3). Shear stress, τ, is defined per area of the surface on which it is applied. Since the deformation in shear is a function of distance from the plane on which the shear is applied, shear strain (ε_s) is measured by the angular deformation of the material:

$$\varepsilon_s = \frac{\delta}{h} = \tan \gamma \tag{5-4}$$

For small deformations, that is, γ near 0 so that $\tan \gamma \simeq \gamma$, a shear modulus ($G$) can be defined:

$$\tau = G\gamma \tag{5-5}$$

Bending deformations also are important, particularly in elongated objects that bear tangential loads (Figure 5.3). If a force F is applied at the end of a symmetrical beam of length L, and the material is isotropic and linearly elastic, the deflection due to bending is

$$\delta = -\frac{FL^3}{3EI} \tag{5-6}$$

where E is Young's modulus and I is moment of inertia for the cross-sectional area. The stress within the material depends on the distance from the central axis, y:

$$\sigma_x = -\frac{My}{I} \tag{5-7}$$

where M is the bending moment (equal to FL at the end of the beam in Figure 5.3). If $M > 0$, the negative sign indicates that the stress is compressive for $y > 0$ and tensile for $y < 0$. Torsional forces also produce stress within materials. The shear stress due to torsion is

$$\tau = \frac{Tr}{J} \tag{5-8}$$

where J is the radial moment of inertia and T is the torque.

5.2 Elementary Fluid Mechanics

5.2.1 Basics and Definitions

A fluid deforms continuously under the action of a shearing stress. Two classes of fluids can be defined: incompressible fluids, in which the density is constant; and compressible fluids, in which the density (ρ) is a function of pressure. Most liquids are incompressible at pressures near atmospheric; pure water has a density of 999 kg/m^3 at 15°C and 993 kg/m^3 at 37°C; blood has a density of 1,060 kg/m^3. Gases are much less dense than liquids and cannot always be assumed incompressible; air has a density of 1.22 kg/m^3 at 15°C and 1 atm.

When a fluid is at rest—that is, in the absence of shearing stresses—the fluid is said to be in hydrostatic equilibrium. A force balance on an element of a stationary incompressible fluid (Figure 5.4) yields the following relationship:

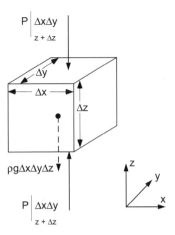

Figure 5.4. Force balance on a volume element in a fluid at rest. Forces acting in the z-direction (parallel to gravitational force) are shown.

$$\frac{\mathrm{d}p}{\mathrm{d}z} = -\rho g \tag{5-9}$$

where g is the acceleration due to gravity ($9.80665\,\mathrm{m/s^2}$). This differential equation can be used to calculate the difference in pressure between any two spatial locations in a stationary fluid. If the fluid is incompressible, the expression must be integrated with density as a function of position.

Viscosity is a material property related to the resistance to "flow" or deformation of a fluid. Consider a fluid entrapped between two parallel plates (Figure 5.5). If the bottom plate is held stationary and the top plate is moved to the right with a constant velocity v_0 by application of a tangential force F, the fluid within the gap will be subjected to a shearing stress that produces fluid motion. The force applied to the plate is uniformly transmitted over the entire area of plate/fluid contact; therefore, the tangential shear stress is equal to F/A, where A is the cross-sectional area of the plate. Experimentally, the shear stress is proportional to the velocity of the upper plate v_0 and the gap distance h:

$$\tau \propto \frac{v_0}{h} \tag{5-10}$$

More precisely, the shear stress is equal to a constant multiplied by the first derivative of the velocity with respect to distance normal to the moving plate:

$$\tau_{xhy} = \eta \frac{\mathrm{d}v_x}{\mathrm{d}y} \tag{5-11}$$

where τ_{xy} is the viscous shear stress in the x-direction exerted on a fluid surface of constant y. This quantity, τ_{yx}, is also the viscous flux of x-momentum (ρv_x) in the y-direction. The negative sign must be included because viscosity has a

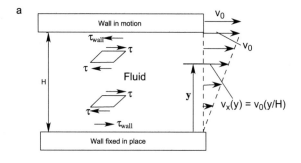

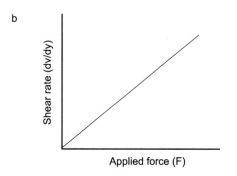

Figure 5.5. Viscosity in a fluid between two parallel plates in relative motion. (a) Schematic diagram showing movement of the upper plate and velocity profile within the fluid. (b) Variation of shear rate with applied force.

positive value ($\eta > 0$) and the momentum flux is positive in the direction of decreasing velocity.

The shear stress and the velocity gradient (also called the shear rate) are proportional, with the constant of proportionality $-\eta$, where η is the viscosity of the fluid. For some fluids, Equation 5-11 holds over a wide range of shear rates with constant η (as in Figure 5.5b); these are called *Newtonian* fluids. The value of the viscosity η is a property of the fluid being a function of fluid phase composition, temperature, and pressure. Water is a Newtonian fluid; at body temperature ($37°C$) the viscosity of water is 0.75 cp (centipoise; 1 cp $= 0.01$ g/cm-s) and that of plasma is 1.2 cp. Whole blood has a viscosity of 3.0 cp, provided that the shear rate is sufficiently high so that red cell aggregates do not form (see discussion on blood cell aggregation in Chapter 8). At lower shear rates, the viscosity of blood is a function of shear rate and blood composition.

5.2.2 Kinematics of Fluid Flow

One is often interested in knowing the velocity of flow within a fluid subjected to shearing stresses. Fluid motion can be described through the use of mathematical expressions of the basic principles of conservation of mass, momentum, and energy. These conservation equations can be derived for a particular system of interest or, alternately, can be developed generally and then applied to a particular system. The latter approach requires consideration of a characteristic infinitesimal volume element; Figure 5.6 illustrates the conservation of total mass in a rectangular coordinate system.

The rate of change in mass of the volume element is equal to the net rate of mass addition to the volume element, which can only occur by fluid flow through one of the six boundaries:

$$\frac{\partial}{\partial t}(\rho)\Delta x \Delta y \Delta z = \rho v_x|_x \Delta y \Delta z - \rho v_x|_{x+\Delta x}\Delta y \Delta z + \rho v_y|_y \Delta x \Delta z$$

$$- \rho v_y|_{y+\Delta y}\Delta x \Delta z + \rho v_z|_z \Delta x \Delta y - \rho v_z|_{z+\Delta z}\Delta x \Delta y$$

(5-12)

Dividing each term by the volume yields

$$\frac{\partial \rho}{\partial t} = \left[\frac{\rho v_x|_x \Delta y \Delta z - \rho v_x|_{x+\Delta x}\Delta y \Delta z}{\Delta x \Delta y \Delta z}\right] + \left[\frac{\rho v_y|_y \Delta x \Delta z - \rho v_y|_{y+\Delta y}\Delta x \Delta z}{\Delta x \Delta y \Delta z}\right]$$

$$+ \left[\frac{\rho v_z|_z \Delta x \Delta y - \rho v_z|_{z+\Delta z}\Delta x \Delta y}{\Delta x \Delta y \Delta z}\right]$$

(5-13)

In the limit, as the volume element becomes infinitesimal, the three terms on the right-hand-side become partial derivatives:

$$\frac{\partial \rho}{\partial t} = \left[\frac{\partial(\rho v_x)}{\partial x}\right] + \left[\frac{\partial(\rho v_y)}{\partial y}\right] + \left[\frac{\partial(\rho v_z)}{\partial z}\right]$$

(5-14)

which can be written in more compact notation as

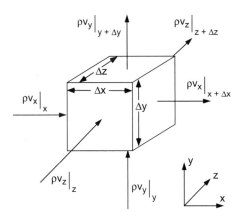

Figure 5.6. Balance of total mass on a volume element within a fluid in motion, illustrated for a rectangular coordinate system. The rate of mass flow through each boundary of the volume element is determined from the local density and velocity perpendicular to the boundary.

$$\frac{\partial \rho}{\partial t} = -\nabla \cdot (\rho \bar{v}) \qquad (5\text{-}15)$$

or expanded to allow inclusion of the substantial derivative of density:

$$\frac{D\rho}{Dt}\left[= \frac{\partial \rho}{\partial t} + \rho \bar{v} \right] = -\rho \nabla \cdot \bar{v} \qquad (5\text{-}16)$$

In the special case of an incompressible fluid, the density is not a function of time or position and the mass balance equation can be simplified:

$$0 = \nabla \cdot \bar{v} \qquad (5\text{-}17)$$

The conservation equation for momentum is somewhat more difficult to obtain, but can be derived by a similar procedure (for more details, see [4, 5]):

$$\frac{\partial(\rho v_x)}{\partial t} = -\left(\frac{\partial(\rho v_x v_x)}{\partial x} + \frac{\partial(\rho v_y v_x)}{\partial y} + \frac{\partial(\rho v_z v_x)}{\partial z} \right) - \left(\frac{\partial \tau_{xx}}{\partial x} + \frac{\partial \tau_{yx}}{\partial y} + \frac{\partial \tau_{zx}}{\partial z} \right) - \frac{\partial p}{\partial x} + \rho g_x$$

$$(5\text{-}18)$$

Equation 5-18 gives the expression for conservation of momentum in the x-direction; similar expressions are obtained in the y- and z-directions [4,5]. These three component expressions can be written as a single, more compact vector expression:

$$\frac{\partial(\rho \bar{v})}{\partial t} = -\nabla p + \rho \bar{g} - \bar{\nabla} \cdot \bar{\tau} - \nabla \cdot \rho \bar{v} \bar{v} \qquad (5\text{-}19)$$

To use this differential equation, we need a constitutive equation that relates the individual elements of the stress tensor ($\bar{\tau}$) to gradients in the velocity field. This constitutive equation relates local rates of movement in the fluid (that is, velocity) to local stress and therefore depends on the physical properties of the fluid of interest. For a Newtonian fluid, the constitutive equation is

$$\left. \begin{aligned}
\tau_{xx} &= -2\eta \frac{\partial v_x}{\partial x} + \frac{2}{3}\eta \left[\frac{\partial v_x}{\partial x} + \frac{\partial v_y}{\partial y} + \frac{\partial v_z}{\partial z} \right] \\[2mm]
\tau_{yy} &= -2\eta \frac{\partial v_y}{\partial y} + \frac{2}{3}\eta \left[\frac{\partial v_x}{\partial x} + \frac{\partial v_y}{\partial y} + \frac{\partial v_z}{\partial z} \right] \\[2mm]
\tau_{zz} &= -2\eta \frac{\partial v_z}{\partial z} + \frac{2}{3}\eta \left[\frac{\partial v_x}{\partial x} + \frac{\partial v_y}{\partial y} + \frac{\partial v_z}{\partial z} \right] \\[2mm]
\tau_{xy} &= \tau_{yx} = -\eta \left(\frac{\partial v_x}{\partial y} + \frac{\partial v_y}{\partial x} \right) \\[2mm]
\tau_{yz} &= \tau_{zy} = -\eta \left(\frac{\partial v_y}{\partial z} + \frac{\partial v_z}{\partial y} \right) \\[2mm]
\tau_{zx} &= \tau_{xz} = -\eta \left(\frac{\partial v_x}{\partial z} + \frac{\partial v_z}{\partial x} \right)
\end{aligned} \right\} \qquad (5\text{-}20)$$

For a Newtonian fluid, the equation for conservation of momentum (Equations 5-19 and 5-20) reduces to

$$\rho \frac{D\bar{v}}{Dt} = -\nabla p + \eta \nabla^2 \bar{v} + \rho \bar{g} \tag{5-21}$$

The velocity field can be determined by solution of Equations 5-17 through 5-21 in certain situations. In the simple system illustrated in Figure 5.5, velocity varies with position in the fluid, but velocity only occurs in the tangential direction, v_x, and is only a function of distance normal to the moving plate y. Therefore, the conservation of mass equation (Equation 5-14) provides no useful information in this system. Conservation of momentum does provide interesting information; the equation for conservation of x-momentum (that is the x-component of Equation 5-21) reduces to

$$0 = -\frac{dp}{dx} + \eta \frac{d^2 v_x}{dy^2} + \rho g_x \tag{5-22}$$

In most cases of interest for tissue engineering, the effect of gravity is small relative to the pressure drop (alternately, depending on the orientation of the parallel plates with respect to the gravitational field, the x-component of the gravitational vector may be equal to zero); the third term on the right-hand side of Equation 5-22 can therefore be neglected. Dropping the third term in Equation 5-22 requires that the other two terms exactly balance:

$$\frac{dp}{dx} = \eta \frac{d^2 v_x}{dy^2} \tag{5-23}$$

But there is no hydrostatic pressure drop in the x-direction in this situation, which leads to a simple solution for the functional form of the velocity profile:

$$v_x = Ay + B \tag{5-24}$$

The values for the velocity in the x-direction are known at the boundaries v_0 at $y = 0$, $v_x = 0$ and at $y = H$, $v_x = v_0$. Therefore, the constants A and B can be evaluated:

$$v_x = v_0 \left(\frac{y}{H} \right) \tag{5-25}$$

This linear profile for velocity as a function of distance from the stationary plate is shown in Figure 5.5.

5.2.3 Example: Flow Through a Cylindrical Tube

Consider an additional example of relevance to tissue engineering (Figure 5.7). The formation of functional blood vessels within tissues is one of the fundamental problems of tissue engineering; blood flow through tissues is essential for oxygen transport to cells within the tissue mass. Mechanically, blood vessels in tissue serve as conduits for the flow of blood. Blood moves at varying velocity through individual tissues within the body via an interconnected and

a

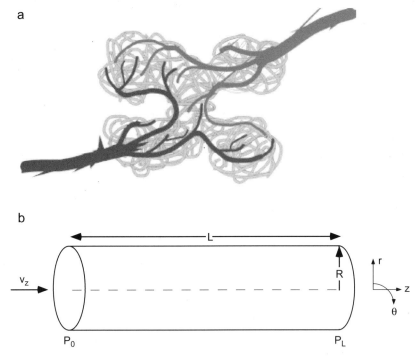

b

Figure 5.7. Fluid flow through a blood vessel. (a) The development of vasculature within a growing tissue is a key problem in tissue engineering. Adapted from a drawing on the Carnegie Mellon University Bone Tissue Engineering Initiative website (http://www-2.cs.cmu.edu/People/tissue/tutorial.html). (b) The flow of blood through a capillary, vein, or artery can be modeled as an incompressible fluid flowing through a cylindrical tube.

highly branched network of cylindrical vessels. Therefore, the flow of an incompressible fluid within a cylindrical vessel is of central importance to the biophysics of the circulatory system and to our understanding of vascular tissue engineering.

Well-behaved flow through a cylindrical tube (Figure 5.7) occurs only in the axial direction ($\bar{v} = v_z(r)\hat{k}$), where v_z is a function of radial distance r from the tube centerline. The z-component of the conservation of momentum equation, Equation 5-21, in cylindrical coordinates, is

$$\rho\left(\frac{\partial v_z}{\partial t} + v_r\frac{\partial v_z}{\partial r} + \frac{v_\Theta}{r}\frac{\partial v_z}{\partial \theta} + v_z\frac{\partial v_z}{\partial z}\right)$$

$$= -\frac{\partial p}{\partial z} + \eta\left[\frac{1}{r}\frac{\partial}{\partial r}\left(r\frac{\partial v_z}{\partial r}\right) + \frac{1}{r^2}\frac{\partial^2 v_z}{\partial^2 r} + \frac{\partial^2 v_z}{\partial^2 z}\right] + \rho g_z$$

(5-26)

This equation can be simplified by the following assumptions, which apply reasonably well to blood flows in most vessels in humans:

- steady flow ($\partial v_z / \partial t = 0$);
- flow only in axial direction ($v_r = v_\theta = 0$);
- gravitational forces are negligible ($g_z \simeq 0$).

These assumptions can be used to simplify Equation 5-26:

$$\frac{\partial p}{\partial z} = \eta \frac{1}{r} \frac{\partial}{\partial r}\left(r \frac{\partial v_z}{\partial r}\right) \tag{5-27}$$

The term on the left-hand side of Equation 5-27 (that is, the pressure gradient) is only a function of z, whereas the term on the right-hand side (that is, the second derivative of the velocity component in the z-direction with respect to r) is only a function of r. These two terms can be equal only if they are both equal to a constant, which we will temporarily call K. Therefore, Equation 5-27 can be separated into two ordinary differential equations:

$$\left.\begin{array}{c} \dfrac{dp}{dz} = K \\[2em] \eta \dfrac{1}{r}\dfrac{d}{dr}\left(r\dfrac{dv_z}{dr}\right) = K \end{array}\right\} \tag{5-28}$$

If the pressure drop over the length of the vessel is known, the value of the constant K corresponding to this physical situation can be determined. For example, if the pressures at the inlet and outlet of the vessel are known,

$$p = p_0 \quad \text{at} \quad z = 0; \qquad p = p_L \quad \text{at} \quad z = L \tag{5-29}$$

then the solution to the first part of Equation 5-28 is

$$p = p_0 + \left(\frac{P_L - P_0}{L}\right)z \tag{5-30}$$

Therefore, the value of K in this case is $(P_L - P_0)/L$. The second part of Equation 5-28 can be solved, subject to the following boundary conditions on velocity:

$$v_z = 0 \quad \text{at} \quad r = R; \qquad \frac{\partial v_z}{\partial r} = 0 \quad \text{at} \quad r = 0 \tag{5-31}$$

to yield

$$v_z = \frac{(P_0 - P_L)R^2}{4\eta L}\left(1 - \frac{r^2}{R^2}\right) \tag{5-32}$$

This parabolic dependence of local velocity on radial position (Figure 5.8) is characteristic of Hagen–Poiseuille flow (named in honor of Jean Leonard Marie Poiseuille and Gotthilf Heinrich Ludwig Hagen). Poiseuille (a physiologist) and Hagen (an engineer) independently published the first systematic measurements of pressure drop within flowing fluids in simple tubes in 1839 and 1840.

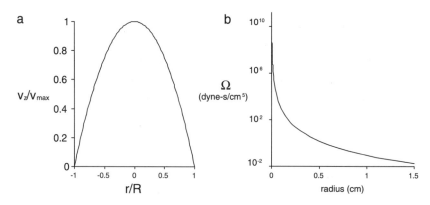

Figure 5.8. Velocity profile through a cylindrical vessel. (a) The velocity varies with the radial distance from the vessel centerline, as in Equation 5-37. (b) The overall resistance of the vessel to flow is a strong function of the vessel radius.

Equation 5-32 can be integrated over the vessel cross-section to obtain an overall rate of blood flow:

$$Q = \int_0^{2\pi} \int_0^R v_z(r)r\,dr\,d\theta = \frac{(P_0 - P_L)\pi R^4}{8\eta L} \tag{5-33}$$

which provides—by analogy to the resistance of electrical circuits ($\Delta V = i\Omega$)—the overall resistance of a cylindrical vessel to flow:

$$\Omega = \frac{\Delta p}{Q} = \frac{8\eta L}{\pi R^4} \tag{5-34}$$

The resistance to flow is a strong function of vessel radius: $\Omega \propto R^{-4}$. As blood vessels become smaller the resistance to flow increases dramatically (Figure 5.8). One consequence of the branching pattern of blood vessels is that the majority of the overall resistance to blood flow resides in the smallest vessels; in the human circulatory system, the majority of the pressure drop ($\sim 80\%$) occurs in arterioles and capillaries. This natural consequence of the physics of fluid flows is exploited in regulation of blood flow to organs of the body. Local blood flow to a tissue is controlled by constriction and dilation of the arterioles delivering blood to that tissue. Since the greatest overall resistance is provided by arterioles, and because individual arterioles have muscular walls which permit them to adjust their diameter, and therefore their resistance (Equation 5-34), the proportion of blood flow arriving at the tissue served by an arteriole can be regulated with precision.

5.3 Mechanical Properties of Biological Fluids and Gels

The preceding two sections describe the mechanical behavior of idealized elastic materials and incompressible fluids, respectively. Real materials sometimes behave like one of these idealized models. On the other hand, bio-logical materials, which are frequently complex in composition, can exhibit complex behaviors that resemble aspects of both the elastic material and an incompressible fluid, but are also unlike either of these idealized models. Materials that exhibit both viscous and elastic natures are called viscoelastic.

5.3.1 Models of Viscoelastic Materials

Consider, first, the behavior of biological tissues such as skin and muscle. Although these materials are rich in water, which is a fluid at body tempera-ture, they also have characteristics of an elastic solid: for example, they retain their shape without a containing vessel. Ideal elastic materials—that is, materi-als that are deformed to less than the elastic limit—deform instantaneously. Although they may deform very rapidly after loading, biological materials often continue to deform slowly after the initial period, exhibiting a behavior called creep (Figure 5.9). When this same material is rapidly deformed, the force required to maintain this deformation decreases gradually; this process is called stress relaxation.

Ideal elastic materials are modeled as springs; their behavior can be pre-dicted by Hooke's law (Equation 5-1). Another element—one that slowly elongates upon application of a force—must be added to model the changes that occur during creep and stress relaxation. Continuous deformation after

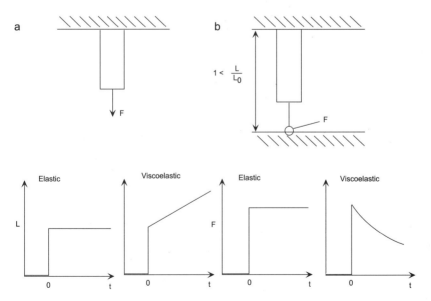

Figure 5.9. Comparison of elastic and viscoelastic behavior. Typical responses of elastic and viscolelastic materials to (a) application of a constant load and (b) application of a constant elongation.

loading is a characteristic of fluids; the rate of deformation is determined by the viscosity of the fluid, as in Equation 5-11. A dashpot, or piston within a cylinder is the mechanical analog for viscosity; the piston slowly moves through the cylinder at a rate that is determined by friction between the surfaces, in response to an applied load. By combining elastic (that is, spring) and viscous (that is, dashpot) elements, models that predict aspects of the behavior of real viscoelastic materials can be developed (Figure 5.10).

   Deformation of viscoelastic materials depends on the total history of applied force. If $F(t)$ is a function describing the history of applied force on a material, then, over a small time interval $d\tau$, the change in applied force is given by $(dF/dt)|_\tau d\tau$. The change in deformation at time t, $dU(t)$, can be expressed in terms of a history, or creep, function, $c(t - \tau)$:

$$dU(t) = c(t - \tau)\frac{dF}{dt}\bigg|_\tau d\tau \qquad (5\text{-}35)$$

This expression can be integrated to obtain the total deformation as a function of time t:

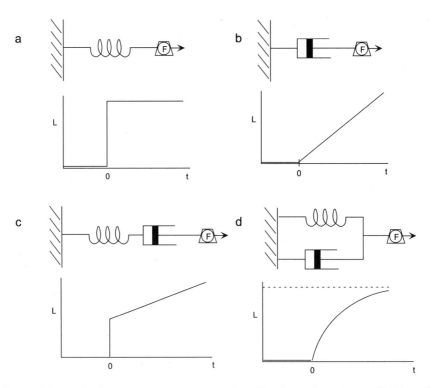

Figure 5.10. Behavior of spring–dashpot models. The elongation after application of a constant load to (a) spring, (b) dashpot, (c) spring and dashpot in series (Maxwell solid), and (d) spring and dashpot in parallel (Voigt solid).

$$U(t) = \int_0^t c(t - \tau) \frac{\mathrm{d}F}{\mathrm{d}t}\bigg|_\tau \mathrm{d}\tau \qquad (5\text{-}36)$$

The relaxation function $k(t - \tau)$, the inverse of the creep function, can be defined in a similar way:

$$\mathrm{d}F(t) = k(t - \tau) \frac{\mathrm{d}U}{\mathrm{d}t}\bigg|_\tau \mathrm{d}\tau \qquad (5\text{-}37)$$

The relaxation function $k(\cdot)$ can be interpreted as the force which must be applied to produce a unit step increase in deformation; the creep function $c(\cdot)$ can be interpreted as the elongation which results from a unit step increase in applied force. In general, the state of the material at the present time depends only on the previous history, so that one may assume $c(0) = 0$ and $k(0) = 0$. The challenge is to find the creep or relaxation function that describes a viscoelastic material of interest.

It is often useful to compare the behavior of real materials with that of idealized models. A simple elastic material, for example, can be compared to a perfectly elastic spring, as shown in Figure 5.10a. The behavior of the perfectly elastic material is provided by Equation 5-1, which can also be written in the form

$$F = \mu U \qquad (5\text{-}38)$$

where F is the total force applied to the material and U is the instantaneous displacement of the material, as defined in Equations 5-35 through 5-37. All of the behavior of the perfectly elastic material is contained in Equation 5-38, which is identical to the equation describing a spring (where F is the force applied to the spring, U is the displacement, and μ is the spring constant). When a force is applied to a spring, the spring instantaneously deforms to the length prescribed by Equation 5-38 (this deformation is illustrated in Figure 5.10a). Similarly, a viscous liquid can be compared to another idealized mechanical object, the dashpot (Figure 5.10b). The dashpot behaves like a simple viscous liquid:

$$F = \eta \frac{\mathrm{d}U}{\mathrm{d}t} \qquad (5\text{-}39)$$

which is similar to Equation 5-11. When a force is applied to a material that behaves like a viscous liquid, it deforms continuously; the deformation of the material will continue for as long as the force is applied.

5.3.2 Example: Creep Function for a Maxwell Solid

Many materials do not behave like perfect springs or dashpots. When a fixed load is applied, the material might deform with time (like a dashpot), reaching some ultimate deformation that is not exceeded (like a spring). Models of materials can be constructed by combining springs and dashpots in different combinations; the Maxwell model and the Voigt model are illustrated in Figures 5.10c and 5.10d respectively. A Maxwell solid behaves like a spring and a dashpot in series; it will deform instantaneously, like a spring, but the deformation will continue at some steady rate, like a dashpot. The total rate of deformation at any time, therefore, depends on the characteristics of both the spring and the dashpot:

$$\frac{dU}{dt} = \frac{1}{\mu}\frac{dF}{dt} + \frac{1}{\eta}F \tag{5-40}$$

where the initial elongation depends only on the force applied at time 0: $U(0) = F(0)/\eta$. Recall that the creep function can be interpreted as the deformation that results from a step change in force; the unit step change can be described mathematically as

$$F(t) = H(t), \qquad \text{where} \qquad H(t) = \begin{cases} 1 & \text{when} & t \geq 0 \\ 0 & \text{when} & t < 0 \end{cases} \tag{5-41}$$

The total deformation at time t can be obtained by integration of Equation 5-40, giving

$$U(t) = \int_{-\infty}^{t} \left(\frac{1}{\mu}\frac{dF}{dt} + \frac{F}{\eta}\right) dt \tag{5-42}$$

which, in the case where the force is a unit step change, becomes

$$U(t) = \int_{-\infty}^{t} \left(\frac{1}{\mu}\delta(t) + \frac{H(t)}{\eta}\right) dt = \frac{1}{\mu} + \frac{t}{\eta} \tag{5-43}$$

where the delta function, $\delta(t)$, is the first derivative of the step function:

$$\delta(t) = \begin{cases} 1 & \text{when} \quad t = 0 \\ 0 & \text{elsewhere} \end{cases} \tag{5-44}$$

The creep function is defined by Equation 5-35. When the applied force is a unit step change, so that the first derivative of F is equal to the delta function, Equation 5-35 reduces to

$$U(t) = \int_{0}^{t} c(t-\tau)\delta(\tau)d\tau = c(t) \tag{5-45}$$

Comparison of Equations 5-43 and 5-45 yields a functional form for the creep function of a Maxwell model:

$$c(t) = \frac{1}{\mu} + \frac{t}{\eta} \tag{5-46}$$

or, more generally, given that the value of the creep function $c(0)$ is known at $t = 0$:

$$c(t - \tau) = \left(\frac{1}{\mu} + \frac{t - \tau}{\eta}\right)H(t - \tau) \tag{5-47}$$

Similar approaches can be used to find the relaxation function for a Maxwell model or the creep/relaxation functions for other model materials (see Exercises 5.3 and 5.4).

5.3.3 Rheological Properties of Biological Fluids and Gels

The deformation character of a biological fluid is often a critical determinant of its function. In blood, for example, the viscosity determines the overall resistance to flow through a vessel (Equation 5-34) and, therefore, the amount of work that must be supplied by the heart to move blood through the circulatory system. A number of methods for determining rheological properties of a fluid (that is, the deformation response of a fluid to applied stresses) have been developed. One common method is capillary viscometry, in which the fluid is forced by pressure through a capillary of known dimensions; the viscosity of the fluid is then calculated from Equation 5-34.

Another common method is cone-and-plate viscometry, in which the fluid is confined between two surfaces as shown in Figure 5.11. In this apparatus the plate is rotated with a constant angular velocity Ω and the cone held stationary. The torque required to hold the cone, T, is measured; this torque is related to the viscosity of the fluid that fills the gap between the surfaces. If the fluid is Newtonian, the shear rate imposed on the fluid is given by

$$\dot{\gamma} = \frac{\Omega}{\tan \alpha} \tag{5-48}$$

where α is the angle between the cone and the plate and $\dot{\gamma}$ is the shear rate. The shear stress τ is calculated from the torque T:

$$\tau = \frac{3T}{2\pi R^3} \tag{5-49}$$

where R is the radius of the cone.

This steady flow approach works for measuring the rheological properties of many fluids, even fluids that are structurally complex, such as blood. When blood is placed between the cone and the plate, the viscosity can be measured as a function of shear rate (Figure 5.11b). The viscosity of blood decreases with increasing shear rate. At low shear rates, $\dot{\gamma} < 0.1 \text{ s}^{-1}$, red blood cells within the blood form aggregates called rouleaux (see Figure 8.2) that resist flow. As the shear rate increases, the flow breaks the aggregates into individual cells, causing a decrease in the bulk viscosity. The complex rheological behavior of blood appears to be due to the aggregation of red cells as well as the deformability of individual cells, which is also a function of shear rate.

In some biological materials, however, the structure of the material is irreversibly altered by the simple shear flow process illustrated above; we might be interested, however, in the material's behavior with small deformations. Consider, for example, a polymer solution in which the concentration of

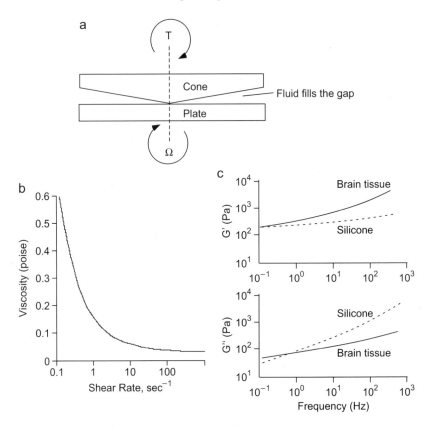

Figure 5.11. Cone-and-plate viscometry. The viscometer (a) can be used to measure the rheological behavior of blood (b) and of gels or tissues (c). Panel c was redrawn from [28].

polymer is above the gel point; that is, the concentration of polymer is high enough that polymer chains within the solution are connected (either chemically by crosslinks or physically by entanglements) into a large unit that spans the entire sample. A continuous shear flow, such as the one created by rotating the plate at a constant angular speed, would alter the structure of the gel phase by disrupting connections between the polymer chains. In biological gels, such as those formed from collagen, it is these polymer–polymer interactions that create the biologically important behavior of the material; therefore, measurements of viscosity in simple shear flow would not be relevant to the biological function. In these cases, the cone-and-plate rheometer can be operated in an oscillatory shear mode by oscillating the plate over small angles; the material between the plates is therefore exposed to a limited range of strains. The shear dependence of the response of the material can be measured by oscillating the plate at different frequencies. For example, a collagen gel sample might be subjected to oscillatory shear by rotating the plate at 2% strain with a frequency ranging from 0.1 to 100 rad/s [6].

In oscillatory shear measurements, a sinusoidally varying shear field of frequency ω is imposed on the material by oscillating the plate; the amplitude of the resulting torque and the phase angle between the imposed shear and resulting torque on the cone are then measured. The stress response (τ) is also oscillatory but shifted from the imposed shear by an angle ϕ:

$$\tau = \tau_{max} \cos(\omega t - \phi) \qquad (5\text{-}50)$$

where τ_{max} is the maximum value of the shear response. This stress can be decomposed into in-phase and out-of-phase terms:

$$\tau = -\eta' \gamma_{max} \omega \cos(\omega t) - \eta'' \gamma_{max} \omega \sin(\omega t) = -G'' \gamma_{max} \cos(\omega t) - G' \gamma_{max} \sin(\omega t) \qquad (5\text{-}51)$$

where γ_{max} is maximum strain, η' and η'' are the two dynamic viscosity coefficients, and G' and G'' are the storage and loss moduli, respectively. The value of G', related to the stress in phase with strain, provides information about the elasticity of the gel. The loss modulus, G'', related to the stress out-of-phase with the strain, is a measure of the dissipated energy in the system [7]. As an example of results obtained by this method, the response, measured from a model material (silicone) and brain tissue, is shown in Figure 5.11c.

5.4 Mechanical Properties of Cells

5.4.1 Mechanical Behavior of Blood Cells

Cells are complex, deformable objects. Red blood cells are slightly larger than the smallest capillaries and therefore must deform in order to move through the circulation (Table 5.2). White cells are substantially larger and less deformable than red cells; therefore, they can have a larger impact on blood flow properties than one would predict from their abundance. As will be discussed in Chapter

Table 5.2
Characteristics of Blood Cells

Cell type	Shape	Characteristic dimensions (μm)	Volume (μm^3)	Cell fraction	Cortical tension (mN/m)
Red cell (erythrocyte)	Biconcave disc	7.7 × (1.4 to 2.8)	96	0.997	
Platelet	Biconcave disc	2 × 0.2	5 to 10	0.007	
Neutrophil	Spherical	8.2 to 8.4	300 to 310	<0.002	0.024 to 0.035
Lymphocyte	Spherical	7.5	220	<0.001	0.06
Monocyte	Spherical	9.1	400	<0.0005	0.035

Data obtained from [8].

10, the mechanical properties of white cells have a profound influence on their fate in the circulation after infusion. A reduction in the deformability of white cells may also play a role in certain diseases, such as leukemia and diabetes, in which the microcirculation can be impaired. The mechanical properties of red and white blood cells have been well studied and are reviewed in [8].

The mechanical properties of many cells—including blood cells—have been directly measured by aspiration into a micropipette (Figure 5.12). The properties of the cell are deduced from the deformations observed as the cell is pulled into the pipette under gentle pressure [9, 10]. For example, in one method, the suction pressure is gradually increased to a critical pressure, $\Delta p_{critical}$, at which a small hemispherical section of the cell is pulled into the pipette. Laplace's law permits calculation of cell cortical tension, T, from the critical pressure:

$$T = \frac{\Delta p_{critical} R_p R_c}{2(R_c - R_p)} \tag{5-52}$$

where R_p is the radius of the micropipette and R_c is the radius of the cell [11]. Similarly, the overall viscosity of a cell can be measured by aspirating the whole cell into a larger micropipette ($\sim 4\,\mu m$ radius for neutrophils) and comparing the time course for cell movement through the pipette lumen to numerical models of individual cell deformation [11].

Other techniques have been used to measure the mechanical properties of individual cells, by deforming them between parallel plates, for example, or by applying smaller mechanical probes such as microneedles [12] and atomic force microscopes [13].

5.4.2 Mechanical Properties of the Cytoskeleton

The intracellular fluid, or cytoplasm, is a much more complicated fluid than plasma. Plasma, or the acellular fraction of blood, is a concentrated protein solution that behaves as a Newtonian fluid with a viscosity of 1.2 cP (or 1.2 mPa-s) at 37°C. The simplest cytoplasm is probably found in red blood cells, which have no nucleus or internal organelles. Red cell cytoplasm is a

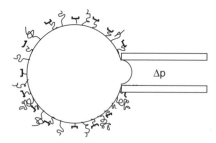

Figure 5.12. Micropipette aspiration to determine cellular mechanics. Gentle suction can be used to deform cells under controlled conditions for evaluation of mechanical properties.

concentrated hemoglobin solution; individual cells contain between 290 and 390 g/L of hemoglobin, which has a viscosity of between 4.2 to 17.2 cP [8].

The basic elements of the cytoskeleton were introduced in Section 3.3.1, in which the shape of a cell was associated with protein filaments in the cytoplasm. The three most important protein filaments are illustrated in Figure 3.12: actin microfilaments, microtubules, and intermediate filaments. These filaments have intrinsic mechanical properties. They can be characterized by a persistence length, which is related to the stiffness of the filament (Table 5.3). In some cases, the mechanical properties of individual filaments have been measured directly, although the measurements are difficult and a clear picture of filament mechanics is not yet available. But it is clear that the three main filaments differ greatly in mechanical properties: actin microfilaments are flexible but unable to withstand tensile forces; microtubules are stiffer than actin filaments but still have poor tensile strength; intermediate filaments are more flexible than actin and stronger under tension [14].

Within the cytoplasm, individual filaments aggregate into bundles; bundling greatly enhances the mechanical strength of the system. In addition, once the ability to bundle and unbundle filaments is regulated, the local mechanical properties of the cytoplasm can be controlled via assembly and disassembly of filaments. Many cytoplasmic constituents participate in the filament assembly process; actin filaments, for example, are crosslinked by at least four different agents (α-actinin, spectrin, fimbrin, and villin), providing the cell with a variety of tools for dynamically regulating filament assembly. Complex mechanical behavior is observed in simple systems of filaments and filament-binding proteins; in the case of actin filaments and α-actinin, complex rheological behavior is observed in reconstituted samples of purified cytoskeletal elements [15]. In general, solutions of cytoskeletal filaments are viscoelastic and have been characterized using the rheological methods described in in Section 5.3.3.

New methods, such as laser tracking microrheometry [16], offer the potential to study the mechanical behavior of cytoplasm within living cells.

5.4.3 Influence of Mechanical Forces on Cell Structure and Function

Cells respond to forces by deformation, as described above. It has also long been known that cell behavior (such as growth control) is dependent on cell

Table 5.3
Characteristics of Cytoskeletal
Filaments

Filament	$L_p(\mu m)$
Actin microfilament	18
Intermediate filament	2
Microtubule	6,000

Data obtained from [14].

shape [17], which suggests that the mechanical forces that act to deform cells (and therefore alter cell shape) can also influence the biochemical function of cells.

Cells of the vascular system are constantly exposed to the forces provided by blood flow and, therefore, it has been logical to study these cells for the impact of fluid shear forces on cell function. It is now well established that shear stress can 1) influence the morphology and orientation of cultured vascular cells; 2) induce changes in signal transduction systems and secondary messengers; 3) influence metabolite secretion; and 4) regulate gene expression (see review [18]). Similarly, mechanical forces that are provided through mechanisms other than from fluid flow—such as stretching of a deformable substrate on which cells are attached—can also influence cell function. Molecular mechanisms for mechanotransduction—that is, conversion of the mechanical force into a biological signal—are not clearly established, but it is likely that multiple mechanisms are involved, since cells encounter mechanical forces from many different sources. Mechanical forces can influence cellular function within tissues, as well; for example, the expression of genes in cells within brain slices is differentially regulated by controlled mechanical strains [19].

5.5 Mechanical Properties of Tissues

The mechanical properties of engineered tissues are often critical for their function (recall Figure 2.1 and related discussion). This section briefly reviews the mechnical behavior of tissues by focusing on the mechanical properties of bone, soft tissues, and tissue-engineered materials. The role of biomechanics in the evaluation of tissue-engineered materials has been reviewed [20].

5.5.1 Bone

Bone is a hard (that is, mechanically strong) tissue that is composed of a mineral phase (60%), a collagen-rich matrix (30%), and water (10%) [21]. The mineral phase appears to provide the stiffness to bone, while the matrix phase provides other properties that are still not well defined [21]. Bone has two typical architectures, cortical (or compact) bone and cancellous (or trabecular) bone, which differ in microscopic structure and mechanical properties (Table 5.1). The dense, rigid cortical architecture is found in long bones whereas the cancellous architecture, which is more porous and oriented, is found in the ribs, spine, and epiphysis. A comprehensive review of those biomechanical properties of bone that are relevant for tissue engineering is available [21].

5.5.2 Soft Connective Tissues

Soft connective tissues surround our organs, provide structural integrity, and protect them from damage. In most soft connective tissues—such as articular cartilage, tendons, ligaments, dermis of skin, and blood vessels—cells are sparsely distributed within an extracellular matrix that provides the mechanical property of the tissue. The molecular constituents of extracellular matrix are reviewed in Chapter 6 (see Section 6.4). In contrast to bone, which is a rigid material, soft connective tissues are typically flexible and deformable (Table 5.1).

Soft tissues are often viscoelastic, behaving like a reinforced composite material in which the structure and orientation of the fiber-reinforcing phase (often collagen and elastin fibers) determines the bulk mechanical behavior [22]. Figure 5.13 shows schematically the behavior of skin—a typical soft tissue that consists predominantly of connective tissue and shows an orientation parallel to the skin surface. With small tensile deformations (phase I in Figure 5.13), the tissue behaves as an elastic material; microscopically, collagen fibers within the tissue are deforming without stretching or bringing about large changes in structure. As the strain increases (phase II), collagen fibers become deformed, straightening in the direction of the strain and increasing the stiffness of the skin. With increased loads, in deformations that are just less than the ultimate tensile strength (phase III), the collagen fibers are individually aligned in the direction of the applied load, and stretched. This illustration demonstrates some of the complexity of the interplay between mechanical forces, tissue structure, and tissue function. Figure 5.13 shows that molecular architecture is influenced by strain; the functional properties of the tissues are also influenced by these changes.

5.5.3 Tissue-Engineered Materials

Many tissue-engineered materials consist of a population of cells embedded into a three-dimensional extracellular matrix. Chapter 1 illustrated this concept

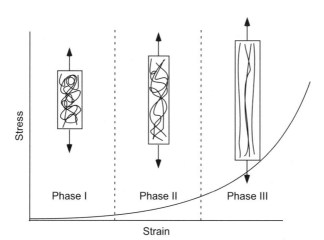

Figure 5.13. Mechanical behavior of soft tissues. The mechanical behavior of soft tissues is illustrated schematically for skin, in which fibers that are oriented parallel to the skin surface provide a nonlinear relationship between stress in the material and deformation. Redrawn from [22].

as a natural extension of conventional cell culture, in which cells are maintained in a three-dimensional environment that permits interaction of cells with the matrix material and with other cells (Figure 1.1).

In Chapter 2, the use of hybrid materials—containing both cells and matrix components, which might be natural or synthetic polymers—for tissue repair was also introduced (Figure 2.3). When cells are embedded into a matrix material, they can interact with the matrix. This interaction may change the functional state of the cells, but they may also alter the physical properties of the matrix by changing the amount or orientation of the matrix materials or by exerting forces on components of the matrix that serve to orient or disrupt the overall architecture.

This phenomenon has been studied in model cell culture systems, sometimes called tissue equivalents [23] or reconstituted model tissues [24], in which cells are suspended within a tissue-like extracellular matrix. When fibroblasts are cultured within a collagen matrix, for example, the cells will attach to and then deform collagen fibers; this action can be observed macroscopically because the mechanical action of the cells causes the gel material to change shape and, in the particular case of fibroblasts in collagen, become more compact. The dynamics of the compaction process reveal the action of cells within the bulk material (Figure 5.14). Usually a lag period is observed first, in which the matrix is forming around the cells. During the early phase of compaction, which usually lasts for the first 24 hours of culture, the cells form attachments to the matrix material and begin to contract it slowly; strains during this phase are typically small, ~10% [25]. Over the first week or two in culture, the cells will steadily compact the matrix materials by a process of adhesion to fibers and mechanical contraction by the cells;

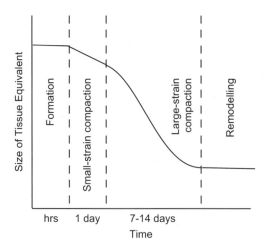

Figure 5.14. Dynamic compaction of a tissue equivalent. Cells can be suspended within a matrix material to produce a three-dimensional tissue equivalent, which will undergo mechanical and geometric changes during maintenance in culture.

strains during this phase can be 50 to 90% [26]. In the final phase, there is no further compaction of the material, but it can become substantially stiffer due to the action of the cells, which may secrete additional matrix proteins or cause crosslinking of existing matrix materials. The extent and the time course of compaction depend on the density of cells in the material, the type of cells that are suspended, and the nature of the material and extra-cellular environment. In all stages of this process, the cells may be modifying the matrix (by stiffening it, for example) and, at the same time, the matrix may be inducing changes in the structure and function of the entrapped cells (as described in Section 5.4.3).

5.5.4 Example: Compression of Cellular Aggregates

Some of these mechanical principles can be illustrated with a practical example of importance to tissue engineering. (The importance of cellular aggregates in tissue engineering will be elaborated in Chapter 8.) As described in Chapter 3, cellular aggregates and tissue fragments have been powerful models for developmental biology. Force relaxation experiments on embryonic tissue fragments, which are allowed to round-up into spherical aggregates in culture, show a characteristic behavior (Figure 5.15a); in response to a fixed deformation, the aggregate exerts a resisting force which declines with a rapid initial rate, followed by a slow, more persistant relaxation [27]. This relaxation is similar to the behaviors illustrated in the spring and dashpot models of Figure 5.10—especially the behavior in panel c (rapid initial response and persistent continuing response) and panel d (slow approach to some limiting response). But the behavior here is more complicated in that two rates of relaxation, or characteristic time constants, are observed.

The simplest model that can incorporate all of the behaviors observed in the dynamics response of living tissue segments to compression is the Kelvin model (Figure 5.15b). In this model, a third element—the slide wire, indicated in the figure with its parameter σ—is used to indicate the equilibrium shape of the aggregate under the compressive force. A force balance on the elements shown in Figure 5.15b yields

$$F + \left(\frac{\eta_1}{\mu_1} + \frac{\eta_2}{\mu_2}\right)\frac{dF}{dt} + \frac{\eta_1\eta_2}{\mu_1\mu_2}\frac{d^2F}{dt^2} = \sigma U_0 \qquad (5\text{-}53)$$

which can be solved to obtain

$$F = (\sigma + \mu_1 e^{-\mu_1 t/\eta_1} + \mu_2 e^{-\mu_2 t/\eta_2})U_0 \qquad (5\text{-}54)$$

This model was compared to force relaxation behavior observed in tissues taken from different regions of the embryo; the mechanical behavior of the living tissue depends on composition (Table 5.4).

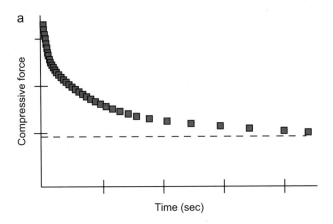

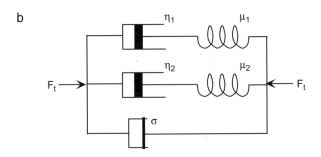

Figure 5.15. Compression of cellular aggregates formed from embryonic tissues. Stress relaxation during compression of the cellular aggregate: experimental data (a) and mechanical model (b). Adapted from [27].

Table 5.4
Viscoelastic Properties of Embryonic Tissues

Tissue Type	μ_1 (dyne/ cm)	η_1 (dyne- s/cm)	η_1/μ_1 (s)	μ_2 (dyne/ cm)	η_2 (dyne- s/cm)	η_1/μ_1 (s)	σ (dyne/ cm)
Neural retina	3.4	7.3	2.2	2.1	55	27	1.6
Liver	4.0	7.6	1.9	2.3	50	23	4.6
Heart	5.1	9.5	1.9	2.5	66	26	8.5
Limb	8.6	24	2.7	7.7	340	45	20

Values for the parameters of the Kelvin model were obtained by measuring force relaxation in aggregates from embryonic tissues. Original data reported in [30].

Summary

- For small strains, many solid materials deform elastically; the mechanical properties of these are similar to those of an ideal spring and can be described by an elastic modulus E.
- Fluids deform continuously under the action of a shearing force; for Newtonian fluids, the viscosity, or ratio of shear force to shear rate, is a constant.
- The physics of fluid flow can be quantified for certain geometries. In the case of steady laminar flow through a cylindrical tube—which is an important flow in biological systems—the behavior of the flow is well described and predictable.
- Many biological materials exhibit both elastic and viscous properties; these materials are called viscoelastic. Mechanical models that combine purely elastic and purely viscous components can sometimes be used to predict their deformation behavior.
- Rheology, or the study of deformations in materials, can be used to analyze the mechanical behavior of biological fluids and gels. Examination of the rheological properties often gives insight into the molecular properties of the material.
- Cells exhibit complex mechanical behaviors and respond in complicated ways to mechanical forces.
- The mechanical properties of many tissues are important for their biological function; the development of methods for biomechanical analysis is an important part of tissue engineering.

Exercises

Exercise 5.1

In a radial flow detachment assay (a device for measuring cell adhesion to a surface, which is discussed in more detail in Chapter 6), cells attached to a planar, cylindrical surface are exposed to a steady fluid flow which originates at the center of the surface $(r = 0)$ and flows toward the outer edge $(r = R)$. Assuming laminar flow through the gap between two stationary surfaces, one containing the adherent cells and the other a uniform height (h) above it, show that the shear stress at the surface depends on radial position from the center: $S = 3Q\mu/\pi rh^2$, where Q is the volumetric flow rate and μ is the fluid viscosity.

Exercise 5.2 (provided by Song Li)

Consider the optimum design of vascular network.

a) Read Fung, Y. C. *Biodynamics: Circulation*, Sections 3.1–3.4 [3].

b) Look for anatomy pictures or data on blood vessel bifurcations in literature. Measure the diameters and branch angles (or quote the data). Are the theoretical results in reasonable agreement with empirical observations?

Exercise 5.3

Use the approach outlined in the chapter to fill in the missing formulas in Table 5.5.

Exercise 5.4 (provided by Song Li)

Derive the creep function and relaxation function for a standard linear solid (Kelvin model), which is shown in Figure 5.16.

Exercise 5.5 (provided by Song Li)

Is soft tissue elastic or viscoelastic? Is the stress–strain relationship linear or nonlinear for soft tissues? What is quasi-linear viscoelasticity?

Exercise 5.6

Assume that the aorta can be modeled as a viscoelastic solid using the Maxwell model with coefficients μ and η. The pressure inside the aorta varies with time according to the function: $P(t) = P_0 \sin \omega t$. The length of the vessel is constant, L, and the radius of the vessel is R_0 when $P = P_0$. How does the radius of the vessel vary with time?

Exercise 5.7

Derive Equation 5-9 from the information provided on forces in Figure 5.4.

Table 5.5
Creep and Relaxation Functions for Models of Viscoelastic Materials

Model	Creep Function, $c(t - \tau)$	Relaxation function, $k(t - \tau)$
Maxwell (Figure 5.10c)	$c(t - \tau) = \left(\dfrac{1}{\mu} + \dfrac{t - \tau}{\eta}\right) H(t - \tau)$	?
Voigt (Figure 5.10d)	?	?
Standard linear model (Figure 5.16)	?	?

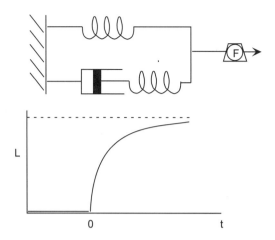

Figure 5.16. Kelvin model of viscoelastic materials.

References

1. Fung, Y.-C., *Biomechanics: Mechanical Properties of Living Tissues*, 2nd ed. New York: Springer-Verlag, 1993.
2. Ozkaya, N. and M. Nordin, *Fundamentals of Biomechanics: Equilibrium, Motion, and Deformation*, 2nd ed. New York: Springer-Verlag, 1999.
3. Fung, Y.C., *Biodynamics: Circulation*, 2nd ed. New York: Springer-Verlag, 1997, 571 pp.
4. Bird, R.B., W.E. Stewart, and E.N. Lightfoot, *Transport Phenomena*. New York: John Wiley & Sons, 1960, 780 pp.
5. Welty, J.R., C.E. Wicks, and R.E. Wilson, *Fundamentals of Momentum, Heat, and Mass Transfer*, 3rd ed. New York: John Wiley & Sons, 1984.
6. Kuntz, R.M. and W.M. Saltzman, Neutrophil motility in extracellular matrix gels: mesh size and adhesion affect speed of migration. *Biophysical Journal*, 1997, **72**, 1472–1480.
7. Prud'homme, R.K., Rheological characterization, in *Electronic Materials Handbook*. Ohio: ASM International, 1989.
8. Waugh, R.E. and R.M. Hochmuth, Mechanics and deformability of hematocytes, in J. D. Bronzino (ed.), *The Biomedical Engineering Handboook*. Boca Raton, FL: CRC Press, 2000, pp. 32-1–32-13.
9. Evans, E. and P. La Celle, Intrinsic material properties of the erythrocyte membrane indicated by mechanical analysis of deformation. *Blood*, 1975. **45**, 29–43.
10. Evans, E. and R. Hochmuth, A solid–liquid composite model of the red cell membrane. *Journal of Membrane Biology*, 1977, **30**, 351–362.
11. Tsai, M.A., R.E. Waugh, and P.C. Keng, Passive mechnical behavior of human neutrophils: effects of colchicine and paclitaxel. *Biophysical Journal*, 1998, **74**, 3282–3291.
12. Felder, S. and E.L. Elson, Mechanics of fibroblast locomotion: quantitative analysis of forces and motions at the leading lamellas of fibroblasts. *Journal of Cell Biology*, 1990, **111**, 2513–2526.

13. Rotsch, C.,K. Jacobson, and M. Radmacher, Dimensional and mechanical dynamics of active and stable edges in motile fibroblasts investigated by using atomic force microscopy. *Proceedings of the National Academy of Sciences, USA*, 1999, **96**, 921–926.

14. Bray, D., *Cell Movement*, 2nd ed. New York: Garland Publishing, 2001, 372 pp.

15. Sato, M., W. Schwarz, and T. Pollard, Dependence of the mechanical properties of actin/a-actinin gels on deformation rate. *Nature*, 1987, **325**, 828–830.

16. Yamada, S.,D. Wirtz, and S.C. Kuo, Mechanics of living cells measured by laser tracking microrheology. *Biophysical Journal*, 2000, **78**, 1736–1747.

17. Folkman, J. and A. Moscona, Role of cell shape in growth control. *Nature*, 1978, **273**, 345–349.

18. Patrick, C.W., R. Sampath, and L.V. McIntire, Fluid shear stress effects on cellular function, in J.D. Bronzino (ed.). *The Biomedical Engineering Handbook*. Boca Raton, FL: CRC Press, 2000, pp. 114-1–114-20.

19. Morrison, B., et al., Dynamic mechanical stretch of organotypic brain slice cultures induces differential genomic expression: relationship to mechanical parameters. *Journal of Biomechanical Engineering*, 2000, **122**, 224–230.

20. Butler, D.L., S.A. Goldstein, and F. Guilak, Functional tissue engineering: the role of biomechanics. *Journal of Biomechanical Engineering*, 2000, **122**, 570–575.

21. Athanasiou, K.A., et al., Fundamentals of biomechanics in tissue engineering of bone. *Tissue Engineering*, 2000, **6**(4), 361–381.

22. Holzapfel, G.A., Biomechanics of soft tissue, in *Handbook of Material Behavior*. J. Lemaitre (ed.), San Diego, CA: Academic Press, 2000.

23. Barocas, V.H. and R.T. Tranquillo, Biphasic theory and in vitro assays of cell–fibril mechanical interactions in tissue-equivalent gels, in V.C. Mow (ed.), *Cell Mechanics and Cellular Engineering*. New York: Springer-Verlag, 1994, pp. 1–25.

24. Wakatsuki, T., et al., Cell mechanics studied by a reconstituted model tissue. *Biophysical Journal*, 2000, **79**, 2353–2368.

25. Barocas, V.H., A.G. Moon, and R.T. Tranquillo, The fibroblast-populated collagen microsphere assay of cell traction force. Part 2. Measurement of the cell traction coefficient. *Journal of Biomechanical Engineering*, 1995, **117**(2), 161–170.

26. Moon, A. G. and R. T. Tranquillo, Fibroblast-populated collagen microsphere assay of cell traction force: Part 1. Continuum model. *AIChE Journal*, 1993, **39**, 163–177.

27. Beysens, D.A., G. Forgacs, and J. A. Glazier, Embryonic tissues are viscoelastic materials. *Canadian Journal of Physics*, 2000, **78**, 243–251.

28. Brands, D.W.A., Predicting brain mechanics during closed head impact. Eindhoven: Technische Universiteit Eindhoven, 2002.

29. Ratner, B., et al. (eds.), *Biomaterials Science: an Introduction to Materials in Medicine*. San Diego, CA: Academic Press, 1996.

30. Forgacs, G., et al., Viscoelastic properties of living embryonic tissues: a quantitative study. *Biophysical Journal*, 1998, **74**, 2227–2234.

6

Cell Adhesion

I am a kind of burr; I shall stick.

William Shakespeare, *Measure for Measure*, act 4, scene 3

The external surface of the cell consists of a phospholipid bilayer which carries a carbohydrate-rich coat called the glycocalyx (Figure 6.1); ionizable groups within the glycocalyx, such as sialic acid (N-acetyl neuraminate), contribute a net negative charge to the cell surface. Many of the carbohydrates that form the glycocalyx are bound to membrane-associated proteins. Each of these components— phospholipid bilayer, carbohydrate-rich coat, membrane-associated protein—has distinct physicochemical characteristics and is abundant. Plasma membranes contain ~50% protein, ~45% lipid, and ~5% carbohydrate by weight. Therefore, each component influences cell interactions with the external environment in important ways.

Cells can become attached to surfaces. The surface of interest may be geometrically complex (for example, the surface of another cell, a virus, a fiber, or an irregular object), but this chapter will focus on adhesion between a cell and a planar surface (Figure 6.2). The consequences of cell–cell adhesion are considered further in Chapter 8 (Cell Aggregation and Tissue Equivalents) and Chapter 9 (Tissue Barriers to Molecular and Cellular Transport). The consequences of cell–substrate adhesion are considered further in Chapter 7 (Cell Migration) and Chapter 12 (Cell Interactions with Polymers).

Since the growth and function of many tissue-derived cells required attachment and spreading on a solid substrate, the events surrounding cell adhesion are fundamentally important. In addition, the strength of cell adhesion is an important determinant of the rate of cell migration, the kinetics of cell–cell aggregation, and the magnitude of tissue barriers to cell and molecule transport. Cell adhesion is therefore a major consideration in the development of methods and materials for cell delivery, tissue engineering, and tissue regeneration.

The most stable and versatile mechanism for cell adhesion involves the specific association of cell surface glycoproteins, called receptors, and complementary molecules in the extracellular space, called ligands [1]. Ligands may exist freely in the extracellular space, they may be associated with the extracellular matrix, or they may be attached to the surface of another cell (Figure

151

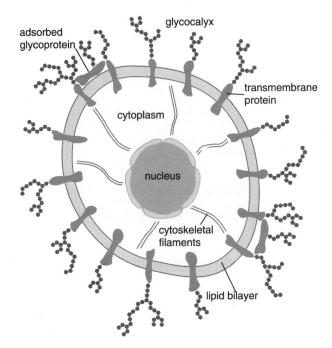

Figure 6.1. Schematic diagram of a simplified animal cell (adapted from Panel I-1 and Figure 6-40 of [28]). The cell is surrounded by a glycocalyx, which consists of carbohydrates on a transmembrane and absorbed proteins. Transmembrane proteins can interact with elements of the filamentous cytoskeleton, providing a mechanism for the transmission of extracellular information to the nucleus.

6.3). Cell–cell adhesion can occur by homophilic binding of identical receptors on different cells, by heterophilic binding of a receptor to a ligand expressed on the surface of a different cell, or by association of two receptors with an intermediate linker. Cell–matrix adhesion usually occurs by heterophilic binding of a receptor to a ligand attached to an insoluble element of the extracellular matrix.

This section begins with a summary of the forces involved in cell adhesion; more detailed analysis is available elsewhere [2–6]. For a review of mathematical models for cell adhesion, see Section 6.2 of [1]. A monograph on the nature of intermolecular forces, and their participation in complex events such as cell adhesion, is also available [7].

6.1 Mechanics of Cell Adhesion

6.1.1 Physical Forces During Cell Adhesion

A cell approaching a surface is subject to attractive and repulsive forces (Figure 6.4); the magnitude of each force is a function of the separation distance

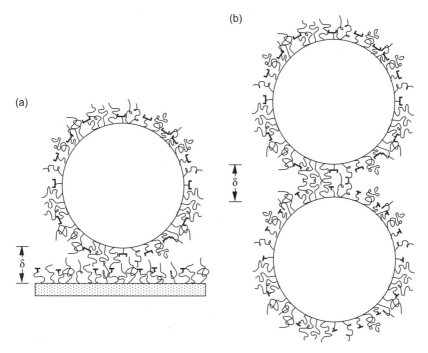

Figure 6.2. Schematic diagram of a cell approaching a surface (a) or another cell (b). As the cell approaches the surface, it encounters repulsive steric stabilization forces which may eventually be overcome by the attractive van der Waals forces, electrostatic forces, or the forces resulting from receptor–ligand interactions.

between the cell and the surface. The balance of forces will determine whether the cell will adhere to the surface—a process that is often followed by cell spreading, migration, and growth—or remain non-adherent and floating above the plane of the surface. Electrostatic, steric stabilization, and van der Waals forces do not require specific interactions between cell surface molecules and complementary ligands on the surface. For a cell approaching another cell, the electrostatic forces are usually repulsive, because the surfaces of both cells carry a net negative charge (Figure 6.1). For a cell approaching a surface, the electrostatic forces can be either attractive or repulsive, depending on the charge associated with the surface: for example, a poly(L-lysine) surface, which has a positive charge from the many primary amine groups, can support the non-specific adhesion of many types of cells. Steric stabilization forces result from an osmotic imbalance developed in the gap region between cell and surface. As water is forced out of this region, cell surface macromolecules in the narrow gap become concentrated, resulting in an osmotic difference that pulls water into the gap and generates a repulsive force; this force can become large as the gap becomes small (Figure 6.2). Cell surface molecules become compressed during close approach, contributing further to the repulsive force. Van der Waals forces, the result of charge interactions between polarizable but

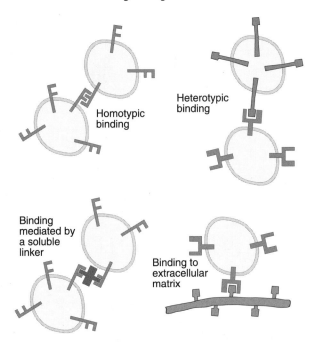

Figure 6.3. Types of cell adhesion (adapted from Figure 14-64 of [28]). Cell–cell binding can occur by the association of identical receptors (homophilic binding), by the association of complementary receptors (heterophilic binding), or through the cooperation of a multifunctional molecule dissolved in the extracellular space. Cell–matrix binding involves the association of a cell surface molecule with a complementary ligand on the matrix.

uncharged molecules, are attractive. These forces dominate at large separation distances (> 200 Å), but are less important as the separation distance becomes small (Figure 6.4).

Cell–cell and cell–surface adhesion occurs at separation distances of ~100–300 Å. During cell adhesion, cell surface receptors interact with ligands on the opposing surface to produce specific cell adhesion forces (Figure 6.4); the molecules involved in adhesion are described in the subsection to follow. These specific interactions are vital to cell–cell and cell–surface adhesion. Without this additional interaction, only weak cell adhesion could occur: the attractive van der Waals forces shown in Figure 6.4 result in an adhesion force of ~1000 dyn/cm², greater than the shear forces that occur in venules (1–10 dyn/cm² [8]) but less than the shear forces in the arterial circulation (10,000 dyn/cm²) or contractile forces in tissues (1000–100,000 dyn/cm² [9]). Equally important, the unique complement of receptor molecules expressed on a cell surface provides selectivity to cell adhesion by modulating the extent to which a cell can adhere to another cell or surface. Receptor–ligand bonds can function to promote adhesion because the overall interaction potential (in the absence of ligand binding) is usually repulsive [10].

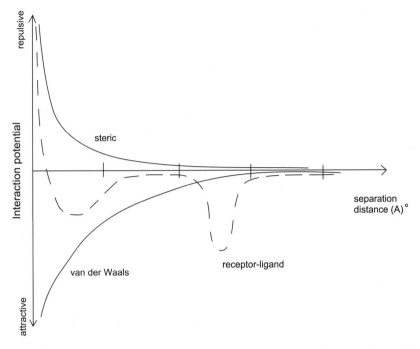

Figure 6.4. Magnitude of non-specific forces important in cell adhesion. The graph shows how the various forces vary with separation distance, similar to Figure 6-17 in [1], which was reprinted from [4]. The continuous curves show each of the forces individually and the dashed curve shows the sum of the forces acting on the cell, including the receptor–ligand interaction.

The specific interactions involved in cell adhesion depend on the reversible association of protein receptors in the cell membrane and complementary ligands on the surface:

$$L + R \underset{k_r}{\overset{k_f}{\rightleftharpoons}} L-R \tag{6-1}$$

where R denotes a receptor molecule, L a ligand, L–R a receptor–ligand complex, and k_f and k_r are the first-order reaction rate constants for the forward and reverse reactions (that is, association and dissociation), respectively. The affinity of the receptor–ligand pair is determined by the equilibrium association or binding constant, K_a:

$$K_d = \frac{1}{K_a} = \frac{C_L C_R}{C_{L-R}} = \frac{k_r}{k_f} \tag{6-2}$$

where concentrations and constants are defined as in Chapter 4 (Equations 6-1 and 6-2 are identical to Equations 4-1 and 4-2). As is most frequently the case, the dissociation constant will be used to characterize receptor–ligand affinity in this book; it is important to note, however, that the association constant is used in some sources.

This formalism for describing ligand–receptor interactions was introduced in Chapter 4 in the context of growth factor, hormone, and nutrient binding to the cell surface. A major difference between hormone binding and cell adhesion ligand binding is the affinity of the molecular interactions. The importance of any particular receptor–ligand pair in cell adhesion depends on the relative abundance of the receptor and ligand molecules in the cell–surface contact area and the affinity of the receptor–ligand association. The affinity is represented by the dissociation constant, which is numerically equal to the ligand concentration required to achieve 50% receptor binding, as described quantitatively in Chapter 4 (Figure 6.5; recall the assumptions in this simple model: univalent binding, total receptor number is constant, ligand is present in excess). Typically, K_d varies between 10^{-6} (low affinity) to 10^{-12} M (high affinity) for receptor–ligand interactions (Table 6.1). Interestingly, for cell adhesion receptors and ECM ligands, such as the integrin/fibronectin binding pair, the dissociation constant can be quite low: $K_d \simeq 10^{-6}$ to 10^{-7} M.

To predict the strength of specific cell adhesion by multiple non-covalent bonds, the tensile strength of receptor–ligand bonds has been estimated. In the simplest calculation, the strength of an affinity bond, F, is assumed to be related to the standard free energy ΔG_0 and the bond length δ: $F = \Delta G_0/\delta$ [11, 12]. The free energy of the standard state, ΔG_0, is determined from the binding constant by

$$\Delta G_0 = (kT)\ln(K_a/K_0) \tag{6-3}$$

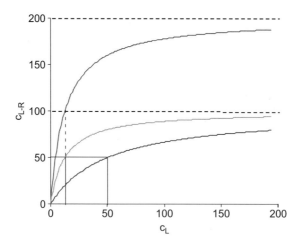

Figure 6.5. Variation in receptor binding with ligand concentration: see equations presented in Chapter 4 (especially Equation 4-7). Three sets of parameters are indicated: for the top line $K_d = 12.5$ and $R_T = 200$; for the middle line $K_d = 12.5$ and $R_T = 100$; for the bottom line $K_d = 50$ and $R_T = 100$.

Table 6.1
Binding Affinity for Cell Adhesion Receptors

Ligand	Receptor	K_a (M^{-1})	K_d (M)	Reference
Integrins				
Fibrinogen	αIIbβ3	7.0×10^6	1.4×10^{-7}	[39]
RGDS	Fibroblast cell surface	6×10^5	1.7×10^{-6}	[40]
cHarGD	αIIbβ3	1×10^8	1×10^{-8}	[41]
Cadherin				
Cadherin	Cadherin		N.A.	see [48, 49]
β-Catenin	α-Catenin	1×10^7	1×10^{-7}	[42]
Ig family				
Phosphacan	N-CAM/Ng-CAM	1×10^{10}	1×10^{-10}	[43]
Neurocan	N-CAM/Ng-CAM	1×10^9	1×10^{-9}	[44]
Selectins				
GlyCAM-1	L-selectin (CD62L)	9.3×10^3	1.1×10^{-4}	[45]
sLe^x	E-selectin (CD62E)	7.2×10^5	1.4×10^{-6}	Reported in [45]
sLe^x	P-selectin (CD62P)	7.8×10^6	1.3×10^{-7}	Reported in [45]
P-selectin glycoprotein ligand-1	P-selectin (CD62P)	3.1×10^6	3.2×10^{-7}	[46]
Other systems, for comparison				
Biotin	Avidin	10^{15}	10^{-15}	

K_d is the dissociation constant. Phosphacan and neurocan are proteoglycans. Abbreviations: N.A., not available; R, arginine; G, glycine; D, aspartic acid; S, serine; Har, homoarginine.

where K_a is the binding constant of the receptor–ligand pair, K_0 is the binding constant of the standard state (1 M^{-1}), k is Boltzmann's constant, and T is the absolute temperature. The bond length, which is difficult to determine experimentally, is assumed to be greater than the size of the individual weak bonds within the binding site (~1 Å) and less than the size of the binding site itself (~10 Å). From typical values of the binding constant and bond length, bond strengths can be estimated as 6 to 120 μdyn/molecule (see Table 6.2). A more complete consideration of bond strength employing multi-step models of receptor–ligand binding—including translational diffusion, rotational diffusion, and an activation barrier—suggests that the probable range of tensile strengths is

Table 6.2
Typical Tensile Strengths for Affinity Bonds

δ (Å)	K_a (M^{-1})	ΔG_0 (J/mol)	F (μdyn/molecule)
10	10^6	35,600	6
1	10^{12}	71,200	120

After [13].

larger (6 to 250 μdyn) and that the "average" bond has a tensile strength of 40 μdyn [13].

With only one of these "average" bonds per μm^2 of cell–surface contact (that is, bonds are spaced ∼1 μm apart on the surface), an overall resisting force of 4,000 dyn/cm^2 would be produced by specific binding; this force is comparable in magnitude to the total non-specific forces (see Figure 6.4). This simple calculation of the total tensile strength of the multiple receptor–ligand adhesion systems assumes that the force tending to separate the cells is applied quickly, so that all of the bonds break simultaneously [13]. In reality, individual affinity bonds are forming and breaking continuously; the lifetime of any one bond is limited by fluctuations in thermal energy. This normal turn-over in binding for individual receptor–ligand pairs leads to a decrease in the tensile strength of the population of bound receptors when the separating force is applied slowly (that is, over periods of time equal to or greater than the lifetime of individual bonds, ∼1 to 1,000 ms). For the "average" bond described above, this effect decreases the tensile strength by a factor of ∼4 to ∼10 μdyn/bond.

The forward and reverse rate constants (Equation 6-1) depend on the chemical interactions between the two species, as well as the rate at which a receptor–ligand pair can achieve the necessary physical proximity for the chemical association to occur. As in the case of soluble ligand binding to the cell surface (see Chapter 4), receptor–ligand association and dissociation can be either reaction- or diffusion-limited [1]. In addition, receptors have mechanical properties that influence their dynamic behavior. A commonly used model supposes that the receptor–ligand bond is a spring with constant σ and equilibrium length λ [14]. This model predicts that the forward and reverse rate constants depend on x, the bond length:

$$k_f(x) = k_f^0 \exp\left[-\sigma_{ts}\frac{(x-\lambda)^2}{2kT}\right] \tag{6-4}$$

$$k_r(x) = k_r^0 \exp\left[-(\sigma-\sigma_{ts})\frac{(x-\lambda)^2}{2kT}\right] \tag{6-5}$$

where σ_{ts} represents the transition state spring constant. Cells that are adherent to a surface resist detachment because multiple receptor–ligand bonds maintain the association. If a sufficient force is applied to the cell, those bonds should all break and the cell detach. Dembo et al. [14] extend the adhesion model to predict that the critical tension for detachment, T_m, depends on the affinity of the receptor–ligand interaction:

$$T_m = \frac{kTN_t}{1+\cos\theta_m}\ln\left[1+\frac{1}{K_d}\right] \tag{6-6}$$

where N_t is the density of receptors and θ_m is the angle between the cell membrane (hence, the detachment force) and the surface. Experimental data on detachment of receptor-coated beads from a ligand-coated surface support this functional dependence [15].

New technology is also permitting measurement of the adhesion forces due to single bonds. For example, an atomic force microscope cantilever was used to measure the adhesion force between avidin and biotin [16]. The measured adhesion forces appeared in integral multiples of 160 ± 20 pN and 85 ± 15 pN (16 and 8.5 µdyne) for biotin and iminobiotin, respectively. The surface force apparatus is capable of measuring 10 nN changes in force between precisely positioned surfaces; two lipid surfaces containing lipid anchored biotin were brought into close proximity with an intervening liquid layer containing the multivalent biotin-binding protein, avidin, which was initially associated with one of the surfaces [17]. Even at long range (>100 Å), the streptavidin produced attractive forces that were $\sim 10\times$ greater than the van der Waals forces. These long-range forces, attributed to hydrophobic interactions between the exposed surfaces of biotin and streptavidin, may be important in guiding diffusible membrane receptors to their complementary ligand targets during cell–surface approach.

The discussion in this section has not considered the role of cell deformation and membrane mechanics in cell adhesion; reviews on this subject are available.

6.1.2 Experimental Methods for Measuring Cell Adhesion

Since cell adhesion is critically important in many physiological and biotechnological situations, a number of different techniques for quantifying the extent and strength of cell adhesion have been developed. The simplest methods for quantifying the extent of cell adhesion to a surface involve three steps (Figure 6.6a): i) sedimentation of cells onto a surface, ii) incubation of the sedimented cells in culture medium for some period of time, and iii) detachment of loosely adherent cells by removal of the culture medium and repeated washing, usually under conditions that are controlled to the extent that is possible. The extent of cell adhesion, which is a function of the conditions of the experiment, is determined by quantifying either the number of cells that remain associated with the surface (the "adherent" cells) or the number of cells that were extracted with the washes. In many cases, the adherent cells are further categorized on the basis of morphological differences (that is, extent of spreading, formation of actin filament bundles, presence of focal contacts, etc.). This technique is simple, rapid, and requires only equipment that is found in most laboratories. This type of measurement is therefore common. Unfortunately, it is difficult to quantify the fluid mechanical force that is provided to dislodge the non-adherent cells. Since it is difficult to control all of the variables determining the force applied to detach the cells, it is difficult to compare results obtained from different laboratories using this same technique.

This disadvantage can be overcome by using a centrifuge to provide a reproducible detachment force. The technique described above is modified slightly: following the incubation period, the plate is inverted and subjected

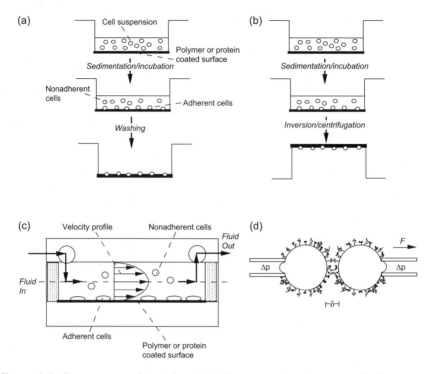

Figure 6.6. Common experimental methods for measuring the extent of cell adhesion: (a) sedimentation-detachment assay; (b) centrifugation assay; (c) fluid flow chambers; (d) micropipette assays.

to a controlled detachment force by centrifugation (Figure 6.6b). The extent of cell attachment is then quantified as before. Since the assay is frequently performed in a 96-well microtiter plate, which permits a small number of cells per well, radiolabeled cells are frequently used to permit accurate measurement of the number of attached cells.

Fluid mechanical forces can also be applied to produce cell detachment in a well-controlled and quantifiable manner (Figure 6.6c). In most flow chambers, the fluid is forced between two parallel plates. Prior to applying the flow field, a cell suspension is injected into the chamber, and the cells are permitted to settle onto the surface of interest and adhere. After some period of incubation, flow is initiated between the plates. These chambers have been used to examine a number of phenomena related to cell adhesion, particularly with regard to the forces experienced by leukocytes attaching to endothelial cells in the circulatory systems. A variety of studies have used these chambers to measure the kinetics of cell attachment, cell detachment, and cell rolling on surfaces under conditions of flow.

Usually, the overall flow rate is adjusted so that the flow is laminar ($R_e < 2$), and the flow chamber is designed so that the shear stresses at the wall approximate the shear stresses found in the circulatory system; however, these chambers can be used to characterize cell detachment under a wide range of conditions. When operated with a steady uniform flow, the velocity profile within the flow chamber is given by [18]:

$$v_y = v_{\text{max}}\left[1 - \left(\frac{x}{a}\right)^2\right] = \frac{3}{4}\frac{Q}{ab}\left[1 - \left(\frac{x}{a}\right)^2\right] \tag{6-7}$$

where v_y is the velocity in the y-direction (along the axis of the flow chamber), v_{max} is the maximum velocity in the y-direction, which occurs at the centerline, Q is the volumetric flow rate of fluid through the channel, a is the half-height of the channel, and b is the width of the channel. The detachment force at the surface, which detaches the cells, can be estimated from the fluid shear stress at the wall, τ:

$$\tau = -\mu \frac{\mathrm{d}v_y}{\mathrm{d}x}\bigg|_{x=a} = \frac{3}{2}\frac{\mu Q}{2a^2 b} \tag{6-8}$$

where μ is the viscosity of the fluid. By adjusting the flow rate through the channel, with all of the other parameters maintained constant, the force tending to detach cells from the surface can be controlled by the investigator.

Radial flow detachment chambers have also been used to measure forces of cell detachment [19]. Because of the geometry of the radial flow chamber, where cells are attached uniformly to a circular plate and fluid is circulated from the center to the periphery of the chamber along radial paths, the fluid shear force experienced by the attached cells decreases with radial position from the center to the periphery. Therefore, in a single experiment, the influence of a range of forces on cell adhesion can be determined.

Finally, micropipettes are frequently used to measure directly the forces of cell–cell or cell–surface adhesion (Figure 6.6d). Cells are manipulated by holding them with micropipettes; slight suction inside the pipette allows the experimenter to hold the cells. Usually, this technique is used to measure cell–cell adhesion by holding two cells in two pipettes and carefully moving the cells together. Since the manipulators that are used to move the pipettes can be calibrated to monitor the force required for motion, the adhesive forces can be measured directly. Variations on this basic approach have been used to measure a wide range of important forces including the forces of adhesion between cells, forces involved in membrane deformation [20], forces exerted by motile cells such as sperm [21], forces exerted by growing or motile cell processes [22], and forces exerted by the macromolecular assemblies involved in cell motion, such as actin filaments [23].

6.2 Cell Junctions

Binding of cell surface receptors to complementary ligands is a principal mechanism for initial association of cells with other cells and with matrix. This mechanism of biological recognition is particularly important during development of the embryo; cells proliferate, migrate, and use specific binding signals to localize in the developing organism. In the adult organism, stability of the cell–cell or cell–matrix assembly is enhanced by the formation of specialized contact regions called cell junctions. Through these junctions, cells in tissue are linked to one another and to their surrounding extracellular matrix.

Three types of junctions are found in tissues: tight cell junctions, anchoring cell junctions, and communicating cell junctions. Tight cell junctions and anchoring cell junctions create mechanically stable tissues from individual cells. Communicating cell junctions, such as gap junctions, provide a mechanism for regulated exchange of molecules between adjacent cells. In gap junctions in the liver, aqueous channels are created by a coordinated assembly of twelve transmembrane proteins called connexins: six connexin molecules are contributed by each cell. The channel permits the passage of small molecules (molecular weight <1,200) from the cytoplasm of one cell to the other (see [24] for a review).

6.2.1 Tight Junctions

Epithelial cells are sealed together, via tight junctions, into a continuous sheet that forms the barrier surface of all mucosal tissues such as the intestinal, reproductive, and respiratory tracts. The tight junction is composed primarily of interconnected transmembrane proteins, contributed equally by both cell partners, which proceed continuously across the space between adjacent cells (Figure 6.7). In this arrangement, tight junctions act as barriers to the passage of small molecules in the extracellular space. Since the permeability of tight junctions decreases logarithmically with protein density in the junction, tissues can have junctional complexes of different structure that permit the diffusion of molecules of a specific size or charge; some tight junctions are so dense that they are essentially impermeable. Within the plasma membrane, tight junctions also act as physical barriers which confine transmembrane proteins involved in carrier-mediated transport to specific regions of the cell (for example, the apical and basolateral surfaces, Figure 6.7). In this way, tight junctions facilitate the transfer of water-soluble molecules, such as proteins or glucose, from the lumen of the gut into the blood, and even permit transport against a concentration gradient.

6.2.2 Anchoring Junctions

Cells are mechanically attached to another cell or an extracellular matrix protein over discrete regions called anchoring junctions. Anchoring junctions serve as mechanical links between cells, as well as points of intersection of cell scaffolding proteins (that is, cytoskeletal filaments) and the plasma membrane. Each junction contains intracellular attachment proteins, which form the physical connection between the cytoskeleton and the membrane, and transmembrane linker proteins, which tether the external face of the membrane to a complementary protein on an adjacent cell or matrix (Figure 6.7). Cellular

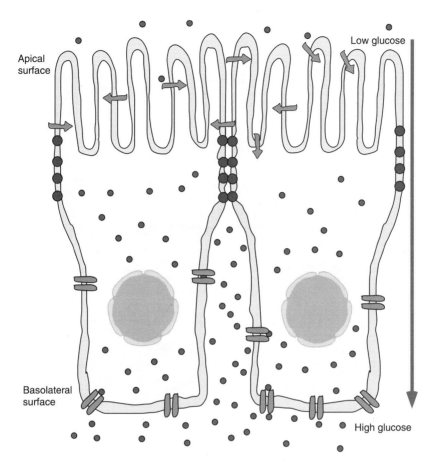

Figure 6.7. Tight junctions form a barrier to the movement of molecules in the space between adjacent cells. The junction is formed by arrays of interlocking protein particles (dark grey circles), contributed by both of the neighboring cells. The junction prevents the diffusion of water-soluble molecules as well as membrane proteins in the extracellular space. The presence of tight junctions creates segregated domains in each cell, with glucose active transport proteins (short grey arrows) confined in the apical domain and glucose facilitated transport channels (grey tunnels) confined in the basolateral domain. Tight junctions enable transport of glucose up a concentration gradient by segregating functional transport proteins in the membrane and prohibiting the back diffusion of glucose through the gaps between cells.

attachment occurs when the extracellular domain of the transmembrane linker protein associates with an extracellular matrix molecule or the extracellular domain of a transmembrane linker protein on another cell. Adheren junctions, desmosomes, and hemidesmosomes are distinct types of anchoring junctions that differ in function, as well as in composition of the junctional complex (Figure 6.8 and Table 6.3).

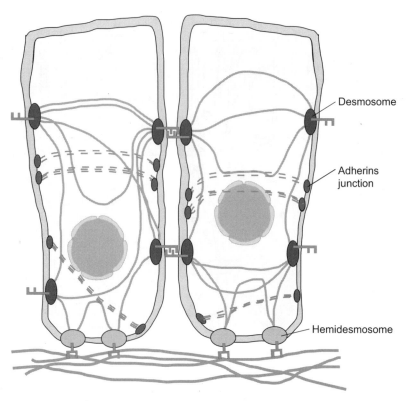

Figure 6.8. Schematic diagram of cells containing a variety of anchoring junctions. Adherens junctions connect actin filaments (dashed lines) to form a contractile adhesion belt. Desmosomes provide a linkage of intermediate filament bundles between cells. Hemidesmosomes connect intermediate filament termination with extracellular matrix. Anchor junctions are also characterized by the protein receptor, represented here as cadherins (𝔽) and integrins (𝕐).

Table 6.3
Summary of Characteristics of Anchoring Junctions

Junction Type	Transmembrane Protein	Extracellular Ligand	Intracellular Linkage (Accessory Proteins)
Adherens	Cadherin	Cadherin	Actin filaments (catenins)
Desmosomes	Cadherin	Cadherin	Intermediate filaments (desmoplakin, plakoglobin)
Hemidesmosomes	$\alpha_6\beta_4$ Integrin	ECM protein	Intermediate filaments
Focal contact	Integrin	ECM protein	Actin filaments (α-actinin, talin, vinculin)

Adapted from [28].

Adherens junctions connect actin filaments, which are intracellular contractile cytoskeletal elements, in one cell to either an extracellular matrix molecule or the extracellular domain of a transmembrane linker protein on another cell. In cell-to-cell adhesion, the transmembrane linker proteins are cadherins. In cell–matrix adhesion, the transmembrane linker proteins are members of a family of cell–surface matrix receptors called integrins.

Adherens junctions occur in several forms in mammalian tissue. Epithelial sheets have continuous belt-like junctions, or adhesion belts, which occur just below the tight junction between adjacent cells. Adhesion belts, formed from contractile actin filaments, generate folding movements in sheets of cells during tissue morphogenesis. In other cells, focal contacts, which are punctate attachment sites, occur on the surface of cells that are associated with extracellular matrix. Focal contacts form in specialized regions of the plasma membrane that coincide with the termination sites of actin filament bundles. The contacts function as mechanical anchors, but they are also capable of translating signals from the extracellular matrix to the cytoskeleton. This signaling capability is an essential element in the regulation of cell functions such as survival, growth, morphology, movement, and differentiation.

Desmosomes provide an indirect link from the intermediate filaments of one cell to those of another. Intermediate filaments are assemblies of fibrous protein (for example, vimentin, keratin, or desmin) that form a rope-like intracellular network; these filaments are responsible for much of the structural framework of the cell. The extracellular domain of cadherin receptors form the link from one cell to another. The physiological importance of desmosomes can be observed in patients with pemphigus, a serious skin disease that involves the destruction of desmosomes between epithelial cells. Patients develop scattered bullae, or blisters, that rupture easily leaving denuded areas of skin and creating, in the worst cases, risk of severe infection and life-threatening fluid loss.

Hemidesmosomes connect the basal surface of epithelial cells and intermediate filaments in the cytoplasm to an underlying thin sheet of extracellular matrix called the basal lamina. The basal lamina therefore separates the epithelium from connective tissue. The transmembrane linker proteins mediating this type of adhesion are integrins.

6.3 Cell Adhesion Receptors

When the net interaction potential between a cell and a surface is attractive, the two can approach one another and become stably associated. This initial association usually involves the formation of specific receptor–ligand bonds. Further maturation of cell–cell or cell–matrix contact involves receptor–ligand bonds that accumulate in specialized junctional complexes, which are described briefly in the previous section. Over the past several decades, a variety of receptor–ligand systems for cell–cell and cell–matrix binding have been identified and characterized (Figure 6.9).

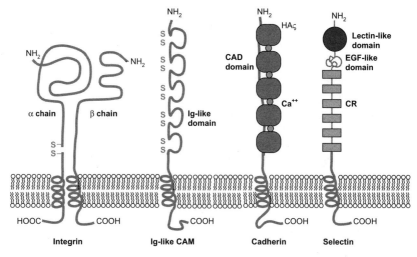

Figure 6.9. Schematic diagrams of the four major families of cell adhesion receptors. (a) The fibronectin receptor is shown as an example of the two subunit integrin family of membrane proteins. Other integrins may differ slightly in the processing of the a subunit (i.e., some integrins do not have the disulfide-linked gap region). Structure from [29]. (b) N-CAM is a member of the immunoglobulin superfamily, which contains immunoglobulin-like domains. Various forms of N-CAM differ in their cytoplasmic region. In fact, some N-CAMs are directly linked to the membrane lipid with no transmembrane or cytoplasmic region. Structure based on [30]. (c) Cadherins are involved in homophilic recognition in cell adhesion. Structure based on [31]. (d) ELAM-1 is a member of the selectin family of cell adhesion receptors. These proteins are characterized by the lectin-like binding domain near the N terminus, which is followed by an EGF-like domain and a number of consensus repeats (CR) that are similar to complement-binding proteins. ELAM-1 has six CR regions; Mel-14 has two; CD62 has nine. Structure based on [32] and [33].

6.3.1 Integrins

The integrin family of cell surface molecules is involved in cell adhesion and cell motility. Integrin-mediated cell adhesion is usually associated with cell–matrix interactions, but certain integrins (particularly those on white blood cells) play an essential role in cell–cell adhesion as well. All integrins are heterodimeric membrane proteins consisting of non-covalently associated α and β subunits; different homologs of the subunits are identified by a numerical suffix (α_1, α_2, α_3,..., β_1, β_2, ...). Each member of the integrin family can be characterized by the combination of subunits involved: for example, $\alpha_1\beta_1$ binds to collagen and laminin, $\alpha_5\beta_1$ binds to fibronectin, and the β_2 integrins bind to ligands on cell surfaces. Integrin binding is Ca^{++}-dependent.

In cell–matrix binding, the extracellular domain of the integrin receptor binds to an extracellular matrix protein and the cytoplasmic integrin domain binds to the protein cytoskeleton (Figure 6.10). Integrin receptors therefore provide a critical connection between the extracellular and intracellular envir-

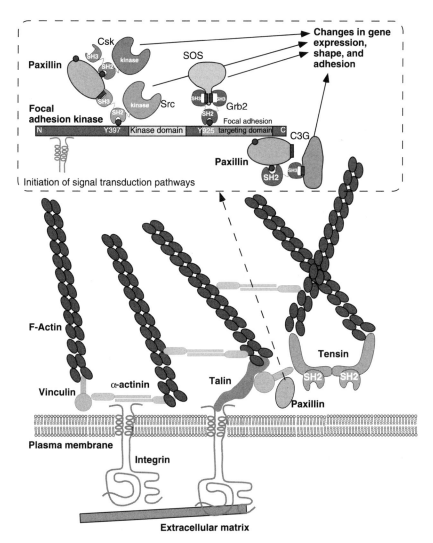

Figure 6.10. Cytoplasmic proteins and cell adhesion: association of cytoplasmic proteins (tensin, talin, vinculin, α-actinin, and F-actin) and extracellular proteins with the cytoplasmic and extracellular domains of a transmembrane integrin receptor. The inset shows a hypothetical model for signal transduction based on focal adhesion kinase (FAK). The model includes tyrosine kinases (Src and Csk), adapter proteins (Grb2 and Crk), and guanine nucleotide exchange factors (SOS and C3G). Binding occurs through SH2 (Src homology 2) domains, which bind to proteins containing a phosphotyrosine (dark circles), and SH3 (Src homology 3) domains, which bind to proteins containing a proline-rich peptide motif (dark rectangles). The diagram was adapted from a variety of sources [1, 27, 28, 34].

onments. Certain aspects of integrin binding are conserved among a variety of extracellular matrix proteins. For example, several matrix proteins (fibronectin, collagen, vitronectin, thrombospondin, tenascin, laminin, and entactin) contain the three amino acid sequence Arg-Gly-Asp (RGD), which is critical for cell binding. Integrin–ECM binding can be reduced, and sometimes eliminated, by addition of dissolved RGD peptides, which compete for the integrin receptor site and, hence, encourage dissociation of the integrin–matrix bond. In addition, cells will adhere to immobilized peptides containing the RGD sequence. RGD is not the only sequence involved in the interaction of integrin with matrix proteins; collagens contain many RGD sequences, but soluble RGD does not alter cell binding to collagen. In addition, different integrins bind selectively to different proteins at RGD-containing sites, suggesting that binding is also influenced by polypeptide domains adjacent to the RGD domain but specific to each protein.

Cell adhesion domains are often associated with the termination points for filaments of the cytoskeleton (Figure 6.8). In the case of integrin-mediated cell adhesion, the association point is an integrated assembly of cytoplasmic proteins, such as vinculin and talin (Figure 6.10). The composition of the analogous protein assembly in hemidesmosomes, which connects the integrin–ECM complex to intermediate filaments, is unknown. However, the β-subunit of the integrin involved in hemidesmosomes, $\alpha_6\beta_4$, has an unusually long cytoplasmic tail, which may interact directly with intermediate filament proteins or facilitate assembly of accessory proteins.

6.3.2 Cadherins

The cadherin receptors are $\sim$700 residue transmembrane proteins that mediate cell–cell adhesion though homophilic binding. Binding of cadherins is Ca^{++}-dependent and ubiquitous: cadherins can be identified in almost all vertebrate cells and account for the Ca^{++} dependence of solid tissue form. In the absence of extracellular Ca^{++}, the cadherins are subject to rapid proteolysis and, therefore, loss of function. The best-characterized cadherins are E-cadherin (found predominantly on epithelial cells), P-cadherin (found on cells of the placenta and skin) and N-cadherin (found on nerve, lens, and heart cells). These molecules have common structural features including five extracellular repeats (CAD domains), Ca^{++} binding regions, a membrane-spanning region, and a cytoplasmic domain (Figure 6.9). Each of the CAD domains has structural similarity, although not sequence homology, with the immunoglobulin folds. Each CAD domain contains an HAV (His-Ala-Val) motif that is important for binding; the specificity of each cadherin appears to be determined by the residues flanking this HAV region.

The affinity of cadherin–cadherin binding is not known, but the available evidence suggests that the affinity of individual bonds is low ($K_d \simeq 64\,\mu m$) [48, 49]. In adherens junctions, the cytoplasmic tail of cadherins interacts with the actin cytoskeleton through the proteins α-catenin and β-catenin, which form a coordinated assembly. The interaction of the cytoplasmic catenin complex with cadherin appears to enhance cadherin–cadherin affinity. Other proteins, such as desmoplakin and plakoglobulin, are associated with cadherin–intermediate filament contact in desmosomes [25].

6.3.3 Ig-like Receptors

Members of the immunoglobulin-like (Ig-like) family of cell surface receptors mediate cell–cell adhesion via a Ca^{++}-independent process. The best studied of these receptors are cell adhesion molecules in the nervous system (for example, neural cell adhesion molecule, N-CAM, and L1). All members of this family have structural similarities to immunoglobulins (Figure 6.9); in addition, N-CAM has structural similarities to extracellular matrix molecules such as fibronectin. N-CAM functions in cell adhesion and neurite outgrowth, predominantly by homophilic binding.

Both cadherins and Ig-like receptors are present on the surfaces of cells during development, and probably provide signals for cell assembly into organized structures. However, cell adhesion mediated by cadherins is much stronger than that mediated by Ig-like proteins; overexpression of cadherins, but not Ig-like receptors, leads to abnormalities in embryo development. These observations suggest that the Ig-like proteins provide fine control over cellular attachments, which are dominated by cadherins.

6.3.4 Selectins

The selectins contain a carbohydrate-binding lectin domain (Figure 6.9) and are transiently expressed during the inflammatory response. These cell adhesion receptors are usually expressed on the surface of endothelial cells, where the lectin domain recognizes specific oligosaccharides expressed on the surface of neutrophils. Neutrophils then bind to endothelial cells at the site of inflammation and roll along the blood vessel surface, until other adhesion mechanisms initiate vessel wall transmigration into and participation in the local inflammatory response.

6.4 Extracellular Matrix

The extracellular space contains a three-dimensional array of protein fibers and filaments (Figure 6.11) which are embedded in a hydrated gel of glycosaminoglycans (GAGs). Extracellular proteins and polysaccharides are secreted locally by cells and assemble to form a scaffold that supports cell attachment, spreading, proliferation, migration, and differentiation. Cells influence the chemistry of the matrix by secretion of protein and polysaccharide elements, but they also modify the physical characteristics of the matrix by release of modifying enzymes or by application of physical forces. This section reviews the properties of molecular constituents of extracellular matrix.

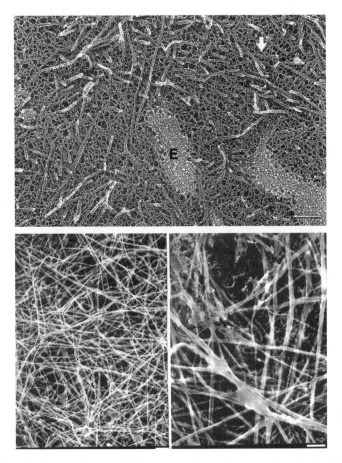

Figure 6.11. Structure of extracellular matrix. Top: electron micrograph of the extracellular matrix of ear cartilage showing collagen fibers and elastin (E) fibers. The arrowhead indicates point of attachment to collagen filaments in plane below the section. Bar = 0.2 μm. From [35]. Bottom left: scanning electron micrograph of a reconstituted collagen gel (0.4 mg/mL collagen) formed from type I collagen extracted from rat tail tendons. Bar = 1 μm. Right: identical to image on left, but with 40 μg/mL of heparin added during reconstitution. Notice that the presence of heparin causes assembly of the collagen fibers into larger structures. Bar = 1 μm. Bottom photos by Rebecca Kuntz Willits and Jeanne Chun.

6.4.1 Glycosaminoglycans and Proteoglycans

GAGs are high-molecular-weight polysaccharides, which are usually highly sulfated and, therefore, negatively charged. Each GAG is a poly(disaccharide), with sugar residues A and B (Table 6.4) repeated in a regular pattern, $-(-A-B-)_n-$ (Figure 6.12). Most GAGs also contain other sugar components, such as D-xylose, which create additional complexity in the linear chemical structure. GAGs are unbranched, relatively inflexible, and highly soluble in water; they adopt random coil conformations that occupy large volumes in

Table 6.4
Characteristics of Glycosaminoglycans (GAGs)

GAG	M.W. (kDa)	Sugar A	Sugar B	Sulfates	Links to Protein	Other Sugars	Tissue Distribution
Hyaluronic Acid	4 to 8,000	D-glucuronic acid	N-acetyl-D-glucosamine	–	–	–	Connective tissues, skin, vitreous body, cartilage, synovial fluid
Chondroitin sulfate	5 to 50	D-glucuronic acid	N-acetyl-D-galactosamine	+	+	+	Cartilage, cornea, bone, skin, arteries
Dermatan sulfate	15 to 40	D-glucuronic acid or L-iduronic acid	N-acetyl-D-galactosamine	+	+	+	Skin, blood vessels, heart
Heparan sulfate	5 to 12	D-glucuronic acid or L-iduronic acid	N-acetyl-D-glucosamine	+	+	+	Lung, arteries, cell surfaces, basal laminae
Heparin	6 to 25	D-glucuronic acid or L-iduronic acid	N-acetyl-D-glucosamine	+	+	+	Lung, liver, skin, mast cells
Keratan sulfate	4 to 19	D-galactose	N-acetyl-D-glucosamine	+	+	+	Cartilage, cornea, intervertebral disc

Adapted from [28].

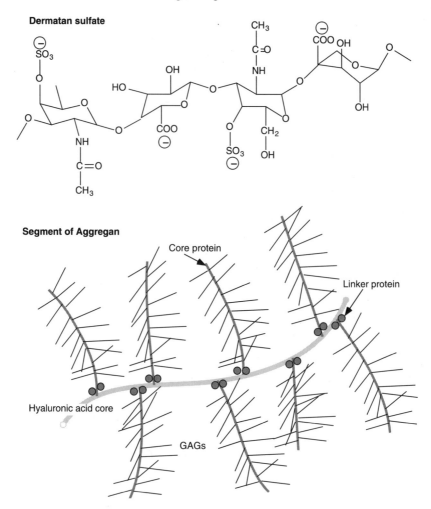

Figure 6.12. Structure of glycosaminoglycans. Top: chemical structure of repeated disaccharide of the GAG dermatan sulfate (protons are not indicated in this schematic diagram). Bottom: schematic diagram of the aggrecan proteoglycan complex showing the relationship between the core and linker proteins, GAGs (straight black lines) and hyaluronic acid (grey).

aqueous medium. Because individual chains are extended and interact with each other to form additional structure, GAGs form hydrated gels at low GAG concentration. Counterions in the aqueous phase surrounding the GAG chain, principally Na^+, create osmotic forces which pull water into the gel. Because of this property, tissues that are high in GAG content, such as cartilage, have high resistance to compressive stress.

Hyaluronic acid is an abundant polysaccharide that is unusual among the GAGs because it is unsulfated, not covalently attached to protein, and free of other sugar groups. Hyaluronic acid is present during embryogenesis, and is frequently associated with tissues undergoing repair. In both of these situations, the presence of hyaluronic acid appears to facilitate cell migration through the extracellular matrix, perhaps by modulating the level of hydration in the tissue.

With the exception of hyaluronic acid, GAGs are covalently attached to a protein; this macromolecular complex is called a proteoglycan (Table 6.5). Proteoglycans can have extremely high sugar contents, up to 95% by weight. The diversity of the core protein structure is compounded by the potential for linkage to combinations of GAGs of different chain length, making proteoglycans a highly heterogeneous group of molecules. Proteoglycans often have an additional level of structural organization in tissues: for example, the individual proteoglycans in aggrecan are arranged systematically around a hyaluronic acid core (Figure 6.12). This structural versatility translates into a variety of functions in tissues: proteoglycans serve as reservoirs of biological activity by binding of growth factors, as size- and charge-selective filters in the glomerulus, and as mediators of adhesion on cell membranes.

6.4.2 Proteins

Proteins in the extracellular space are either of the structural type (for example, collagen, elastin) or the adhesive type (for example, laminin, fibronectin).

Collagen is the most abundant protein found in the extracellular space and is secreted by chondrocytes, fibroblasts, and other cell types. Several chemically distinct forms of collagen have been identified, each of which contains the same basic macromolecular unit: an alpha helical chain formed by the interaction of three polypeptides (Figure 6.13). These polypeptide chains are 1000 amino acids in length and are specific to each type of collagen. The most common forms of collagen found within the extracellular space are types I, II, III, and

Table 6.5
Characteristics of Proteoglycans

Proteoglycan	M.W. of Core Protein (kDa)	Type of GAG	Number of GAGs	Tissue Distribution
Aggregan	210	Chondroitin sulfate Keratan sulfate	~130	Cartilage
Decorin	40	Chondroitin sulfate Dermatan sulfate	1	Connective tissues
Syndecan-1	32	Chondroitin sulfate Heparan sulfate	1-3	Fibroblast and epithelial cell surfaces

Adapted from [28].

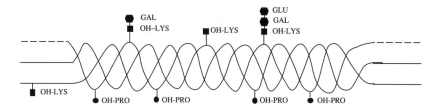

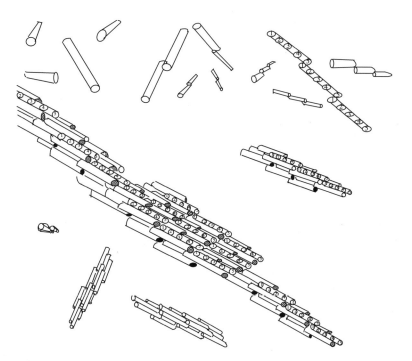

Figure 6.13. Structure of collagen. Procollagen molecules are produced by cells and secreted. The collagen triple helix is produced by enzymatic cleavage in the extracellular environment. Collagen molecules assemble into fibrils and fibers by an orderly arrangement that is stabilized by crosslinking between individual molecules.

IV. Following secretion into the ECM, molecules of collagen types I, II, and III organize into larger fibrils which are 10 to 300 nm in diameter (Figure 6.13). These fibrils are stabilized by crosslinks which connect lysine residues within or between adjacent collagen molecules. In some tissues these fibrils become further organized, forming larger collagen fibers several micrometers in diameter. Fibrillar collagens interact with cells through integrin receptors on cell surfaces. Cell differentiation and migration during development are influenced by fibrillar collagens.

In contrast to the fibrillar collagens, collagen type IV forms a mesh-like lattice that constitutes a major part of the mature basal lamina, the thin mat separating epithelial sheets from other tissues. Collagen type IV interacts with cells indirectly by binding to laminin, another major component of the basal lamina (Table 6.6).

Fibronectin is a dimeric glycoprotein composed of similar subunits, each containing 2500 amino acids (Figure 6.14). The two similar polypeptide chains are linked by disulfide bonds at the carboxyl termini and folded into a number of globular domains. The biological activities of certain polypeptide domains within the fibronectin macromolecule have been defined by observing the properties of fibronectin fragments. Fibronectin binds to collagen and heparin; this binding contributes to the organization of the extracellular matrix. Integrin receptors on cell surfaces bind to a fibronectin domain containing the tripeptide sequence RGD. It appears that complete cellular adhesion also requires the participation of another region on fibronectin, the "synergy" region on the amino terminus side of the RGD-containing region. A second cell binding region on fibronectin, the IIICS region, contains sequences permitting the adhesion of specific cell types. Usually fibroblasts do not adhere to the IIICS region, but other cells (for example, neural cells and lymphocytes) do. Cellular interactions with fibronectin have been shown to affect cell morphology, migration, and differentiation.

Laminin is a large cross-shaped protein composed of three polypeptide subunits: α, β, and γ (Figure 6.15). At least twelve different heterotrimeric

Table 6.6
Characteristics of the Four Major Types of Collagen

Type	Molecular Formula	Polymerized Form	Features	Distribution
I	$[\alpha1(I)]_2\alpha2(I)$	Fibril	Low hydroxylysine and carbohydrate, broad fibrils	Skin, tendon, bone, ligaments, cornea, internal organs (accounts for ~90% of body collagen)
II	$[\alpha1(II)]_3$	Fibril	High hydroxylysine and carbohydrate, thinner fibrils than type I	cartilage, intervertebral disc, notochord, vitreous body
III	$[\alpha1(III)]_3$	Fibril	High hydroxyproline, low hydroxylysine and carbohydrate	Skin, blood vessels, internal organs
IV	$[\alpha1(IV)]_2\alpha2(IV)$	Basal lamina	Very high hydroxyproline, high carbohydrate, retains procollagen extension peptides	Basal laminae

This table reproduced from [36], Table 14-3 (p. 810).

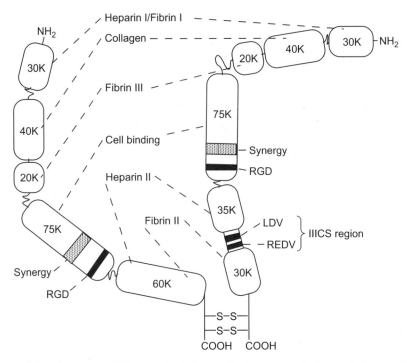

Figure 6.14. Structure of fibronectin. Fibronectin is composed of two similar 2500 amino acid peptide chains, linked by two disulfide bonds near the carboxy termini. The numbers on each domain indicate the approximate molecular weight. Regions for collagen, heparin, fibrin, and cell binding have been identified on each of the chains. The cell binding region contains the tripeptide sequence –RGD– as well as an additional region that appears to function synergistically with the RGD sequence in cell adhesion. The alternatively spliced region, IIICS, provides short peptide sequences that permit cell-specific adhesion. Diagram adapted from [36] and [37].

laminins are found in mammals. These different isoforms are created by assembly of one each from the five known α, three known β, and three known γ chains; the particular isoform is specified by the chains that constitute it: for example, laminin-1 contains α1, β1, and γ1 and laminin-5 contains α3A, β3, and γ2. In the long arm of laminin, the three subunits form a coiled-coil α-helical domain. The existence of homologous forms of laminin, which have different distributions within the adult and the embryo, suggests that these laminin isoforms may have different functions as well. Some of the mechanisms that underlie functional divversity are known. Laminin-1 has an important role in neurite growth and cell migration; laminin-5 is highly adhesive for epithelial cells; and laminin-11 is known to be a stop signal for Schwann cells [26].

   Laminin contains binding sites for cell attachment and other binding sites that promote neurite outgrowth. Regions that promote cell attachment, heparin binding, and neurite outgrowth have been identified and involve the specific peptide sequences RGD, YIGSR, IKVAV on the α chain. Several

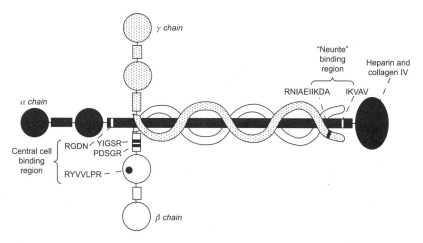

Figure 6.15. Schematic diagram of the structure of laminin. The extracellular matrix protein laminin has three subunits: α (400,000 Da), β (215,000 Da), and γ (205,000 Da). The three polypeptide subunits are linked by disulfide bonds to form ~800,000 Da protein that is widely distributed throughout mammalian tissues, associated predominantly with basement membranes. Adapted from Figure 1 of [38] and Figure 4-5 of [37].

integrin receptors ($\alpha_6\beta_1$, $\alpha_3\beta_1$) have been implicated in cell interactions with laminin, but the IKVAV region appears to interact with non-integrin receptors.

Elastin is a hydrophobic, nonglycosylated protein composed of 830 amino acids. After secretion into the ECM, extended elastin molecules form cross-linked fibers and sheets which can stretch and relax upon deformation (Figure 6.11). Elastin is found in abundance in tissues that undergo repeated stretching, such as the blood vessels.

Tenascin, a multiunit glycoprotein of 1.9×10^6 daltons, has both cell adhesive and anti-adhesive properties. While it is confined primarily to the nervous system in adults, it is present in embryonic tissues and may be involved in modulating cell migration during embryogenesis. Tenascin is composed of six polypeptide chains, some containing the RGD sequence, which are disulfide-linked to produce a windmill-shaped complex.

The intact form of *vitronectin*, a 75,000 dalton monomer, is proteolytically converted into 65,000 and 10,000 dalton fragments. These molecules are present in the blood (0.2–0.4 g/L) and in certain tissues, usually associated with fibronectin. Vitronectin contains the RGD tripeptide sequence and can promote the attachment of many cell types, presumably through integrin receptors other than the common fibronectin binding integrin.

Thrombospondin is a trimer consisting of three identical 140,000 dalton subunits that is presumed to be important in control of cell growth. The cell adhesion activity of thrombospondin is associated with a heparin-binding domain and an RGD sequence. Certain regions can also interact with collagen, laminin, and fibronectin.

Entactin (nidogen) is a protein of 150,000 daltons that is found in basement membranes, where it is strongly associated with laminin. Almost all laminin preparations contain entactin, which is associated stoichiometrically with the laminin central cell-binding region. Entactin contains the RGD sequence and a region that permits self-association.

6.4.3 Function of Extracellular Matrix

The composition and structure of extracellular matrix in a particular tissue is related to its function. In general, the extracellular matrix of connective tissue consists of collagen and/or elastin fibers coursing through a GAG-rich ground substance in which mesenchymal cells, such as fibroblasts, migrate. Protein fibers give the tissue tensile strength (collagen) and elasticity (elastin), while the GAG gel resists compression; mesenchymal cells secrete protein and carbohydrates, facilitate organization of the matrix structure, and infiltrate into damaged tissue to initiate wound healing. Epithelial tissues are typically organized around basal laminae; these thin gel layers are rich in collagen IV and laminin. When present on one face of a cell monolayer, a basal lamina can induce cell polarity. For example, columnar epithelial cells in the intestine rest on a basal lamina that induces differentiation of the cell surface into basal and apical domains. The development and maintenance of polarity is essential for intestinal tissue function, for example (see Figure 6.7).

Modularity and self-assembly are important concepts in extracellular matrix function. Many extracellular matrix molecules can self-assemble into larger units, as in the cases of collagen (Figure 6.13) and laminin. Self-assembly allows molecular units to form larger structures, such as basement membrane, which present an array of sites for cell binding. Since many extracellular matrix molecules also have binding sites that recognize other extracellular matrix molecules, heterogeneous membranes can be formed that have spatially-arranged binding regions, with different regions specialized to recognize cells with different receptors (Figure 6.16a).

Extracellular matrix interactions with cells are critically important in the developing organism. The extracellular matrix composition varies with time and location during embryogenesis (Figure 6.16b). Changes in composition are produced by protein secretion from embryonic cells. Cell-derived matrix cues provide guides for cell migration and assembly into specialized tissues. When these cues are missing, as when fibronectin-rich segments of tissue are removed or transplanted during development, mesodermal cells cannot migrate properly during the early stages of gastrulation. Similar experiments (in the case of fibronectin, for example, using microinjection of anti-fibronectin antibodies, using adhesion-blocking RGD-peptides, or using embryos with the fibronectin gene eliminated) have defined the critical importance of matrix composition in cell migration, cell differentiation, and normal progression through almost every stage of animal development.

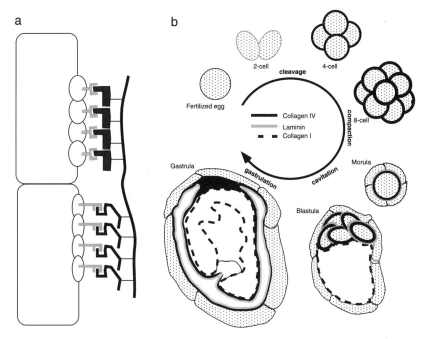

Figure 6.16. Distribution of ECM: (a) the modular, self-assembled nature of ECM permits spatial patterning of adhesive components; (b) a highly schematic diagram of the distribution of collagen (types I and IV), fibronectin, and laminin during the early stages of mouse development. Collagen IV is the first protein to appear during development; fibronectin on the inner blastocoel surface is critical for migration of mesodermal cells during gastrulation; collagen I does not appear until after implantation.

6.5 Cell Adhesion and Intracellular Signaling

The previous sections cataloged properties of cell adhesion receptors and extracellular matrix proteins, and presented a simplified description of cell interactions with their surrounding environment. Non-specific forces bring cells in proximity of a surface; receptor–ligand interactions add strength and specificity to binding; stabilization is often produced by the development of specialized junctional complexes. Specific cell binding is accomplished with transmembrane receptors: cell–cell binding is typically mediated by cadherins, while cell–matrix binding is mediated by integrins.

Receptor extracellular domains are continuous with cytoplasmic domains, which are often linked to the filamentous cytoskeleton. In this way, binding at the cell surface is united with intracellular signal transduction and metabolic pathways. For example, focal contacts have an important function as anchors for cells, but they also relay signals from the extracellular matrix into the cytoplasm. The focal contact region is rich in a variety of proteins with enzymatic activity, such as focal adhesion kinase (FAK) and

Src, the tyrosine kinase encoded by the *src* gene (Figure 6.10). These kinases phosphorylate other proteins, including components of the cytoskeleton; phosphorylation modulates binding activity, providing sites for association of additional proteins, and localizing powerful enzymatic activities to the adhesion site.

Considerable experimental evidence supports the following model for integrin-mediated signal transduction [27] (Figure 6.10 inset): integrin–ECM binding promotes FAK autophosphorylation of the Tyr residue at position 397, which stimulates Src binding. Once bound, Src catalyzes additional phosphorylation (at the Tyr residue 925), creating a binding site for the Src homology 2 (SH2) domain of Grb2, which presents proline-rich polypeptide motifs that facilitate SOS binding (through the Src homology 3 [SH3] domains). This regulated cascade of kinase activity produces an assembly of activated proteins at the focal adhesion site; these proteins mediate cell shape and cell migration by modulating local assembly of the cytoskeleton as well as binding affinity of the integrin extracellular domains. In addition, important intracellular signal transduction proteins, such as Ras and Rho, are activated. Ras and Rho are members of the GTPase super-family: Ras activates proteins that control cell growth and differentiation, whereas Rho influences actin stress fiber assembly. Although many elements of the overall process are poorly understood at present, it is clear that integrin binding has consequences beyond adhesion: binding of integrins to ECM can influence cell processes as vital and complex as growth and movement. Similar mechanisms are present in cadherin-mediated adhesion complexes as well.

Summary

- Cell adhesion occurs within the background of attractive and repulsive forces: electrostatic and van der Waals forces bring a cell into proximity with a surface, and steric stabilization forces resist approach.
- Biological cell adhesion requires the formation of specific chemical bonds between receptors on the cell and ligands on the surface.
- Cell adhesions can mature into junctional complexes—such as anchoring, tight, and gap junctions—which produce molecular connectivity among populations of cells.
- Biological adhesion is regulated by families of cell surface receptors with shared characteristics.
- The extracellular matrix, a complex assortment of biopolymers, provides attachment sites for cells. In addition, extracellular matrix molecules contribute to the mechanical properties of tissues and adhesion at the cell surface can lead to intracellular signals that regulate cell function and behavior.

Exercises

Exercise 6.1

Show that Equation 6–2 can be rewritten in a linearized form ($y = Mx + B$), where x is the bound ligand concentration [R–L] and y is the ratio of bound: free ligand ([R–L]/[L]). Assume that the total number of receptors is constant (R_T) and sufficient ligand molecules are present in solution so that binding does not appreciably change the overall ligand concentration.

Exercise 6.2

Write a step-by-step protocol for an experimental technique to measure:

a) the concentration of cell adhesion molecules present on a surface
b) the number of receptor molecules present in the cell population (molecules/cell).

Exercise 6.3

Using the result from Exercise 6.1, find the dissociation constant and total receptor number for the following data. Assume the cell density is 10^6 cells/mL.

[L] (μM)	0.01	0.1	0.3	0.9	1.8	3	8	16	32
[R–L] (μM)	0.016	0.15	0.35	0.6	0.8	0.92	0.97	1	1.1

How well does the model (Equation 6–2) describe this experimental data?

Exercise 6.4

Consider the schematic diagram of a cell interacting with a surface (Figure 6.2, panel a). List all of the variables that you expect to influence cell adhesion. Separate these variables into three categories: (1) properties of the cell population; (2) properties of the surface; and (3) properties of the fluid phase surrounding the cells and surface.

Exercise 6.5

An adherent cell is exposed to shear forces from buffered water flowing in a parallel plate flow chamber. The gap thickness is 250 μm and the channel width is 14 mm. The flow rate is adjusted so that the wall shear stress varies from 0.25 to 4 dyn/cm^2.

a) Calculate the volumetric flow rate that is required to achieve each value of shear stress in the table on page 182.
b) Calculate the force experienced by an "average" endothelial cell attached to the surface of the lower plate. Make and justify whatever assumptions are necessary to perform this calculation.

c) How much would you expect the force experienced by the cell to vary with position in the flow chamber?

d) How much would you expect the force experienced by the cell to vary with cell shape and pattern of attachment?

Shear stress at the wall (dyn/cm^2)	0.25	0.5	1	2	4
Volumetric flow rate (cm^3/s)					
Force on adherent cell (dyn/cell)					

Exercise 6.6 (provided by Linda G. Griffith)

Platelets were isolated from two different individuals (P1 and P2). Prior to injection in the flow chamber, the platelets are activated by incubating them with type IV collagen. The surface of the flow chamber (identical to the one shown in Figure 6.6c) is coated with fibrinogen. A platelet suspension from the first individual is injected into the chamber and the cells are then given time to settle onto the surface and adhere. A fluid is then sent through the plates at a volumetric flow rate Q. The velocity profile between the parallel plates assumes a parabolic form and produces a homogeneous wall shear stress which approximates the shear stress experienced by the platelets adhered to the chamber surface. The entire chamber is located on the stage of an inverted microscope. A CCD camera, mounted on the microscope, along with a recorder, is used to take snapshots of the viewing area. Videotaped data frames are analyzed to determine the total number of adherent platelets. This experiment is repeated for increasing flow rates. The data obtained for platelets from each individual are:

	Total of Adherent Platelets	
Q (L/min)	P1 (cells/cm^2)	P2 (cells/cm^2)
6	802	26
12	740	19
120	362	6
360	112	3
600	22	0

a) Graph the total number of adherent cells (cells/cm^2) as a function of wall shear stress (dyn/cm^2). Assume the width of the flow chamber is 2 cm and the viscosity of the fluid flowing through the chamber is 2.7×10^{-3} N-s/m^2.

b) Hypothesize as to the difference between the platelets taken from P1 and P2, knowing that the second individual, P2, requires a prolonged time for a simple cut to heal.

c) Briefly describe at least three experiments to test the hypothesis given in part b).

Exercise 6.7 (provided by Song Li)

Search the literature and find a research article on the use of peptides derived from extracellular matrix in tissue engineering. Write a brief review (less than a page) of this article. The review should indicate the hypothesis or aim of the work. Address whether that hypothesis was proven or disproven. Describe the experimental procedures and results. Discuss the future directions and whether the applications of the peptides are cell or tissue specific.

Exercise 6.8 (provided by Linda G. Griffith)

Type IV collagen forms the basic two-dimensional network of all basal laminae. Alport syndrome is a hereditary disease characterized by progressive renal failure, neurosensory hearing loss, and ocular abnormalities. Families with this disease are consistently found to have mutations in genes that code for type IV collagen α3 and α4 chains or in an X-linked gene that codes for Type IV collagen α5 chain. Figure 6.17 shows the results of a western blot analysis done on kidney cells from four separate patients already diagnosed with Alport syndrome. In this western blot the primary Ab was against the type IV collagen α5 chain. The molecular weight of the functional type IV collagen α5 chain is ~180 kD. Explain the significance of the bands in each lane (patient 1, 2, 3, and 4). Keep in mind that all four patients have been diagnosed with Alport syndrome but have different genetic backgrounds.

Exercise 6.9 (provided by Linda G. Griffith)

A cardiovascular products company has hired you to consult on a new bioartificial heart valve. Currently, heart valve replacements are made from titanium alloys or biocompatible polymers; unfortunately, each type of replacement wears out over time. The company has been trying to make a cell-and-matrix

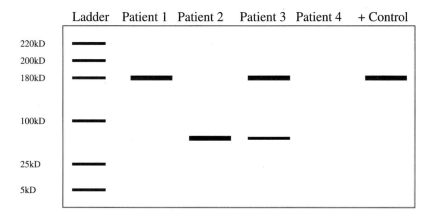

Figure 6.17. Western blot analysis.

heart valve that will integrate with cardiac tissue and keep itself in good repair just like a natural heart valve. The company has had no problems making a matrix in the proper shape and seeding it with cells, and they claim to have solved any immune rejection issues. However, they have one problem: the replacement does not hold up under the high fluid forces of flow through a heart valve. They want to know if using a stronger matrix or introducing extra integrin molecules into the cell membranes will allow their tissue replacement to withstand cardiac stresses.

Data: Peak flow velocity through a heart valve: $v \simeq 5\,\text{m/s}$; viscosity of blood: $\mu \simeq 5\,\text{cP} = 5 \times 10^{-3}\,\text{Pa-s}$. Flow with a velocity v, in a medium of viscosity μ, exerts a viscous force on a sphere of radius R given by $F = 6\pi R\mu v$; consider a cell to be a $10\,\mu\text{m}$ sphere.

a) From your readings and the discussion of extracellular matrix molecules in class, what kind of molecules would you recommend that they use to build a heart valve? Keep in mind that the valve must be thin, flexible, and able to withstand high forces.

b) Given the matrix composition you recommended in part a), what kind of adhesion molecules (for example, α2 vs. α5 integrins) would you expect to best help in keeping the cells attached to the membrane? (Hint: see [47], Table 22–2, for help.)

c) One of the recurring themes in cell adhesion is multiple weak interactions. The attachment strength of a single integrin molecule is on the order of $10\,\text{pN}$. How many integrin molecules per cell would be needed to bind your matrix to resist the detachment force?

d) A normal endothelial cell maintains a few thousand integrin molecules on its surface, each of which has a K_d of about $10^{-7}\,\text{mol/L}$. The proportion of bound integrins is given by the equation:

$$\frac{n_{\text{bound}}}{n_{\text{unbound}}} = \frac{C_{\text{matrix sites}}}{K_d}$$

How many total integrin molecules would be required to achieve the number of bound integrins you calculated in part c)? You will have to estimate the concentration of integrin-binding sites in the matrix you proposed in part a).

e) Does this seem like a reasonable amount of integrin to express on a cell membrane? Would you recommend that the company go ahead with its plan to make cells that express high levels of integrin, or would you recommend a different strategy?

Exercise 6.10

Construct two new tables (analogous to Table 6.3) that list all of the (a) extracellular matrix molecules and (b) cell adhesion receptors described in this chapter. In each case, think carefully about the column headings that you will use to define each of the molecules. Using biology textbooks or current papers from the literature, find at least one extracellular matrix molecule and one cell adhesion receptor that are not discussed directly in the chapter, and show their relationship to the other known molecules.

Exercise 6.11

Using the methods presented in Chapter 5 (Section 5.2), derive Equations 6-7 and 6-8.

References

1. Lauffenburger, D.A. and J.J. Linderman, Receptors: models for binding, trafficking, and signaling. New York: Oxford University Press, 1993, 365 pp.
2. Vogler, E., Thermodynamics of short-term cell adhesion in vitro. *Biophysical Journal*, 1988, **53**, 759–769.
3. Torney, D., M. Dembo, and G. Bell, Thermodynamics of cell adhesion II. Freely mobile repellers. *Biophysical Journal*, 1986, **49**, 501–507.
4. Bell, G., M. Dembro, and P. Bongrand, Cell adhesion. Competition between nonspecific repulsion and specific bonding. *Biophysical Journal*, 1984, **45**, 1051–1064.
5. Hammer, D. and D. Lauffenburger, A dynamical model for receptor-mediated cell adhesion to surfaces. *Biophysical Journal*, 1987, **52**, 475–487.
6. Ward, M.D. and D.A. Hammer, A theoretical analysis for the effect of focal contact formation on cell-substrate attachment strength. *Biophysics Journal*, 1993, **64** (March), 936–959.
7. Israelachvili, J., *Intermolecular and Surface Forces: with Applications to Colloidal and Biological Systems*. New York: Academic Press, 1985.
8. Lawrence, M.B., et al., Effect of venous shear stress on CD18-mediated neutrophil adhesion to cultured endothelium. *Blood*, 1990, **75**, 227–237.
9. Felder, S. and E.L. Elson, Mechanics of fibroblast locomotion: quantitative analysis of forces and motions at the leading lamellas of fibroblasts. *Journal of Cell Biology*, 1990, **111**, p. 2513–2526.
10. Hammer, D.A. and M. Tirrell, Biological adhesion at interfaces. *Annual Reviews of Materials Science*, 1996, **26**, 651–691.
11. Zhurkov, S.N., *International Journal of Fracture Mechanics*, 1965, **1**, 311–323.
12. Bell, G.I., Models for the specific adhesion of cells to cells. *Science*, 1978, **200**, 618–627.
13. Baltz, J.M. and R.A. Cone, The strength of non-covalent biological bonds and adhesions by multiple independent bonds. *Journal of Theoretical Biology*, 1990, **142**, 163–178.
14. Dembo, M., et al., *Proceedings of the Royal Society London, Series B*, 1988, **234**, 55–83.
15. Kuo, S. and D. Lauffenburger, Relationship between receptor/ligand binding affinity and adhesion strength. *Biophysical Journal*, 1993, **65**, 2191–2200.
16. Florin, E.-L., V.T. Moy, and H.E. Gaub, Adhesion forces between individual ligand–receptor pairs. *Science*, 1994, **264**, 415–417.
17. Leckband, D.E., et al., Long-range attraction and molecular rearrangements in receptor–ligand interactions. *Science*, 1992, **255**, 1419–1421.

18. Lawrence, M., L. McIntire, and S. Eskin, Effect of flow on polymorphonuclear leukocyte/endothelial cell adhesion. *Blood*, 1987, **70**, 1284–1290.
19. Cozens-Roberts, C., J. Quinn, and D. Lauffenburger, Receptor-mediated adhesion phenomena: model studies with the radial-flow detachment assay. *Biophysical Journal*, 1990, **58**, 107–125.
20. Evans, E., New membrane concept applied to the analysis of fluid shear- and micropipette-deformed red blood cells. *Biophysical Journal*, 1973, **13**, 941–954.
21. Baltz, J., D. Katz, and R. Cone, Mechanics of sperm–egg interaction at the zona pellucida. *Biophysical Journal*, 1988, **54**(October), 643–654.
22. Lamoureux, P., R. Buxbaum, and S. Heideman, Direct evidence that growth cones pull. *Nature*, 1989, **340**, 159–162.
23. Kishino, A. and T. Yanagida, Force measurements by micromanipulation of a single actin filament by glass needles. *Nature*, 1988, **334**, 74–76.
24. Kumar, N.M. and N.B. Gilula, The gap junction communication channel. *Cell*, 1996, **84**, 381–388.
25. Chitaev, N.A., et al., Molecular organization of the desmoglein–plakoglobulin complex. *Journal of Cell Science*, 1998, **11**(14), 1941–1949.
26. Colognato, H. and P.D. Yurchenco, Form and function: the laminin family of heterotrimers. *Developmental Dynamics*, 2000, **218**, 213–234.
27. Clark, E.A. and J.S. Brugge, Integrins and signal transduction pathways: the road taken. *Science*, 1995, **268**, 233–239.
28. Alberts, B., et al., Molecular Biology of the Cell, 3rd ed. New York: Garland Publishing, 1994.
29. Ruoslahti, E., Integrins as receptors for extracellular matrix, in E.D. Hay, ed., *Cell Biology of Extracellular Matrix*. New York: Plenum, 1991.
30. Cunningham, B., et al., Neural cell adhesion molecule: structure, immunoglobulin-like domains, cell surface modulation, and alternative RNA splicing. *Science*, 1987, **236**, 799–806.
31. Overduin, M., et al., Solution structure of the epithelial cadherin domain responsible for selective cell adhesion. *Science*, 1995, **267**, 386–389.
32. Bevilacqua, M.P., et al., Endothelial leukocyte adhesion molecule 1: an inducible receptor for neutrophils related to complement regulatory proteins and lectins. *Science*, 1989, **243**, 1160–1165.
33. Springer, T., Adhesion receptors of the immune system. *Nature*, 1990, **346**, 425–434.
34. Longhurst, C.M. and L.K. Jennings, Integrin-mediated signal transduction. *Cellular and Molecular Life Sciences*, 1998, **54**, 514–526.
35. Mecham, R.P. and J. Heuser, Three-dimensional structure of extracellular matrix in elastic cartilage as viewed by quick-freeze, deep etch electron microscopy. *Connective Tissue Research*, 1990, **24**, 83–93.
36. Alberts, B., et al., *Molecular Biology of the Cell*, 2nd ed. New York: Garland Publishing, 1989, 1218pp.
37. Yamada, K.M., Fibronectin and other cell interactive glycoproteins, in E.D. Hay, ed., *Cell Biology of Extracellular Matrix*. New York: Plenum Press, 1991, pp. 111–146.
38. Sephel, G.C., B.A. Burrous, and H.K. Kleinman, Laminin neural activity and binding proteins. *Developmental Neuroscience*, 1989, **11**, 313–331.
39. Palecek, S.P., et al., Integrin–ligand binding properties govern cell migration speed through cell–substratum adhesiveness. *Nature*, 1997, **385**, 537–540.
40. Pierschbacher, M.D. and E. Ruoslahti, Cell attachment activity of fibronectin can be duplicated by small synthetic fragments of the molecule. *Nature*, 1984, **309**, 30–33.

41. Suehiro, K., J.W. Smith, and E.F. Plow, The ligand recognition specificity of β3 integrin. *Journal of Biological Chemistry*, 1996, **271**(17), 10365–10371.

42. Koslov, E.R., et al., α-catenin can form asymmetric homodimeric complexes and/or heterodimeric complexes with β-catenin. *Journal of Biological Chemistry*, 1997, **272**(43), 27301–27306.

43. Milev, P., et al., Interactions of the chondroitin sulfate proteoglycan phosphacan, the extracellular domain of a receptor-type protein tyrosine phosphatase, with neurons, glia, and neural cell adhesion molecules. *Journal of Cell Biology*, 1994, **127**(6), 1703–1715.

44. Friedlander, D.R., et al., The neuronal chondroitin sulfate proteoglycan neurocan binds to the neural cell adhesion molecules Ng-CAM/L1/NILE and N-CAM, and inhibits neuronal adhesion and neurite outgrowth. *Journal of Cell Biology*, 1994, **125**(3), 669–680.

45. Nicholson, M.W., et al., Affinity and kinetic analysis of L-selectin (CD62L) binding to glycosylation-dependent cell-adhesion molecule—1. *Journal of Biological Chemistry*, 1998, **273**(2), 763–770.

46. Mehta, P., R.D. Cummings, and R.P. McEver, Affinity and kinteic analysis of P-selectin binding to P-selectin glycoprotein ligand—1. *Journal of Biological Chemistry*, 1998, **273**(49), 32506–32513.

47. Lodish, H., et al., *Molecular Cell Biology*. New York: W.H. Freeman, 1995.

48. Chappuis-Flambent, S., et al., Multiple cadherin extracellular repeats mediate homophilic binding and adhesion. *Journal of Cell Biology*, 2001, **154**, 231–243.

49. Sivasankar, S., B. M. Gumbiner and D. Leckband. Direct measurements of multiple adhesive alignments and unbinding trajectories between cadherin extracellular domains. *Biophysical Journal*, 2001, **80**, 1758–1768.

7

Cell Migration

And their feet move
rhythmically ...

Sappho

I thought I could see a kind of motion ahead of me.

Joseph Conrad, *Heart of Darkness*

Cell migration is crucial to the life of unicellular and multicellular organisms. Unicellular organisms migrate to find food and avoid predators; this migration can occur by swimming through a fluid, which is achieved by flagellar or ciliary beating (exemplified by *E. coli* or *Paramecium*, respectively), or crawling along a surface (as in amoebae). In multicellular organisms, migration of a particular cell population is often a component of complex multicellular behaviors including tumor invasion and metastasis [1], embryogenesis [2], angiogenesis [3], and immune responses [4] (Figure 7.1 and Table 7.1). In both cases, the speed and pattern of migration are determined by the nature of the cell and by chemicals (both soluble and surface-bound) in the environment. Since cell migration is critical in the formation or regeneration of tissues, a clearer understanding of the dynamics of cell migration would greatly enhance our ability to design materials and processes for tissue engineering.

7.1 Overview of Cell Migration

Cell migration is a fundamental mechanism for forming of structures within developing embryos. Accordingly, the migration of cells during embryogenesis is under exquisite control; development of tissue structure and cell migration are interdependent. Chapter 3 discussed limb regeneration in salamanders, a process in which positional gradients of cell adhesion influence cell migration and, ultimately, tissue structure. Similarly, the rate and migration of myogenic cells from the somitic mesoderm is influenced by the presence of local signals in the form of diffusible factors and extracellular matrix composition. These local signals are also produced by cells, with the result that cells throughout the developing limb (which are present in a particular arrangement or tissue struc-

188

a   INFLAMMATION

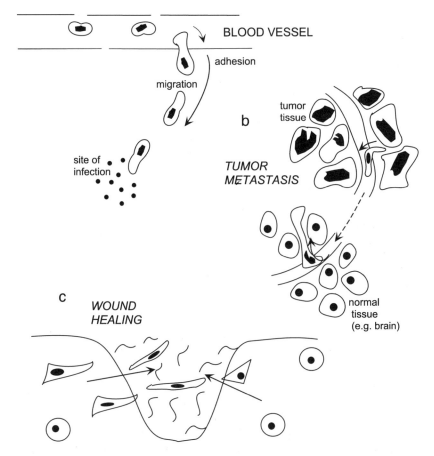

Figure 7.1. Cell migration is an essential step in many physiological processes. (a) Neutrophils transmigrate through the blood vessel wall and invade the tissue space; (b) tumor cells in the circulation can migrate into tissues distant from the original tumor site; (c) fibroblasts migrate into wound sites to initiate healing.

ture) control and coordinate the migration of myogenic cells by secretion of activating factors and expression or organization of extracellular matrix molecules [5]. A better understanding of the mechanisms underlying cell migration in the embryo, and the strategies that nature uses to control migration, will almost certainly provide inspiration for tissue engineering.

Cell migration underlies many important physiological functions in adults. For example, the immune system, with its widely dispersed ensemble of B and T cells, relies heavily on the coordinated migration of individual cells to patrol the body and to provide opportunities for cell–cell interaction. Cell migration is an essential—and perhaps unavoidable—consequence of treatments that depend on transplantation of cells or tissues. A recent study of magnetically

Table 7.1
Importance of Cell Migration

Type of Migrating Cell	Role of Migrating Cell
Neutrophils	Phagocytosis of bacteria
Lymphocytes	Destruction of infected cells
Macrophages	Antigen presentation
Endothelial cells	Angiogenesis
Epidermal cells and fibroblasts	Wound healing
Tumor cells	Metastasis
Neurons and axons	Development and regeneration in the nervous system
Embryonic cells	Embryogenesis

Many cells in the body are motile. Several cells types are listed above, together with their role in human physiology.

labeled oligodendrocyte progenitors by magnetic resonance imaging (MRI) demonstrated that cells migrate to cover a region > 8 mm in size during the first 10 days after injection into the spinal cord [6]. Some cell migration is desirable in many situations, such as this example of cell transplantation within the spinal cord; dispersion of cells within the nervous system leads to distribution of their capacity to myelinate. However, cell migration may cause side effects or loss of function at the transplantation site. In the neurotransplantation example, where cells are intended to function locally in the tissue, migration is counterproductive if all of the transplanted cells leave the local site. In the more general case, cell migration to distant sites after organ transplantation may lead to microchimerism (see Section 10.3)—the appearance of cells from the transplanted tissue at low levels in organs throughout the patient—that influences subsequent immune responses to the transplanted tissue.

In summary, cell migration enables normal fetal development and circulation of certain cells to occur throughout life. In tissue engineering, cell migration may be desirable or dangerous, depending on the application; in either case, our ability to understand and manipulate cell migration will be a critical component of our ultimate success.

7.2 Experimental Observations on Cell Motility

7.2.1 Common Experimental Techniques

The physiological significance of cell migration has motivated numerous experimental studies [7, 8], beginning with the seminal time-lapse studies of Comandon [9]. In general, structural complexity and lack of transparency make it difficult to study migration of cells within multicellular organisms. However, modern imaging methods can permit observation of cell movement within living tissues. Fluorescent dyes can be used to label cells, which can then be tracked by time-lapse microscopy [10–12] or conventional microscopy after sectioning [13] or collection of tissue samples [14]. New microscopy techniques—including two-photon imaging [15, 16]—are enabling the visualization of structures that were previously difficult to image within thick specimens. Green fluoresent proteins (GFPs) can be introduced into specific cell populations to permit tracking of cell lineages during development and migration [10]. Lymphocytes and other phagocytic cells will ingest superparamagnetic particles, enabling visualization of cell position within the body by magnetic resonance imaging [17]. MRI techniques can now be performed with sufficient resolution ($\sim 1\ \mu m$) to allow tracking of cell movements during embryogenesis [18] or after transplantation [6]. Immunological or genetic markers—either natural [14, 19] or introduced by transfection [20]—can be introduced into cells for tracking; this is usually accomplished by sectioning tissue to identify the position of the marked cell. When most of these techniques are applied in animals, the movement of a sub-population of labeled cells is recorded; to date, most of these analyses have been descriptive. Time-lapse techniques permit quantitative analysis of individual cell movements; these continuous records of cell movement in the native tissue are providing insight into the mechanisms of cell migration.

Historically, most studies of cell migration involve cell culture methods that attempt to replicate specific aspects of the natural cell environment. Most experimental methods for characterizing cell motility can be placed into one of two categories (Figure 7.2). In visual assays or single-cell assays, the movements of a small number of cells are observed individually [21–23]. Population techniques involve the observation of the collective movements of a group of

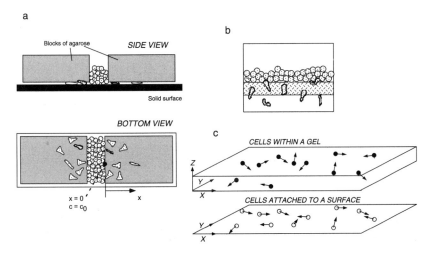

Figure 7.2. Schematic diagram of common cell migration assay systems. (a) In the under-agarose assay, a cell suspension is placed in a well of semisolid agarose; motile cells crawl on the solid substrate underneath the agarose. (b) In the filter assay, a cell suspension is placed on a filter with small pores; motile cells crawl through the pores of the filter material to the other side, where they are detected. (c) In direct visualization assays, the paths of movement of many individual cells are directly observed for cells migrating on surfaces and within solid gels.

cells [24–26]. The experimental details, advantages, and limitations of these assays have been reviewed [27]. In both measurements, cell motility can be quantified in terms of intrinsic cell motility parameters [22, 28–31], which are described in more detail in the sections that follow. One such parameter, the random motility coefficient (μ), characterizes the migration of cells in isotropic environments. Although each individual technique is self-consistent and reproducible, experimentally measured motility coefficients can vary significantly between different assay systems [30]. This variation suggests that methods that mimic the host environment may be most useful for predicting cell behavior *in vivo*.

The simplest and most commonly used migration assays present cells with an environment that is significantly different from that encountered by cells in an organism. For example, many assay systems require cells to be attached to a two-dimensional substrate, while in tissues motile cells are frequently dispersed in three dimensions. Also, in most assays, motile cells contact glass, tissue culture polystyrene, cellulose ester, or cellulose acetate filters; the native extracellular matrix (ECM), however, is a complex gel of biopolymers, with collagen being the most abundant.

In recent years, three-dimensional cell culture techniques have been developed to more closely simulate tissues [32–36]. Of the few studies that have addressed cell motility in these situations [37–42], most have involved plating a cell suspension on top of a collagen gel and subsequently following the infiltration of the gel by the cells. Most typically, infiltration is measured by following the leading front distance of the cell population as a function of time. While much information can be gained from these studies, the time course of infiltration is usually on the order of hours or days. Furthermore, measurement of the leading front distance provides an accurate description of the behavior of the fastest moving cells rather than the entire cell population.

7.2.2 Cell Polarity

Migrating cells in culture look as if they are moving in a particular direction (Figure 7.3). The characteristic shape—which depends on cell type—is due to the internal arrangement of cytoskeletal components, the pattern of adhesion sites between the cell and the surface, and the movement of membranes around the cell periphery (Figure 7.4). The "front" region of the cell (that is, the edge that faces the direction of cell movement) is called the leading edge or lamellipodium and the "rear" region is called the uropodium. Both of these regions are relatively stable during periods when the cell is moving forward in a straight line, without turning; this period, which is called the persistence time P, is critical to the overall pattern of movement of the cell. The development of a polarized morphology, with a front and rear region that are morphologically distinct (Figure 7.3) and biochemically distinct (Figure 7.4), is an early event in the migration of many cells, including leukocytes [43].

Cell movement is initiated by active membrane protrusion in the lamellipodial region. In fibroblasts, the leading edge of the cell protrudes and retracts

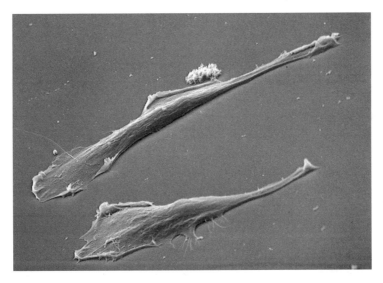

Figure 7.3. Fibroblast migration on a surface: many tissue-derived cells, such as the fibroblast shown here, migrate after attachment to a solid surface. The cells have a noticeable polarity, with a broad leading edge that faces the current direction of migration. (Photograph courtesy of Guenter Albrecht-Buehler.)

in a cyclic fashion, with a peak velocity of 50–60 nm/s ($\sim 3\,\mu\text{m/min}$) and an average net speed of 5.5 nm/s ($\sim 0.3\,\mu\text{m/min}$) [44], which is approximately equal to the speed of forward motion for the whole cell (Table 7.2). Other edges of the cell are relatively stationary. The leading edge is considerably thinner (in the direction normal to the substrate) and stiffer than other edges of the cell. This membrane activity is probably related to actin polymerization and actin fiber rearrangement within the peripheral membrane. In the region of active movement, the membrane sweeps over an area of the substrate; during this process, cell adhesion molecules in the membrane have an opportunity to bind to counterligands on the substrate. If binding occurs, a new site of adhesion may be formed and subsequently stabilized by the participation of additional receptor–ligand binding pairs.

Cells crawl across a substrate through a repetitive process of lamellipodial searching, adhesion at a new surface site, and detachment from an old site. As the leading edge of the membrane moves forward, the cell stretches because it is constrained by previous adhesion sites (Figure 7.5). Tension in the cell increases, due to this slow stretching and to active contractions of cytoskeletal elements in the cell. Eventually, if the cell is to move forward, the adhesions at the trailing edge of the cell must release, causing the stretched cell to relax with an overall advance in the location of the cell center-of-mass.

This mechanistic model of cell migration predicts that cell migration speed should be optimal at intermediate substrate adhesiveness [45]. When adhesion is too weak, new attachment sites cannot form at the leading edge; when

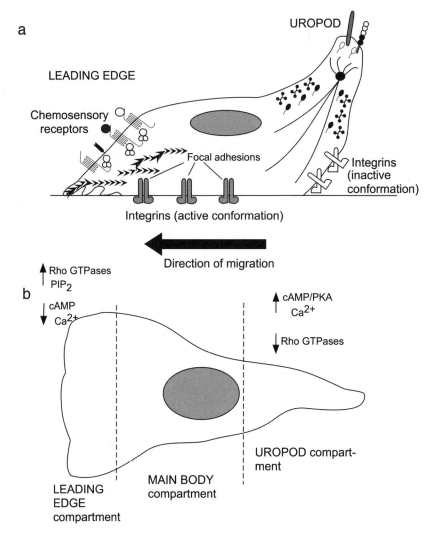

Figure 7.4. Mechanisms for development of polarity in leukocytes (adapted from [43]). The polarized morphology of leukocytes results in the formation of distinct front and rear regions with different biochemical compositions, membrane compositions, and functions. (a) Side view, indicating the distribution of cell surface molecules and cytoskeletal elements. (b) Top view, detailing the biochemical compartments within a migrating cell.

adhesion is too strong, old attachments sites cannot release at the rear. This prediction has been confirmed experimentally (Figure 7.6). Molecular biological tools and engineering analysis allow quantification of these mechanisms. Using cells with genetically engineered integrin receptors, the speed of cell migration was shown to depend on the number of receptor–ligand bonds between the cell and the substrate (which depends on both receptor number

Table 7.2
Typical Cell Speeds and Persistence Times

Cell Type	P (min)	S (μm/min)	μ (cm^2/s)
Neutrophils	1–4	20	30×10^{-9}
Macrophages	30	2	10×10^{-9}
Fibroblasts	60	0.5	1.2×10^{-9}
Endothelial cells	300	0.4	
Smooth muscle cells	240–300	0.5	6.2×10^{-9}
Neurons on laminin [74]		1–3	
Cerebellar granule cell neurons migrating on astroglial fibers [75]	Saltatory	~ 1 (with pauses and long breaks) 0.05 – 0.3 (when observed over several hours)	
Cerebellar granule cell neurons migrating on laminin-coated or astroglial membrane-coated glass fibers [76]	Saltatory	~ 0.1	

The variables are defined in the text: P is the persistance time, S is the speed of migration, and μ is the random motility coefficient.

in the cell and ligand density on the surface) and the affinity of each bond [46]. These experimental results confirm the predictions of a mathematical model that relates cell motile speed to the strength of cell–substrate adhesion (Figure 7.7). The model also predicts the influence of rheology and intracellular force generation on motile speed.

7.2.3 Patterns of Migration in Cell Populations

The motion of individual cells in culture can be tracked by time-lapse optical microscopy. When observed over a sufficiently long time in a uniform environment (that is, one without spatial gradients in properties of the fluid or solid phase), the migratory path of each cell appears to be random and bears a striking similarity to the random paths of particles in Brownian motion (Figure 7.8). Characterization of the speed of cell migration is therefore often performed by analogy with the methods for characterizing the speed of particles in Brownian motion, which is reviewed and applied in the next subsections.

Random Migration. A solute particle in Brownian motion moves as a result of collisions with other particles that constitute the solvent phase; momentum is transferred to the Brownian particle by each collision. A particle, therefore, moves with a velocity $\overline{V}$ until another collision causes it to change directions and move with new velocity $\overline{V}'$. Changes in direction are instantaneous and

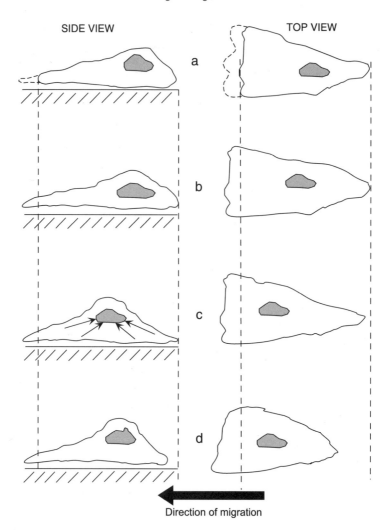

Figure 7.5. Mechanism of cell migration along a flat surface. For surface-attached cells, such as fibroblasts, migration occurs by a sequence of events: (a) protrusion of the lamellipodium at the forward edge of the cell; (b) formation of new adhesion sites at the forward edge; (c) accumulation of tension within the cell; and (d) release of adhesion sites at the trailing edge. Compare this schematic diagram to the photograph of the cells in Figure 7.3.

random, since the collisions occur from all directions with equal probability. The time between directional changes, or the time between collisions, depends on the density of molecules in the fluid. The average time between collisions can be estimated from the average distance the particle travels between collisions (called the mean free path) and the average speed $|\overline{V}|$. For oxygen at standard temperature and pressure, the mean free path is 1.6×10^{-5} cm (1600 Å) and the average time between collisions is 4×10^{-10} s [47] (p. 422).

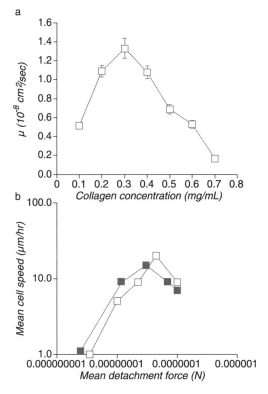

Figure 7.6. Cell motile speed has an optimum. The speed of random migration was measured for neutrophils migrating through a three-dimensional collagen gel (a) and for CHO cells migrating along a fibronectin-coated surface (b). Experimental results are redrawn from [56] and [46].

In a liquid, the higher particle density makes these times and distances even smaller. Therefore, the movement of a collection of Brownian particles is typically characterized by the rate of increase in the mean-squared displacement over observation times that are very long with respect to the mean free path interval. As described in the appendix section of this chapter, this behavior can in general be completely characterized by a diffusion coefficient D, which accounts for dispersion of the particle population that results from this process of repeated collision and random directional change.

Migratory paths of cells are similar to those of particles in Brownian motion. But do they result from the same underlying mechanism? The Stokes–Einstein equation provides a quantitative relationship between the rate of dispersion due to thermal fluctuations (that is, the diffusion coefficient D) and drag due to viscosity on the diffusing particle [48]:

$$D = \frac{k_{\mathrm{B}}T}{6\pi\eta a} \tag{7-1}$$

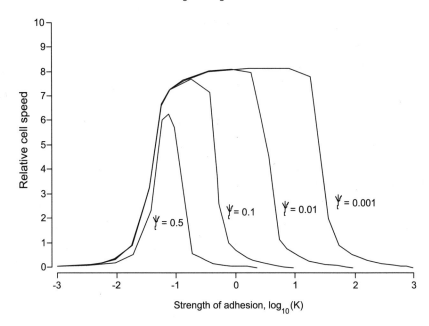

Figure 7.7. The characteristics of cell migration agree with mathematical models such as the model predictions from Figure 4 of [45]. The variable K is related to the strength of cell–substrate adhesion and ψ is a property of the cell population which depends on the rheological properties of the cell and the efficiency of force generation (see [45] for details).

where k_B is Boltzmann's constant, T is absolute temperature, a is the particle radius, and η is the viscosity of the fluid. This expression can be used to estimate the diffusion coefficient for particles of different sizes (Table 7.3). Neutrophils migrate through a collagen gel ~ 20 times faster than you would expect them to diffuse in water, in spite of the fact that the collagen gel is considerably more viscous than water. This rapid motility requires metabolic activity from the cell; dead or fixed cells can still move as Brownian particles (with the diffusion coefficient predicted by Equation 7-1), but they cannot migrate through a gel or over a surface.

Although the migratory path of a cell shares many similarities with the motion of Brownian particles, there are also important differences. The most striking difference is the observation that cells move in the same direction—at nearly constant speed—when observed over short experimental time intervals. The duration of the interval varies with cell type, but is generally on the order of one minute for rapidly moving cells such as neutrophils. This difference is sensible; cells do not move by instantaneous momentum transfer from other particles, but rather by a sequence of events involving attachment, contraction of intracellular fiber systems, and detachment (Figure 7.6). These processes are not instantaneous but require extensive rearrangement of internal cell structures as well as binding reactions between the cell surface and the substratum.

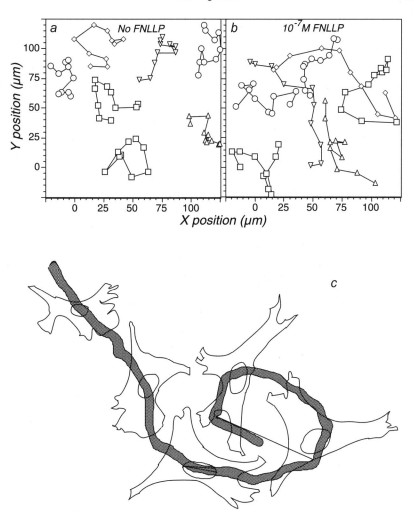

Figure 7.8. Pattern of migration for motile cells. This figure illustrates the migration of cells attached to surfaces and cells suspended in gels. In panels (a) and (b), each symbol represents a neutrophil that is migrating through a collagen gel. The position of the symbol represents the (x, y) position of the cell at a specific point in time; intervals of 1.5 min separate each symbol along the connected paths. The cell population was either not exposed (a) or exposed (b) to an agent that leads to faster migration. In panel (c), the characteristic changes in cell shape, as well as the position of the cell center of mass, are shown for a fibroblast migrating on a tissue culture surface (redrawn from [71]).

Changes in direction occur randomly, probably due to the stochastic nature of the membrane adhesions and cytoskeletal contraction events, but substantial changes in direction occur only after many small, random perturbations have accumulated. The migratory path looks like Brownian motion only if it is viewed as a series of "snapshots" of particle position taken at suitably long

Table 7.3
Diffusion Coefficients for Particles Estimated from Stokes–Einstein Equation

	Radius (μm)	D (10^{-7} cm^2/s)
Particle diffusion		
O_2 in water	0.00018	200
Protein in water	0.003	5
Neutrophil in water	5	0.005
Migration		
Neutrophil in 3D collagen gel	5	0.1
Fibroblast on glass surface	5–10	0.01
Pigmented retinal cell in neural aggregate	∼5	0.00005

See also [56, 73].

intervals (as shown in Figure 7.8). Higher resolution observations reveal steady forward motion and continuous directional changes; for many cells, the physical part of the cell at the leading edge remains constant, even as the cell turns. These observations suggest that cell migration occurs by a different physical process than the collision–run–collision process that yields Brownian motion.

In spite of these fundamental differences, studies of cell migration profit by comparison of cell movement with the statistical process of Brownian motion. Therefore, the physics of Brownian motion—or the statistics of a random walk process—are introduced in the next section (and a short background section is included at the end of this chapter).

Directed Migration.   Cells respond to their environment; rates of migration depend on the composition of the local environment. Receptors on cell membranes bind to soluble factors (such as hormones, nutrients, and growth factors) and surface-bound factors (such as the ECM molecules reviewed in Chapter 6). If the environment contains uniform concentrations of diffusible and immobilized chemicals, cell migration is usually random. However, if spatial variations are present, cells are capable of detecting these gradients and changing their migration behavior. This process of moving in response to gradients is called taxis and is critical to the regulation of almost every biological event that involves cell movement.

A variety of cell responses can lead to taxis: enhanced turning towards the stimulus (topotaxis), increased cell speed when the cell is oriented towards the stimulus (orthotaxis), or decreased turning when the cell is oriented towards the stimulus (klinotaxis). Cell movement is influenced by spatial gradients of dissolved chemicals (chemotaxis), cell adhesion (haptotaxis), light (phototaxis), and other signals. Certain agents cause chemokinesis, a change in the kinetics of cell random migration that does not require a gradient but depends on the total concentration of an agent in the environment; chemokinesis is further classified into orthokinesis (due to variations in cell speed) and klinokinesis (due to variations in cell persistence time). Chemokinetic changes can lead to overall cell accumulation at a stimulus site; for example, an agent that decreases cell speed will cause cells to accumulate at the site of maximum concentration (since cells that arrive at that spot are unable to move away).

7.3 Quantitative Methods for Describing the Movement of Individual Cells

7.3.1 Random Migration of Cells

The pattern of random migration of cells on a surface differs from Brownian motion: cell motions are usually observed at time intervals that are less than the time required for the cell to make a significant directional change. Observation times are relatively much longer than for particles in Brownian motion; the time between direction changes for albumin is $\tau = 4 \times 10^{-12}$ s (see Appendix of this Chapter), much smaller than the times relevant for cell movement. Cell migration is an example of a persistent random walk; at short observation times the cell appears to persist in whatever direction it is currently migrating, but at long observation times the migration is random (that is, similar to Brownian motion). If migrating cells were behaving as particles in a random walk, the mean squared displacement would increase linearly with time (as shown in Equation 7A-12 at the end of the chapter):

$$\langle d^2(t) \rangle = 4\mu t \qquad (7\text{-}2)$$

where μ is the random motility coefficient for the cell population and $d_i(t)$ is the displacement of an individual cell at time t: $\bar{d}_i(t) = \bar{r}_i(t) - \bar{r}_i(0)$ with $\bar{r}_i$ the position of the cell in some appropriate coordinate system.

Equation 7-2 is written to describe the random motion of cells on a two-dimensional surface. A persistent random walk can be described by a modified form of Equation 7-2, which accounts for the persistence in directional migration observed at short times:

$$\langle d^2(t) \rangle = 4\mu(t - P + Pe^{-t/P}) \qquad (7\text{-}3)$$

where P is the persistence time, which is related to the time between significant changes in direction for a migrating cell (Figure 7.8c). These two relationships (Equations 7-2 and 7-3) are shown in Figure 7.9.

The persistent random walk model was first applied to the migration of fibroblasts on a tissue culture surface [22]. The dynamics of Brownian motion were simulated by a simple random walk model in which particles change position suddenly and randomly; Brownian motion is more correctly described by considering fluctuations that arise in particle velocity instead of position [49]. The persistent random walk model can be developed from the Langevin equation (see [50] for a more complete description of this equation and its use in modeling Brownian particles):

$$dv(t) = -\beta v(t) dt + dW(t) \qquad (7\text{-}4)$$

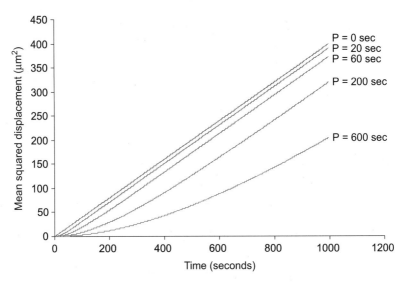

Figure 7.9. Mean-squared displacement for persistent random walks. The figure shows several plots of mean-squared displacement versus time, calculated from Equation 7-3, with the persistence time increasing over the range 0 to 600 s.

where $v(t)$ is the cell velocity and $W(t)$ is the stochastic Weiner process (that is, Gaussian random noise with a mean value of zero and a variance αdt). This differential equation specifies the two forces that contribute to changes in cell speed: cell speed is decreased by drag, a deterministic force that is proportional to cell speed with a characteristic coefficient β, and cell speed is influenced by a stochastic driving force that is characterized by the Weiner process. For one-dimensional movement of a population of cells whose velocities are described by this stochastic differential equation, it is possible to demonstrate that the mean squared displacement and mean squared speed of the population are [51]:

$$\langle d^2(t)\rangle^{1D} = \frac{\alpha}{\beta^3}(\beta t - 1 + e^{-\beta t}) \tag{7-5}$$

$$\langle S^2\rangle^{1D} = \frac{\alpha}{2\beta} \tag{7-6}$$

where d is the displacement of a cell after time t and S is the cell velocity, $v(t)$. As before, the bracketed terms on the left-hand sides of Equations 7-5 and 7-6 indicate mean squared quantities for the cell population. This description can be extended to higher dimensions by using the Pythagorean theorem:

$$\langle d^2(t)\rangle^{2D} = \langle d^2(t)\rangle^{1D} + \langle d^2(t)\rangle^{1D} = 2\frac{\alpha}{\beta^3}(\beta t - 1 + e^{-\beta t}) \tag{7-7}$$

$$\langle d^2(t)\rangle^{3D} = 3\frac{\alpha}{\beta^3}(\beta t - 1 + e^{-\beta t}) \tag{7-8}$$

$$\langle S^2 \rangle^{2D} = \langle S^2 \rangle^{1D} + \langle S^2 \rangle^{1D} = \frac{\alpha}{\beta} \tag{7-9}$$

$$\langle S^2 \rangle^{3D} = \frac{3\alpha}{2\beta} \tag{7-10}$$

It is more convenient to replace α and β, which describe the variance of statistical fluctuations and resistance to cell motility, respectively, by other terms that are related to more easily measured phenomena: that is, the cell speed, S_n = root mean square speed for n-dimensional migration, from Equations 7-6, 7-9, and 7-10:

$$S_n = \sqrt{\langle S^2 \rangle^{nD}} = \sqrt{\frac{n\alpha}{2\beta}} \tag{7-11}$$

and the persistence time:

$$P = \frac{1}{\beta} \tag{7-12}$$

With these terms defined, Equations 7-5, 7-7, and 7-8 can be written in the more general form:

$$\langle d^2(t) \rangle^{nD} = 2(S_n)^2 P\left(t - P + Pe^{-t/P}\right) \tag{7-13}$$

Finally, the random motility coefficient is defined from Equation 7-13:

$$\mu = \frac{\alpha}{2\beta^2} = \frac{(S_n)^2 P}{n} \tag{7-14}$$

so that the expressions for mean square displacement become

$$\langle d^2(t) \rangle^{nD} = 2n\mu(t - P + Pe^{-t/P}) \tag{7-15}$$

When $t \gg P$, Equation 7-15 reduces to 7-2 (and analogous equations for one- and three-dimensional random walks). For time scales that are large compared to the persistence time of a cell, the random migration of cells in a uniform environment can be described using the mathematical methods developed for molecular diffusion, which are reviewed in a number of texts [52–54].

This stochastic differential equation, Equation 7-4, can also be used as the basis of computer simulations of cell migration [55]. Using this approach, the pattern of migration for a small population of cells with the desired speed and persistence (S and P) can be simulated. This method is useful for visualizing the influence of cell motility parameters (S, μ, and P) on patterns of migration (Figure 7.10). It can also be used to test statistical methods for estimating motility parameters from experimental data [56].

The persistent random walk model has been used to characterize the rate of migration for a variety of cells; some examples are listed in Table 7.2. In general, the persistence time increases as the cell speed decreases. The average distance traveled between directional changes is approximately $S \times P$, or the mean free path length. The observation that S and P are reciprocally related is

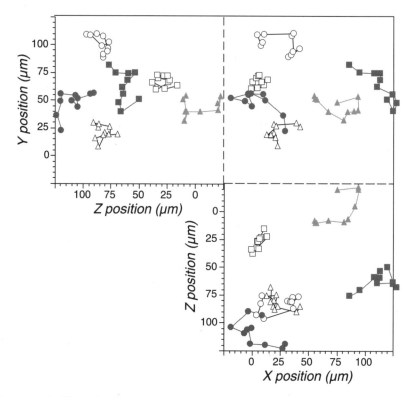

Figure 7.10. Migration paths for cells simulated using the stochastic differential equation. See text for details on the simulation procedure (more details are provided in [45]). This diagram shows several individual cells (each cell represented by a different symbol) migrating in a three-dimensional space.

reasonable, since the mean free path length must be optimal for cells to move productively: if $S \times P$ were too low, the cell would get nowhere, and if $S \times P$ were too high, the cell would move too far in the wrong direction.

7.3.2 Chemotaxis

Chemotaxis is the directed migration of cells in response to a gradient of a chemical signaling agent, or chemoattractant. Since migrating cells have a polarized morphology (that is, the front and rear of a migrating cell can be distinguished), a simple method for assessing the strength of a chemo-attractant is to observe the percentage of cells that are migrating in the "correct" direction; usually, the "correct" direction is up the gradient, towards higher concentrations of the agent. The strength of a chemo-attractant depends on the absolute concentration of the attractant and the steepness of the gradient (Figure 7.11). In general, the activity of a chemo-attractant increases with concentration up to some optimal value, above

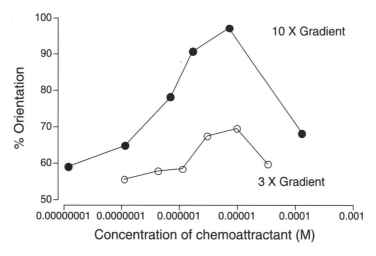

Figure 7.11. Orientation of neutrophils in a gradient of the peptide fMMM (redrawn from [23]). For a gradient applied in one dimension, as in this example, 50% of randomly migrating cells will be moving in the "correct" direction.

which the activity decreases; for formylated peptides, the concentration of optimal activity is $\sim 10^{-6}$ to 10^{-5} M.

The chemotactic movement of a population of cells can be characterized by the chemotactic index, CI:

$$CI = \frac{\langle d \rangle}{L_{\text{path}}} \left\{ 1 - \frac{P(1 - e^{-t/P})}{t} \right\}^{-1} \tag{7-16}$$

where $\langle d \rangle$ is the straight-line distance traveled towards the attractant source and L_{path} is the total distance traveled. For observation times that are large compared to the persistence time, that is, $t \gg P$, this expression reduces to:

$$CI = \frac{\langle d \rangle}{L_{\text{path}}} \tag{7-17}$$

The chemotactic index is equal to zero for perfectly random migration and one for perfectly directed migration. Computer simulations, similar to the ones described earlier for cells moving in persistent random walks but with a selected bias added to either the speed or direction of migration, have been used to study patterns of random migration in the presence of chemoattractants. These simulations have yielded insight into the mechanisms of signaling during directed migration [55, 57].

How do cells recognize the presence of chemoattractants? What mechanism does a cell use to determine the direction of a chemical gradient? These questions are not fully answered [58], but are best understood in bacterial cells, amoebae, and leukocytes from mammals. A bacterium swims by coordinated rotation of helical protein complexes called flagella [59]. Flagellar rotation is generated by a motor which connects each flagellum to the cell wall; energy for rotation is provided by a proton flux across the plasma membrane. Since flagella are helical, clockwise and counter-clockwise rotation can produce different outcomes. In *E. coli*, when all of the flagella (each one is a left-handed helix) are rotating counter-clockwise, the cell is propelled smoothly forward through the fluid medium with all the flagella moving as a coordinated unit (Figure 7.12a). During clockwise rotation, the individual flagella pull the cell body in different directions, leading to rapid changes in cell direction; the cell appears to be tumbling (Figure 7.12b). The direction of flagellar rotation changes during a period of cell migration; when observed over time, the cell alternates between smooth swimming (running) and tumbling. At the end of a tumble, the cell is most likely to be pointed in a different direction than it was prior to the tumble. Chemoattractant chemicals act by modifying the frequency of clockwise rotation or tumbling; when a cell experiences increasing chemoattractant concentration (that is, when it is swimming up a chemical gradient), the frequency of tumbling decreases. Chemoattractants exert their effects by binding to receptors in the periplasmic space (Table 7.4); receptor binding activates an internal signal, involving a cascade of phosphorylation of proteins of the Che family (Figure 7.12).

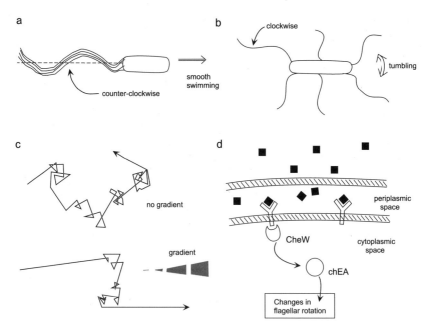

Figure 7.12. Mechanism of chemotaxis in *E. coli* bacterial cells (diagram adapted from Chapter 18 of [59]). The left-handed *E. coli* flagella produce (a) smooth forward swimming by counter-clockwise rotation, and (b) tumbling by clockwise rotation. (c) Chemoattractants modify the relative frequency of tumbles, producing net movement toward the source. (d) Chemoattractants act through a signal transduction pathway.

Table 7.4
Chemicals that Stimulate Directed
Cell Movement

Cell	Attractant	Receptor
E. coli	Serine	*Tsr* protein
	Aspartate	*Tar* protein
	Glucose	*Trg* protein
	Dipeptides	*Tap* protein

Some of the chemicals that can
attract bacterial cells are listed.

Bacterial cells detect the presence of chemical gradients by moving and sampling concentration at different places. This is a sensible strategy for small (1 μm), rapidly moving cells, since detection by another mechanism—such as comparing concentration at two different locations on the cell at the same moment in time—would be difficult. Amoebae and leukocytes, however, are substantially larger, so other mechanisms are possible. In fact, leukocytes appear to extend pseudopodia in the correct direction (that is, up the gradient) even before they initiate motion, suggesting that sensing is independent of motion (and time).

Chemotaxis in leukocytes and other eukaryotic cells is regulated by a G protein-linked receptor with seven membrane-spanning regions (Figure 7.13). Binding of a chemoattractant leads to a conformational change in the receptor, which activates the G protein by causing the binding of GTP and the release of GDP. The activated G protein stimulates activity of adenylyl cyclase (or another effector enzyme), causing generation of the second messenger cAMP. Cells move in the direction of highest concentration of chemoattractant, but the receptor protein and G protein β subunit remain uniformly distributed throughout the cell surface. The generated signal, which eventually leads to an accumulation of actin-binding proteins at the leading edge of the cell, must become spatially localized at some step in the signal transduction pathway between G protein activation and actin-binding protein accumulation. The most recent evidence suggests that binding of proteins with a pleckstrin homology (PH) domain to the G-protein β subunit is an important step in localization.

7.4 Quantitative Methods for Describing the Movement of Cell Populations

The previous section described methods for observing and quantifying the migration of individual cells. When cells are delivered to an organism, as in the cell delivery or tissue engineering applications considered here, we are usually more interested in the fate of a large number of cells than in the variations in behavior of individuals. This chapter therefore presents mathe-

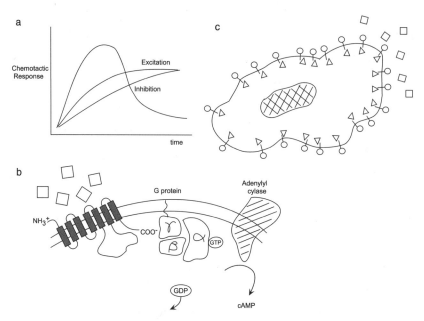

Figure 7.13. Chemotaxis signal transduction in leukocytes (information taken from [58, 72]). (a) Typical behavior of chemotaxis: the presence of a chemoattractant activates an excitation signal and a slower inhibition signal. The overall response is proportional to the difference between these signals; this model suggests that the difference gets smaller with time, hence the response to a constant concentration gradient is transient. (b) A common class of G protein-linked receptors has seven transmembrane domains. The trimeric G protein transduces the signal to an effector enzyme, such as adenylyl cyclase, which generates the second messenger cAMP. (c) Both receptors (circles) and G proteins (triangles) are uniformly distributed on the cell surface during chemotaxis; actin-binding proteins accumulate at the leading edge.

matical techniques that can be used to describe the movement of cell populations. To the degree that it is possible, these models of cell population behavior will be written in terms of the same parameters that were used to describe individual cell behavior. The development of quantitative methods for describing the movement of populations of randomly migrating cells is largely due to the efforts of Lauffenburger and his colleagues, who have developed a systematic and rigorous approach for analyzing cell motility and a variety of receptor-mediated phenomena in cells. That approach is reviewed in [60], and in the references that are provided in the text below.

7.4.1 Mathematical Descriptions of Cell Fux

Consider the movement of a population of cells in one dimension (higher dimensionality is harder to treat; see [61, 62]), following a derivation provided earlier [63]. At some time in every spatial location, assume some fraction of the cells are moving in the $(+)$ direction, described by a number density n^+ and local velocity v^+, and the remainder are moving in the $(-)$ direction, with number density n^- and local velocity v^- (Figure 7.14). The total cell density at this location, c, is equal to $n^+ + n^-$ and the local net cell flux, J, is

$$J = v^+ n^+ - v^- n^- \tag{7-18}$$

In general, cell speed is a function of local conditions but not the direction of migration, so that $v^- = v^+$, which simplifies the cell flux equation:

$$J = v(n^+ - n^-) \tag{7-19}$$

By considering a cell balance over a characteristic volume element—the region indicated by Δx in Figure 7.14, for example—conservation equations can be written for the $(+)-$ and $(-)$-moving cells. The usual conservation expression (accumulation $=$ in out $+$ generation $-$ loss) can be applied to the volume element indicated in Figure 7.14 for cells moving in the $(+)$ direction:

$$(+)\text{direction}: \frac{\partial n^+}{\partial t} + \frac{\partial}{\partial x}(vn^+) = p^- n^- - p^+ n^+ \tag{7-20}$$

and for cells moving in the $(-)$ direction:

$$(-)\text{direction}: \frac{\partial n-}{\partial t} + \frac{\partial}{\partial x}(vn-) = -p^- n^- + p^+ n^+ \tag{7-21}$$

where p^+ is the probability (cells/second) that a $(+)$-moving cell will begin moving in the $(-)$ direction and p^- is the probability that a $(-)$-moving cell will begin moving in the $(+)$ direction. By summing the conservation equations for the $(+)$ and $(-)$ moving cells, the usual expression for conservation of species is obtained:

$$\frac{\partial c}{\partial t} = -\frac{\partial J}{\partial x} \tag{7-22}$$

Equation 7-22 is analogous to the expression describing conservation of mass for diffusing molecules. For example, substitution of Fick's law (Equation 7A-16, see section at end of chapter) and substitution of the variable a to denote molecular concentration (since c is used to refer to cellular concentrations in this chapter) give a second-order differential equation for molecular concentration:

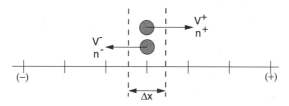

Figure 7.14. Simple coordinate system for derivation of equations for cell migration.

$$\frac{\partial d}{\partial t} = D_a \frac{\partial^2 a}{\partial x^2} \qquad (7\text{-}23)$$

Solutions to this partial differential equation give concentrations of an agent as a function of time and position. (See the related sections on "Diffusion of soluble signals" in Chapter 3, pp. 55–59 and "Ligand diffusion and binding" in Chapter 4, pp. 86–87) A solution requires knowledge of the geometry of the environment (this knowledge provides boundary conditions on concentration a) and the initial state of the system. Consider the situation indicated in Figure 7.15, in which a chemical is introduced at high concentration into one end of a tube filled with an unstirred gel. The appropriate boundary and initial conditions are: $a = a_0$ at $x = L$; $a = 0$ for x far from $x = L$ (that is, as $x \rightarrow \infty$); and $a = 0$ at $t = 0$. With these conditions, Equation 7-23 has the following solution:

$$a = a_0 \left\{ 1 - \mathrm{erf}\left(\frac{L - x}{\sqrt{4 D_a t}} \right) \right\} \qquad (7\text{-}24)$$

This equation can be used to examine the changes in agent concentration over time, as shown in Figure 7.15.

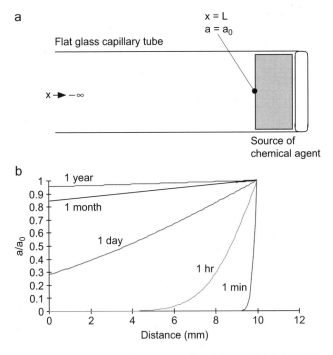

Figure 7.15. Diffusion of a chemical agent predicted from Fick's law. The figure shows the diffusion of a chemical agent with diffusion coefficient $5 \times 10^{-6}\,\mathrm{cm}^2/\mathrm{s}$ into a semi-infinite medium. The concentration of the agent at the position $L = 10\,\mathrm{mm}$ is maintained at the initial concentration a_0.

In the context of cell migration, the conservation equation (Equation 7-22) can be used to describe the overall movements of a population of cells, provided that an appropriate expression is available to relate the local cell flux to position, which accounts correctly for the prevailing conditions in the local environment. That is, an expression for the functional dependence of J on cell concentration, chemoattractant concentration, and any other important variable must be known. The expression for the local cell flux can be obtained by examining the difference between the $(+)$ and $(-)$ conservation equations provided in Equations 7-20 and 7-21:

$$\frac{\partial J}{\partial t} - v^{-1}J\frac{\partial v}{\partial t} = -J(p^* - p^-) - v\frac{\partial}{\partial x}(vc) - vc(p^+ - p^-) \quad (7\text{-}25)$$

This expression provides a means for evaluating the change in local cell flux. It is important to notice that the local flux will change with time, even if the local conditions (as determined by p^+, p^-, and v) remain constant with time. Equation 7-25 can be compared with Fick's law (Equation 7A-16). Assuming that local conditions are constant—that is, that v, p^+, and p^- are independent of time and spatial location—reduces Equation 7-25 to

$$\frac{\partial J}{\partial t} = -J(p^+ - p^-) - v\left(v\frac{\partial c}{\partial x} + c\frac{\partial v}{\partial x}\right) - vc(p^+ - p^-) \quad (7\text{-}26)$$

Equation 7-26 suggests that the time constant for changes in J is $\sim (p^+ + p^-)$, a quantity that is related to the persistence time defined for individual cell movements in the previous section (see Equation 7-3). As before, this persistence of migration is the result of the finite rate at which a cell can change either speed or direction of migration.

Substitution of Equation 7-25 into the total cell balance, Equation 7-22, yields a differential equation describing the complete evolution of cell population migration with time. Although complete, the resulting hyperbolic partial differential equation is cumbersome. In most cases of interest to tissue engineering, changes in cell position occur over a time scale that is large compared to the persistence time of the cell. In those situations, changes in local cell flux with time can be neglected by assuming $\partial J/\partial t = 0$; the flux expression reduces, with some rearrangement, to

$$J = -\left\{\frac{v^2}{(p^+ + p^-) - v^{-1}\frac{\partial v}{\partial t}}\right\}\frac{\partial c}{\partial x} - \left\{\frac{v\frac{\partial v}{\partial x}}{(p^* + p^-) - v^{-1}\frac{\partial v}{\partial t}}\right\}c$$
$$+ \left\{\frac{v(p^- - p^+)}{(p^+ + p^-) - v^{-1}\frac{\partial v}{\partial t}}\right\}c \quad (7\text{-}2)$$

which becomes more manageable with the definition of a modified persistence time T_p, the random motility coefficient μ (see Equation 7-14), and the chemotactic velocity V_c:

$$T_{\mathrm{p}} = \left[*(p^{+} + p^{-}) - v^{-1}\frac{\partial v}{\partial t} \right]^{-1} \tag{7-28}$$

$$\mu = T_{\mathrm{p}}v^{2} \tag{7-29}$$

$$V_{\mathrm{c}} = T_{\mathrm{p}}v(p^{-} - p^{+}) \tag{7-30}$$

Substitution of these parameters into the flux expression, Equation 7-27, leads to the following simplified flux expression:

$$J = -\mu\frac{\partial c}{\partial x} + V_{\mathrm{c}}c - \frac{1}{2}\left[\frac{\partial \mu}{\partial x} - \mu\frac{\partial \ln T_{\mathrm{p}}}{\partial x} \right]c \tag{7-31}$$

This expression distinguishes three factors that influence the flux during cell migration. The flux due to dispersion from random cell motility is proportional to the gradient of the total cell concentration (first term on right-hand-side of Equation 7-31). Since cell speed or persistence time may be functions of position—due to the presence of chemokinetic factors, for example—there is an additional contribution to flux from chemokinesis (third term on right-hand-side of Equation 7-31). Finally, spatial variations in the directional change probabilities (p^{+} and p^{-}) also may contribute to the local flux; this phenomena is called chemotaxis (second term on right-hand side of Equation 7-31). In a completely uniform environment, the second and third terms in Equation 7-31 are negligible, and the flux expression reduces to a familiar form:

$$J = -\mu\frac{\partial c}{\partial x} \tag{7-32}$$

which is analogous to the flux expression for molecular diffusion (compare to Equation 7A-16). The preceding derivation relates the underlying mechanistic description of cell motile behavior to the dynamics of the movement of cell populations. A different analysis, based on stochastic properties of individual cells, is also available [64].

A commonly used expression for the chemotactic movement of a cell population was developed by Keller and Segal [77]:

$$J_{\mathrm{c}} = -\mu\frac{\partial c}{\partial x} + \chi c\frac{\partial a}{\partial x} \tag{7-33}$$

where a is the concentration of a chemotactic agent, and χ is the chemotaxis coefficient. This equation was developed empirically, but it has been applied fruitfully to a number of experimental situations. Unlike the expression derived above, Equation 7-31, this empirical expression does not predict all of the behaviors observed in real cell populations, in particular: (1) that responses must asymptotically approach a limiting population flux as the stimulant gradient becomes large (because the speed of cell movement is finite); and (2) that temporal gradients of stimulants can influence cell migration. In addition, Equation 7-33 does not help identify the proper functional dependence of chemoattractant concentration (a) on μ and χ.

Another commonly used model of cell flux during chemotaxis was developed by Alt [61]. This model can be obtained from Equation 7-31 by replacing the modified persistence time, T_p, with the persistence time P and expending the spatial derivatives of μ and P in terms of the attractant concentration a:

$$J = -\mu \frac{\partial c}{\partial x} + V_c c - \frac{1}{2}\left[\frac{\partial \mu}{\partial a} - \frac{\mu}{P}\frac{\partial P}{\partial a}\right] c \frac{\partial a}{\partial x} \qquad (7\text{-}34)$$

Assuming that the random motility coefficient is only a function of a, and that the persistence time is a constant, yields

$$J = -\mu \frac{\partial c}{x} + V_c c - \frac{1}{2}\frac{d\mu}{da} c \frac{\partial a}{\partial x} \qquad (7\text{-}35)$$

The chemotactic velocity, V_c, is the net velocity of cell movement towards the source of the chemoattractant. V_c is related to the speed of cell migration, v, and the fraction of cells that are moving towards the source, f:

$$V_c = vf - v(1 - f) = \phi v \qquad (7\text{-}36)$$

where ϕ is the orientation bias, a number between 0 and 1, which is numerically equal to $2f - 1$. Orientation bias is a function of the local gradient of the chemoattractant (as in Figure 7.11). The cell is able to sense this gradient because attractant molecules bind to receptors on the cell surface; therefore, the orientation bias is a function of the chemical gradient as well as the affinity of attractant binding to cell receptors. One model for cell detection of an attractant gradient is shown in Figure 7.16; the orientation can be characterized quantitatively by analogy with expressions commonly encountered in the study of receptor–ligand binding (see [60] and Chapter 4):

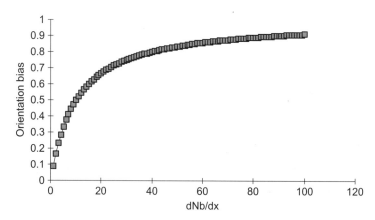

Figure 7.16. Variation of orientation bias for cells migrating within a gradient of soluble chemoattractant a. The orientation bias is plotted versus the first derivative of the number of bound receptor molecules. The functional form of Equation 7-37 is used.

$$\phi = \frac{\chi_0\left(\dfrac{\partial N_b}{\partial x}\right)}{1 + \chi_0\left(\dfrac{\partial N_b}{\partial x}\right)} = \frac{\chi_0\left(\dfrac{dN_b}{da}\dfrac{\partial a}{\partial x}\right)}{1 + \chi_0\left(\dfrac{dN_b}{da}\dfrac{\partial a}{\partial x}\right)} \tag{7-37}$$

where χ_0 is a coefficient denoting the chemotactic sensitivity and N_b is the number of cell surface receptors for the attractant that are occupied by the chemoattractant ligand, which is a function of the local concentration of chemoattractant, a. The chemotactic sensitivity provides a measure of cell responsiveness to the particular attractant; when the spatial gradient of bound receptors is equal to $1/\chi_0$, the orientation bias reaches half of its maximum value (Figure 7.16). A similar expression can be used to model the dependence of receptor occupancy on local chemoattractant concentration:

$$N_b = \frac{N_T a}{K_d + a} \tag{7-38}$$

where N_T is the total number of receptors on the cell surface and K_d is the dissociation constant, a quantitative measure of the affinity of attractant–receptor binding ($N_b = N_T/2$ when $a = K_d$). The derivative of N_b with respect to attractant concentration is easily obtained:

$$\frac{dN_b}{da} = \frac{N_T K_d}{(K_d + a)^2} \tag{7-39}$$

When the concentration gradient of chemoattractant is small, so that $\chi_0(\partial N_b/\partial x)$ is much less than 1, the denominator in Equation 7-37 becomes equal to 1. Substitution of these simplified Equations 7-38 and 7-39 into the cell flux expression, Equation 7-35, yields

$$J = -\mu\frac{\partial c}{\partial x} + \chi_0\left(\frac{dN_b}{da}\frac{\partial a}{\partial x}\right)vc - \frac{1}{2}\frac{d\mu}{da}c\frac{\partial a}{\partial x} \tag{7-40}$$

which can be further simplified by defining the chemotaxis coefficient, χ:

$$\chi = \frac{\phi}{\partial a/\partial x}v = \chi_0\frac{dN_b}{da}v \tag{7-41}$$

with the result

$$J = -\mu\frac{\partial}{\partial x} + \chi c\frac{\partial a}{\partial x} - \frac{1}{2}\frac{d\mu}{da}c\frac{\partial a}{\partial x} \tag{7-42}$$

which reduces to the form proposed by Keller and Segal [77], Equation 7-33, when the random motility coefficient is not a function of chemoattractant concentration (that is, when $d\mu/da = 0$).

7.4.2 Solutions to the Equations for Migration of Cell Populations

Substitution of the constitutive equation for the cell flux (Equation 7-42) into the conservation equation (7-22) yields

$$\frac{\partial c}{\partial t} = \mu \frac{\partial^2 c}{\partial x^2} + \frac{\partial}{\partial x}\left[\chi c \frac{\partial a}{\partial x}\right] - \frac{1}{2}\frac{\partial}{\partial x}\left[\frac{d\mu}{da}c\frac{\partial a}{\partial x}\right] \tag{7-43}$$

This equation can be solved to provide a description of the movement of a cell population when random migration, chemotaxis, and chemokinesis are all important.

Migration in a Uniform Environment. For migration in a uniform environment, with no gradients in chemoattractant concentration, Equation 7-43 reduces to a familiar differential equation:

$$\frac{\partial c}{\partial t} = \mu \frac{\partial^2 c}{\partial x^2} \tag{7-44}$$

which is analogous to Fick's second law for molecular diffusion (Equation 7-23). The following boundary and initial conditions are appropriate for describing a linear under-agarose assay (Figure 7.2a):

$$
\begin{array}{llll}
c = c_0 & \text{at} & x = 0 & t > 0 \\
c = 0 & \text{at} & x \to \infty & t > 0 \\
c = 0 & \text{at} & 0 \le x < \infty & t = 0
\end{array}
\tag{7-45}
$$

Therefore, Equation 7-44 can be solved subject to the conditions in Equation 7-45 to yield cell concentration profiles:

$$c = c_0 \ \text{erfc}\left(\frac{x}{2\sqrt{\mu t}}\right) \tag{7-46}$$

where c_0 is the concentration of cells at the edge of the agarose well and erfc is the complement of the error function (erfc $[x] = 1 - \text{erf}[x]$, see Appendix). In this situation, cell concentration varies with time; eventually, the cell concentration rises throughout the local environment (Figure 7.17). The time that is required for cell dispersion over a distance of 10 to 100 μm (such as is shown in

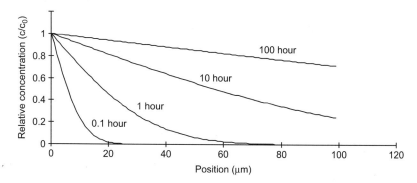

Figure 7.17. The cell concentration that results from random migration in a uniform environment for 0.1, 1, 10, and 100 hours. The migrating cell population is characterized by a random motility coefficient of 10^{-9} cm^2/s.

Figure 7.17) depends on the random motility coefficient. For a value of μ that has been measured for fibroblasts (Table 7.2), dispersion over this distance takes several hours when it occurs strictly by random migration.

Migration with Chemotaxis.   To examine the movement of a cell population in the presence of a chemical gradient, consider the simple configuration illustrated in Figure 7.18. Cells are initially confined to a region at one end of the one-dimensional system ($x < 0$), and the chemoattractant is initially confined to a region at the opposite end ($x > L$). All of the terms in the cell flux equation are potentially important in this experimental situation. Equation 7-43 can be expanded to obtain

$$\frac{\partial c}{\partial t} = \mu \frac{\partial^2 c}{\partial x^2} - \left[\chi - \frac{1}{2}\frac{d\mu}{da}\right]\left[c\frac{\partial^2 a}{\partial x^2} + \frac{\partial c}{\partial x}\frac{\partial a}{\partial x}\right] - \left[\frac{d\chi}{da} - \frac{1}{2}\frac{d^2\mu}{da^2}\right]c\left(\frac{\partial a}{\partial x}\right)^2 + \frac{d\mu}{da}\frac{\partial c}{\partial x}\frac{\partial a}{\partial x}$$

$$(7\text{-}47)$$

This equation can be solved subject to the same boundary and initial conditions listed in Equation 7-45, as long as migrating cells do not reach the chemoattractant reservoir during the period of observation.

To solve Equation 7-47 subject to these conditions, the dependence of both μ and χ on concentration of chemoattractant, a, must be known. The dependence of μ on a can be determined experimentally by measuring cell motility in uniform concentrations of a—by using the under-agarose assay described in the previous subsection, for example—and obtaining numerical values of μ for each concentration. The values of μ can be obtained by comparing experimental data to cell migration patterns predicted by models such as Equation 7-46. Alternatively, the paths of individual cells migrating within uniform environ-

Flat glass capillary tube

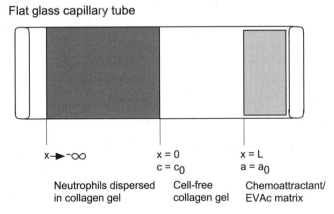

$x \longrightarrow -\infty$	$x = 0$	$x = L$
	$c = c_0$	$a = a_0$
Neutrophils dispersed in collagen gel	Cell-free collagen gel	Chemoattractant/ EVAc matrix

Figure 7.18. A simple experimental assay system for examining the migration of a cell population in the presence of a gradient of a chemoattractant (see [65]). A three-dimensional gel (composed, for example, of collagen) contains a suspension of motile cells at one end and a reservoir of chemoattractant at the opposite end.

ments of chemoattractant can be followed using time-lapse video techniques and subsequently compared to Equation 7-15 for estimation of μ and P. Either of these techniques will provide experimental evidence for the dependence of μ on chemoattractant concentration.

Figure 7.19 shows the random motility coefficient for neutrophils suspended in collagen gels as a function of concentration of a chemotactic peptide; random motility coefficients were determined by time-lapse video-microscopy of individual cells migrating in a uniform environment. This experimental data, $\mu(a)$, can be fit to an appropriate function for determination of the derivatives—$d\mu/da$ and $d^2\mu/da^2$—which are needed to evaluate Equation 7-47 (see [65] for an example of this procedure).

The functional dependence of χ on the chemoattractant concentration can be estimated by referring to the definition of χ provided in Equation 7-41. Substituting expressions for the cell speed (Equation 7-14) and the variation in the number of bound receptors with attractant concentration (Equation 7-39) yields

$$\chi = \chi_0 N_{T,0} f(a) \frac{K_d}{(K_d + a)^2} \sqrt{\frac{2\mu}{P}} \qquad (7\text{-}48)$$

where the function $f(a)(= N_T/N_{T,0})$ is introduced to account for changes in receptor number due to the presence of chemoattractant a. These changes might be due to receptor up- or down-regulation, which often occurs in the presence of ligand binding. Appropriate derivatives of χ with respect to attractant concentration can be evaluated from Equation 7-48.

To complete the mathematical description of chemotaxis, the spatial variation in chemoattractant concentration a must be supplied. For the system

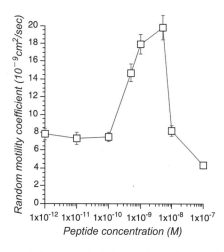

Figure 7.19. Random motility coefficient for neutrophils as a function of chemoattractant concentration (from [65], Figure 3.5). The random motility coefficient for neutrophils migrating in gels of 0.4 mg/mL rat tail collagen was measured as a function of FNLPNTL concentration.

shown in Figure 7.18, the variation in chemoattractant concentration is provided by Equation 7-24; the geometries of the vessels with respect to agent diffusion are identical (see Figures 7.18 and 7.15). Recall that Equation 7-24 was obtained from the equation for conservation of mass, solved subject to appropriate boundary and initial conditions.

Equation 7-24 can be differentiated to obtain the first and second derivatives of a with respect to x, which are required for solution of Equation 7-47:

$$\left.\begin{array}{l} \dfrac{\partial a}{\partial x} = \dfrac{a_0}{\sqrt{\pi D_a t}} \exp\left[-\dfrac{(L-x)^2}{4D_a t} \right] \\[20pt] \dfrac{\partial^2 a}{\partial x^2} = \dfrac{(L-x)a_0}{(D_a t)^{3/2}\sqrt{4\pi}} \exp\left[-\dfrac{(L-x)^2}{4D_a t} \right] \end{array}\right\} \tag{7-49}$$

In summary, cell density profiles as a function of time for the configuration shown in Figure 7.18 can be obtained by solving Equation 7-47 subject to the conditions in Equation 7-45. Equation 7-48 is used to obtain χ and derivatives; Equation 7-49 is used for derivatives of a; and an experimentally determined functional form is used for $\mu(a)$ (as illustrated in Figure 7.19).

This approach was used by Parkhurst to predict cell density profiles for neutrophils migrating within a collagen gel (0.4. mg collagen/mL) in the presence of the chemoattractant peptide FNLPNTL [65]. The parameters used in solving the equations are listed in Table 7.5. In separate experiments, the diffusion coefficient for the peptide through the collagen gel was determined to be 5×10^{-6} cm^2/s. The equations were solved by a finite difference technique to yield estimates for cell density and chemoattractant concentration as a function of time and position within the gel. Typical model results, obtained by selecting values for model parameters L and a_0, are shown in Figure 7.20.

A similar approach has been applied to the chemotaxis of rat alveolar macrophages in response to gradients of C5a, a proteolytic fragment of the complement protein C5 that is chemoattractant for macrophages [31]. To obtain estimates of all of the parameters required to solve these equations, and to compare the description obtained by monitoring cell population movements with characterizations of individual cell motility, two different types of experiment were performed: random motility coefficients and chemotaxis coefficients were obtained by time-lapse microscopy of individual cells; and cell concentration profiles were obtained by an under-agarose assay, in which a population of cells is permitted to migrate from a localized source under a gel containing a gradient of diffusible C5a.

7.5 Mean Time to Capture

The equations for mean time to capture provide an alternative method of analysis that is useful for analyzing cell migration in some situations. Assume that a migrating cell is initially at position (x, y) on a two-dimensional

Table 7.5
Chemotaxis Coefficient as a Function of Concentration for
Neutrophils Migrating in FNLPNTL

a (M)	$\log_{10}\left(\dfrac{a}{K_d}\right)$	μ $(10^{-9}\ \text{cm}^2/\text{s})$	P (min)	f^a	χ $(\text{cm}^2/\text{s-M})$
0	$-\infty$	7.7 ± 0.6	0.8 ± 0.5	1	5350
10^{-11}	-1.78	7.3 ± 0.7	0.8 ± 0.6	1	5040
10^{-10}	-0.78	7.5 ± 0.5	0.6 ± 0.4	0.86	3330
5×10^{-10}	-0.08	15 ± 1.0	1.0 ± 0.4	0.54	1190
10^{-9}	0.22	18 ± 1.1	1.0 ± 0.4	0.43	496
5×10^{-9}	0.92	20 ± 1.4	1.0 ± 0.5	0.25	24
10^{-8}	1.22	8.2 ± 0.6	0.13 ± 0.5	0.2	3.5
10^{-7}	2.22	4.3 ± 0.3	0.25 ± 0.4	0.2	0.03

Adapted from [65], assuming $K_d = 6 \times 10^{-10}$ M and $N_{T0} = 50,000$. P
and μ were determined experimentally, as in Figure 7.19. Estimates
for χ were obtained from Equation 7-64, using values of f that were
estimated as described by Tranquillo et al. [57].
[a]The following function works for rabbit neutrophils in the presence
of the chemoattractant peptide fNLLP [66]:

$$
f = \begin{cases}
1 & \text{when} & \log_{10}\left(\dfrac{a}{K_d}\right) < -1.3 \\[2ex]
0.093\left[\log_{10}\left(\dfrac{a}{K_d}\right)\right]^2 - 0.37\log_{10}\left(\dfrac{a}{K_d}\right) + 0.51 & \text{when} & -1.3 < \log_{10}\left(\dfrac{a}{K_d}\right) < 1.2 \\[2ex]
0.2 & \text{when} & 1.2 < \log_{10}\left(\dfrac{a}{K_d}\right)
\end{cases}
$$

grid (Figure 7.21). The migrating cell moves by random migration from its
initial location (x, y) until it encounters a site belonging to a locus of sites of
interest, called absorbing sites, where it is captured; this process of release,
random migration, and capture requires some period of time, w, which depends
on the initial position. If this process is repeated many times for a population
of migrating cells, the mean time to capture for the population can be obtained
from the differential equation [67]

$$-1 = \mu\nabla^2 W \tag{7-50}$$

where μ is the random motility coefficient and $W(x, y)$ is the mean time to
capture for a population of cells that originate at position (x, y). This differential equation follows from the discrete equation obtained for migration
between sites on a square lattice. If the distance between sites is δ and the
time required for the particle to move from one site to another is Δt:

$$W(x, y) = \Delta t + \frac{1}{4}[W(x + \delta, y) + W(x - \delta, y) + W(x, y + \delta) + W(x, y - \delta)] \tag{7-51}$$

because a cell initially at position (x, y) is equally likely to be at any of the four
sites $(x \pm \delta, y \pm \delta)$ after Δt. Equation 7-50 follows directly from Equation 7-51

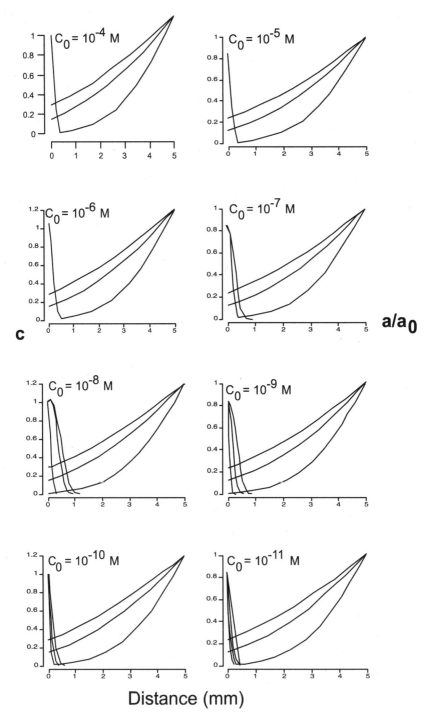

Figure 7.20. Model predictions for cell density profiles within collagen gels in the presence of chemoattractant gradients. Cell density profiles and chemoattractant concentration profiles were predicted using Equation 7-63 and the parameter values are provided in Table 7.5.

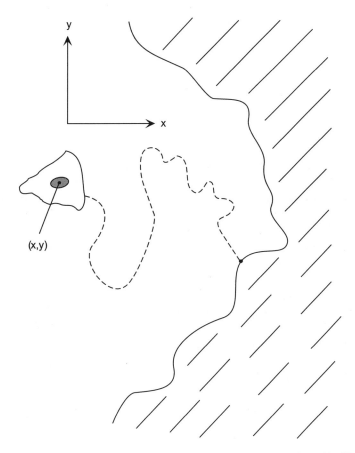

Figure 7.21. Illustration of time to capture for a migrating cell. The cell will move randomly until it encounters an adhesive boundary.

in the limit as the lattice spacing becomes vanishingly small, and using the definition that μ is equal to $\delta^2/4\Delta t$ (Equation 7-2).

Boundary conditions are needed to complete the solution of Equation 7-50. The locus of capture positions (x^*, y^*) must satisfy: $W(x^*, y^*) = 0$. Other boundaries in the system cannot be crossed by migrating cells, but also do not capture the cell. These reflecting boundaries must satisfy $\hat{n} \cdot \nabla W = 0$

Consider the situation in which a cell is initially released at a site that is a distance L from a location where it will be captured. For purposes of illustration, assume that this is a lymphocyte that is migrating through the interstitial space until it enters a lymph vessel. The differential equation for this capture, in one dimension, is

$$-1 = \mu \frac{d^2}{dx^2} W(x) \tag{7-52}$$

which is easily solved, subject to the boundary conditions $(dW/dx)_{x=0} = 0$, and $W(L) = 0$ to give

$$W(x) = \frac{L^2 - x^2}{2\mu} \tag{7-53}$$

The cell is released at $x = 0$ and therefore has a mean time to capture of $L^2/2\mu$.

7.6 Coordination of Cell Migration

In the previous discussion, the migration of cells occurred independently; migrating cells were assumed to be incapable of communicating with each other or influencing the migration of other cells. However, groups of cells sometimes move with coordination. Chain migration, for example, appears to move large numbers of precursor cells to the appropriate position in the brain [68]; this process occurs during development but also, for some kinds of cells, after birth and into adulthood.

There is some evidence that cell–cell communication is an important aspect of the coordinated movements of cell populations. For example, cell–cell communication that is mediated by gap junctions can influence the rate of migration of neural crest cells [20]; reductions in gap junctions—achieved by genetic or pharmacologic means—reduced the rate of migration. Perhaps this cell–cell communication operates to control the pathway for neural crest migration during development. Alternatively, gap junction communication provides a mechanism for communities of cells to share information relevant to migration of the entire population.

Summary

- Cell migration is fundamental to the processes of life. It is an important force in shaping the embryo during development and is essential for the physiological function of adults. Cell migration is an important feature of many approaches to tissue engineering
- The kinetics of random cell migration are analogous to molecular dispersion by diffusion, although the persistence time for cell migration is often comparable to the observation time.
- Cell migration can be biased by molecules in the environment. Chemotaxis, the directed migration of cells in response to a chemical gradient, allows cells to regulate their speed and direction of movement in response to the environment.
- The migration of individual cells can be analyzed quantitatively by comparison with statistical models of random walks.
- The migration of populations of cells can be analyzed by the solution of partial differential equations that are similar to the equations that

engineers frequently use to analyze heat transfer and molecular diffusion. In many cases, the coefficients in these equations are not constant, so solution of the differential equation requires a clear understanding of properties of the environment (such as gradients of chemoattractant molecules) and properties of the cell (such as its responsiveness to chemoattractant chemicals).

Appendix: Additional Information on Brownian Motion and Random Walks

Brownian motion occurs by the random movement of individual molecules; molecular motion is generated by thermal energy. The velocity of particle motion depends on absolute temperature, T [48]:

$$\left\langle \frac{mv_x^2}{2} \right\rangle = \frac{k_B T}{2} \tag{7A-1}$$

where v_x is the velocity of the particle on one axis, m is the mass of a particle, and k_B is Boltzmann's constant ($k_B T = 4.14 \times 10^{-14}$ g-cm^2/s^2 at 300 K). The root-mean-square (r.m.s.) velocity can be found from

$$v_{rms} = \sqrt{\langle v_x^2 \rangle} = \sqrt{\frac{kT}{m}} \tag{7A-2}$$

A moderate-sized protein ($\sim$70,000 daltons) has an r.m.s. velocity of 6 m/s at 300 K. Since air and water have different molecular densities, the number of collisions per second—and hence the rate of overall dispersion—differs for these fluids.

Brownian motion can be reproduced by a statistical process called a random walk. In this process, a particle moves with constant velocity and changes direction randomly at a fixed interval. Berg provides a useful introduction to the random walk and biological systems [69]. Whitney provides a complete, tutorial introduction to random processes, including the random walk [49].

In the simplest random walk, a particle is constrained to move along a one-dimensional axis. During a small time interval τ, the particle can move a distance δ which depends on the particle's velocity v_x: $\delta = v_x \tau$. At the end of each period τ, the particle changes its direction of movement, randomly moving to either the right or the left. In an unbiased random walk, right or left turning occurs with equal probability. At each step in the walk, a new direction is chosen randomly and does not depend on the particle's previous history of movement. If a large number of identical particles, each moving according to these simple rules, begin at the origin of the coordinate system at $t = 0$, one-half of the particles will be at position $-\delta$ and the other half will be at $+\delta$ at the end of the first interval τ. Individual particles are specified by an index i; the position of each particle after $n - 1$ time intervals is designated $x_i(n - 1)$. The position of particle i after n intervals is

$$x_i(n) = x_i(n-1) \pm \delta \tag{7A-3}$$

The mean particle position can be predicted by averaging Equation 7A-3 over the ensemble of particles to obtain

$$\langle x(n) \rangle - \frac{1}{N}\sum_{i=1}^{N} x_i(n-1) + \frac{1}{N}\sum_{i=1}^{N}(\pm\delta) \tag{7A-4}$$

upon substitution of Equation 7A-3. For an unbiased random walk, the second term on the right-hand side of Equation 7A-4 is zero, since an equal number of particles will move to the right ($+\delta$) and to the left ($-\delta$), which produces

$$\langle x(n) \rangle = \langle x(n-1) \rangle \tag{7A-5}$$

The average position of the collection of particles is independent of time.

Although random migration does not change the average position of the ensemble, it does tend to spread the particles over the axis. The extent of spread can be determined by examining the mean-square displacement of the particle ensemble, $\langle x^2(n) \rangle$:

$$\langle x^2(n) \rangle = \frac{1}{N}\sum_{i=1}^{N}(x_i^2(n-1) \pm \delta)^2 \tag{7A-6}$$

Expansion of the summation yields

$$\langle x^2(n) \rangle = \langle x^2(n-2) \rangle + \delta^2 \tag{7A-7}$$

Since the mean-square displacement is initially 0, Equation 7A-7 indicates that the mean-square displacement increases linearly with the number of steps in the random walk:

$$\langle x^2(n) \rangle = n\delta^2 \tag{7A-8}$$

Since the total elapsed time t is equal to $n\tau$, the mean-square displacement also increases linearly with time:

$$\langle x^2(t) \rangle = \left(\frac{\delta^2}{\tau}\right)t \tag{7A-9}$$

The r.m.s. displacement, x_{rms}, increases with the square root of time:

$$x_{rms} = \langle x^2(t) \rangle^{1/2} = \sqrt{2Dt} \tag{7A-10}$$

Equation 7A-10 is the defining equation for the diffusion coefficient D:

$$D = \delta^2/2\tau \tag{7A-11}$$

Experimental measurements, obtained by measuring the rate of spreading of particles in solution, suggest that D for a protein of moderate size (albumin: 68,000 dalton) at 300 K is $\sim 8 \times 10^{-7}\,cm^2/s$. Since v_x is the particle velocity between changes of direction, which is equal to δ/τ, the distance between direction changes δ can be estimated as $2D/v_x$; for albumin, with $v_x = v_{rms} = 600\,cm/s$, this yields a value for δ of $3 \times 10^{-9}\,cm$ (or 0.3 Å, small compared to the diameter of albumin, which is $\sim 60\,\text{Å}$) and a time between direction changes τ of $4 \times 10^{-12}\,\text{s}$.

This analysis can be extended to two- and three-dimensional random walks by assuming that particle motion in each dimension is independent. The mean-square displacement and r.m.s. displacement for higher dimension random walks become

$$\langle r^2 \rangle_{2D} = 4Dt \qquad \text{or} \qquad \langle r^2 \rangle_{2D}^{1/2} = \sqrt{4Dt} \qquad (7A\text{-}12)$$

$$\langle r^2 \rangle_{3D} = 6Dt \qquad \text{or} \qquad \langle r^2 \rangle_{3D}^{1/2} = \sqrt{6Dt} \qquad (7A\text{-}13)$$

The rate of movement of particles at any particular location can be estimated. During a single step in the random walk, which occurs over the time interval τ, the net rate of particle movement between two adjacent positions x and $x + \delta$ is $N(x)/2 - N(x + \delta)/2$, where $N(\cdot)$ gives the number of particles at a given location; half of the particles at position x will move to the right (ending at $x + \delta$) and half of the particles at $x + \delta$ will move to the left (ending at x). The particle flux j_x is defined as the net rate of particle movement per unit area, or

$$j_x = -\frac{1}{2A\tau}[N(x + \delta) - N(x)] \qquad (7A\text{-}14)$$

Rearranging slightly gives

$$j_x = -\frac{\delta^2}{2r}\left[\frac{C(x + \delta) - C(x)}{\delta}\right] \qquad (7A\text{-}15)$$

where $C(x)$ is the concentration of particles at a given location, $N(x)/A\delta$. The limit of Equation 7A-15 as δ goes to zero is

$$j_x = -D\frac{\partial C}{\partial x} \qquad (7A\text{-}16)$$

where the diffusion coefficient D is defined as in Equation 7A-11. Particles move toward locations with lower concentration; the flux of particles is directly proportional to the concentration gradient. This expression is often called Fick's law [70].

Exercises

Exercise 7.1 (provided by Christine Schmidt)

You work in a research lab. You hypothesize that a particular protein (NOB protein) is involved in the migration of dermal fibroblast cells, and thus is involved in wound healing of skin. To determine whether NOB protein is playing a role in the migration of these fibroblast cells, you have planned a series of experiments.

    a) First, you want to see whether NOB protein is found in higher levels in the fibroblasts that are actively migrating than in the cells that are not migrating. To do this, your supervisor suggests that you isolate all the proteins from the cells and run these proteins on a polyacrylamide gel (SDS gel electrophoresis). You stain these proteins with Coomassie blue to visualize all the proteins. You then transfer these proteins from the gel to a nitrocellulose membrane and blot with an antibody that binds specifically to the NOB protein (Western analysis). Results are shown in Figure 7.22a. The molecular weight marker bands are of the following sizes: 15, 25, 40, and 100 kDa What is the *approximate* molecular weight (in kDa) of NOB protein?

b) From these results, does the NOB protein likely play a role in fibroblast migration? Why or why not?

c) Next, your supervisor suggests that you look at the spatial distribution (localization) of the NOB protein within the migrating dermal fibroblast cells. What technique will you use to specifically localize the NOB protein to a particular part of the cell? Explain and justify.

d) You find that the NOB protein localizes to protrusions at the front of the cell that only extend when the cell is actively moving forward. In

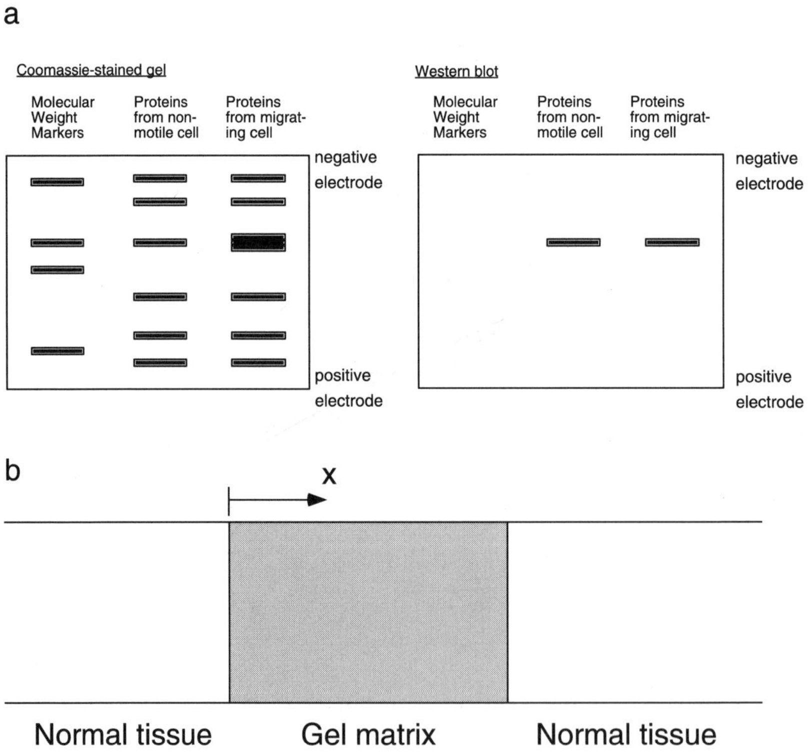

Figure 7.22. Western blot analysis for Exercise 7.1(a) and experimental setup for Exercise 7.5(b).

fact, your analysis suggests that the NOB protein binds to the prominent cytoskeleton protein found in these protrusions. Which cytoskeleton protein is most likely NOB binding?

e) You next want to determine whether NOB is associated with the adherens junctions that are found in the protrusions and which serve to link the internal cytoskeletal structure of the fibroblast to the surrounding components of the dermis. What is most likely the identity of the transmembrane protein found in these adherens junctions?

Exercise 7.2

Cells were uniformly distributed within a three-dimensional hydrogel and observed by light microscopy. Using time-lapse video imaging and computer image analysis, the location of each cell within the field of view was determined at discrete intervals over a 15-min period. The (x, y) coordinates provided below give positions as a function of time for 8 individual cells.

a) Determine the random motility coefficient and persistence time for these cells.
b) What kind of cells do you think they are?

Cell 1		Cell 2		Cell 3		Cell 4	
x	y	x	y	x	y	x	y
91.23	12.42	9.96	25.46	109.29	23.18	12.25	41.64
86.07	3.24	-2.94	68.3	122.19	23.18	22.57	39.6
102.84	-4.92	-4.23	59.12	111.87	31.34	23.86	55.92
109.29	1.2	4.8	48.92	108	30.32	27.73	70.2
119.61	18.54	3.51	29.54	89.94	24.2	34.18	56.94
117.03	-1.86	20.28	32.69	3.81	31.34	41.92	54.9
115.74	0.18	46.08	38.72	93.81	43.58	56.11	31.44
113.16	1.2	53.82	34.64	102.84	44.6	66.43	23.28
110.58	4.26	84.78	32.6	95.1	47.66	78.04	33.48
108	6.3	88.65	14.24	96.39	50.72	62.56	45.72

Cell 5		Cell 6		Cell 7		Cell 8	
x	y	x	y	x	y	x	y
109.34	113.04	72.68	67.22	-4.76	-23.7	11.49	74.94
119.66	114.06	71.39	75.38	2.98	-4.32	34.71	81.06
124.82	116.16	7.52	86.6	13.3	-11.46	32.13	95.34
113.21	106.92	77.84	96.8	33.94	-18.6	25.68	94.32
104.18	111	84.29	72.32	17.17	-7.38	25.68	102.48
105.47	99.78	90.74	54.98	0.4	-6.36	8.91	95.34
97.73	106.92	107.51	41.72	-4.76	2.82	-11.73	104.52
91.28	107.94	110.09	39.68	-11.21	13.02	-11.73	104.52
99.02	103.86	103.64	47.84	-22.82	-9.42	-10.44	102.48
105.47	114.06	106.22	46.82	-3.47	-1.26	-11.73	105.54

Exercise 7.3 (provided by Keith Gooch)

Fibroblasts are initially seeded with a uniform distribution on tissue-culture plastic. A chemoattractant, A, is added to the right side of the flask so that a linear concentration gradient is maintained for all time. On one graph, sketch the number of cells N as a function of position x on the graph at steady state. On a second graph, sketch the flux of the cell population, J_{cells}, as a function of position at steady state. Assume that cell migration can be modeled by the equation $J_{cells} = -\mu(dN/dx) + B(dA/dx)N$; and that the chemotaxis coefficient B is a constant.

Exercise 7.4

Consider an under-agarose assay wherein a population of cells is initially placed in a cylindrical well $(r = R_A)$ at the center of a round cell culture plate $(r = R_B)$. Cells attach uniformly to the surface in the region $r > R_A$ and migrate along the surface in the region $R_A < r < R_B$.

a) If the concentration of cells at the agarose boundary $(r = R_A)$ is assumed constant throughout the experiment, find an expression for the expected cell density as a function of time and radial position.
b) If the random motility coefficient for the cell population under study is 1×10^{-8} cm^2/s, the persistence time is 90 s, and RA is 5 mm, fill in the table below, where each cell in the table contains the normalized cell concentration (C/C_0) at the indicated time and position.

	$T = 12$ hr	$T = 24$ hr	$T = 72$ hr
$r = 5.1$ mm			
$r = 6$ mm			
$r = 8$ mm			
$r = 10$ mm			

c) What is the minimum value for R_B so that the expression derived in a) can be safely applied to this experiment?
d) You have just demonstrated how to apply this simple cell culture geometry for determining random motility coefficients. How could you adapt this method to allow experimental determination of chemotaxis?

Exercise 7.5

A polymeric material, similar to the gel matrix described in Exercise 7.2, is implanted into a wound site. The geometry of the site is indicated in Figure 7.22b. The total length of the matrix is 10 cm and its cross-section is 5 cm × 5 cm. Assume that cell migration is only possible through the interfaces between normal tissue and gel matrix that are indicated (that is, only migration in the *x*-direction must be considered). Assume that the normal tissue contains $\sim 10^7$ motile cells per mL.

a) If cells attempt to crawl into the matrix, and if the population of cells has a random motility coefficient μ of 1×10^{-9} cm^2/s, find an equation for the concentration density of cells within the matrix as a function of time.

b) Plot the cell concentration within the gel matrix as a function of position at 1 day, 1 month, and 1 year after implantation (assume that there is no cell proliferation).

c) On the basis of the cell concentration profiles prepared for part a), estimate the time required for the first cells to reach the midline of the matrix. Estimate the time required for the matrix to become "filled" with cells; provide your own definition for "filled."

d) Assume that the "normal tissue" on the left-hand-side of the gel matrix is replaced by a controlled-release device which steadily releases a 30,000 molecular weight protein that stimulates cell migration. Assume that this agent is "chemokinetic" only, in that it increases cell speed (as shown in Figure 7.19), but does not induce chemotaxis. Develop a quantitative model for the concentration of this protein within the gel matrix. Use this model, together with an appropriate model for cell migration, to predict the degree of enhancement in cell migration provided by release of the chemokinetic agent.

e) What is the optimal concentration of protein to include in the polymer?

Exercise 7.6

Consider three foreign objects, symmetrically placed on a circular track of radius R as shown in Figure 7.23a. Each object is separated by a distance $2\pi R/3$ measured along the track circumference. A phagocytic cell is initially

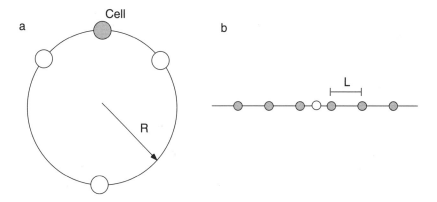

Figure 7.23. Diagram for Exercises 7.6(c) and 7.7(b).

on the track at the exact midpoint between two of the foreign objects. The cell moves randomly with a characteristic random motility μ, but is confined to always move along the track circumference. Assume that as soon as the cell encounters a foreign object, it instantaneously consumes it. Further assume that the persistence time is much shorter than the time required to move between objects on the track.

How long will it take for the cell to ingest all of the objects?

Exercise 7.7

Assume a phagocyte is placed on a linear track as shown in Figure 7.23b. The track also has multiple foreign objects, each separated by a distance L. The phagocyte (open circle) is initially placed at the midpoint between two foreign objects (closed circles).

a) Using the mean capture time equation, calculate the mean time required to capture four foreign objects. Assume that when the cell collides with the foreign object it takes time t_p for the object to be phagocytosed.
b) Assuming that the phagocyte has just consumed the nth foreign object, is there a general expression for the time to consume the $(n+1)$th foreign object?

Exercise 7.8 (provided by Song Li)

Given a peptide, how do you determine whether this peptide has a chemotaxis and/or haptotaxis effect on cell migration? Describe your experimental approach.

References

1. Poste, G. and I. Fidler, The pathogenesis of cancer metastasis. *Nature*, 1980, **283**, 139–146.
2. Trinkhaus, J.P., Cells into Organs. *The Forces that Shape the Embryo*, 2nd ed. Englewood Cliffs, NJ: Prentice-Hall, 1984.
3. Carmeliet, P. and R.K. Jain, Angiogenesis in cancer and other diseases. *Nature*, 2000, **407**, 249–257.
4. Wilkinson, P.C. and J.M. Lackie, The adhesion, migration, and chemotaxis of leukocytes in inflammation, in H.Z. Movat, ed., *Inflammatory Reaction*. Berlin: Springer-Verlag, 1979, pp. 47–88.
5. Ewan, K.B.R. and A.W. Everett, Migration of myogenic cells in the developing limb. *Basic and Applied Myology*, 1997, **7**(2), 131–135.
6. Bulte, J.W.M., et al., Neurotransplantation of magnetically labeled oligodendro-cyte progenitors: magnetic resonance tracking of cell migration and myelination. *Proceedings of the National Academy of Sciences*, 1999, **96**(26), 15256–15261.
7. Bellairs, R., A. Curtis, and G. Dunn, eds., *Cell Behavior*. Cambridge, UK: Cambridge University Press, 1982.

8. Lackie, J.M., *Cell Movement and Cell Behavior*. London: Allen & Unwin, 1986.
9. Comandon, J., Phagocytose in vitro des hematozaires du calfat (enregistrement cinematographique). *Compt. Rend. Soc. Biol.* (Paris), 1917, **80**, 314–316.
10. Okada, A., et al., Imaging cells in the developing nervous system with retrovirus expressing modified green fluorescent protein. *Experimental Neurology*, 1999, **156**(2), 394–406.
11. Kulesa, P.M. and S.E. Fraser, Neural crest cell dynamics revealed by time-lapse video microscopy of whole embryo chick explant cultures. *Developmental Biology*, 1998, **204**(2), 327–344.
12. Kulesa, P.M. and S.E. Fraser, Cell dynamics during somite boundary formation revealed by time-lapse analysis. *Science*, 2002, **298**, 991–995.
13. Sheen, V.L. and J.D. Macklis, Targeted neocortical death in adult mice guides migration and differentiation of transplanted embryonic neurons. *Journal of Neuroscience*, 1995, **15**, 8378–8392.
14. Andrade, W.N., M.G. Johnston, and J.B. Hay, The relationship of blood lymphocytes to the recirculating lymphocyte pool. *Blood*, 1998, **91**(5), 1653–1661.
15. Denk, W., D.W. Piston, and W.W. Webb, Two-photon molecular excitation in laser-scanning microscopy, in J.B. Pawley, ed., *Handbook of Biological Confocal Microscopy*. New York: Plenum Press, 1995, pp. 445–458.
16. Williams, R.M., D.W. Piston, and W.W. Webb, Two-photon molecular excitation provides intrinsic 3-dimensional resolution for laser-based microscopy and micro-photochemistry. *FASEB Journal*, 1994, **8**(11), 804–813.
17. Schoepf, U., et al., Intracellular magnetic labeling of lymphocytes for *in vivo* trafficking studies. *Biotechniques*, 1998, **24**(4), 642.
18. Jacobs, R.E., et al., Looking deeper into vertebrate development. *Trends in Cell Biology*, 1999, **9**(2), 73–76.
19. Bonney, E.A. and P. Matzinger, The maternal immune system's interaction with circulating fetal cells. *Journal of Immunology*, 1997, **158**(1), 40–47.
20. Huang, G.Y., et al., Gap junction-mediated cell–cell communication modulates mouse neural crest migration. *Journal of Cell Biology*, 1998, **143**, 1725–1734.
21. Allan, R.B. and P.C. Wilkinson, A visual analysis of chemotactic and chemokinetic locomotion of human neutrophil leukocytes: use of a new assay with *Candida albicans* as gradient source. *Experimental Cell Research*, 1978, **111**, 191–203.
22. Gail, M. and C. Boone, The locomotion of mouse fibroblasts in tissue culture. *Biophysical Journal*, 1970, **10**, 980–993.
23. Zigmond, S.H., Ability of polymorphonuclear leukocytes to orient in gradients of chemotactic factors. *Journal of Cell Biology*, 1977, **75**, 606–616.
24. Nelson, R.D., P.G. Quie, and R.L. Simmons, Chemotaxis under agarose: a new and simple method for measuring chemotaxis and spontaneous migration of human polymorphonuclear leukocytes and monocytes. *Journal of Immunology*, 1975, **115**, 1650–1656.
25. Cutler, J.E., A simple *in vitro* method for studies on chemotaxis. *Proceedings of the Society for Experimental Biology and Medicine*, 1974, **147**, 471–474.
26. Boyden, S.V., The chemotactic effect of mixtures of antibody and antigen on polymorphonuclear leukocytes. *Journal of Experimental Medicine*, 1962, **115**, 453–466.
27. Wilkinson, P., J. Lackie, and R. Allan, Methods for measuring leukocyte locomotion, in N. Catsimpoolas, ed., *Cell Analysis*. New York: Plenum Press, 1952, pp 145–194.

28. Dunn, G.A., Characterizing a kinesis response: time averaged measures of cell speed and directional persistence. *Agents & Actions Supplement*, 1983, **12**, 14–33.
29. Lauffenburger, D., Measurement of phenomenological parameters for leukocyte motility and chemotaxis. *Agents & Actions Supplement*, 1983, **12**, 34–53.
30. Buettner, H.M., D.A. Lauffenburger, and S.H. Zigmond, Measurement of leukocyte motility and chemotaxis parameters with the Millipore filter assay. *Journal of Immunological Methods*, 1989, **123**, 25–37.
31. Farrell, B., R. Daniele, and D. Lauffenburger, Quantitative relationships between single-cell and cell-population model parameters for chemosensory migration responses of alveolar macrophages to C5a. *Cell Motility and the Cytoskeleton*, 1990, **16**, 279–293.
32. Bell, E.B., B. Ivarsson, and C. Merrill, Production of a tissue-like structure by contraction of collagen lattices by human fibroblasts with different proliferative potential. *Proceedings of the National Academy of Sciences USA*, 1979, **75**, 1274–1278.
33. Schor, S., T. Allen, and C. Harrison, Cell migration through three-dimensional gels of native collagen fibres: collagenolytic activity is not required for the migration of two permanent cell lines. *Journal of Cell Science*, 1980, **46**, 171–186.
34. Schor, S., A. Schor, and G. Bazill, The effects of fibronectin on the migration of human foreskin fibroblasts and Syrian hamster melanoma cells into three-dimensional gels of native collagen fibres. *Journal of Cell Science*, 1981, **48**, 301–314.
35. Elsdale, T. and J. Bard, Collagen substrate for studies of cell behavior. *Journal of Cell Biology*, 1972, **54**, 626–637.
36. Richards, J., et al., Method for culturing mammary epithelial cells in a rat tail collagen gel matrtix. *Journal of Tissue Cultue Methods*, 1983, **8**, 31–36.
37. Wilkinson, P., A visual study of chemotaxis of human lymphocytes using a collagen-gel assay. *Journal of Immunological Methods*, 1985, **76**, 105–120.
38. Haston, W., J. Shields, and P. Wilkinson, Lymphocyte locomotion and attachment on two-dimensional surfaces and in three-dimensional matrices. *Journal of Cell Biology*, 1982, **92**, 747–752.
39. Haston, W. and P. Wilkinson, Visual methods for measuring leukocyte locomotion. *Methods in Enzymology*, 1988, **162**, 17–38.
40. Brown, A., Neutrophil granulocytes: adhesion and locomotion on collagen substrata and in collagen matrices. *Journal of Cell Science*, 1982, **58**, 455–467.
41. Schor, S., Cell proliferation and migration on collagen substrata *in vitro*. *Journal of Cell Science*, 1980, **41**, 159–175.
42. Grinnell, F., Migration of human neutrophils in hydrated collagen lattices. *Journal of Cell Science*, 1982, **58**, 95–108.
43. Sanchez-Madrid, F. and M. Angel del Pozo, Leucocyte polarization in cell migration and immune interactions. *EMBO Journal*, 1999, **18**(3), 501–511.
44. Rotsch, C., K. Jacobson, and M. Radmacher, Dimensional and mechanical dynamics of active and stable edges in motile fibroblasts investigated by using atomic force microscopy. *Proceedings of the National Academy of Sciences USA*, 1999, **96**, 921–926.
45. DiMilla, P.A., K. Barbee, and D.A. Lauffenburger, Mathematical model for the effects of adhesion and mechanics on cell migration speed. *Biophysical Journal*, 1991, **60**, 15–37.
46. Palecek, S.P., et al., Integrin–ligand binding properties govern cell migration speed through cell-substratum adhesiveness. *Nature*, 1997, **385**, 537–540.

47. Levine, I.N., *Physical Chemistry*. New York: McGraw-Hill, 1978.
48. Einstein, A., A new determination of molecular dimensions. *Annalen der Physik*, 1906, **19**, 289–306 (in German).
49. Whitney, C.A., *Random Processes in Physical Systems*. New York: John Wiley & Sons, 1990.
50. Boon, J.P. and S. Yip, *Molecular Hydrodynamics*. New York: Dover Publications, 1980.
51. Doob, J., The Brownian movement and stochastic equations. *Annals of Mathematics*, 1942, **43**, 351–369.
52. Crank, J., *The Mathematics of Diffusion*. 2nd ed. Oxford: Oxford University Press, 1975.
53. Carslaw, H.S. and J.C. Jaeger, *Conduction of Heat in Solids*, 2nd ed. Oxford: Oxford University Press, 1959.
54. Saltzman, W.M., *Drug Delivery: Engineering Principles for Drug Therapy*. New York: Oxford University Press, 2001.
55. Tranquillo, R. and D. Lauffenburger, Stochastic model of leukocyte chemosensory movement. *Journal of Mathematical Biology*, 1987, **25**, 229–262.
56. Parkhurst, M.R. and W.M. Saltzman, Quantification of human neutrophil motility in three-dimensional collagen gels: effect of collagen concentration. *Biophysical Journal*, 1992, **61**, 306–315.
57. Tranquillo, R., D. Lauffenburger, and S. Zigmond, A stochastic model for leukocyte random motility and chemotaxis based on receptor binding fluctuations. *Journal of Cell Biology*, 1988, **106**, 303–309.
58. Parent, C.A. and P.N. Devreotes, A cell's sense of direction. *Science*, 1999, **284**, 765–770.
59. Bray, D., Cell Movement. New York: Garland Publishing, 1992.
60. Lauffenburger, D.A. and J.J. Linderman, *Receptors: Models for Binding, Trafficking, and Signaling*. New York: Oxford University Press, 1993.
61. Alt, W., Biased random walk models for chemotaxis and related diffusion approximations. *Journal of Mathematical Biology*, 1980, **9**, 147–177.
62. Othmer, H., S. Dunbar, and W. Alt, Models of dispersal in biological systems. *Journal of Mathematical Biology*, 1988, **26**, 263–298.
63. Rivero, M., et al., Transport models for chemotactic cell populations based on individual cell behavior. *Chemical Engineering Science*, 1989, **44**, 2881–2897.
64. Dickinson, R.B. and R.T. Tranquillo, Transport equations and indices for random and biased cell migration based on single cell properties. *SIAM Journal of Applied Mathematics*, 1995, **55**(5), 1419–1454.
65. Parkhurst, M.R., Leukocyte migration in mucus and interaction with mucosal epithelia: potential targets for immunoprotection and therapy, in *Chemical Engineering*. Baltimore, MD: Johns Hopkins University Press, 1994.
66. Tranquillo, R.T., Phenomenological and fundamental descriptions of leukocyte random motility and chemotaxis. PhD Thesis, University of Pennsylvania, 1986.
67. Berg, H. and E. Purcell, Physics of chemoreception. *Biophysical Journal*, 1977, **20**, 193–219.
68. Lois, C., J.-M. Garcia-Verdugo, and A. Alvarez-Buylla, Chain migration of neuronal precursors. *Science*, 1996, **271**, 978–981.
69. Berg, H.C., *Random Walks in Biology*. Princeton, NJ: Princeton University Press, 1983.
70. Fick, A., *Ueber Diffusion. Annalen der Physik*, 1855, **94**, 59–86.

71. Dunn, G.A. and A.F. Brown, A unified approach to analyzing cell motility. *Journal of Cell Science Supplement*, 1987, **8**, 81–102.
72. Lodish, H., et al., *Molecular Cell Biology*. New York: W.H. Freeman, 1995.
73. Saltzman, W.M., et al., Antibody diffusion in human cervical mucus. *Biophysical Journal*, 1994, **66**, 508–515.
74. Calof, A.L. and A.D. Lander, Relationship between neuronal migration and cell–substratum adhesion: laminin and merosin promote olfactory neuronal migration but are anti-adhesive. *Journal of Cell Biology*, 1991, **115**(3), 779–794.
75. Hatten, M.E. and C.A. Mason, Mechanisms of glial-guided neuronal migration *in vitro* and *in vivo*. *Experientia*, 1990, **46**, 907–916.
76. Fishman, R.B. and M.E. Hatten, Multiple receptor systems promote CNS neural migration. *Journal of Neuroscience*, 1993, **13**(8), 3485–3495.
77. Keller, E.F. and L.A. Segel, Model for chemotaxis. *Journal of Theoretical Biology*, 1971, **30**, 225.

8

Cell Aggregation and
Tissue Equivalents

> ... what could it be but the kingly voice of the Aggregate itself.
>
> Thomas Pynchon, *Gravity's Rainbow*

Development of an individual from a fertilized egg involves a rich choreography of cell division, cell movement, and cell shape change. Cells replicate, interact with their surroundings, and move individually and in coordination. Development produces a multicellular organism in which cells are organized into cooperative communities. Adult tissues and organs are orderly ensembles of cells—usually the ensemble contains more than one type of cell—in which both ensemble architecture and dynamic interactions between individual cells are critical for proper function (Figure 8.1).

Tissues are collections of cells, united for a common function. Tissues that differ in function also differ in architecture, that is, in the shape and arrangement of cells. Even in the absence of other information, this observation could lead one to speculate on the power of the influence of cell–cell interactions on tissue development and function. It is well known that selective cell adhesion is a fundamental mechanism underlying mammalian development (see Chapter 3). But cell adhesion and cell–cell communication are essential throughout the lifetime of an organism. The previous three chapters described the biophysical processes of division, adhesion, and motility and introduced some of the molecular mechanisms that cells use to interact with, and learn about, their environment. This chapter considers the relationship of cell adhesion to cell aggregation, or the formation and maintenance of cell communities. The role of cell adhesion in circulation and trafficking of cells throughout the body is discussed in Chapter 10.

8.1 Overview and Significance

A community is often more effective than the sum of its members. This is abundantly evident in biological systems; swarms of bees and colonies of ants are more effective than their numbers suggest because bees and ants can

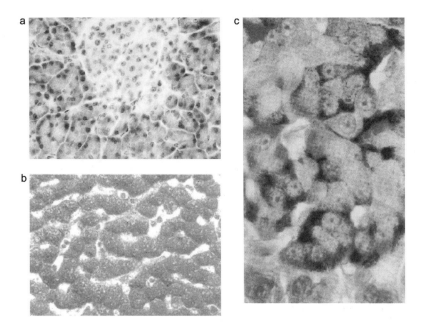

Figure 8.1. Cell aggregation within the pancreas and liver (adapted from [51]): (a) islet of Langerhans; (b) liver (stained for glycogen deposits); (c) islet of Langerhans (high magnification, stained to differentiate different endocrine cell types).

act in coordination. Synergistic activity in multicomponent biological systems requires information exchange between units and control mechanisms to guide a unit response.

Cell aggregates are communities of cells that are organized in a specific three-dimensional architecture. The preferred aggregation pattern within a particular tissue or organ has important consequences with regard to tissue function. Certain architectures produce essential physical properties; the barrier properties of skin and intestinal mucosa are produced by cell assembly into stratified layers and the filtration of blood is accomplished efficiently by the tuft-like arrangements of glomerular capillaries within Bowman's capsule. Other arrangements are important because they optimize cell–cell contact, as in the liver, or segregate tissues into different functional regions, as in the lymph nodes or thymus. Some tissue architectures are so complex that they are difficult to describe completely, but they are nonetheless important to the function of the tissue; for example, the network arrangement of cells in the nervous system is critical for its function.

Aggregate formation is essential during development, but it occurs throughout life. Aggregation can result from simple biophysical processes. Red blood cells form aggregates, called rouleaux, at low flow rates, due to the presence of proteins such as fibrinogen. This microscopic behavior affects the macroscopic behavior of whole blood; at low shear rates the cells assemble into stacks, which increases the viscosity of the blood (Figure 8.2).

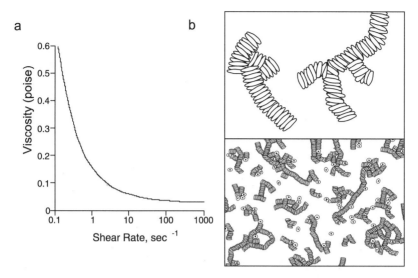

Figure 8.2. Aggregation characteristics of red blood cells influence their rheological behavior (adapted from Cooney, see chapter on blood rheology [47]). (a) Viscosity changes with shear rate for red blood cell suspensions (under certain conditions) and whole blood. (b) The change in viscosity is related to the shear-dependent aggregation of red cells into rouleaux.

Our understanding of cooperative behavior in cell aggregates derives largely from studies of aggregated cells in culture. Tissues frequently perform functions that are more efficient, or even qualitatively different, than the function performed by an individual cell. This increase in efficiency can result from cell–cell communication, and it often requires contact between cells in the population. For example, adult hepatocytes form spheroids under a variety of conditions, such as when cultured on positively charged polystyrene surfaces [1]; in this case, each 100–150 µm diameter spheroid contains ~100 hepatocytes in a typical cuboidal morphology. In the spheroid state, the cells synthesize little DNA but maintain high levels of albumin secretion. This situation is reversed when spheroids are disaggregated by culture on collagen-coated plates; cells in monolayer culture exhibit a transient increase in DNA synthesis and a decrease in albumin secretion.

Cells from fetal nervous tissue, when dissociated and maintained in culture, will reorganize to form multicellular structures; the architecture of the structure can be varied by controlling the culture conditions [2]. Embryonic chicken optic lobe neurons attach to the poly-L-lysine-coated surface and exhibit distinct and reproducible patterns of migration and aggregation on the culture dish. The neurons attach to the culture surface and form fasciculating processes [3]. Other neurons migrate along these processes, apparently by attaching to the surface, and migrate towards the cell body, where an aggregate of cell bodies is formed. Over the course of ~ 4 days in culture, aggregates of ~ 30–80 µm diameter are formed. The size of the aggregates is presumably related to the rate of cell migration; aggregate size can be increased by the addition of a purified ganglioside mixture and inhibited by the addition of a monoclonal antibody that specifically binds certain gangliosides. Similar observations of migration-dependent aggregation have been reported in three-dimensional cultures of the neuron-like PC12 cell cultures [4].

Cell aggregates within tissues are often composed of more than one cell type, which provides more opportunities for structural complexity. In the pancreas, cells within islets of Langerhans are not randomly organized (Figure 8.3a). The typical three-dimensional arrangement of cells is not maintained in islets from diabetic animals, which suggests that the local organization of cells is related to the function of the tissue. Disassociated islet cells form aggregates in culture, and several studies have shown that the function of the aggregates is

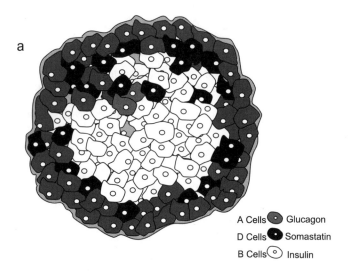

a

A Cells ⊙ Glucagon
D Cells ● Somastatin
B Cells ○ Insulin

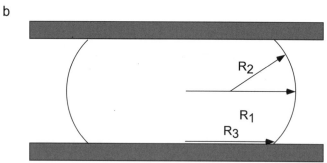

b

R_2

R_1

R_3

Figure 8.3. Organization of cells within the islet of Langerhans. (a) A pancreatic islet contains multiple cell types with specialized biochemical functions. The organization of different cells within an aggregate is not random; the figure shows how cells are organized within a typical islet (redrawn from [48]). (b) Method for measuring the properties of aggregates by controlled compression between two parallel plates.

related to its cellular organization [5–7]. In culture, aggregation begins after ~5–6 hours, when small aggregates (2–4 cells) are formed. After 24 hours much larger aggregates (~100 cells) are observed; after several days the diameter of the aggregates can reach several hundred micrometers. The reformed aggregates secrete insulin and respond to glucose by increasing insulin production, but the overall function of the aggregate depends on the architecture that it achieved in culture [5–7]. For example, dissociated cells will reorganize into cellular aggregates containing B cells and non-B cells. When allowed to aggregate in the presence of tumor necrosis factor-α (TNF-α), the cellular organization and function within the aggregate is altered. These effects are reversible: the normal segregated morphology is recovered when TNF-α is removed. Since the adhesive properties of individual cells also change when incubated in TNF-α, this suggests that the change of aggregate morphology is related to adhesive properties of the individual cells. The formation of cell assemblies in culture mimics, in many ways, the architecture of a fully developed islet.

Cell aggregates are often essential model systems for studying the process of tissue development. For example, aggregated cells from the retina provide a powerful model for studying the development of the layered structure of retinal tissue [8]. In the case of the retina, the complex structure of normal tissue is produced in stages involving cell sorting (which is described more fully in the next section) as well as growth and differentiation of groups of cells within the aggregate.

8.2 Cell Aggregation and Cell Sorting

Cell aggregates are important tools in the study of tissue function, permitting correlation of cell–cell interactions with cell differentiation, viability, and migration, as well as subsequent tissue formation. The aggregate morphology permits re-establishment of cell–cell contacts normally present in tissues; therefore, cell function and survival are frequently enhanced in aggregate culture [6, 9–12]. To employ cell aggregates in this manner, techniques for controlling the formation of aggregates from specific cells of interest must be developed.

8.2.1 Methods for Cell Aggregation

Aggregates are usually formed by incubating cells in suspension, using gentle rotational stirring to disperse the cells. This procedure was first described by Moscona, who formed cell suspensions in medium containing 10% serum [13]. Neural retinal cells from a 7-day chick embryo formed several large aggregates (300–1,000 μm in diameter) after 24 hr in culture with a typical histological arrangement; liver cells from a 7-day chick embryo formed 1–2 large spherical aggregates of ~1.5 mm diameter; limb bud mesoblasts from 4-day embryos formed many smaller aggregates (50–300 μm diameter); mesonephros from a 7-day embryo formed heterogeneous aggregates of 20–900 μm diameter; other cell types were also examined. Mixtures of heterologous cells sort in the aggregate into homogeneous regions, as observed with other aggregation methods. In this rotary suspension system, cell concentration can influence the size of cell aggregates obtained, with aggregate diameter increasing with increasing concentration and decreasing with increasing rotational speed (although aggregation of some cells is not sensitive to these experimental variables). In general, the ability of cells to aggregate decreases with temperature, such that no aggregation is observed below 15°C.

While this simple method is suitable for aggregation of many cells, serum or serum proteins must be added to promote cell aggregation in many cases [14], thus making it difficult to characterize the aggregation process and to control the size and composition of the aggregate. Alternately, large aggregates can be formed by gentle centrifugation of a cell suspension to form a condensed pellet which will subsequently "round-up" into a spherical aggregate during suspension culture [15]. Specialized techniques can be used to produce aggregates in certain cases, principally by controlling cell detachment from a solid substratum. For example, stationary culture of hepatocytes above a non-adherent surface [11, 12] or attached to a temperature-sensitive polymer substratum have been used to form aggregates. None of these techniques, however, allow the investigator to adjust the affinity of the cell–cell interactions or to control these interactions on the molecular level. To accomplish this, water-soluble derivatives of poly(ethylene glycol) (PEG) have been produced in which the amino terminus of either RGD or YIGSR was covalently coupled to carboxyl termini on the linear PEG chain. These synthetic molecules can enhance the aggregation of cells in suspension [16], and suggest new methods for molecular control of the cell aggregation process.

8.2.2 Cell Sorting

When two or more cell types are assembled into aggregates, the initial distribution of cell type can change after aggregate formation. Often, the cells of different types will congregate into regions or layers. This phenomenon was presented in Chapter 3; cell-sorting behavior has provided important clues into the mechanisms that cells use to form segregated communities and patterns during development.

One of the most striking aspects of cell sorting is its analogy to the spreading of immiscible liquids. Intermixing cell populations and immiscible liquids share several fundamental characteristics: both are collections of many cohesive mobile subunits. In liquid systems, cohesion between molecules is essential for maintaining its condensed nature. When two immiscible liquids (that is, two liquids whose subunits prefer to adhere to their own kind of molecule rather than the other) are contacted, the liquids will separate into two phases with one phase surrounding the other (Figure 8.4).

This separation or sorting process in a liquid is a natural consequence of the minimization of free energy. A single liquid phase—consisting of a single type of mobile cohesive subunits—will form a sphere at equilibrium. The spherical arrangement maximizes contact between cohesive units by leaving the

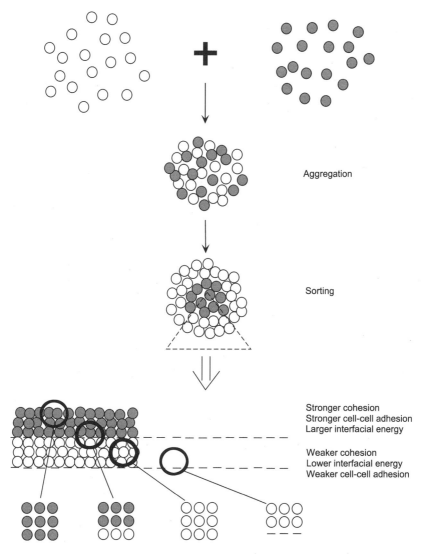

Figure 8.4. Cells within aggregates sort into regions of similar cell adhesion characteristics. The characteristics of cell sorting appear to follow many of the physical principles that govern the behavior of immiscible liquid phases. The liquid with the highest surface tension, reflecting the largest cohesive forces between molecules, will form an internal phase surrounded by the liquid with lower surface tension.

minimum number of units in "undesirable" surface positions where they are sacrificing contact with other cohesive partners. The sphere geometry minimizes surface/volume ratio: subunits within the sphere are surrounded by identical subunits; subunits at the surface experience a different environment since they contact both of the other subunits and a separate phase. When subunits of two immiscible liquids are dispersed, they will sort into spherical phases in which the less cohesive liquid surrounds the other; that is, the less cohesive liquid will "spread" over the other liquid.

Steinberg and his colleagues have shown that cultured cells exhibit a property similar to surface tension—or cohesiveness—that can be used to predict sorting behavior (recall the discussion in Chapter 3 and review Figures 3.13 and 3.14) [17]. The "surface tension" within a cell aggregate can be measured by compressing the aggregate and observing its deformation behavior (recall also the example in Chapter 5). When a cellular aggregate is compressed between two parallel plates, it adopts the configuration shown in Figure 8.3b. The surface tension of this aggregate can be obtained from Laplace's equation

$$\frac{F_{c,\text{equil}}}{\pi R_3^2} = \sigma\left(\frac{1}{R_1} + \frac{1}{R_2}\right) \tag{8-1}$$

where $F_{c,\text{equil}}$ is the equilibrium value of the compressive force applied to the plates, and the radii are defined as in Figure 8.3b.

The surface tension σ in Equation 8-1 provides an estimate of the interfacial tension between the aggregate and the liquid medium that surrounds the aggregate. Surface tension has been measured for aggregates formed from a variety of embryonic tissues, and it varies with the tissue: the interfacial tension was 1.6×10^{-5} N/cm for aggregates of neural retinal cells and 20×10^{-5} N/cm for aggregates of limb bud cells [17]. If the aggregate is composed of cells of a single type, then one can infer the level of cohesion between individual cells from the overall equilibrium surface tension σ. Dimensional analysis suggests that σ is proportional to $N \times J$, where N is the number of cell adhesion molecules forming the bond between adjacent cells (per unit contact area) and J is the effective binding energy of each bond [18]. Assuming the same cell adhesion pairs (and therefore the same energy per bond) for each of the embryonic tissues, which is probably not a good assumption, this simple analysis suggests that the neural retinal cells have about 10 times the number of active cell adhesion molecules per unit area as the limb bud cells.

8.3 Models of Cell Aggregation

8.3.1 Model Development

Cell aggregates are cell communities in which the individual members are in direct cell–cell contact with other members. Aggregates can grow directly, by division of member cells, or indirectly, by migration and "joining" of new cells from outside (Figure 8.5). The rate of aggregate growth by division is directly related to the rate of division; if division is responsible, cell number within an aggregate should follow the growth kinetics of the cell population (see Chapter 4). This section considers the alternate situation in which cells join an aggregate by migration from outside the community. What is the rate of aggregate growth in this situation?

a

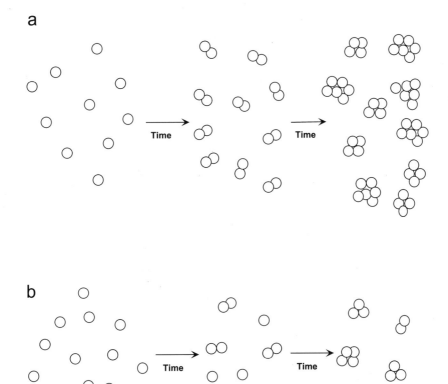

b

Figure 8.5. Mechanisms for aggregate growth: aggregate size can grow by a variety of mechanisms. For example, the aggregate size may increase in size because of cell division within the aggregates (panel a) or because new cellular units are being added to the aggregates, without any increase in total cell number (panel b).

Migration-driven aggregates grow because two small aggregates (or single cells) collide and adhere to one another. Collisions between two particles, one of volume v_i and another of volume v_j, result in a larger particle of volume v_k:

$$v_k = v_i + v_j \tag{8-2}$$

If collision or adhesion introduces interstitial space between the particles, then the total volume after collision may be larger than v_k. If N_{ij} is the rate of collision between particles of size i and j, the rate of formation of particles of size k is given by:

$$\frac{dn_k}{dt} = \frac{1}{2} \sum_{i=1, j=k-i}^{i=k-1} N_{ij} - \sum_{i=1}^{\infty} M_{ik}; \qquad \text{for} \qquad k = 2, L\ldots, \infty \tag{8-3}$$

where n_k is the number of particles of size k, with volume v_k, per volume. The total number of elementary particles is assumed constant, so that the number of particles containing a single unit (n_1) is found by mass balance:

$$n_{\text{total}} = \sum_{i=1}^{\infty} i n_i \qquad (8\text{-}4)$$

where n_{total} is the number of elementary particles introduced into the system initially. The factor 1/2 is included with the first summation in Equation 8-3 because collisions of particles of size i and j are counted twice. Assuming the collision frequency N_{ij} is first order in n_i and n_j [19], the collision frequency becomes

$$N_{ij} = \beta(v_i, v_j) n_i n_j \qquad (8\text{-}5)$$

where β is the collision frequency function, which depends on the physical mechanisms controlling particle collision. Substitution of Equation 8-5 into Equation 8-3 yields a set of coupled differential equations:

$$\frac{dn_k}{dt} = \frac{1}{2} \sum_{\substack{i=1, j=k-i}}^{i=k-1} \beta_{ij} n_i n_j - \sum_{i=1}^{\infty} \beta_{ik} n_i n_k; \qquad \text{for} \qquad k = 2, \ldots, \infty \qquad (8\text{-}6)$$

If the collision frequency terms—$\beta(v_i, v_j)$ or β_{ij}—are known, the evolution of aggregates up to N in size—$n_1(t), n_2(t), \ldots, n_N(t)$—can be found by solving the $N-1$ differential equations implied in Equation 8-6 together with Equation 8-4. Initial conditions—$n_1(0), n_2(0), \ldots, n_N(0)$—are needed to fully specify the problem.

In completely unmixed systems, particle motion is Brownian, so the rate of Brownian diffusion controls the collision frequency. Even in well-mixed systems, an unstirred layer near the particle surface provides a resistance to collision. In these cases, collision frequency depends on the rate of particle diffusion through the unstirred layer. A model for the dynamics of Brownian collision was first developed by Smoluchowski [20]. For this calculation, a spherical coordinate system is centered on a single particle and is assumed to move with the particle. The concentration of particles, assumed to be of type i (i-particles), surrounding the central particle, is n_i within the bulk (Figure 8.6).

The rate of particle diffusion towards the central particle is determined by considering a mass balance around the central particle, which yields the usual transient diffusion equation

$$\frac{\partial n}{\partial t} = \frac{1}{r^2} \frac{\partial}{\partial r} \left[D r^2 \frac{\partial n}{\partial r} \right] \qquad (8\text{-}7)$$

where n is the concentration of particles surrounding the central particle and D is the characteristic diffusion coefficient for the particles. The initial and boundary conditions are

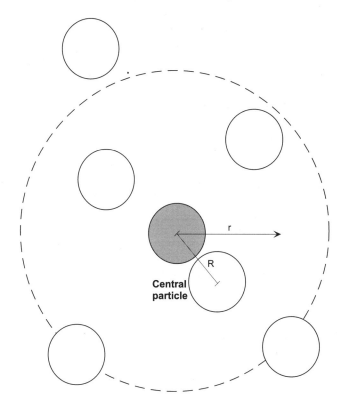

Figure 8.6. Model for particle collision frequency in Brownian aggregation. To calculate the collision frequency, a spherical coordinate system is centered on a central particle. The coordinate system is assumed to move with the central particle, so that only diffusive transport of other particles from the bulk to the surface of the central particle needs to be considered.

$$
\left.
\begin{aligned}
n &= n_i & \text{at} &\quad t = 0 & \text{for} &\quad r > R \\
n &= 0 & \text{at} &\quad r = R & \text{for} &\quad t > 0 \\
n &= n_i & \text{at} &\quad r \to \infty & \text{for} &\quad t > 0
\end{aligned}
\right\} \tag{8-8}
$$

where R is an interaction distance at which the central particle and the diffusing particles will collide and stick (see Figure 8.6). The differential equation, 8-7, can be solved subject to these conditions, producing

$$
n = n_i \left(1 - \frac{R}{r} \operatorname{erfc}\left[\frac{r - R}{2\sqrt{Dt}} \right] \right) \tag{8-9}
$$

which reduces to the following at steady state:

$$
n = n_i \left(1 - \frac{R}{r} \right) \tag{8-10}
$$

The time required to reach steady state depends on the characteristics of the system. Figure 8.7a shows the change in particle concentration with position as a function of time for a system in which the central particle is 10 µm in radius and the diffusion coefficient is 10^{-7} cm^2/s; in this case, it takes about 1000 seconds to achieve steady state.

The rate of collision can be calculated from the flux of i-particles that reach the interaction distance:

$$j|_{r=R} = -D \frac{\partial n}{\partial r}\Big|_{r=R} = -\frac{Dn_i}{R} \tag{8-11}$$

To determine the total number of collisions, Equation 8-11 is multiplied by the surface area and the total number of central particles, assumed of type j (j-particles):

$$N_{ij} = -(4\pi R^2)j|_{r=R}n_j = 4\pi D R n_i n_j \tag{8-12}$$

This derivation has assumed that the central particle is motionless with respect to the diffusing particles that surround it. In fact, the central particle is also diffusing, so that the diffusion coefficient D in Equation 8-12 is the sum of the tracer diffusion coefficient of i-particles, D_i, and the tracer diffusion coefficient of j-particles, D_j. This diffusion coefficient can be estimated by assuming that the particles obey the Stokes–Einstein equation:

$$D_{ij} = D_i + D_j = \frac{k_B T}{6\pi \eta r_i} + \frac{k_B T}{6\pi \eta r_j} \tag{8-13}$$

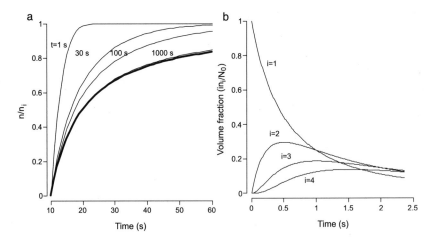

Figure 8.7. Evolution of aggregate size distribution. (a) Variation in concentration in the vicinity of the central particle. The curves indicate Equation 8-9 for various times (1, 30, 100, and 1000 s) with a diffusion coefficient of 10^{-7} cm^2/s. The thick line shows the corresponding steady-state solution from Equation 8-10. (b) A simplification ($r_i = r_j$) was assumed to permit solution of Equation 8-14, subject to the initial condition that all N_0 particles were singly dispersed. See [49] for details.

where k_B is Boltzmann's constant, T is absolute temperature, and η is the viscosity of the fluid surrounding the particles. The interaction distance R is usually assumed to be equal to the distance between the particle centers on contact:

$$R = r_i + r_j \tag{8-14}$$

Substituting Equations 8-12 to 8-14 into the governing equation for aggregate growth, 8-3, yields

$$\frac{dn_k}{dt} = \frac{k_B T}{3\eta} \left\{ \sum_{i=1,j=k-i}^{i=k-1} n_i n_j (r_i + r_j) \left(\frac{1}{r_i} + \frac{1}{r_j} \right) - 2n_k \sum_{i=1}^{\infty} n_i (r_i + r_k) \left(\frac{1}{r_i} + \frac{1}{r_k} \right) \right\} \tag{8-15}$$

Figure 8.7b shows an approximate solution for $i = 1$ to 4, assuming that all of the particles are singly dispersed at $t = 0$.

This balance equation approach for calculating the size evolution of aggregating colloidal particles has been tested under a variety of conditions [19].

8.3.2 Examples of Applications of Aggregation Models

These flocculation equations have been modified to analyze the formation of hepatocyte aggregates in two-dimensional culture. Experimentally, hepatocytes were maintained on a non-adhesive surface; cells rest on the surface and move due to the presence of vibrations and thermal motions in the fluid (Figure 8.8). When two hepatocytes collide, they aggregate. To analyze experimental data, Equation 8-6 was solved with collision frequencies obtained using a two-dimensional analog of the diffusion equation. A similar approach has been used to analyze the aggregation of microcarriers within slowly rotating bioreactors [21].

For tissue engineering applications, it is useful to consider a simpler situation in which cells are suspended within a gel, such that cell migration through the gel matrix—rather than Brownian motion in a fluid—controls the rate of collision. In this case, single cells move in a pattern very similar to Brownian motion with the diffusion coefficient replaced by a random motility coefficient μ (see Equation 7-32 and related discussion). If we assume that only single cells can move, and that aggregates containing two or more cells are immotile, the equations can be greatly simplified. The reader is encouraged to explore this situation by completing Exercise 8.1.

8.4 Cell-Populated Tissue Equivalents

Since the early twentieth century scientists have used cell and tissue culture to systematically test hypotheses regarding cell behavior in the body [22]. For example, cells cultured in chemically defined media were used to iden-

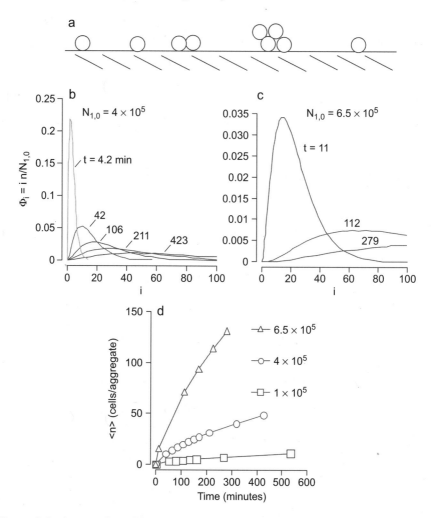

Figure 8.8. Aggregation of hepatocytes upon a non-adherent surface. (a) Hepatocytes were cultured on non-adhesive surfaces; cell aggregation occurred during subsequent culture. (b, c) Numerical simulation of the balance equations yielded size distributions which shift to the right with increasing time. Here, the *y*-axis indicates the density function or the fraction of the total number of cells that are included in aggregates of size *i*. The solution is shown for two different initial densities in (b) and (c). (d) The mean aggregate size depends on the initial concentration of hepatocytes on the surface. For more details, see [50].

tify growth factors and minimum essential nutrients for cultured cells [23–25]. Similarly, the role of extracellular matrix (ECM) in modulating cell behavior was studied in cultured cells attached to solid substrates with adsorbed ECM proteins [26, 27]. Cells within tissues encounter a complex chemical and physical environment that is quite different from commonly used culture conditions: each cell is surrounded by a matrix of hydrated macromolecules (as described in Section 6.4); each cell can contact other cells of the same or different type (as described in the previous sections of this chapter); each cell is bathed in an aqueous medium containing soluble factors that provide signals for growth and differentation (as described in Chapter 4). By culturing cells under conditions that are similar to those found in tissues, specific issues concerning the relationship between cell function and tissue structure can be isolated and studied. In addition, as we will see in later chapters of this book, *in vitro* methods for growing cells in tissue-like environments may have direct applications in organ regeneration and tissue engineering.

Cell aggregation is one method for re-establishing cell–cell contact and a more "natural" three-dimensional structure. But it is also possible to create three-dimensional cell-tissue-like structures by suspending individual cells within a semi-solid medium such as agarose or collagen gel. In these materials (which are sometimes called cell-populated tissue equivalents or engineered tissue constructs), cell concentration (or density) can be changed by the investigator, with concomitant changes in the number of cell–cell interactions. In addition, extracellular matrix materials can be added into the interstitial spaces between cells in the three-dimensional culture.

Many previous investigators have used three-dimensional cell culture methods to simulate the chemical and physical environment of tissues [28–35]. Many cell types—including white blood cells, fibroblasts, pancreatic cells, and epithelial cells—have been cultured in gels containing ECM components. Most of these previous studies were descriptive, but a few engineering analyses of cell behavior in three-dimensional environments are now available [36–39]. For example, Figures 7.2c, 7.6, and 7.8 illustrate the migration of neutrophils through a three-dimensional collagen matrix.

The mechanical behavior of three-dimensional tissue equivalents has been studied in detail. The basic mechanical aspects of tissue equivalents were introduced in Chapter 5 (see Section 5.5.3). For example, predictive mechanical models of tissue equivalents can be developed from biphasic models [40], and the deformation of individual cells within a skeletal muscle tissue construct can be examined by finite element models [41].

One important use of tissue equivalents is for the creation of models of tissue structure that can not be accomplished in conventional culture. For example, in early work on tissue equivalents, tissue models were produced by suspension of active fibroblasts within gels of collagen [33] and the formation of three-dimensional tissue structures was examined by suspending mammary epithelial cells within collagen gels [35, 42]. Recently, tissue equivalents have been used to study the role of environmental cues and gene expression in the development of mature vascular networks [43]. Pituitary cells have been reaggregated in serum-free medium to estimate the rate of diffusion of macromolecules in the three-dimensional tissue [44]. The resulting aggregates are several hundred micrometers in diameter. The diffusion coefficient of FITC-BSA within the aggregates was estimated by FRAP (Table 8.1).

Table 8.1
Diffusion of FITC-BSA in Pituitary Cell Aggregates

Preparation	Diffusion Coefficient $(10^{-7}\,\text{cm}^2/\text{s})$
Aggregates from 14-day-old female rats	1.33 ± 0.31
Aggregates from adult female rats	2.45 ± 0.55
Aggregates enriched in folliculo-stellate cells from adult female rats	1.85 ± 0.77
Free in solution	Range 6.00–6.45

Data collected from [44].

Of course, these cell-populated tissue equivalents may also be useful as precursors for use in tissue engineering. Tissue-engineered skin can be produced by suspending dermal cells within gels [45]; this technique is a precursor to tissue engineering products such as Dermagraft (Advanced Tissue Sciences), which is discussed more completely in Chapter 13.

Summary

- Tissues are collections of cells that are organized into structures; the aggregation of cells into multicellular units can be a precursor for tissue assembly.
- Cells cultured within aggregates are often different in function to cells cultured as monolayers.
- The final architecture of a cellular aggregate is determined by rearrangement of cells within the aggregate (that is, cell sorting), by proliferation, and by differentiation of cells. Many of the features of sorting can be explained by defining a "surface tension" for cells within an aggregate.
- The kinetics of aggregation can be predicted by modeling the steps that lead to aggregate growth; one common model assumes that diffusion determines the rate of particle–particle collision, which is a prerequisite for aggregate growth.
- Cells suspended within gels can be used as model tissues or tissue equivalents. These materials are useful for modeling the biological events underlying tissue formation; they also can serve as the basis for tissue engineering products.

Exercises

Exercise 8.1

How do individual cells come together to form functional tissue? Describe a mechanism of mimicking this process *in vitro* for a tissue-engineered device.

Exercise 8.2

Assume that cells are suspended within gel at a density of 10^7 cells/mL; assume that the cells in the gel are identical—with regard to cell motility—to the cells used in Exercise 7.2. Further assume that all of the cells migrate within the three-dimensional gel and that, when any two cells collide, they stick together. Aggregated cells (cell clumps consisting of two or more attached cells) do not migrate.

a) Show how the equations for colloidal flocculation can be applied to this situation. Please be sure to write all the assumptions required.
b) Calculate the aggregate size distribution (that is, the number of aggregates per mL for aggregates containing 2, 3, 4, etc. cells) after 1 hr, 6 hr, and 24 hr.
c) Estimate the mean aggregate radius at each of these times.

Exercise 8.3 (provided by Linda Griffith)

Embryonic stem cells, which are derived from the inner cell mass of embryos (recall Chapter 3), are both promising and controversial. They can proliferate extensively in certain conditions. These growth conditions can be altered to possibly induce the differentiation of these stem cells into almost all of the tissues of the body. These cells, therefore, are exceptionally interesting to tissue engineers, as they may some day represent an easily expanded source of tissue for just about any application. When murine embryonic stem cells are induced to differentiate, they ball up into multicellular aggregates known as embryoid bodies (EBs). Gassman et al. [46] have characterized the oxygen consumption rate of these EBs, and have given preliminary evidence that reduced oxygen concentration within the center of these bodies may be responsible for the ingrowth of new blood vessels (angiogenesis).

a) Find an expression for the concentration profile within the sphere in terms of radius R, oxygen consumption rate Q_{O_2} (in mol/(cm^3-s)), the radial coordinate r, the diffusion coefficient D_{O_2}, and the surface concentration C_0.
b) Using the Henry's law constant, convert the concentration profile to partial pressures (the same form as given by Gassman et al. on page 2868—Gassman uses α for the Henry's law constant).
c) The oxygen profile within an EB, as determined by Gassman et al., is shown in Figure 8.9. What is $P_O(s)$, the surface partial pressure of oxygen, approximately?
d) For an EB of 880 µm, using the P_{O_2} profile shown in Figure 8.9b to determine the oxygen consumption rate, find V_{O_2} in mol/(cm3-s). (Hint: for this problem, you will need to estimate the data from the paper. Then, using a polynomial fitting program, fit your partial pressure profile you derived in a) to the P_{O_2} curve to obtain the oxygen consumption rate.) Assume D_{O_2} is 2.3×10^{-5} cm^2/s.

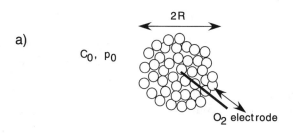

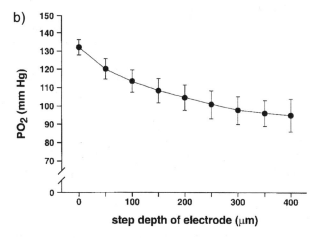

Figure 8.9. Information for Exercise 8.3: (a) an oxygen electrode is inserted into a cell aggregate, permittivity measurement of oxygen concentration as a function of position in the aggregate (b).

References

1. Yuasa, C., et al., Importance of cell aggregation for expression of liver functions and regeneration demonstrated with primary cultured hepatocytes. *Journal of Cellular Physiology*, 1993, **156**, 522–530.
2. Mahoney, M.J. and W.M. Saltzman, Cultures of cells from fetal rat brain: methods to control composition, morphology, and biochemical activity. *Biotechnology and Bioengineering*, 1999, **62**, 461–467.
3. Greis, C. and H. Rosner, Migration and aggregation of embryonic chicken neurons *in vitro*: possible functional implication of polysialogangliosides. *Developmental Brain Research*, 1990, **57**, 223–234.
4. Baldwin, S.P., C.E. Krewson, and W.M. Saltzman, PC12 cell aggregation and neurite growth in gels of collagen, laminin, and fibronectin. *International Journal of Developmental Neuroscience*, 1996, **14**, 351–364.
5. Ablamunits, V.G., et al., Islet-cell aggregates: structure and insulin-producing activity during *in vitro* culture. *Byulleten' Eksperimental'noi Biologii i Meditsiny*, 1990, **110**, 650–653.

6. Cirulli, V., P.A. Halban, and D.G. Rouiller, Tumor necrosis factor-α modifies adhesion properties of rat islet B cells. *Journal of Clinical Investigation*, 1993, **91**, 1868–1876.

7. Rouiller, D.G., V. Cirulli, and P.A. Halban, Differences in aggregation properties and levels of the neural cell adhesion molecule (NCAM) between islet cell types. *Experimental Cell Research*, 1990, **191**, 305–312.

8. Layer, P.G., et al., Of layers and spheres: the reaggregate approach in tissue engineering. *Trends in Neurosciences*, 2002, **25**(3), 131–134.

9. Matthieu, J., et al., Aggregating brain cell cultures: A model to study brain development, in A. Minkowski and M. Monset-Couehard (eds.), *Physiological and Biochemical Basis for Perinatal Medicine*. Basel: Karger, 1981, pp. 359–366.

10. Peshwa, M.V., et al., Kinetics of hepatocyte spheroid formation. *Biotechnology Progress*, 1994, **10**, 460–466.

11. Koide, N., et al., Continued high albumin production by multicellular spheroids of adult rat hepatocytes formed in the presence of liver-derived proteoglycans. *Biochemical and Biophysical Research Communications*, 1989, **161**, 385–391.

12. Parsons-Wingerter, P. and W.M. Saltzman, Growth versus function in three-dimensional culture of single and aggregated hepatocytes within collagen gels. *Biotechnology Progress*, 1993, **9**, 600–607.

13. Moscona, A.A., Rotation-mediated histogenic aggregation of dissociated cells. A quantifiable approach to cell interactions *in vitro*. *Experimental Cell Research*, 1961, **22**, 455–475.

14. Matsuda, M., Serum proteins enhance aggregate formation of dissociated fetal rat brain cells in an aggregating culture. *In Vitro Cellular & Developmental Biology*, 1988, **24**, 1031–1036.

15. Foty, R.A., et al., Liquid properties of embryonic tissues: measurement of interfacial tensions. *Physical Review Letters*, 1994, **72**, 2298–2301.

16. Dai, W., J. Belt, and W.M. Saltzman, Cell-binding peptides conjugated to poly(ethylene glycol) promote neural cell aggregation. *Bio/Technology*, 1994, **12**, 797–801.

17. Foty, R.A., et al., Surface tensions of embryonic tissues predict their mutual envelopment behavior. *Development*, 1996, **122**(5), 1611–1620.

18. Beysens, D.A., G. Forgacs, and J.A. Glazier, Embryonic tissues are viscoelastic materials. *Canadian Journal of Physics*, 2000, **78**, 243–251.

19. Friedlander, S., Collision and Coagulation, Chapter 7 in *Smoke, Dust and Haze: Fundamentals of Aerosol Behavior*. New York: John Wiley & Sons, 1977, pp. 175–208.

20. Smoluchowski, M., Versuch einer mathematischen Theorie der Koagulationskinetik kolloider Losungen. *Z. Physik Chem.*, 1917, **92**(9), 129–168.

21. Muhitch, J.W., et al., Characterization of aggregation and protein expression of bovine corneal endothelial cells as microcarrier cultures in a rotating-wall vessel. *Cytotechnology*, 2000, **32**, 253–263.

22. Harrison, R.G., Observations on the living developing nerve fiber. *Proceedings of the Society for Experimental Biology and Medicine*, 1907, **4**, 140–143.

23. Ham, R.G., Clonal growth of mammalian cells in a chemically defined, synthetic medium. *Proceedings of the National Academy of Sciences USA*, 1965, **53**, 288–293.

24. Loo, D., et al., Extended culture of mouse embryo cells without senescence: inhibition by serum. *Science*, 1987, **236**, 200–202.

25. Eagle, H., Amino acid metabolism in mammalian cell cultures. *Science*, 1959, **130**, 432–437.

26. Ingber, D., J. Madri, and J. Folkman, Endothelial growth factors and extracellular matrix regulate DNA synthesis through modulation of cell and nuclear expansion. *In Vitro Cellular and Developmental Biology*, 1987, **23**, 387–394.

27. Ben-Ze'ev, A., et al., Cell–cell and cell–matrix interactions differentially regulate the expression of hepatic and cytoskeletal genes in primary cultures of rat hepatocytes. *Proceedings of the National Academy of Sciences USA*, 1988, **85**, 2161–2165.

28. Haston, W. and P. Wilkinson, Visual methods for measuring leukocyte locomotion. *Methods in Enzymology*, 1988, **162**, 17–38.

29. Noble, P.B. and M.D. Levine, *Computer-assisted Analyses of Cell Locomotion and Chemotaxis*. Boca Raton, FL: CRC Press, 1986.

30. Grinnell, F., Migration of human neutrophils in hydrated collagen lattices. *Journal of Cell Science*, 1982, **58**, 95–108.

31. Brown, A., Neutrophil granulocytes: adhesion and locomotion on collagen substrata and in collagen matrices. *Journal of Cell Science*, 1982, **58**, 455–467.

32. Schor, S., T. Allen, and C. Harrison, Cell migration through three-dimensional gels of native collagen fibres: collagenolytic activity is not required for the migration of two permanent cell lines. *Journal of Cell Science*, 1980, **46**, 171–186.

33. Bell, E.B., B. Ivarsson, and C. Merrill, Production of a tissue-like structure by contraction of collagen lattices by human fibroblasts with different proliferative potential. *Proceedings of the National Academy of Sciences USA*, 1979, **75**, 1274–1278.

34. Chen, J., E. Stuckey, and C. Berry, Three-dimensional culture of rat exocrine pancreatic cells using collagen gels. *British Journal of Experimental Pathology*, 1985, **66**, 551–559.

35. Yang, J., et al., Sustained growth and three-dimensional organization of primary mammary tumor epithelial cells embedded in collagen gels. *Proceedings of the National Academy of Sciences USA*, 1979, **76**, 3401–3405.

36. Parkhurst, M.R. and W.M. Saltzman, Quantification of human neutrophil motility in three-dimensional collagen gels: effect of collagen concentration. *Biophysical Journal*, 1992, **61**, 306–315.

37. Dickinson, R.B., J.B. McCarthy, and R.T. Tranquillo, Quantitative characterization of cell invasion *in vitro*: formulation and validation of a mathematical model of the collagen gel invasion assay. *Annals of Biomedical Engineering*, 1993, **21**, 679–697.

38. Moghe, P.V., R.D. Nelson, and R.T. Tranquillo, Cytokine-stimulated chemotaxis of human neutrophils in a 3-D conjoined fibrin gel assay. *Journal of Immunological Methods*, 1995, **180**, 193–211.

39. Ranucci, C.S., et al., Control of hepatocyte function on collagen foams: sizing matrix pores toward selective induction of 2D and 3D cellular morphogenesis. *Biomaterials*, 2000, **21**, 783–793.

40. Barocas, V.H. and R.T. Tranquillo, Biphasic theory and *in vitro* assays of cell–fibril mechanical interactions in tissue-equivalent gels, in V.C. Mow (ed.), *Cell Mechanics and Cellular Engineering*. New York: Springer-Verlag, 1994, pp. 1–25.

41. Breuls, R.G.M., et al., Predicting local cell deformations in engineered tissue constructs: a multilevel finite element approach. *Journal of Biomechanical Engineering*, 2002, **124**, 198–207.

42. Yang, J., et al., Primary culture of human mammary epithelial cells embedded in collagen gels. *Journal of the National Cancer Institute*, 1980, **65**, 337–341.

43. Schechner, J.S., et al., *In vivo* formation of complex microvessels lined by human endothelial cells in an immunodeficient mouse. *Proceedings of the National Academy of Sciences*, 2000, **97**(16), 9191–9196.

44. Allaerts, W., et al., Evidence that folliculo-stellate cells do not impede the permeability of intercellular spaces to molecular diffusion in three-dimensional aggregate cell cultures of rat anterior pituitary. *Endocrinology*, 1990, **127**, 1517–1525.

45. Bell, E., et al., Recipes for reconstituting skin. *Journal of Biomechanical Engineering*, 1991, **113**, 113–119.

46. Gassman, M., et al., Oxygen supply and oxygen-dependent gene expression in differentiating embryonic stem cells. *Proceedings of the National Academy of Sciences USA*, 1996, **93**, 2867–2872.

47. Cooney, D.O., *Biomedical Engineering Principles: An Introduction to Fluid, Heat and Mass Transport Processes*. New York: Marcel Dekker, 1976.

48. Orci, L. and R.H. Unger, Functional subdivision of islets of langerhans and possible role of D cells. Lancet, 1975, December 20, 1243–1244.

49. Vold, R.D. and M.J. Vold, *Colloid and Interface Chemistry*. San Diego, CA: Addison-Wesley, 1983.

50. Parsons-Wingerter, P., Cooperativity in hepatocyte culture from cell–cell and cell–substrate interactions. PhD Thesis, Department of Chemical Engineering. Johns Hopkins University, Baltimore, MD, 1992.

51. Fawcett, D.W. and R.P. Jensh (ed.), *Bloom & Fawcett: Concise Histology*. Philadelphia, PA: Lippincott Williams and Wilkins, 1997.

9

Tissue Barriers to Molecular and Cellular Transport

Canst thou remember
A time before we came unto this cell?

William Shakespeare, *The Tempest*, act 1, scene 2

Previous chapters have revealed the importance of molecular diffusion in tissue engineering. Molecules—and gradients of molecules—may represent the underlying mechanism of tissue induction and pattern formation (Chapter 3); growth factors—and the rate of delivery of growth factors to a cell surface—can influence the rate of cell proliferation (Chapter 4); chemoattractants can influence the rate and pattern of cell migration within a tissue space (Chapter 7). To think quantitatively about these processes, it is often helpful to think about molecular concentrations and the spatial variations in concentration that produce diffusion fluxes. This idea has been illustrated earlier in the book for specific examples such as bicoid gradient formation in the insect embryo (Section 3.3.4) and ligand diffusion to the cell surface (Section 4.3.2). Some of the basic concepts of molecular transport are also reviewed in Appendix B.

But tissues are often heterogeneous structures, formed by the assembly of cells and the accumulation of matrix materials in the extracellular space. The heterogeneous composition of tissues can have a dramatic influence on local rates of molecular movement through the tissue; capillary endothelial cells prevent the diffusion of intravascular proteins into the tissue interstitial space, for example. This chapter discusses this concept and provides quantitative methods for evaluating rates of molecular movement between tissue spaces that are separated by diffusive barriers. In addition, the last section of the chapter shows how this same analysis may be useful when thinking about rates of cellular movement between tissue compartments.

In multicellular organisms, thin lipid membranes serve as semipermeable barriers between aqueous compartments (Figure 9.1). The plasma membrane of the cell separates the cytoplasm from the extracellular space; endothelial cell membranes separate the blood within the vascular space from the rest of the tissue. Properties of the lipid membrane are critically important in regulating

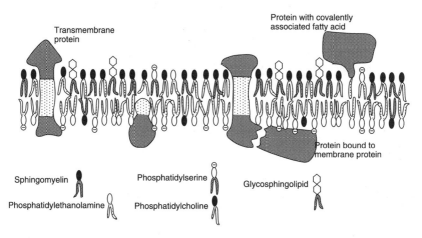

Figure 9.1. Model of cell membranes as lipid bilayers with associated proteins. This composite diagram was assembled from diagrams in a variety of sources. For this, and many of the figures in this chapter, a similar figure appeared previously in Chapter 5 of [15].

the movement of molecules between aqueous spaces. While certain barrier properties of membranes can be attributed to the lipid components, accessory molecules within the cell membrane—particularly transport proteins and ion channels—control the rate of permeation of many solutes. Transport proteins permit the cell to regulate the composition of its intracellular environment in response to extracellular conditions.

Cells assemble into tissue structures (described in Chapter 8) that are stabilized by cell adhesion (introduced in Chapter 6). Stabilized assemblies of cells can be used to separate organs and tissues into distinct compartments; multicellular barriers then impede the movement of molecules between body compartments. For example, a continuous monolayer of endothelial cells separates the vascular compartment (containing plasma and blood cells) from the tissue interstitial space. Some cells circulate throughout the body. To move from the vascular compartment into tissue these cells must also cross this multicellular barrier.

9.1 Mobility of Lipids and Proteins in the Membrane

The cell membrane contains lipid, protein, and carbohydrate molecules (recall Figure 6.1 in Chapter 6). The lipid composition varies between membranes for different cells. In addition, the outermost monolayer of lipids, called the outer leaflet, has a different lipid composition from the inner leaflet. Lipids and accessory molecules are distributed throughout a phase that, because of its slight thickness, is roughly two-dimensional. Most lipid and protein molecules are mobile in the plane of the membrane. Protein mobility was first observed by the redistribution of labeled proteins in the membranes of two cells after fusion (Figure 9.2). Molecular mobility confers essential properties to the membrane.

A number of biophysical techniques have been used to measure rates and patterns of molecular motility. One of the most powerful of these approaches is fluorescence photobleaching recovery (FPR) (Figure 9.2b). In FPR, a focused laser is used to photobleach molecules within a small defined volume of tissue; fluorescent molecules from adjacent regions of tissue subsequently diffuse into the bleached volume, causing the fluorescence intensity to increase with time. The time interval for recovery depends on the diffusion coefficient and the size of the bleached region ($t = L^2/D$); the size is usually small ($< 1\ \mu m$) and is adjusted so that recovery occurs within a fraction of a minute. Over this short interval, elimination can usually be neglected and D is obtained by adjusting solutions to the diffusion equation to fit the measured intensity recovery curve.

These biophysical techiques reveal that the plasma membrane is a dynamic structure. How do molecules move across this barrier? As described in more

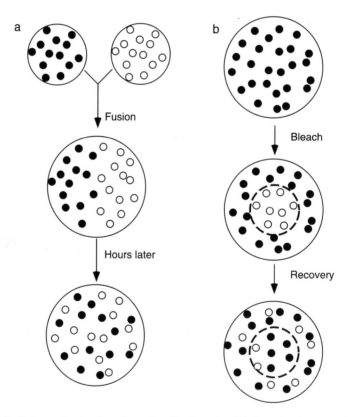

Figure 9.2. Schematic showing the redistribution of labeled molecules after fusion and after photobleaching: (a) protein mobility after cell fusion; (b) protein redistribution after photobleaching.

detail below, the mechanisms and therefore the rate of movement depend on characteristics of the molecule. Small lipid-soluble molecules can diffuse through the lipid-rich bilayer, but larger or more water-soluble molecules must find other paths for transport.

9.2 Permeation of Molecules through Membranes

9.2.1 Permeation through Lipid Bilayers

The permeation of low molecular weight nonelectrolytes through lipid membranes has been studied extensively. In a typical experiment, a tracer molecule is added to a cell suspension and the rate of accumulation of tracer within the cell is measured. Using tracer solutes with a range of physicochemical properties, the permeability k_s (cm/s) of nonelectrolytes is determined as a function of the oil:water partition coefficient. The oil:water partition coefficient is a convenient measure of the relative solubility of a solute within a membrane. A reasonable estimate of the permeability of a solute can frequently be obtained by comparison with experimental measurements for solutes that cover a range of partition coefficients (Figure 9.3). The partition coefficient appears to be the single best indicator for permeability of nonelectrolytes, although there is con-

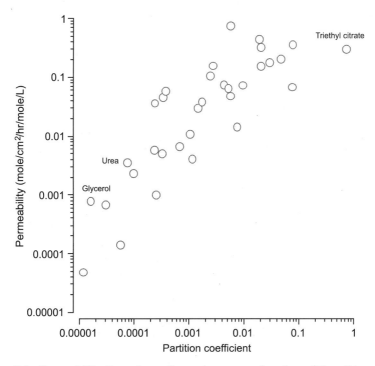

Figure 9.3. Permeability through a cell membrane as a function of the olive oil:water partition coefficient (from [1]).

siderable variability in the permeability of compounds with similar partition coefficients (Figure 9.3).

A closer inspection of the definition of membrane permeability suggests additional methods to correlate the permeability with other properties of the diffusing species. The permeability, called k_s or P, is related to the equilibrium partition coefficient K, the diffusion coefficient in the membrane, D_m, and the thickness of the membrane L:

$$P = k_s = \frac{KD_m}{L} \tag{9-1}$$

This definition of the permeability arises from the equation for steady-state flux through the membrane, N:

$$N = P(c_0 - c_L) \tag{9-2}$$

where c_0 and c_L are concentrations of the solute in the external phase on either side of the membrane. (N is the molar flux of solute defined with respect to a fixed coordinate system; see Appendix B for background information.) Diffusion through polymers is often empirically correlated by power-law expressions. This analysis leads to another correlation for permeability as a function of partition coefficient and molecular weight:

$$P = P_0 K M_w^{-s_m} \tag{9-3}$$

where P_0 is equal to D_m^0/L and the coefficients s_m and D_m^0 are determined by characteristics of the membrane. This expression suggests that nonelectrolytes of various molecular weight diffusing through cell membranes behave like solutes diffusing through a polymer film [1]; this correlation agrees well with experimental data, including the permeation of molecules into erythrocytes (Figure 9.4). For nonelectrolytes of molecular weight less than 200, permeability decreases with increasing molecular weight; compounds with molecular weight over 300 are essentially excluded from the membrane. Charged molecules do not partition into lipid bilayers; ions therefore have a very low permeability in the erythrocyte membrane. The low intrinsic permeability of ions underlies the ability of membranes to support an electrical potential difference, which is discussed more fully in Section 9.2.3.

Solute permeability is also a function of membrane composition. The rate of permeation of doxorubicin, measured through artificial lipid bilayers composed of cholesterol and phospholipids, changes substantially with composition. This is an important finding, since cells have distinct membrane compositions. In addition, the composition of the individual leaflets of a membrane can vary, which suggests the possibility of asymmetric passive transport (i.e., permeabilities that differ depending on the direction of transport, out-to-in or in-to-out).

9.2.2 Permeation through Porous Membranes

In the previous section, the permeation of solutes through uniform lipid membranes was discussed; however, cell membranes and cellular barriers are not

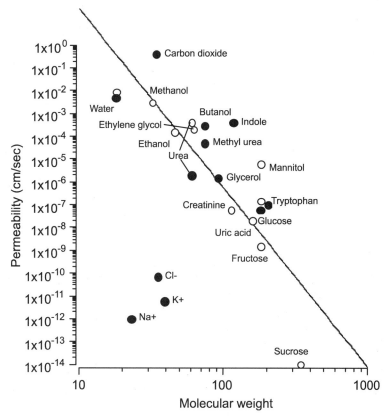

Figure 9.4. Permeability of membranes to small molecules. The figure shows permeability P (cm/s) for a variety of molecules in red blood cells (open circles) and lipid vesicles (closed circles).

perfectly uniform (Figure 9.1). Proteins interrupt the continuous lipid membrane and provide an additional pathway for the diffusion of water-soluble molecules. Protein channels in the membrane, for example, permit the selective diffusion of certain ions. In the blood vessel wall, water-filled spaces between the adjacent endothelial cells provide an alternate path for transport.

Figure 9.5 illustrates a useful model for diffusion of water-soluble molecules through aqueous pores in a membrane. In this model, the pore space is assumed to consist of a monodisperse ensemble of straight cylindrical pores. The transport of solutes through this hypothetical porous material can be analyzed by consideration of the dynamics of a single spherical particle through this idealized cylindrical pore. In many systems of biological interest, the radius of the diffusing particle, r_s, is almost as large as the radius of the pore, r_0. The movement of the particle is therefore hindered in comparison with the movement of the particle in an unbounded fluid [2-5]. One of the advantages associated with models of transport in this highly idealized geometry is

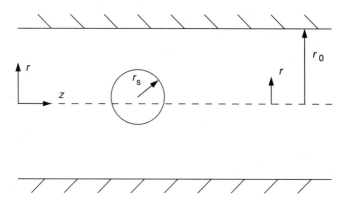

Figure 9.5. Hindered transport through porous membranes: schematic diagram of model for hindered transport of a spherical particle in a cylindrical pore.

that model predictions can be tested experimentally, using membranes with straight cylindrical pores and size-fractionated spherical solutes. More detail is provided in the review by Deen [2].

The key parameters used in describing hindered transport through cylindrical pores are illustrated in Figure 9.5. A critical parameter is the ratio of the solute radius to the pore radius, $\lambda = r_s/r_0$. As λ approaches 1, the pore walls become an increasingly important obstacle for particle transport. In the limit as λ approaches 0, the fluid within the pore can be considered unbounded from the perspective of the particle. Between these two limiting cases, when $0 < \lambda < 1$, lie a number of situations of biological interest, such as permeation of water-soluble compounds through the aqueous pores in a capillary wall. The total steady-state flux through the pore can be determined:

$$\langle N_z \rangle = \frac{WV_0c_0\left[1 - \left(\dfrac{c_L}{c_0}\right)e^{-Pe}\right]}{1 - e^{-Pe}} \tag{9-4}$$

where $\qquad Pe = \dfrac{WV_0L}{HD_\infty}; \qquad W = \Phi K_c; \qquad H = \Phi K_d$

which is obtained using the boundary conditions $\langle c \rangle_0 = \Phi c_0$ at $x = 0$ and $\langle c \rangle_L = \Phi c_L$. The concentrations c_0 and c_L are averaged across the pore cross-section, Pe is the Peclet number (which is a measure of the relative importance of bulk flow to diffusion), V_0 is the bulk fluid velocity, Φ is a partition coefficient between the bulk fluid and the fluid in the pore, and W and H are hydrodynamic coefficients that depend on the details of geometry and interactions between the particle and the walls of the pore. This equation reduces to the following simple expressions in the limits for small and large Pe:

$$\langle N_z \rangle = \frac{HD_\infty}{L}(c_0 - c_L) \qquad Pe \ll 1$$

$$\langle N_z \rangle = WV_0 c_0 \qquad Pe \gg 1$$

$$(9\text{-}5)$$

When the Peclet number is small, Equation 9-5 reduces to the familiar expression for membrane permeability (recall Equation 9-2), where the membrane permeability is now $k = HD_\infty/L$. When Pe is large, Equation 9-5 reduces to the expression for ultrafiltration, where the commonly used reflection coefficient is $\sigma = 1 - W$.

The dependences of H and W on λ are shown in Figure 9.6. These hydrodynamic coefficients can be determined by finding the drag on a sphere within a tube and the approach velocity for a sphere in parabolic flow, as described previously for spheres on the tube centerline [5] or distributed throughout the tube [4]. The solid lines in Figure 9.6 indicate values of H and W when spheres are confined to the tube axis:

$$H = (1 - \lambda)^2 [1 - 2.1044\lambda + 2.089\lambda^3 - 0.948\lambda^5]$$

$$W = (1 - \lambda)^2 (1 + \lambda)[1 - \tfrac{2}{3}\lambda^2 - 0.163\lambda^3]$$

$$(9\text{-}6)$$

9.2.3 Facilitated, Active, and Ion Transport across Membranes

Many molecules do not diffuse through lipid bilayers (see Figure 9.4 and notice that sucrose and ions do not permeate). One of the most important functions of accessory molecules in the membrane is to regulate the transport of molecules that do not pass freely through the lipid bilayer. Several classes of accessory

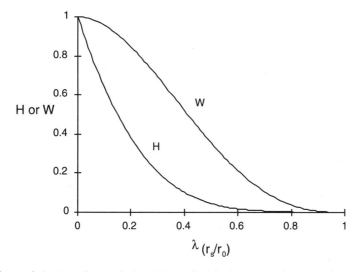

Figure 9.6. H and W calculated for cylindrical pores, using Equation 9-6.

molecules are engaged in membrane transport, as described in the sections that follow.

Facilitated Diffusional Transport. Although the extracellular concentration of glucose is usually higher than the intracellular concentration, the low permeability of the lipid bilayer to glucose prevents passive transport of enough molecules of glucose to support metabolism. Glucose transport proteins in the cell membrane solve this problem by providing aqueous pathways that shuttle glucose through the hydrophobic bilayer. The glucose transporter facilitates glucose permeation by periodic changes in conformation: in one conformation, a glucose binding site is exposed on the extracellular face, whereas in another conformation the binding site is exposed to the intracellular face (Figure 9.7). Conformational changes occur due to natural thermal fluctuations in the membrane; these changes occur whether the glucose binding site is occupied or vacant. As a result of this periodic change in structure, the transport protein permits the passage of glucose (or another molecule that is able to bind to the transporter binding site) without the use of any additional energy. Glucose molecules can move in either direction across the bilayer; the net flux will occur from the region of high to low concentration.

Facilitated transport proteins, such as the glucose transporter, are present in the cell membrane in limited number. As the concentration of the solute increases, the transporter binding sites become saturated and the net rate of solute transport across the membrane decreases (Figure 9.8). The rate of transport via the facilitated transport mechanism can be analyzed by considering binding of the transported solute (S) to the transmembrane carrier protein (C_P), to form a carrier–solute complex (S–C_P):

$$S + C_P \underset{k_{-1}}{\overset{k_1}{\rightleftharpoons}} S-C_P \overset{k_2}{\rightarrow} S^*-C_P \overset{k_3}{\rightarrow} S^* + C_P \tag{9-7}$$

The conformational change of the carrier protein moves the solute from one side of the membrane (a state designated S) to the opposite side (designated S^*), from which it is released. If the rate of release of transported solute is rapid

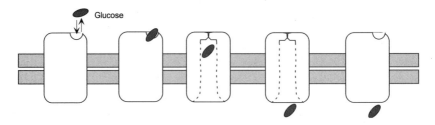

Figure 9.7. Schematic illustration of the mechanism of action of the glucose transport protein, showing the steps involved in glucose transport: recognition of glucose on the external face of the membrane, confirmational change of the transport molecule, and release of glucose.

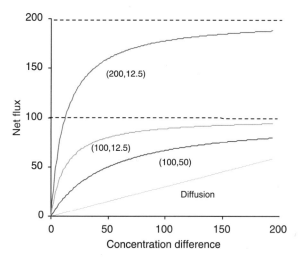

Figure 9.8. Transport proteins in cell membranes. The kinetics of glucose transport protein depends on the affinity of the binding site and the number of transport proteins present. Unlike simple diffusion through the membrane bilayer, facilitated transport systems become saturated as the solute concentration difference increases. In this hypothetical example, the permeability of the membrane in simple diffusion is 0.4 and V_{max} and K_m for facilitated transport are (200,12.5), (100,12.5), and (100,50).

compared to the rate of conformational change ($k_3 >> k_2$), the concentration of solute on the opposite side of the membrane is negligible ($S^* \sim 0$), and binding of solute to carrier is at equilibrium, then the flux of solute across the membrane is given by

$$N_{S^*} = \frac{1}{A}\frac{d[S^*]}{dt} = k_2[SC_P] \tag{9-8}$$

The concentration of the solute–carrier complex is assumed constant (i.e., the rate of formation of the complex is equal to the rate of dissociation), so that

$$k_1[S][C_P] = k_{-1}[SC_P] + k_2[SC_P] \tag{9-9}$$

and the total number of carrier proteins is also assumed constant, C_{TOT}:

$$C_{TOT} = [C_P] + [SC_P] \tag{9-10}$$

Substitution of Equations 9-9 and 9-10 into Equation 9-8 yields

$$N_{S^*} = \frac{k_2 C_{TOT}}{\left(1 + \dfrac{k_{-1} + k_2}{k_1}\dfrac{1}{[S]}\right)} \tag{9-11}$$

which can be simplified by definition of the lumped constants $V_{max} = k_2 C_{TOT}$ and $K_m = (k_{-1} + k_2)/k_1$:

$$N_{S^*} = \frac{V_{max}[S]}{([S] + K_m)} \tag{9-12}$$

A similar derivation is commonly used to describe the kinetics of product formation in enzyme-catalyzed reactions (substitute enzyme for carrier protein and product formation for the conformational change of the carrier protein). Under the assumptions of this simple model, carrier conformational change is the rate-limiting step, so it is reasonable to assume further that k_2 is much less than k_{-1}. In this case, the constant K_m is approximately equal to $K_d = k_{-1}/k_1$, the dissociation constant for the binding of solute to carrier. For this reason, it is common to refer to K_m as the "affinity" of the solute for the carrier (note the analogy to Equation 4-2). V_{max} is the maximum flux due to this carrier-mediated transport, which occurs when all of the carrier binding sites are occupied (Figure 9.8).

Both facilitated and simple diffusion depend on concentration gradients: net solute transport always occurs from high to low concentration. Unlike diffusion, facilitated transport systems are specific, since they depend on binding of the solute to a site on the transport protein. For example, the D-glucose transporter is very inefficient at transporting L-glucose, but it can accommodate D-mannose and D-galactose (Table 9.1).

The neutral amino acid transporter is responsible for movement of neutral amino acids from the blood into the brain; these compounds are not soluble in membranes and therefore would not diffuse into the brain in the absence of a transport system. This transporter is efficient in brain capillaries, but it is found in other tissues as well (Table 9.2). The concentrations of amino acids in the blood are close to the values of K_m for brain capillaries, which suggests that the transporter is near saturation under normal conditions. Because of this, and because the transporter is equally efficient with a number of amino acids, changes in the blood concentration of one neutral amino acid can influence the rate of transport of all the other neutral amino acids.

Active Transport.   Active transport systems are similar to facilitated transport systems; both involve the participation of transmembrane proteins that bind a specific solute (Figure 9.9). In active transport, however, energy is required to drive the conformational change that leads to solute transport. The Na^+/K^+ pump is the best characterized active transport system (Figure 9.9). The pump is an assembly of membrane proteins, with $3\,Na^+$ binding sites on the cytoplasmic surface, $2\,K^+$ binding sites on the extracellular surface, and a

Table 9.1
Specificity of the Glucose
Transporter Protein

	$K_m (mM)$
D-glucose	1.5
L-glucose	> 3,000
D-mannose	20
D-galactose	30

Table 9.2
K_m Values (mM) for Transport of Neutral Amino acids in Tissues

Amino Acid	Intestinal Epithelia	Renal Tubule	Exocrine Pancreas	Red Blood Cells	Liver	Blood–Brain Barrier
Phenylalanine	1			4	4	0.032
Leucine	2			2	6	0.087
Tryptophan		4				0.052
Methionine	5		3	5		0.083
Histidine	6	5				0.16
Valine	3		7	7		0.17

region of ATPase activity on the cytoplasmic surface near the Na^+ binding sites.

Like facilitated transport systems, active transport mechanisms can be saturated. The rates of molecular transport across a typical active transport and facilitated transport system are similar. Both carrier-mediated transport systems have less transport capacity than channel-mediated transport or simple diffusion (Table 9.3).

Ion Transport, Membrane Potentials, and Action Potentials. Lipid bilayers are impermeable to ions and other charged species, but ions such as Na^+ and K^+ are found in abundance in both the extracellular and intracellular environment. Active transport proteins can move ions across membranes, even moving molecules against a concentration gradient. Cells and microorganisms are exquisitely sensitive to changes in their ionic environment; ion movement across membranes is of profound physiological importance.

Ion movement across membranes is regulated by specialized membrane proteins called ion channels (Figures 9.9 and 9.10). Some ion channels are

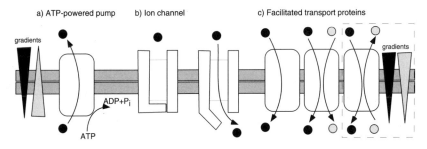

Figure 9.9. Transport proteins in cell membranes: (a) energy-dependent, ATP-powered ion pumps such as the Na/K exchange ATPase; (b) channels, gated or non-gated, which permit diffusion through an aqueous pathway, such as voltage-gated Na channels; (c) passive, facilitated transport systems which can act in uniport, symport, or antiport modes, such as the glucose transporter.

Table 9.3
Characteristics of Membrane Transport Mechanisms

	Restrictions	Capacity (molecules/s)	Example
Simple diffusion	Solubility in membrane With a concentration gradient	∞^a	See Figure 9.3
Channel-mediated transport	Specific channel required With a concentration gradient Gating is possible	10^7–10^8	Na^+ and K^+ channels
Facilitated transport	Specific transport proteins required With a concentration gradient[b]	10^2–10^4	Glucose transporter
Active transport	Specific transport proteins required Energy required	1–10^3	Na^+/K^+ pump

[a] Capacity is limited only by the solubility of solute in the membrane.

[b] Symport and antiport systems can move one of the transported solutes against a gradient.

selective, permitting the permeation of specific ions only. Selectivity is accomplished by a combination of channel characteristics including molecular sieving (which selects for ions of certain size), binding to the protein surface, and stabilization of the non-hydrated ion. Some channels are gated; gated channels exist in multiple states that either permit or exclude ion movement across the membrane. In the open state, conductance (or permeability) to the ion rapidly increases. The closed/open state of the ion channel is regulated by extracellular and intracellular conditions. Some channels are voltage-regulated; others are regulated by ligand binding or mechanical stretching of the membrane.

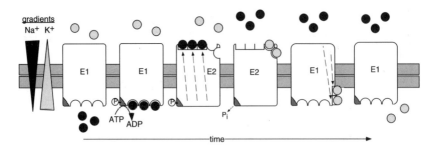

Figure 9.10. Na/K ATPase moves ions across the plasma membrane. Energy-dependent, ATP-powered ion pumps such as the Na/K exchange ATPase.

Most channels behave as simple resistors to current flow: when the channel is open, the current through the channel varies linearly with membrane potential ($\Delta V = IR$). The antibiotic polypeptide gramicidin A forms a cylindrical channel by end-to-end dimerization of two peptides, one in each of the bilayer leaflets. Individual gramicidin channels exhibit a resistance of 8×10^{10} ohms over membrane potentials from -75 to $+75$ mV (by standard convention, the membrane potential is positive if the cell interior is positively charged with respect to the exterior). This electrical resistance can also be expressed as a conductance, the reciprocal of resistance, of 12×10^{-12} siemens (S, where 1 $S = 1$ ohm^{-1}). In other channels, the relationship between voltage and current is nonlinear, such that resistance varies with imposed potential. These channels are rectifying, in that current flow is unequal for $(+)$ or $(-)$ potentials.

The overall potential of a cell membrane depends on the concentrations of ions on each side of the membrane (Figure 9.11) and the permeability of the membrane to each ion. Membrane potential is generated by gradient-driven movement of ions across the membrane. Most cells have intracellular K$^+$ concentrations that are much higher than the extracellular K$^+$ concentration. If the membrane contains channels that permit K$^+$ permeation, ions will diffuse out from the cell into the extracellular environment. This selective permeation creates a separation of charge, because the $(-)$-charged counterions for K$^+$ do not cross the membrane. Therefore, an electrochemical potential develops and increases until, eventually, it balances the concentration driving force, at which point K$^+$ diffusion will cease. For a membrane that is permeable to a single ion, the equilibrium membrane potential E_{ion} is given by the Nernst equation

$$E_{ion} = -\frac{RT}{Z_{ion}F}\ln\left(\frac{C_{in}}{C_{out}}\right) \tag{9-13}$$

where R and F are the gas constant and Faraday's constant, respectively, T is absolute temperature, z is the valence of the ion, and C_{in} and C_{out} are the intracellular and extracellular ion concentrations. The membrane potential is defined so that a $(+)$-ion gradient from inside to out results in a $(-)$ potential across the membrane. Equilibrium potentials for K$^+$ and Na$^+$ at 37°C are -94 mV and $+61$ mV, respectively.

When a membrane is permeable to more than one ionic species, the net membrane potential V_m depends on concentration and permeability:

$$V_m = -\frac{RT}{F}\ln\left(\frac{P_K C_{K^*,in} + P_{Na} C_{Na^*,in} + P_{Cl^-,in}}{P_K C_{K^*,out} + P_{Na} C_{Na^*,out} + P_{Cl} C_{Cl^-,out}}\right) \tag{9-14}$$

Na$^+$, K$^+$, and Cl$^-$ are the most important ions for determining membrane potential in human cells. The importance of each ion in determining the resting membrane potential depends on the permeability of each ion in the membrane; permeability depends on the number of non-gated channels available for that ion. For many mammalian cells, the net membrane potential is ~ -60 mV, which is closer to the equilibrium potential of potassium than that of sodium due to the greater permeability of resting membranes to potassium.

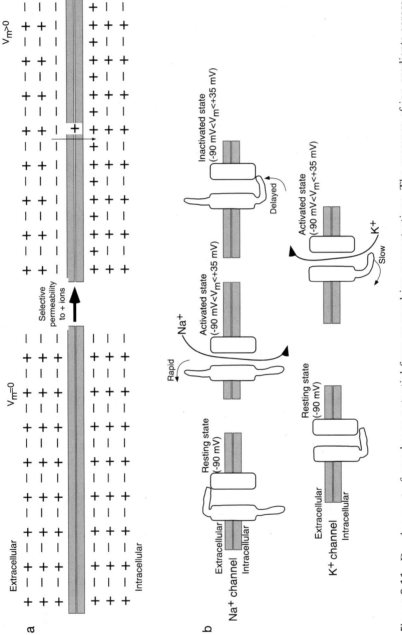

Figure 9.11. Development of membrane potential from unequal ion concentrations. The presence of ion gradients across a membrane leads to a resting membrane potential. The value of the potential depends on the magnitude of the ion gradient and the permeability of the membrane to each ion.

Excitable cells in the nervous system are capable of propagating signals over long distances very rapidly, with no attenuation of the signal as it moves. This remarkable property enables us to respond rapidly to our environment, as when we reflexively withdraw our hand from a flame. These rapidly moving signals are transmitted by changes in membrane potential. Since membrane potential depends on membrane permeability to ions (Equation 9–14), signal movement through tissue occurs via spatial changes in ion conductance. This signaling can be controlled, because ion conductance is regulated by voltage-gated ion channels which can open or close in response to changes in the local membrane potential. Voltage-clamp techniques, first developed in 1949, permit the measurement of ion conductance at fixed membrane potential. When the local potential changes, ion channels open, creating more paths for ion diffusion. Although the potential may change rapidly, changes in conductance occur more slowly; the overall kinetics of conductance change reflect the contributions from many individual ion channels, which open and close at different times.

For a fixed change in membrane potential, voltage-gated Na^+ channels produce more rapid changes in conductance than K^+ channels. This difference in speed of response is essential for signal propagation, as first described by Hodgkins and Huxley (see historical background in [20]). Action potentials—sudden, reversible changes in overall membrane potential—are initiated by local depolarization of the membrane: depolarization occurs when the overall membrane potential becomes slightly less negative than at its resting (polarized) state. A few voltage-gated Na^+ channels open in response to this small depolarization; opening of these few Na^+ channels creates an increase in the inward Na^+ flux through the membrane, which causes further depolarization, which in turn causes more Na^+ channels to open, causing further depolarization. As a result of this cascade, the initial small change in membrane potential suddenly becomes a large change in potential; if enough channels open, the net membrane potential will approach the sodium equilibrium potential given by Equation 9-13 (Figure 9.12). But the sodium equilibrium potential is never achieved, because depolarization also opens voltage-gated K^+ channels which produce an outward flow of K^+ ions. This outward K^+ current tends to return the potential to its former value; since K^+ flux serves to reestablish the polarized state of the membrane, this process is called repolarization. K^+ channels respond more slowly than Na^+ channels but they remain open longer, resulting in a slight hyperpolarization (due to the residual permeability to K^+) at the end of the action potential. For a short period after the action potential, most membranes cannot be depolarized. This refractory state, which reflects the non-responsiveness of Na^+ channels for a brief period after opening, lasts for several milliseconds. Near the end of the refractory period an action potential can be induced, but a greater threshold depolarization is required for initiation.

Other Transport Mechanisms. Passive diffusion, facilitated and active transport, and diffusion through channels account for the majority of molecular

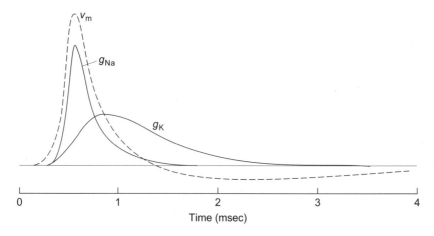

Figure 9.12. The action potential is the result of reversible changes in sodium and potassium conductance. A more complete description is available in [20].

transit across membranes. Several other mechanisms involving membrane-associated proteins are also important in the life of a cell. For example, in Chapter 4 the kinetics of receptor binding, endocytosis, and signal transduction were presented. Receptor-mediated endocytosis is another important mechanism for molecular movement across cell membrane barriers.

9.3 Permeation of Molecules through Cell Layers

9.3.1 Hydraulic Permeability

The movement of water through membranes and cell layers is critical for cell and tissue function. In its simplest formulation, the transmembrane volumetric fluid flux V_w, is given by:

$$V_w = k_m(\Delta P - \Delta \pi) \tag{9-15}$$

where ΔP and $\Delta \pi$ represent hydrostatic $\Delta P = (P_{in} - P_{out})$ and osmotic $\Delta \pi = \pi_{in} - \pi_{out}$) pressure gradients across the membrane. In Equation 9-15, k_m represents the hydraulic permeability of the barrier; it is therefore similar to a mass transfer coefficient for fluid movement across the layer. This equation assumes that the membrane barrier is perfectly impermeable to the solutes that are generating the osmotic driving force. In many cases, the membrane barrier is imperfect; therefore, the osmotic driving force must be adjusted. The reflection coefficient σ, is used to make this correction:

$$\sigma_i = \begin{cases} 1 & \text{membrane is a perfect barrier} \\ (1 - v_i/v_w)_{\sigma=0} & \text{membrane is semipermeable} \\ 0 & \text{membrane is very permeable} \end{cases} \tag{9-16}$$

where v_i and v_w are the velocities of solute and water through the barrier. With this definition, the overall fluid flux can be written as

$$V_w = k_m \left(\Delta P - \sum_{i=1}^{n} \sigma_i RT \Delta C_i \right) \qquad (9\text{-}17)$$

in which the van't Hoff equation for ideal dilute solutions ($\pi = RTC$) has also been used.

9.3.2 Solute Permeation across Tissue Barriers

An alternative definition of solvent and solute flow is based on irreversible thermodynamics and was initially derived by Kedem and Katchalsky (see [6] for a review). J_v is the solvent flow:

$$J_v = L_p S (\Delta P - \sigma \Delta \pi) \qquad (9\text{-}18)$$

where L_p is the hydraulic conductance and S is the surface area. Correspondingly, the flow of solute i can be expressed as

$$J_s = J_v (1 - \sigma) \overline{C}_i + PS \Delta C_i \qquad (9\text{-}19)$$

where $\overline{C}_i$ is the mean intramembrane concentration and P is the permeability of the barrier to solute i. Equation 9-19 accounts for both diffusive transport (defined in Equation 9-2) and convective transport due to solute movement across the barrier. The permeability P is related to the diffusion coefficient (see Equation 9-1) and the thickness of the barrier; therefore, Equation 9-19 can also be written in differential form:

$$J_s = J_v (1 - \sigma) C_i + D_i S \frac{dC_i}{dx} \qquad (9\text{-}20)$$

and integrated from $x = 0$ to $x = L$ (the thickness of the barrier) to yield

$$\text{Clearance } (Cl) = \frac{J_s}{C_{i,\text{plasma}}} = J_v (1 - \sigma_i) \frac{1 - \dfrac{C_{i,\text{interstitial}}}{C_{i,\text{plasma}}} e^{-Pe}}{1 - e^{-Pe}} \qquad (9\text{-}21)$$

where $C_{i,\text{plasma}}$ and $C_{i,\text{interstitial}}$ are solute concentrations on the plasma and interstitial sides of the barrier, respectively, Cl is the solute clearance, and Pe is a modified Peclet number, defined as $J_v (1 - \sigma_i)/PS$. (The concept of clearance is described more fully in Chapter 13, in the context of clearance of solutes during dialysis.) The relationship between filtration rate (J_v) and clearance is shown in Figure 9.13. When Pe is low ($Pe \sim 0$), diffusion of solute across the barrier is the primary mechanism of transport. When the Pe is high ($Pe > 3$), fluid convection is the dominant mechanism of transport, and transport is proportional to the product $J_v (1 - \sigma)$ (dashed line in Figure 9.13).

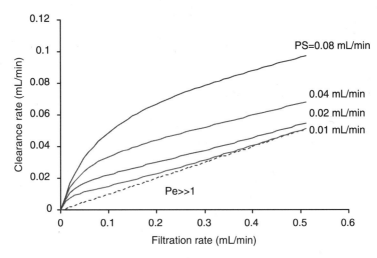

Figure 9.13. Clearance vs. filtration rate for simple homogeneous transport through a tissue barrier. The dashed lines indicate transport in the absence of diffusion ($Pe \gg 1$). Equation 9-21 is plotted for $\sigma = 0.9$ at steady state (i.e., lymphatic clearance is equal to solute flux, see [6]).

9.3.3 Permeation through Endothelial Layers

General Concepts.   The capillary endothelium is the major site of exchange for nutrients, hormones, and proteins between blood and tissues. When the solute is a macromolecule, transport occurs through pores in the endothelium. Capillaries in the general circulation are highly permeable to water and glucose, and nearly impermeable to proteins larger than albumin (Table 9.4). Capillary permeability is qualitatively different from cell membrane permeability: the ratio of glucose to water permeability is 0.6 for a muscle capillary (Table 9.4) and 0.0001 for a cell membrane (Figure 9.4). The enhanced permeability of water-soluble molecules through capillary walls is due to the presence

Table 9.4
Relative Permeability of Muscle Capillaries to Solutes of
Various Molecular Weight

	Molecular Weight	Relative Permeability
Water	18	1
NaCl	59	0.96
Urea	60	0.8
Glucose	180	0.6
Sucrose	342	0.4
Inulin	5000	0.2
Myoglobin	17,600	0.03
Hemoglobin	68,000	0.01
Albumin	69,000	0.001

Data taken from [21].

of water-filled pores that are sufficiently large to accommodate the movement of glucose and sucrose. As the size of the solute increases, permeability through the capillary wall decreases, suggesting that the pores are only slightly larger than albumin, which has a radius of $\sim 35\,\text{Å}$.

Experimental measurements of rates of protein transport suggest that convection and diffusion through large pores (~ 200–$400\,\text{Å}$ radius) are the dominant mechanisms of movement from blood into tissue [6]. However, the pores in the endothelium are not uniform in size. Pores of different radii present different resistances to diffusive and convective transport of macromolecules (see Figure 9.6), and the overall clearance is influenced by these different transport resistances. For a typical protein such as albumin, the overall clearance is equal to the sum of clearance from the different pore populations.

It is possible that some substances move through the capillary wall by transcytosis. The importance of this pathway is not clear, but capillaries in some tissues contain numerous vesicles.

Capillaries in different tissues vary tremendously in their permeability characteristics, as is described in the sections that follow.

Capillaries in the Kidney.   Filtration in the kidney occurs across a specialized capillary in the glomerulus. The glomerular capillary has several layers: a monolayer of endothelial cells that interface with the flowing blood, an acellular basement membrane, and a filtration layer formed by glomerular epithelial cells. The endothelium is fenestrated; that is, there are numerous small holes or fenestrae throughout the continuous endothelium. For example, fenestrated capillaries in the liver allow almost free exchange of proteins across the capillary barrier. These holes are large enough for proteins to pass freely (in contrast to muscle capillaries, which are not fenestrated). Proteins cannot, however, pass easily through the basement membrane, which is an entangled gel of proteins and proteoglycans; protein permeability is low because of the fine mesh within the basement membrane gel and because of the dense negative charge provided by the proteoglycans. The endothelial layer contains slits filled with porous diaphragms that permit the free passage of water; the structure of the diaphragm is still in debate, although the open spacings in the diaphragm are approximately the same size as the albumin molecule. The glomerular capillary, which is designed to permit filtration of large volumes of water, still allows for slow diffusion of macromolecules (Figure 9.14) [7]. Most of the diffusive resistance is due to the presence of small fenestrae and slits in the cellular layers ($\sim 80\%$), but the basement membrane provides a substantial resistance that increases with molecular size. The reduced diffusion coefficient (D/D_∞) decreases from ~ 0.01 to ~ 0.001 over the range of molecular radii shown in Figure 9.14.

Capillaries in the Brain (the Blood–Brain Barrier).   Capillaries in the brain are less permeable than capillaries in other tissues. This limited permeability, which is frequently called the blood–brain barrier, is essential for brain function, since low permeability serves as a buffer that maintains a constant brain extracel-

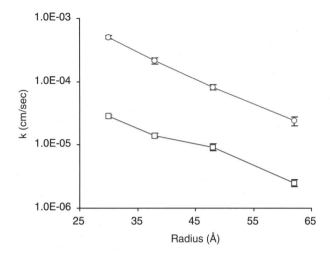

Figure 9.14. Diffusion of Ficoll through the glomerular capillary (from [7]). Diffusion of molecular weight fractions of Ficoll through isolated glomerular capillaries (squares) or capillaries with the cells removed (circles).

lular environment, even at times when blood chemistry is changing. The basis for this lower permeability is the relative paucity of pores in the brain endothelium. Therefore, molecules that move from blood to brain must diffuse through the endothelial cell membranes.

As expected from this observation, the permeability of brain capillaries depends on the size and lipid solubility of the solute. In general, molecules that are larger than several hundred in molecular weight do not permeate into the brain. Empirical relationships between cerebrovascular permeability and the oil:water partition coefficient have been developed [8]:

$$\log_{10} P = 4.30 + 0.866 \log_{10} K \qquad (9\text{-}22)$$

This correlation is useful for rapid estimation of the blood–brain barrier permeability. More accurate estimation can be obtained by examining other physical characteristics of the compound, such as cross-sectional area and critical micellar concentration [9]. Because of the extremely low permeability of brain capillaries to most molecules, brain endothelial cells have a variety of specialized transport systems—including transporters for glucose, amino acids, insulin, and transferrin—that enable essential molecules to move from the blood into the brain extracellular space. A number of useful reviews of the blood–brain barrier are available, including [10].

Capillaries in Tumors.　The blood vessels that develop in tumors are generally more permeable than vessels that develop in normal tissues. As a result, large molecules that would not penetrate through a normal vessel will permeate through a vessel in a tumor. The size cutoff for a vessel can be determined by injecting particles of a known size intravenously, then looking in the interstitial space of the tumor to see whether the particles are extravasated. In one previous study [11], subcutaneous tumors were generally permeable to larger particles than intracranial tumors. The same tumor, when introduced subcutaneously or intracranially, had different permeability characteristics, highlighting the importance of local tissue environment in defining local vascular permeability.

9.3.4 Permeation through Epithelial Barriers

Skin and mucosal surfaces of the gut, respiratory, and reproductive tracts represent a principal barrier against entry of pathogens and molecules encountered in the environment. These multicellular structures are often the most important barrier to the administration of drugs. For example, the oral route of drug administration, which is usually the preferred route, is limited by the extent to which drug molecules can penetrate the epithelial surface of the intestinal tract. The structure, and therefore the barrier characteristics, of epithelial tissues show considerable variability; schematic diagrams of the major types of epithelium are shown in Figure 9.15. The permeability of some compounds through intestinal epithelium is listed in Table 9.5.

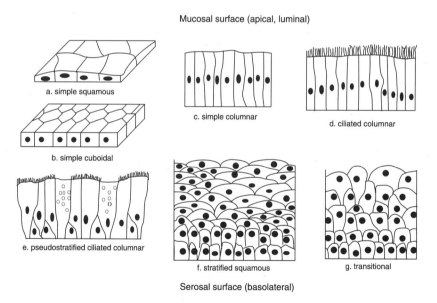

Figure 9.15. Illustration of the structure of epithelial tissue barriers in the body (modified from [16]). Epithelial tissues have a variety of histological patterns: (a) simple squamous, as found in the initial segments of ducts in glands and the alveolus; (b) simple cuboidal, as found in glandular ducts and ovary; (c) simple columnar, as found in stomach, intestines, uterus, and cervix; (d) ciliated columnar, as found in the small bronchi, intestines, and cervix; (e) pseudostratified ciliated columnar with mucus-secreting (goblet) cells, as found in the trachea, large bronchi, and vas deferens; (f) stratified squamous, as found in skin, esophagus, tongue, and vagina; and (g) transitional, as found in the ureter and urinary bladder.

Table 9.5
Permeability of some Carbohydrates through Isolated Intestinal Strips[a]

Carbohydrate	Molecular Weight	Radius of Gyration (Å)	Intestinal Permeability (μmol/g-hr)
Inulin	5,000	14.8	0
Lactose	342	4.4	5
Mannose	180	3.6	19
Ribose	150	3.6	22
Glyceraldehyde	90	2.4	45

[a]Permeability of golden hamster intestinal strips to passively diffusing carbohydrates. Original data from T.H. Wilson, *Intestinal Absorption*, Philadelphia: Saunders, 1962, Table 5, p. 4, as reported in [18].

Different mucosal surfaces differ in permeability. The permeability of nasal, rectal, and vaginal membranes from the rabbit was determined: for mannitol, $P_{nasal} > P_{vaginal} > P_{rectal}$; for progesterone, $P_{nasal} > P_{rectal} > P_{vaginal}$ [12]. Permeability was assessed using electrical resistance and the permeability of epithelial barriers to a water-soluble fluorescent dye, 6-carboxyfluorescein. The rank order of permeabilities was intestinal ~nasal $\geq$ bronchial $\geq$ tracheal > vaginal $\geq$ rectal > corneal > buccal > skin [13].

Permeation through the Skin.   Our skin provides a mechanical barrier that prevents entry of pathogens into our tissues and therefore protects us from infection. Skin also prevents excessive loss of fluid due to evaporation, by regulating the access of water to the body surface. The barrier properties of skin are impressive; although the average person has 1.8 m^2 of exposed skin, insignificant quantities of most compounds enter the body through this surface.

Skin is a keratinized, stratified, squamous epithelium and is therefore a complex multilayer barrier. The outermost layer of the skin, the stratum corneum, appears to be the major barrier to permeation of most compounds. Topical drug application is an effective and simple method for treatment of local skin diseases; drug molecules need only to penetrate locally in relatively small amounts. If systemic delivery is required, however, obstacles abound: overall bioavailability can be limited by the intrinsic permeability of the stratum corneum, by local degradation of drugs during permeation, or by the availability of blood flow to skin at the site of drug application. The overall flux of drug molecules through the skin, J, depends on concentration and permeability:

$$J = \frac{C_{skin} - C_{blood}}{(R_{blood} + 1/P_{sc})} \qquad (9\text{-}23)$$

where c_{skin} and c_{blood} are drug concentrations at the skin surface and in the blood, P_{sc} is the permeability of the stratum corneum, and R_{blood} is the effective resistance to transport through the tissue beneath the stratum corneum. This resistance includes the availability of blood flow, which serves as a reservoir for the drug molecules penetrating through the skin. For permeabilities of the stratum corneum less than $\sim 0.01\,cm/min$, the resistance of the stratum corneum dominates the overall transport.

9.4 Permeation of Cells through Cell Layers

Cells can also move through the tissue barriers formed from other cells. Cells of the immune system circulate through the body by movement in the vascular system, and by crawling across the vascular endothelial barrier to enter tissues. White blood cells also patrol the mucosal surfaces of body by crawling through epithelial barriers; neutrophils cross the intestinal epithelium, for example, to function within the mucus layer outside of the body. When cancer cells metastasize through the bloodstream, they crawl across the endothelium to enter the bloodstream and to exit into a new tissue site (Figure 7.1).

This process of cell movement across a tissue barrier is called transmigration. The role of transmigration in the overall process of cell circulation within the body is discussed in Chapter 10. In this section, the process of transmigration is described briefly and the kinetics of transmigration in some particular systems are illustrated.

9.4.1 Basic Elements of Cell Permeation

The movement of molecules through a tissue barrier is powered by a concentration gradient or by an energy-dependent transport system. In transmigration, the motile cell provides its own power, using mechanisms that are similar to those described in Chapter 7. Movement may still occur down a concentration gradient (i.e., there are fewer cells on the receiving side of the tissue barrier), but it can also be influenced by the presence of gradients of chemoattractants, which create a net movement of cells in a particular direction that is independent of the cell concentration gradient.

The overall event—a motile cell crossing a tissue barrier—can be divided into components, which differ in importance for each particular system. The basic components are margination, adhesion, and transmigration. If a cell is initially within the flowing bloodstream, it must come into contact with the vessel wall as a prelude to transmigration. Margination is the name of this process of cell movement to the outer edge of a flowing bloodstream (it is discussed more completely in Chapter 10). Once the cell is at the vessel boundary, it can adhere to the surface of the tissue barrier (i.e., to the surface of the cells that comprise the barrier) using receptor-ligand mediated adhesion processes. Several modes of adhesion have now been recognized. Cells can exhibit a "rolling" type of adhesion in which the cell is loosely associated with the surface and appears to roll along the barrier, but at a speed which is substantially lower than the speed of the flowing blood. Cells can also experience firm adhesion, in which they are immobilized to a specific site on the tissue barrier. These different modes of adhesion are mediated by different sets of cell adhesion molecules (see Chapter 10). The alternate modes of adhesion also serve different physiological functions: in rolling adhesion, the cell can search or survey a surface for an optimal transmigration site, whereas in firm adhesion the cell is preparing for the transmigration event.

9.4.2 Model Systems for Studying Cell Permeation through Tissue Barriers

The significance of the overall process—margination, adhesion, and transmigration—in the circulation of cells throughout the body is discussed in Chapter 10. Here, attention is focused on the permeation step; that is, the process of transmigration or penetration of a tissue barrier by a motile cell.

A commonly used model system for studying transmigation is illustrated in Figure 9.16. This particular system is used for measuring the ability of inflammatory cells (neutrophils) to cross an intact intestinal mucosa (a monolayer of T84 cells). The intactness of the tissue barrier is usually determined by measuring electrical resistance; any breaks in the barrier would cause an increase in the resistance of the layer. The number of cells that transmigrate across the monolayer is measured, as a function of time, either by collecting the fluid in the reservoir and measuring the cell number or by directly observing the emergence of motile cells from the monolayer, using a microscope.

Characteristic data for neutrophil migration across a confluent endothelial cell monolayer (an experimental model for a blood vessel wall) are shown in Figure 9.17. Cells transmigrate across the barrier, with measurable numbers appearing after 10 min and increasing steadily over the 60 min experiment. As the cells transmigrate, there is a decrease in endothelial resistance, presumably as the neutrophils create gaps in the confluent barrier that permit their transit. In addition, the endothelial barrier becomes leaky to macromolecules such as albumin.

An important observation, which has been made consistently in these systems, is that the act or process of transmigration is accompanied by changes in the permeability to molecules and, sometimes, pathogens. For example, neutrophils that are applied to the basal side of T84 monolayers will increase permeability and permit invasion by *Shigella flexneri*, initially present only on the apical surface. The bacteria induce PMN transmigration (by serving as a chemoattractant), which transiently increases the permeability of the epithelial monolayer. This increased paracellular permeability permits *S. flexneri* to migrate to the basolateral surface of the cells, where they are infective [14].

Summary

- Membranes form selectively permeable barriers that separate aqueous compartments in cells.
- Lipids and proteins are mobile within the membrane phospholipid bilayer.

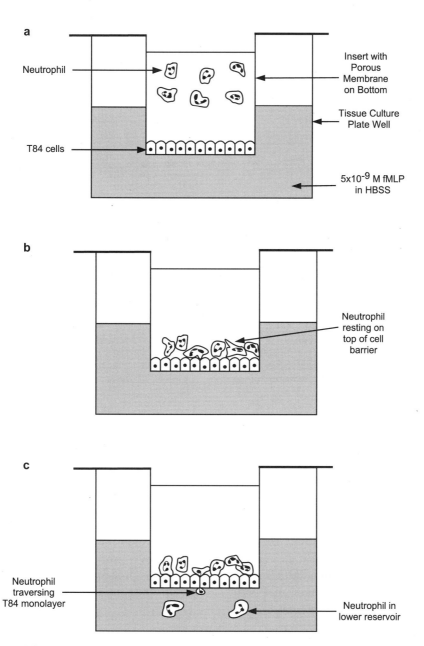

Figure 9.16. Cell culture system for examining leukocyte transmigration across eptihelial cell monolayers. This is a typical experimental system for analysis of transmigration, based on a culture system in which a porous insert is placed into a conventional tissue culture well or dish. (a) A confluent cell monolayer (which represents the tissue barrier) is formed by culturing cells on a porous substrate. Here the T84 cells form the tissue barrier. A population of migrating cells (neutrophils in this case) is added to one side of the tissue barrier and a chemoattractant (fMLP in this case) is added to the opposite side. (b) The migrating cells come into contact with the tissue barrier. (c) Cells that transmigrate across the tissue barrier can be collected or observed in the lower reservoir of the tissue culture apparatus.

281

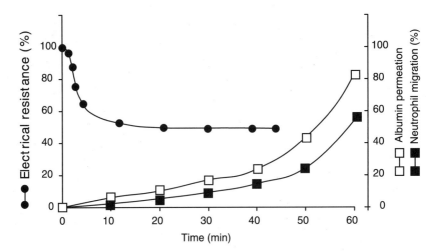

Figure 9.17. Transmigration of neutrophils through a confluent endothelial barrier; the figure illustrates data presented in [17]. An experimental system similar to that of Figure 9.16 was used, in which the confluent monolayer was formed from endothelial cells (instead of epithelial cells, as in Figure 9.16). In addition to measuring the number of neutrophils that crossed the barrier as a function of time, the investigators measured the permeability of the layer to macromolecules (such as albumin) and the electrical resistance.

- Nonelectrolytes permeate membranes by dissolution and diffusion; permeation depends on both molecular size and solubility.
- Solute permeation of porous membranes depends on the size of the solute molecule relative to the pore.
- Specialized proteins within the membrane provide mechanisms for facilitated transport, active transport, and ion transport.
- Movement of molecules across multicellular tissue barriers usually involves a combination of the mechanisms described in this chapter.
- Certain cells can also cross tissue barriers by a process called transmigration. Although the kinetics of this process are less well studied than molecular permeation, transmigration should also yield to quantitative analysis.

Exercises

Exercise 9.1 (provided by Christine Schmidt)

An artificial blood substitute consists of four free hemoglobin molecules connected by diaspirin (a crosslinking agent). If this arrangement is sufficient to transport oxygen through the blood to the tissues, speculate on why the body has evolved a system with hemoglobin inside a membrane structure (the red blood cell).

Exercise 9.2

A micropipette filled with an aqueous solution of a fluorescent dye is inserted into a large body of water. At time $t = 0$, particles of dye are injected into the water at the rate i per second for an infinitesimal period of time dt. The total number of particles injected is $N = idt$.

a) Write the differential equation to describe the subsequent diffusion of tracer molecules in this situation, including boundary and initial conditions.

b) Demonstrate that the following solution satisfies the differential equation obtained in part (a):

$$C(r, t) = \frac{N}{(4\pi Dt)^{3/2}} e^{-r^2/4Dt}$$

c) Determine the comparable solution for the situation in which dye molecules are continuously injected at rate i for the period $t = 0$ to t^*.

Exercise 9.3

a) Using the similarity transform technique, with the similarity variable $\eta = x/2\sqrt{t}$, show how the partial differential equation with an initial condition and two boundary conditions

$$\frac{\partial C}{\partial t} = D \frac{\partial^2 C}{\partial x^2}$$

$$C = 0; \quad t = 0; \quad 0 \le x \le \infty$$
$$C = 0; \quad t > 0; \quad x \to \infty$$
$$C = C_0; \quad t > 0; \quad x = 0$$

reduces to a second-order ordinary differential equation with two boundary conditions.

b) Use the results from part (a) to obtain the solution to the partial differential equation. Non-dimensionalize the time and space variables by defining: $c = C/C_0$, $X = x/L$, and $T = tD/L^2$, where L is some characteristic length scale. Plot the results, using these non-dimensional variables, to indicate how the concentration near a solid interface with constant concentration changes with time.

Exercise 9.4 (provided by Linda G. Griffith)

In the European Union there is strong pressure to eliminate the use of animals in research, and thus there is a major focus on developing tissues that can serve as materials in toxicology tests. The use of alternatives is also being explored in the U.S. Wagner et al. [19] are developing a new tissue-engineered skin called Epiderm for use in testing dermal penetration and toxicity. This skin is made from living human donor cells, grown into a dermal equivalent and an epidermal equivalent in culture. One important assessment is how it compares to normal skin in terms of permeability.

An experiment is conducted in which the skin is placed in a two-chamber diffusion apparatus, where the concentration of model penetrant (flufenamic acid, a lipophilic molecule) is kept at constant values in the source chamber and the sink chamber. The surface area of skin between the two chambers is $2\,cm^2$. The concentration of the amount of penetrant is determined in each chamber as a function of time and used to calculate the amount penetrating as a function of time. In these experiments, the concentration of the penetrant in the source chamber is much greater than that in the sink chamber, so the concentration profile in the skin can be assumed to be steady state after an initial transient. The data, collected in Table 9.6, were all taken in the steady state regime.

It is determined in a separate experiment that the partition coefficient for the penetrant in stratum corneum is 5.6, in epidermis is 1.5, and in dermis is 0.7. On the basis of the table data:

a) calculate the steady-state flux in each case;
b) calculate the diffusion coefficient in each case;
c) How close is the Epiderm to real dermis, and why might it be different?

Exercise 9.5 (provided by Linda G. Griffith)

You are interviewing for a job with a company that is developing a synthetic blood substitute. The company's approach is to encapsulate human recombinant hemoglobin in a special type of polymer membrane to make synthetic red cells. The membrane has a comparable solute permeability to normal erythrocyte membranes (i.e., it allows passage of salts but not most plasma proteins). Why are the researchers bothering to encapsulate the hemoglobin instead of using it directly dissolved in their artificial plasma? What are the implications for the fluid balance between plasma and interstitial fluid if you do not encapsulate the hemoglobin?

Table 9.6
Data for Exercise 9.4

Epidermis, Normal Skin Thickness = 75.2 µm		Stratum Corneum, Normal Skin Thickness = 12.2 µm		Full skin, Normal Skin Thickness = 2910 µm		Epiderm Thickness = 67.3 µm	
Time (hr)	Amount (µg)	Time (hr)	Amount (µg)	Time (hr)	Amount (µg)	Time (hr)	Amount (µg)
5	10	5	10	5	3.5	5	115
10	19	10	20	10	7	10	230
20	38	20	40	20	14	20	460

Data obtained from [19].

Data: hemoglobin content of red cells: $0.335 \, \text{g/mL}$ of red cells; molecular weight of hemoglobin: $68{,}000 \, \text{g/mol}$; erythrocyte volume fraction in blood: $\sim 0.4 \, (40\%)$.

Exercise 9.6 (provided by Linda G. Griffith)

Many soluble secreted peptides that influence cell behavior, such as the fibroblast growth factor (FGF), bind reversibly to components of extracellular matrix, such as heparin, according to

$$\text{FGF}_{\text{solution}} + \text{Heparin}_{\text{fixed in matrix}} \leftarrow \rightarrow \text{F--H}_{\text{fixed complex}}$$

Extracellular matrix is a gel, and heparin is fixed within the gel and does not diffuse. FGF can diffuse freely through the extracellular matrix and bind reversibly to heparin. Such binding is governed by the equilibrium relationship

$$K_d = \frac{C_{\text{FGF}} C_{\text{hep}}}{C_{\text{F--H complex}}}$$

where K_d is the dissociation constant (M), C_{FGF} is the concentration of free (unbound) FGF, C_{hep} is the concentration of free FGF binding sites on heparin, and $C_{\text{F--H complex}}$ is the concentration of FGF bound to heparin. The total concentration of heparin binding sites is the sum of the free heparin binding sites and the complexes: $C_{\text{hep, total}} = C_{\text{hep}} + C_{\text{F--H complex}}$. This problem explores how the binding to heparin might influence transient and steady-state transport properties of FGF in matrix.

a) Consider a situation where a region of extracellular matrix containing FGF at a constant concentration is suddenly exposed to fluid with no FGF. Note that the total concentration of FGF in matrix comprises the sum of free and heparin-bound FGF. Such a situation might happen in a wound, for example. This situation can be modeled as a semi-inifinite slab with a change in surface concentration at time zero. Show that, provided the binding reaction is very fast compared to diffusion, the transient diffusion of free FGF in the matrix is given by

$$\frac{\partial C_{\text{FGF}}}{\partial t} = D_{\text{FGF}} \frac{\partial^2 C_{\text{FGF}}}{\partial x^2} - \frac{\partial C_{\text{F--H complex}}}{\partial t}$$

b) Show that the equation in (a) can be expressed in the more useful form

$$\frac{\partial C_{\text{FGF}}}{\partial t} = \frac{D_{\text{FGF}}}{\left[1 + \dfrac{C_{\text{hep, total}} K_d}{(K_d + C_{\text{FGF}})^2} \right]} \frac{\partial^2 C_{\text{FGF}}}{\partial x^2}$$

What form does this equation take if $C_{\text{FGF}} \ll K_d$? For this limit, calculate the characteristic diffusion times *relative to the case where no heparin is present* (i.e., free diffusion case) for the following situations: $C_{\text{hep, total}} = K_d$; $C_{\text{hep, total}} = 10 K_d$; $C_{\text{hep, total}} = 1000 K_d$. Note that in order to calculate the relative times you do not need the absolute values of any parameters. What are the implications for the presence of heparin on how fast FGF might diffuse out of matrix?

References

1. Lieb, W. and W. Stein, Biological membranes behave as non-porous polymeric sheets with respect to the diffusion of non-electrolytes. *Nature*, 1969, **224**, 240–249.
2. Deen, W.M., Hindered transport of large molecules in liquid filled pores. *AIChE Journal*, 1987, **33**, 1409–1425.
3. Renkin, E.M., Filtration, diffusion, and molecular sieving through porous cellulose membranes. *Journal of General Physiology*, 1954, **38**, 225–243.
4. Brenner, H. and L. Gaydos, The constrained Brownian movement of spherical particles in cylindrical pores of comparable radius. Models of the diffusive and convective transport of solute molecules in membranes and porous media. *Journal of Colloid and Interface Science*, 1977, **58**, 312–356.
5. Anderson, J.L. and J.A. Quinn, Restricted transport in small pores: a model for steric exclusion and hindered particle motion. *Biophysical Journal*, 1974, **14**, 130–150.
6. Rippe, B. and B. Haraldsson, Transport of macromolecules across microvessel walls: the two-pore theory. *Physiological Reviews*, 1994, **74**(1), 163–219.
7. Edwards, A., W.M. Deen, and B.S. Daniels, Hindered transport of macromolecules in isolated glomeruli. I. Diffusion across intact and cell-free capillaries. *Biophysical Journal*, 1997, **72**, 204–213.
8. Rapoport, S., K. Ohno, and K. Pettigrew, Drug entry into the brain. *Brain Research*, 1979, **172**, 354–359.
9. Fischer, H., R. Gottschlich, and A. Seelig, Blood–brain barrier permeation: molecular parameters governing passive diffusion. *Journal of Membrane Biology*, 1998, **165**, 201–211.
10. Pardridge, W.M., ed., *Introduction to the Blood–Brain Barrier: Methodology, Biology, and Pathology*. Cambridge: Cambridge University Press, 1998.
11. Hobbs, S.K., et al., Regulation of transport pathways in tumor vessels: role of tumor type and microenvironment. *Proceedings of the National Academy of Sciences*, 1998, **95**, 4607–4612.
12. Corbo, D.C., J.-C. Liu, and Y.W. Chien, Characterization of the barrier properties of mucosal membranes. *Journal of Pharmaceutical Sciences*, 1990, **79**(3), 202–206.
13. Rojanasakul, Y., et al., The transport barrier of epithelia: a comparative study on membrane permeability and charge selectivity in the rabbit. *Pharmaceutical Research*, 1992, **9**(8), 1029–1034.
14. Perdomo, J.J., P. Gounon, and P.J. Sansonetti, Polymophonuclear leukocyte transmigration promotes invasion of colonic epithelial monolayer by *Shigella flexneri*. *Journal of Clinical Investigation*, 1994, **93**, 633–643.
15. Saltzman, W.M., *Drug Delivery: Engineering Principles for Drug Therapy*. New York: Oxford University Press, 2001.
16. Parkhurst, M.R., Leukocyte migration in mucus and interaction with mucosal epithelia: potential targets for immunoprotection and therapy, in *Chemical Engineering*. Baltimore, MD: Johns Hopkins University Press, 1994.

17. Gautam, N., P. Hedqvist, and L. Lindbom, Kinetics of leukocyte-induced changes in endothelial barrier function. *British Journal of Pharmacology*, 1998, **125**, 1109–1114.
18. Creasey, W.A., *Drug Disposition in Humans: The Basis of Clinical Pharmacology*. New York: Oxford University Press, 1979.
19. Wagner, H., et al., Interrelation of permeation and penetration parameters obtained from *in vitro* experiments with human skin and skin equivalents. *Journal of Controlled Release*, 2001, **75**, 283–295.
20. Kandel, E.R., J.H. Schwartz and T. M. Jessell, eds., *Principles of Neural Science*. New York: McGraw-Hill, 2000.
21. Guyton, A.C. and J.E. Hall, *Textbook of Medical Physiology*. Philadelphia: W. B. Saunders Company, 1996.

Part 3

TISSUE ENGINEERING PRACTICE

10

Cell Delivery and Recirculation

The Spheres themselves by motion do endure,
And they move on by Circulation too.

Katherine Philips, *To my Lucasia, in defense of declared Friendship*

Perhaps the simplest realization of tissue engineering involves the direct administration of a suspension of engineered cells—cells that have been isolated, characterized, manipulated, and amplified outside of the body. One can imagine engineering diverse and useful properties into the injected cells: functional enzymes, secretion of drugs, resistance to immune recognition, and growth control. We are most familiar with methods for manipulating the cell internal chemistry by introduction or removal of genes; for example, the first gene therapy experiments involved cells that were engineered to produce a deficient enzyme, adenine deaminase (see Chapter 2). But genes also encode systems that enable cell movement, cell mechanics, and cell adhesion. Conceivably, these systems can be modified to direct the interactions of an administered cell with its new host. For example, cell adhesion signals could be introduced to provide tissue targeting, cytoskeleton-associated proteins could be added to alter viscosity and deformability (in order to prolong circulation time), and motor proteins could be added to facilitate cell migration.

Ideally, cell fate would also be engineered, so that the cell would move to the appropriate location in the body, no matter how it was administered; for example, transfused liver cells would circulate in the blood and, eventually, crawl into the liver parenchyma. Cells find their place in developing organisms by a variety of chemotactic and adhesive signals, but can these same signaling mechanisms be engaged to target cells administered to an adult organism? We have already considered the critical role of cell movement in development in Chapter 3. In this chapter, the utility of cell trafficking in tissue engineering is approached by first considering the normal role of cell recirculation and trafficking within the adult organism.

10.1 Cell Movement within the Circulatory System

Most cells can be easily introduced into the body by intravenous injection or infusion. This procedure is particularly appropriate for cells that function within the circulation; for example, red blood cells (RBCs) and lymphocytes. The first blood transfusions into humans were performed by Jean-Baptiste Denis, a French physician, in 1667. This early appearance of transfusion is startling, since the circulatory system was described by William Harvey only a few decades earlier, in 1628. Denis used the blood of calves and lambs, choosing the animal that best matched the level of gentleness desired in the recipient. Early experience with transfusion was not entirely successful; Denis transfused blood into several patients, some on multiple occasions, and most experienced side effects such as shock and fever. Denis's procedure was blamed for the death of at least one patient, who was under treatment for madness, but further investigation revealed that the patient died of poisoning by arsenic, which was apparently administered by his abused wife (see an excellent history of blood and politics [1]). Transfusion was not widely used until the early 1900s, after Karl Landsteiner's discovery of blood types.

10.1.1 Circulation of Transfused Blood Cells

The utility of whole blood transfusion is now widely recognized. In addition, the fate of individual cells after introduction from a donor to a host is now well studied. Transfused RBCs circulate for long periods in normal human subjects. When RBCs are transfused into a patient, the cells disappear from the circulation linearly over 110 to 120 days following transfusion (Figure 10.1). When ^{51}Cr-labeled donor cells of type O were transfused into healthy recipients of type A, the persistence of the donor cells in the circulation could be followed by measuring radioactivity levels and products of hemolyzed cells of type O [2]. There were small but significant differences in the life span of the donor cells (life span $= 114 \pm 8$ days for donor 1 cells in three patients; life span $= 129 \pm 5$ days for donor 2 cells in the same three patients), which appeared to be related to the donor. These observations are consistent with the following hypothesis: the population of transfused RBCs has a uniform distribution of ages and each RBC has a finite life span of ~ 120 days.

How are RBCs removed from the circulation? Experimentally, it is difficult to tell a young RBC from an old RBC in a blood sample, but cells do differ in some properties such as membrane rigidity, suggesting that mechanical properties of cells may be an important signal for removal. While the survival curves in Figure 10.1 appear linear, the disappearance appears more curvilinear in other cases, suggesting that either the distribution of ages in the transfused cells is not uniform or cells are subject to a random elimination process.

Other blood-borne cells have a similar fate after transfusion, although the circulation lifetime of these cells varies greatly (Table 10.1). Some cells, such as the cells involved in immunological memory, may persist in the circulation for many decades.

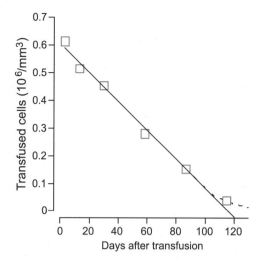

Figure 10.1. Survival of transfused red cells in a male adult. Until elimination of the cells is almost complete, the points fall on a slope which may be linear or slightly curvilinear. If the slope is assumed to be linear, mean cell life, estimated by extrapolation of the line to the time axis, is 114 days. The persistence of a few transfused cells beyond 114 days is due to variation in red cell life-span (redrawn from [4], p. 24).

The lung is an important site for trapping and loss of infused cells. Human lungs contain a tremendous number of capillaries, which carry deoxygenated blood from artery to vein in its passage over the alveolar wall. The average capillary diameter ($\sim 7.5 \pm 2.3\,\mu m$) is about the same size as a neutrophil ($6.8 \pm 0.8\,\mu m$) and a red blood cell ($7.5\,\mu m$). But neutrophils and RBCs differ dramatically in their mechanical properties, as described in Chapter 5; RBCs are more easily deformable. RBCs are therefore able to squeeze through the small lung capillaries more easily than neutrophils. RBCs move across the pulmonary capillary bed in ~ 1 second; transit of neutrophils through the lung capillaries is 60–100 times slower than that of RBCs [3]. Inflammatory

Table 10.1
Persistence of Transfused Cells in the Circulation

	Lifespan (days)	Notes
Red cells	120	
Platelets	8	
Neutrophils	0.3	45–55% are recoverable
Lymphocytes	~ 30	5–8% persist for > 270 days
TIL	Variable	98% disappear within a few hours

Collected from a variety of sources. TIL = tumor infiltrating lymphocyte.

mediators, and other factors that increase cell stiffness, further prolong neutrophil transit time.

Only about 45–55% of the infused granulocytes are recoverable, even after intravenous administration, presumably because the other fraction is marginated in venules throughout the body [4]. Granulocytes that are labelled with ^{3}H-thymidine disappear from the bloodstream with a half-life of 7.6 hours, suggesting a daily production rate of 0.85×10^9/kg. It has been estimated that a 70 kg man has $\sim 4.2 \times 10^{11}$ marrow granulocytes of which 2×10^{10} are circulating ($\sim$ 5% of the total pool) [5]. Small lymphocytes have a life span of $\sim$ 1 month, but 5–8% of the cells have a lifespan of more than 9 months. In humans, some lymphocytes can live for years.

10.1.2 Cell Margination and Interaction with Endothelial Cells

Intravenously injected cells can sometimes find their way into extravascular body compartments. A simple example of blood-cell homing between blood and lymph compartments is shown in Figure 10.2 [6]. When lymphocytes were collected from blood and then injected intravenously, most of the injected cells remained in the blood (Figure 10.2a). In contrast, lymphocytes that were collected from the lymph tissue and then injected intravenously migrated back into the lymph (Figure 10.2a). Although the cells were circulating within the blood vessels immediately after injection in both cases, they were able to migrate out of the circulation and accumulate in other tissue locations; many of these cells can find their way back to their native tissue space (that is, the site where they were found). There are other well-known examples of this control of the fate of circulating cells; for example, infused hematopoeitic stem cells find their way back to the bone marrow.

How are intravenously infused cells able to escape from the blood? As described in Chapter 9, some cells have the remarkable ability to migrate out of the circulatory system into a specific tissue space, such as the skin or brain or heart. Since the blood vessel wall is the physical barrier between blood and tissue, it is logical to assume that control over cell exit from the circulation resides at the vessel wall. But how does interaction with specialized endothelium beds resident in varying tissues determine whether or not a cell will exit the circulation?

Circulating cells can associate with the blood vessel wall as a first step in the process of migrating out of the vessel and into local tissue. The sequential processes of margination, adhesion, and transmigration—which occurs frequently in the post-capillary venules—were described in Section 9.4.1 and are illustrated in Figure 10.3. In lymph nodes and specialized regions of the gut, lymphocytes in the circulation interact with an endothelium specialized for trafficking of lymphocytes; this specialized endothelium is found in post-capillary venules that are called high endothelial venules (HEV). Specialized endothelial cells of the HEV are recognized by lymphocytes through the selective binding interaction of cell adhesion receptors on both cell surfaces. The importance of cell–cell recognition is a common feature in regulation of cell

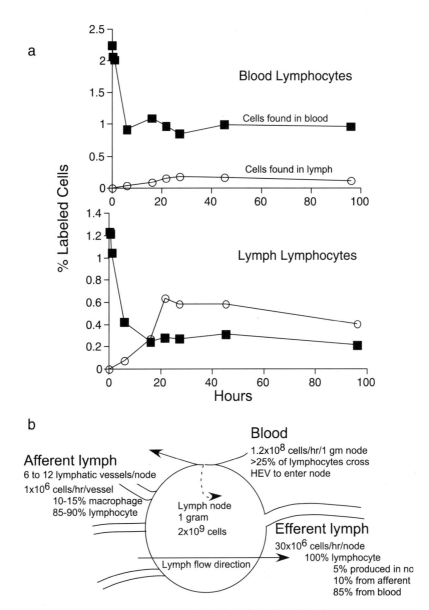

Figure 10.2. Some cells tend to return to their site of origin. (a) Cells were harvested from peripheral blood or lymph and then reinjected back into the circulation [6]. Cells harvested from blood (top panel) were found predominantly in the blood compartment after administration. Cells harvested from lymph (middle panel) tended to go back into the lymphatic system. (b) Traffic of lymphocytes in a typical 1-gram lymph node, redrawn from [43].

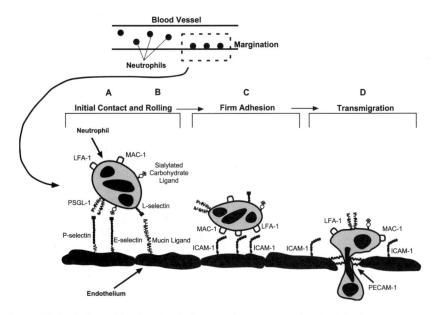

Figure 10.3. Cells within the circulation can become associated with the endothelium of the blood vessel. This process, called margination, occurs in a series of steps involving initial contact between the cell and the endothelial cell, loose adhesion (which is often characterized by the cell "rolling" along the surface), and firm adhesion which is resistant to the forces of the flowing fluid. Firmly attached cells can transmigrate through the vessel wall (see Chapter 9). Cell–cell adhesion molecules are involved with all of these events.

circulation. One part of the answer to the question posed at the end of the last paragraph seems to be this: circulating cells (such as lymphocytes) recognize a local tissue site for transmigration (such as the HEV of the lymph node) by molecular interactions with the specific set of cell adhesion molecules that is expressed on the surface of the local endothelium (such as HEV). This model can explain many of the features essential for control of cell recirculation: tissue sites can be made distinct according to their stage of biological development, their state of inflammation, or the type of immune response (for example, innate or acquired, allergic or inflammatory) which dominates the tissue microenvironment. Specificity is achieved by virtue of the set of receptors that are expressed on the local endothelium, leading to cognate receptor–ligand interactions. This point will be discussed more completely in a later section of this chapter. Control of this process is ongoing since these interactions influence expression of the cell surface receptors that intitially led to tissue recruitment in the first place (for example, chemokine receptors functionally expressed on the leukocyte cell membrane are typically down-regulated following ligand engagement by internalization).

Margination occurs continuously within the vascular system, so that the cells within the vasculature can be subdivided into two populations: the circulating fraction (f_C) and the marginated fraction (f_M) (see [2] for more detail). Individual cells can move between the two populations; that is, cells can become associated with the vessel wall and then return to the circulatory flow. The dynamics of movement of cells from one sub-population to the other can be characterized by rate constants, as illustrated in Figure 10.4; the rate constants describe the movement from the circulating to the marginated fraction, M, or return from the marginated to the circulating fraction, R. In addition, marginated and circulating cells can leave the vasculature to enter tissues; the fraction of cells in the tissue is f_T.

Fluid forces cause some cells to move to the periphery of the vessel cross-section, in position to interact with the endothelium. Certain characteristics of red cells, such as their tendency to aggregate or form rouleaux, cause them to be preferentially concentrated in the center of the vessel, with the result that other cells, such as neutrophils, are forced to the marginal position. Once a cell is at the vessel wall, the process of cell adhesion to the endothelium can be subdivided into phases (Figure 10.3). Primary adhesion, due to receptors on the tips of microvilli on the blood cell, is the initial interaction; firm adhesion, stabilized due to the engagement of integrin receptors, occurs later.

The process of cell adhesion to the vessel wall and transmigration out of the vessel and into the extravascular space is mediated by molecular interactions between the circulating cell and the endothelium. These interactions

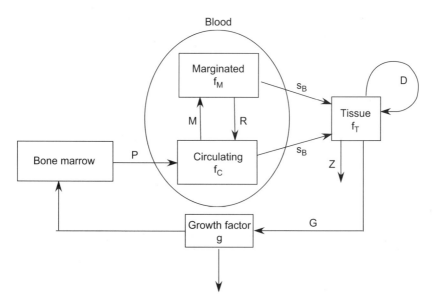

Figure 10.4. Model for cell margination and return. Cells within the circulation can be subdivided into two pools: circulating, C, and marginated, M. This schematic diagram illustrates a model for the fate of monocytes and neutrophils. The model is described in [7].

involve cell adhesion receptors on both the blood-borne cell and the endothelial cell (recall the discussion on adhesion receptors in Chapter 6). Our knowledge of the molecular identity of these receptors has increased dramatically in recent years, in part due to the explosion of genetic information available. For example, chemokines are a large family (over 50 members and growing) of small proteins (typically under 100 amino acids) with a degree of sequence homology that has permitted many of them to be discovered by cloning "in silico" (that is, by computer-based bioinformatics rather than the traditional laboratory approach). Although our list of the key players continues to grow with each discovery, the biological significance of these molecular ligands and their interactive roles under normal and pathological circumstances require definition.

One very interesting point regarding the circulating immune system is that normally there is a constitutive recirculation of lymphocytes between blood and tissue, referred to as immunosurveillance. For example, naïve T cells on the prowl for non-self or altered self antigens percolate through lymph nodes in hope of a rendezvous with their cognate antigen. Circulation of T cells through lymph nodes occurs continuously; large numbers of lymphocytes—entering from blood and from afferent lymphatics—move through lymph nodes every hour (Figure 10.2b). When antigen recognition does occur, it leads to T cell activation, which in turn alters the normal pattern of margination such that the activated T cell is now equipped to be efficiently recruited to the site of antigen origin in the periphery (for example, the skin where there is a site of injury and inflammation). Predictable changes in patterns of margination are known to occur in response to infection, organ transplantation, or allergic response. The modulation away from normal patterns of margination, measurable in terms of the fractional distribution of a distinct cellular subpopulation among blood and tissue, closely reflects the character of the perturbations occurring in a biological system.

10.1.3 Models for Cell Traffic Throughout the Body

Pharmacokinetic models have long been used to describe the dynamics of movement of molecules (particularly drugs or toxins) between tissues within the human body. Similar mathematical methods can be used to describe the fate of cell populations [7, 8]. Consider the case of neutrophils or monocytes, which circulate in the blood but can also marginate to the vessel wall and subsequently transmigrate into a tissue space. A simple mathematical model of blood cell trafficking throughout the body can be constructed [7]; in this model, cells can be in either the circulating, marginated, or tissue-associated state (Figure 10.4). The cells are produced at sites in extravascular tissues (that is, the bone marrow for neutrophils and monocytes) at a rate P; they may proliferate in tissues with a rate constant D; and they are destroyed with a rate constant Z. A model for the marginated, circulating, and tissue-associated cell subpopulations can be formulated from this description:

$$\frac{df_C}{dt} = P + P_g(g) + Rf_M - (M + S_B)f_C \qquad \text{(a)}$$

$$\frac{df_M}{dt} = Mf_C - (R + S_B)f_M \qquad \text{(b)}$$

$$\frac{df_T}{dt} = S_B f_C + S_B f_M + (D - Z)f_T \qquad \text{(c)}$$

$$\frac{dg}{dt} = Gf_T - Kg \qquad \text{(d)}$$

(10-1)

where g is the concentration of a self-stimulating growth factor that encourages cell production; this factor is produced by tissue cells (with a specific production rate G) and is eliminated from the tissue with a rate constant K (equal to $\ln(2)/\text{tissue-half-life}$). Examples of the use of this set of equations for analysis of the extent of leukocyte margination have been presented [7], and are considered further in Exercise 10.1 at the end of the chapter. Importantly, these equations integrate patterns of leukocyte margination with other biologically related processes such as cellular destruction (apoptosis), which is ongoing and serves as a mechanism of cellular turnover that contributes to immune system responsiveness.

Similar pharmacokinetic models have been used to predict the effectiveness of adoptive immunotherapy [8].

10.2 Examples of Cell Trafficking between Body Compartments

10.2.1 Lymphocyte Recirculation

Lymphocytes are an essential element of the immune system, particularly with regard to their role in surveillance and recognition of foreign antigens (see [9]) . Lymphocytes are fantastically efficient at this function because they are continuously recirculating through tissue sites throughout the body—including the peripheral lymphoid organs and sites of likely infection, where foreign antigens are concentrated (Figures 10.2b and 10.5).

The patterns of recirculation are best known for T cells (Figure 10.5b). Naïve T cells (that is, T cells that have not yet responded to a specific antigen) arise from precursors in bone marrow and mature in the thymus before they enter the circulation; circulating human naïve cells can be identified by the presence of a high molecular weight isoform of CD45 (CD45A) on their surface. These circulating cells adhere to endothelial cells of the HEV within lymph nodes by a process involving L-selectin on the T cell and a molecule called peripheral node addressin (PNAd), initiating the first step of cell migration from the circulation into the tissue of the node, known as tethering. PNAd refers to any one of a group of endothelial sialomucins—(CD34, podocalixin, glyocsylation-dependent cell adhesion molecule 1 (GlyCAM-1), and sialyated glycoprotein of 200 kDa (sgp200) [10]. All of these molecules contain a sulfated sialyl-Lewis^X-like motif.

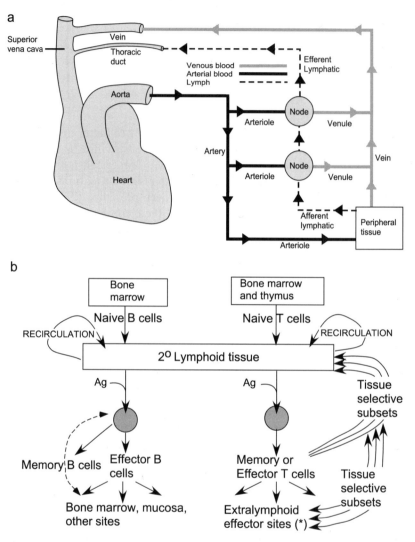

Figure 10.5. Schematic diagram of lymphocyte recirculation thoughout the body.
(a) Lymphocytes follow a typical pattern in their circulation throughout the body.
This pattern of circulation allows cells to observe, or sample, a large volume of the
body, but also to be present for large periods of time within the lymphatic tissue,
where they have more frequent encounters with foreign antigens associated with
antigen-presenting cells. (b) Pathways for circulation and differentiation of B and T
cells of the immune system. All cells move from their site of production, though the
circulatory systems, and eventually into secondary and tertiary tissue sites. (*)
includes skin, lung, intestine, etc.

Recruitment into tissue includes additional steps that follow tethering: rolling, firm arrest, and transmigration across the endothelial vascular lining. During transmigration, the lymphocyte becomes deformed and flattened in order to physically squeeze between the membrane–membrane interface of juxtaposed endothelial cells; the endothelial cells also respond to the act of lymphocyte transmigration by alteration of cytoskeletal structure and distribution of surface molecules. The extravasated cell now travels through the lymph node, which is rich in foreign antigens that have been collected from peripheral tissues (Figure 10.5b). The antigen collection process in the lymph node is also dependent on many of the same migratory mechanisms. Antigen collection involves homing of antigen-laden dendritic cells from the antigen-rich periphery to the lymph node; this migration is guided by a distinct set of cognate binding interactions that are dependent on receptors found on the dendritic cell surface.

The physical localization of the lymphocyte within the lymph node is also dependent upon these interactions. If the T cell does not encounter its antigen within the node, it leaves via an efferent lymphatic vessel which carries the cell back to the venous circulation (Figures 10.2b and 10.5a). Amazingly, a recirculating T cell completes an excursion through the lymph node in approximately 1 hour. Immunoprotection depends upon the daily flux of naïve T cells through the compact, cellularly dense lymph tissue; the flux is high, providing many opportunities for antigen/T cell recognition.

A T cell that encounters an antigen during movement through the lymph tissue becomes activated. Activation causes the cell to enter the cell cycle and to increase the expression of certain surface molecules as well as their affinity for their counter-ligand (Table 10.2). These surface proteins increase cell adhesion to extracellular matrix (ECM) and, therefore, slow cell migration through the

Table 10.2
Surface Proteins Characteristic of T cells during Circulation and Differentiation

	Surface Proteins	Adhesion	Homing Receptors (T cell/Endothelium)
Naïve T cell	CD45A	Lymph node endothelium	L-selectin/ PNAd,GlyCAM-1 LFA-1/?
Activated T cell	CD11aCD18 (LFA-1) CD49dCD29 (VLA-4) CD49eCD29 (VLA-5) CD49fCD29 (VLA-6) CD44	Lymph node extracellular matrix	
Differentiated T cell	CD45RO	Inflammatory endothelium	VLA-4/VCAM-1 LFA-1/ICAM-1,2 CD44/Hylauronate
		Mucosal tissues	$\alpha4\beta7$integrin/MadCAM-1 CD44/?

From [44].

lymph node, which is rich in ECM. Division and differentiation of activated T cells produce effector and memory cells; differentiated progeny retain high levels of expression of adhesion molecules, but these molecules do not exhibit high affinity. The differentiated cells are therefore released from the tissue and return to the circulation. Once in the circulation, however, the cells display a preferential adhesion to the endothelium of inflamed tissues and, therefore, an increased likelihood of migrating from the circulation at tissue sites where T cell effector activity is needed. Because the selective adhesiveness of T cells changes during activation and differentiation, cells at different stages of development have different fates in the body: naïve cells recirculate continuously through peripheral lymph tissue, activated cells commence proliferation and differentiation within the lymph node parenchyma, and memory/effector cells target inflamed tissue sites. This process of selective lymphocyte movement, which occurs in coordination with the activated molecular surface of the vascular endothelium in peripheral tissues, is called homing.

How do T cells recognize particular locations in a tissue? As described above, T cell migration from the circulation occurs preferentially within specialized vessels with protruding endothelial cell walls called HEVs. HEVs were first found in lymph nodes, but are also present in Peyer's patches of the gut. Endothelial cells of the HEV are particularly adhesive to T cells, so that cells passing through these vessels will cling briefly to the endothelium during transit. This brief halting of cell movement (descriptively referred to as "tethering") creates an opportunity for the T cell to roll along the vascular surface and concomitantly sample the repertoire of heparin-bound chemokines present on that surface. This rolling/sampling process can trigger firm T cell adherence to the wall, which leads to extravasation.

Lymphocytes are distinguished by the molecular composition of their outer membranes; some of the distinct molecules of each lymphocyte are involved in the process of recognition of endothelium and homing. Molecules that are involved in this process have been described for a number of different lymphocyte subpopulations (Table 10.3).

10.2.2 Peripheral Blood Stem Cell Infusions

The delivery of extremely high doses of chemotherapy agents can improve the survival of patients with certain kinds of tumors. Unfortunately, high-dose chemotherapy is often associated with devastating toxicity, particularly the suppression of production of normal bone marrow tissue components. But suppressed bone marrow can be repopulated by transfusion of cryopreserved bone marrow stem cells. The infused marrow stem cells may be autologous (harvested from the patient prior to the high dose chemotherapy) or allogeneic (harvested from a donor). Alternatively, marrow stem cells can be obtained from neonatal umbilical cord blood or from peripheral blood following mobilization, a process in which chemotherapy drugs or cytokines are used to induce the release of stem cells from the marrow into the peripheral blood.

Table 10.3
Adhesion Decision Cascades for Lymphocyte Homing

Lymphocytes	Target Destination	Endothelial Cell Adhesion Molecule	Counter-receptor on Lymphocytes			
			Contact	Rolling	Arrest	Diapedesis
Naïve B or T cells	Peyer's patch	MAdCAM MAdCAM-1 ICAM	L-selectin----	----------- -- α4β7 ------	-------------------	LFA1 ------------
Naïve B or T cells	Peripheral lymph node	PNAd ??? ICAMS	L-selectin----	----------- --???---------	-------------------	LFA1 ------------
Skin-homing memory cells	Skin	E-selectin VCAM-1 ICAMs	CLA---------	------- ----- α4β1--	------------------- -----	LFA1 ------------
Nonmucosal memory cells or blasts	Inflamed CNS, heart, others	??? VCAM-1 ICAMs	??? ----------	------- ----- α4β1--	------------------- -----	LFA1 ------------

More detailed information is available in review article [10].

Because of the disadvantages of current techniques for bone marrow harvest, including the complicated and uncomfortable procedure of collecting 1 to 2 L of bone marrow from patients, there is substantial interest in the development of cell culture systems that would permit the expansion of bone marrow outside the body (see [5] for a review of this technology).

10.2.3 T cell Therapies

Great progress has been made over the past two decades in the development of therapies that employ adoptive transfer of activated or engineered T cells [11]. Adoptive transfer of cells has many advantages over vaccine approaches in which a patient's own immune system is stimulated to produce active T cells. In cell transfer therapy, large numbers of cells can be administered; the cells can be activated *ex vivo*, allowing for control of the activation process; the exact cells that are required for therapy can be identified; and the host can be manipulated prior to transfer in order to optimize therapy.

The first evidence that the immune system could be manipulated to treat solid tumors in humans was achieved by high-dose delivery of the cytokine interleukin-2 (IL-2). IL-2 has a diverse spectrum of activities in the immune system, including stimulating the proliferation of activated lymphocytes. High-dose IL-2 led to tumor regression in a fraction of patients with metastatic melanoma (15% of patients experienced regression) and metastatic renal cell cancer (19%). IL-2 has no direct effect on tumor cell growth; the regression must therefore be due to an influence of the cytokine on cytotoxic immune cells. In this case, the IL-2 is acting on cells that already reside in the patient; responses, therefore, are limited only to patients who harbor enough cells that are capable of responding to the cytokine. This approach is also limited by the toxicity of high-dose IL-2 therapy to other cells and tissues in patients.

To further enhance the beneficial activity of IL-2, it can be administered together with an additional population of activated lymphocytes. In this approach, the activity of IL-2 on the patient's immune system is augmented by providing a large number of new cells that are capable of mediating tumour regression. Success of this cell transfer therapy depends on (1) the ability to identify cell populations that will be effective at mediating tumor regression in the patient, and (2) the ability to amplify the cell population *ex vivo*. Often, the precursor cells are collected from within the tumor itself; these cells are called tumor-infiltrating lymphocytes (TILs).

The circulation of lymphocytes after infusion depends on the source of the cells and can be influenced by treatment with cytokines. In an early study, TILs were labeled with ^{111}In (10^{10} cells) and infused together with IL-2 therapy, as tolerated [12]. In these patients TILs disappeared rapidly from the circulation: less than 2% were found after 1–2 hr. Initially, TILs were localized in the lung (30%), liver (30%), and spleen (10%). Liver and spleen levels were stable over seven days, while lung levels dropped to $\sim 10\%$ after one day. Tumor uptake increased over time, with maximum uptake occurring in the period of 48–72 h following infusion; the tumor localization index (ratio of cells in tumor/normal tissue) varied between 1 and 40 over the first 10 days after infusion. Normal, unactivated lymphocytes appear predominantly in the liver, lung, and spleen after infusion, with lung activity clearing within 24 h and liver and spleen activity stable for 96 h. The main differences between normal lymphocytes and TILs are (1) that some TILs remain in the liver for an extended period, and (2) that normal lymphocytes can traffic, but do not accumulate in the skin (whereas the TILs localize to the melanoma sites).

In a report of tumor-infiltrating cell infusions in patients, five patients were treated with TILs that had been transduced with a retroviral gene as a marker [13]. TILs, harvested from resected tumors and propogated in culture, were transduced with the retroviral vector in culture. Up to 2×10^{11} cells were infused into the patient over a 30–60 min period. Infusions of cells were followed by infusion of IL-2 . Cells were found in the circulation of patients for three weeks in all patients (up to two months in two patients). Cells were found at tumor sites up to 60 days following infusion. An example of the number of cells present in the peripheral blood of one of the patients is shown in Figure 10.6.

Other T cell therapies are already available for clinical use. For example, extracorporeal photochemotherapy or photophoresis is used to treat patients with cutaneous T cell lymphoma [14]. In photophoresis, ultraviolet light is focused on the blood of lymphoma patients as it flows through a serpentine-shaped plastic chamber outside of the body. Exposure to the light causes the tumorigenic blood-borne T lymphocytes to enter apoptosis; debris resulting

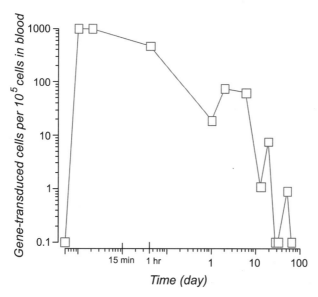

Figure 10.6. TIL cell elimination from the peripheral blood following transfusion into a patient. A semi-quantitative determination of cell number is shown as a function of time following TIL infusion (adapted from Figure 5 of [13]).

from cell death is taken up in part by circulating monocytes. Exposure of monocytes to the plastic surface of the extracorporeal chamber also seems to induce their differentiation to dendritic cells, which are effective in antigen presentation [45]. The monocytes are reintroduced to the blood of the patient; it is believed that immune activation accounts for full or partial recovery in a substantial percentage of cases. It is suspected, but not proven, that this therapy results in the activation of anti-tumor killer T cells that attack the tumorigenic T cell at the site of the skin lesion.

Animal models have also been used to study the fate of transfused cells. For example, mouse natural killer (NK) cells were activated with IL-2 and then injected into the tail vein of mice with the subcutaneous FSaII fibrosarcoma [15]. Positron emission tomography (PET) was used to measure the biodistribution of cells labelled with [11C]methyl iodide for animals that received injections of 10^7 activated NK cells or control (unactivated) cells. Retention of cells within the tumor was increased, compared to control cells, during the first 30–60 min following injection (Table 10.4). It is not clear whether the increased retention at the tumor site is due to increased rigidity of the activated cells, which increases mechanical trapping of cells in the tumor vasculature, or to increased interactions of cells with the tumor endothelium, although the vessels in the tumor appear to be large enough to permit even rigid cells to pass through easily. It is now possible to learn about the molecular details of interaction in systems such as this one; for example, the expression of adhesion molecules and chemokine receptors can be measured on the entrapped cells, using molecular tools such as quantitative RT-PCR.

10.2.4 Tumor Metastasis

In addition to the movement of blood cells out of vessels, migration from the interior of the vessel to the outside has also been observed for other types of cells. One unfortunate example is tumor metastasis; malignant cells sometimes

Table 10.4
Distribution of Activated NK cells Injected into the
Vasculature of a Tumor[a]

	Activated NK cells	Control cells
Tumor	15.3 ± 4.9	3.4 ± 0.2
Lungs	28.3 ± 5.1	21.6 ± 0.9
Liver + spleen	15.3 ± 1.6	17.0 ± 0.6
Other	41.9 ± 3.5	57.9 ± 1.6

[a]Percentage of total injected cells at various sites 30–60 min after injection of 10^7 cells into the tail vein of mice with subcutaneous tumor in the tail. Data from [15]. Retention of activated cells within the tumor is enhanced, but the mechanisms contributing to this enhancement are still unknown.

enter the circulation and then re-emerge from vessels at a distant tissue site. Tumor cell egress from the vasculature has been visualized using the chorioallantonic membrane (CAM) [16, 17], which allows determination of the time course of tumor cell migration from the vasculature after injection (Figure 10.7). Within 2 min of injection, all of the tumor cells were arrested, probably due to size restrictions since the cells are significantly larger ($\sim 20\,\mu m$) than the plexus channels in the CAM ($\sim 9\,\mu m$). In these experiments, there was almost no evidence that tumor cells were arrested due to adhesion to the vessel wall. (The mechanisms responsible for cell arrest are still in debate [18].) Following arrest, the cells may move slowly with the flow within the local vasculature, while undergoing extensive deformation and changes in morphology. The cells could then extravasate from the vessel into the extravascular space; this occurred primarily within the period of 5–10 hr following injection (Figure 10.7). The rate of cell migration into the extravascular space was approximately 1 μm/hr (which is consistent with rates of tumor cell migration, Table 7.2). No cell destruction was observed during the periods of observation, but this may be due to the milder flow conditions in the chick membrane (no white cells in the blood, low-velocity blood flow). The majority of potentially metastatic cells (up to 99%) are destroyed in the mouse lung following injection. In the CAM, cell division did not occur prior to extravasation, but did occur after; the cells tended to divide to form micrometastases around the vessels.

Since cell adhesion receptors mediate the interaction of blood-borne cells with the vessel wall, and since this interaction is essential for transmigration

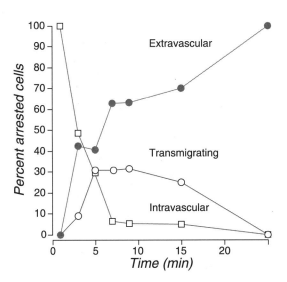

Figure 10.7. Dynamics of transmigration in a model system. The dynamics of tumor cell migration out of the circulatory system can be studied in model systems such as the chick chorioallantoic membrane (CAM). In this experiment, the tumor cells are initially within the blood vessels, but they quickly adhere to vessel walls and transmigrate into the extravascular space.

into tissues, it might be possible to block tissue localization by using agents that block cell adhesion. One early report testing this hypothesis provides evidence for reduction in colonization of the lung of mice with the coadministration of GRGDS, a peptide that should inhibit tumor cell binding to integrin receptors, and B16-F10 murine melanoma cells [19]. Reduction in colonization requires high doses (~ 3 mg) of GRGDS per mouse, which leads to a blood concentration of 3 mM. The low efficiency of this approach may be due to the relative low affinity of blocking peptides with cell adhesion receptors. For example, the affinity of fibronectin for its receptor is $K_d = 0.8 \times 10^{-6}$ M (recall discussion in Chapter 6). Still, at least in some experimental models, it is possible to reduce colonization with high doses of peptide. It is likely that more can be done in this regard in the future by enagaging multiple arms of the immune system; for example, down-regulation of inflammatory mediators (for example, TNF) might be useful as an adjuvant therapy to this blocking peptide strategy.

10.3 Microchimerism

A common method in tissue engineering is the transplantation of cells from a donor into a host. In this chapter so far, we have been considering the introduction of cells by infusion into the circulatory system. It is clear from previous experience that infused cells can enter tissues, and that the dispersion and retention of cells will depend on properties of the transplanted cell population as well as properties of the host. How does this information guide our thinking about the long-term consequences of tissue engineering in human patients?

It is now known that transplanted cells, even when introduced to the host by means other than infusion, can migrate to tissues of the recipient that are distant from their site of introduction and that they can persist at these sites for long periods of time. This new appreciation of the frequency and magnitude of mixing of cells between the donor tissue and the host—a slow process of intermingling that results in a "mixed" state that is called microchimerism— has emerged from observations in two different clinical settings: cells from transplanted solid organs that mix into other tissues of a transplant recipient [20], and cells from a fetus that persist within tissues of the mother [21].

The modern age of organ transplantation began in the middle of the twentieth century (see Chapter 1). It has been known for several decades now that the transplanted organ becomes chimeric: cells from the host migrate into the transplanted organ and function in that environment. For example, reticuloendothelial cells of the host migrate into transplanted livers and replace donor cells, creating a transplanted organ that has abundant cells from the donor (liver parenchymal cells, endothelial cells) and cells from the host (reticuloendothelial cells). It is also well known that the migration of donor immune cells from the transplant can initiate pathological changes in the host through a spectrum of diseases known as graft-versus-host disease (GVHD). But, in 1992, Starzl and his colleagues demonstrated that chimerism after solid organ transplantation is, in fact, systemic [20]. In long-term recipients of liver and kidney transplants, donor cells could be found in the host skin, blood, lymph nodes, heart, and other organs (Figure 10.8).

In microchimeric patients, after solid organ transplantation, many of the systemic donor cells have been identified as antigen-presenting cells. Since this state of microchimerism was found in long-term transplant survivors, it was hypothesized that the microchimeric state was an important step in the dynamics of immune response to a transplanted organ. The patient now has cells from two immune systems (host and donor) and these cells can both be active; if the response of the donor cells dominates, then GVHD can develop, whereas if the response of the host immune system dominates, then organ rejection can occur. Perhaps the microchimeric state represents a piece of an equilibrium condition that is established between immune response of the host and donor, in which a balance has been obtained that produces neither GVHD nor rejection. This balance, which leads to organ acceptance or immunological tolerance, may be facilitated by the cellular events observed in microchimerism. In this hypothesis, immunosuppression therapy, which is given to transplant recipients, may serve as a screen that allows microchimerism to prosper, producing an ultimate state of immune balance in which organ acceptance requires no additional immunosuppressive drugs. One prediction of this hypothesis is that immune tolerance may be enhanced by the intentional introduction of donor leukocytes into the patient. Animal models of rejection and microchimerism after skin grafts suggest that maturity of the host immune system and function of the donor cells are both important variables in the prediction of rejection or tolerance outcomes [22].

Although the overall hypothesis—that microchimerism enhances the process of tolerance—is still controversial [23], it is clear that substantial exchange

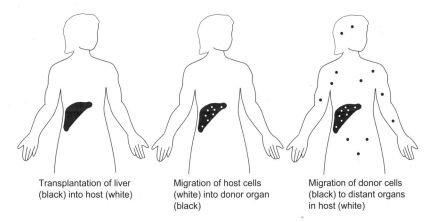

| Transplantation of liver (black) into host (white) | Migration of host cells (white) into donor organ (black) | Migration of donor cells (black) to distant organs in host (white) |

Figure 10.8. Development of microchimerism. After transplantation of a solid organ (here, a "black" liver into a "white" host, left panel), cells from the host can migrate into the donor organ (middle panel) and cells from the organ can migrate into the host (right panel).

of cells can occur between transplanted solid organs and the host. This observation may have important consequences for clinical use of tissue-engineered products. Indeed, in order for graft acceptance to succeed, transplanted organs must become perfused by the recipient's blood, itself an invitation to the exchange of cells.

Cells of fetal origin can persist for long periods (perhaps a lifetime) in the tissues of a mother. Since women experience an increased incidence of a variety of autoimmune diseases (such as systemic sclerosis, primary biliary cirrhosis, and Sjögrens syndrome), it has been hypothesized that the microchimeric state produced by pregnancy may increase the risk for autoimmune diseases. Again, studies on both sides of the hypothesis have been reported and the relation between microchimerism and autoimmune disease remains controversial [22].

10.4 Cell Penetration into Three-Dimensional Tissues

The physics of cell movement through the circulation is well known; the physical forces and chemical components of transmigration across an endothelial barrier are emerging (as outlined in the sections above). But how do cells migrate through a three-dimensional tissue space which is filled with other cells and, potentially, a dense extracellular matrix in the interstitial space?

Some motile cells can migrate through reconstituted extracellular matrix gels, which may reflect the ability of cells to migrate through solid tissues *in vivo*. It is well known that such movement is required physiologically, since, once extravasation occurs, monocytes and T cells must make their way through the ECM guided in part by chemokines produced by the underlying epithelia (for example, keratinocytes in skin) in order to eventually find their way to the afferent lymphatic which leads to the local draining lymph node. Mechanistically, human neutrophils move rapidly within three-dimensional gels of rat tail collagen; the rate of movement depends on the nature of the surrounding gel, in particular on the density of the ECM gel [24] (see Figure 7.6a). This observation may have important implications. In fulfilling their role in the immune response, neutrophils migrate out of capillaries, through tissue, to sites of infection. Perhaps, within the tissue, cell speed is influenced by the level of ECM hydration. The local tissue edema that accompanies inflammation may be a significant factor, modulating the rate of neutrophil infiltration. Similar factors may influence the speed of leukocyte migration—and therefore the efficiency of immune cell surveillance—in mucus secretions. For these reasons, experimental techniques for quantifying cell movement in three-dimensional gels and tissues have been developed as a first step in evaluating the mechanism by which cells migrate through tissues [24, 25]. Much about the process of cell migration through complex media remains unknown; for example, the relationship between the stiffness of the migrating cell—and changes in stiffness due to dynamic changes in the cytoskeletal architecture at the intracellular level—and the rate of cell migration is still unknown.

Motile cells within three-dimensional gels exhibit a random migration process that is similar to cell migration on a surface. In some systems the similarity between the trajectories of motile cells and particles undergoing Brownian motion is striking, suggesting that diffusion might be responsible for the movement that is quantified by direct observation in three-dimensional gels. The diffusion coefficient for a spherical particle in water can be estimated from the Stokes–Einstein equation

$$D_w = \frac{kT}{6\pi\eta r} \tag{10-2}$$

where D_w is the diffusion coefficient of the particle in water, k is Boltzman's constant, T is the absolute temperature, η is the viscosity of water at T, and r is the radius of the particle. For a particle with a radius of 5 μm diffusing in water at 37°C, Equation 10-2 gives D_w of 6×10^{-10} cm^2/s, not much lower than the smallest random motility coefficient measured in common experimental systems (that is, 16×10^{-10} cm^2/s) (Figure 7.6a). But red blood cells, which are similar in size to neutrophils, never move after suspension in a collagen gel, even when the experimental duration is long. Furthermore, if diffusion were responsible for cell movement, the diffusion coefficient would monotonically decrease with increasing collagen concentration due to the increase in viscosity and/or viscoelasticity; however, motility coefficients show a maximum in the random motility coefficient at an intermediate collagen concentration (Figure 7.6a). On the basis of these observations it is reasonable to speculate that the fibers in the gel prevent diffusion of cell-sized particles; there must be some active interaction between cells and ECM fibers that enables these cells to traverse the gel.

Random motility coefficients for human neutrophils within gels of rat tail collagen varied from 1.6 to 13×10^{-9} cm^2/s (Figure 7.6a). How does this compare to the rate of cell migration on a solid surface? Two alternative quantitative assays have previously been employed to estimate this coefficient for neutrophils. Using an under-agarose assay, in which cells are attached to a two-dimensional substrate, μ was $\sim 10^{-8}$ cm^2/s [26], near the maximum observed in this study; using a filter assay, where cells migrate through a three-dimensional mesh of synthetic fibers, μ was $\sim 10^{-9}$ cm^2/s [27], near the minimum observed in collagen gels. While there are potentially important quantitative differences between observed migration rates in these assay systems, it is interesting that these three very different techniques yield similar values for the random motility coefficient.

Several previous reports examining the relationship between adhesion and cell motility on surfaces suggest that the strength of a cell–surface adhesion must be at an optimal level for cell migration (recall discussion in Chapter 7). If the adhesive strength is well above this optimum, cells will become fixed to the surface and hence will not migrate. If cell–surface adhesion falls much below the optimal level, the cell will not be able to gain sufficient traction to translocate across the surface. There is probably also an optimal adhesiveness for neutrophils migrating in three-dimensional materials. In the collagen gel systems, below a concentration of 0.1 mg/mL, most neutrophils rapidly sink through the gel; at concentrations above 0.7 mg/mL, the majority of neutrophils are immobilized (although neutrophils were seen to extend and retract pseudopodia in these high concentration gels, they were unable to make significant displacements from their initial positions). Between these two extremes, neutrophils exhibit maximal motility at a collagen concentration of 0.3 mg/mL (Figure 7.7). Inter-collagen fiber spacing is approximately equal to a neutrophil diameter ($\sim 10\,\mu$m) at 0.1 mg/mL, and decreases as the collagen concentration is raised [28]. These previous results suggest that when the collagen concentration is increased above the optimal level (0.3 mg/mL), the strength of the cell–fiber interactions becomes stronger due to the increased number of collagen fibers surrounding the cell. Analogously, at lower collagen concentrations where there are fewer fibers, the cell–fiber adhesive strength is lower (and the speed of migration can be influenced by adding antibodies against cell adhesion receptors [29]). Both of these situations result in a decrease in the effectiveness with which cells are able to migrate through the gel. Cells in solid tissues experience a more complex environment—they are surrounded by a variety of ECM components as well as adjacent cell surfaces—but some aspects of this mechanism probably act in tissues as well.

How do these results compare to the rates of cell migration in tissues in a living organism? This question is difficult to answer, since there are few reliable, quantitative measurements of the rate of cell migration through a tissue space. In one model system, the rate of migration of pigmented retinal cells within a neural cell aggregate was determined [30]. The rate of cell movement in this situation was much slower than rates of cell movement on surfaces or within three-dimensional ECM gels (Table 10.5).

Cells that have been transplanted into solid tissue can potentially migrate, reducing their effectiveness at the local site and potentially leading to unwanted side effects of the cell delivery. It may also be possible to learn about rates of cell migration in tissues by studying the fates of cells transplanted into a living organ. Neuronal cell transplantation has been an important experimental tool for many years. As early as 1917, pieces of neural tissue were transplanted into defects in the neocortex of adult animals [31] or introduced through cannulae

Table 10.5
Random Motility Coefficient for Cells in Different Experimental Systems

	Motility Coefficient, μ or Diffusion Coefficient, D (cm^2/s)	Reference
Oxygen in water	1×10^{-5}	[41]
Protein in water	1×10^{-7}	[41]
Neutrophil in ECM gel	1×10^{-8}	[24]
Fibroblasts on glass surface	1×10^{-9}	[42]
Pigmented retinal cell in neural aggregate	5×10^{-12}	[30]

[32]. More recently, techniques for the transplantation of dissociated neural tissues have been introduced and studied extensively [33–38]. An excellent review of the technical procedures involved in neural transplantation of tissue pieces, dissociated tissue fragments, and dissociated cell suspensions is available [39].

Cells within the subventricular zone of the lateral ventricle in adult mice continue to proliferate. Using genetically labeled cells from donor transgenic mice, which were transplanted into immunologically identical hosts, as well as endogenous cells labeled with microinjected ^{3}H-thymidine, these proliferating cells were found to migrate into the olfactory bulb [40]. The speed of migration was estimated as $30\,\mu m/hr$ (see Table 7.2 for comparisons). When examined during the period 6– 30 days following transplantation, the cells had migrated up to 5 mm. Although it is difficult to make quantitative comparisons with the rates of migration in model systems, which are more easily quantified, it is clear that cells can migrate long distances after transplantation into a solid tissue.

Summary

- Cells can be introduced into a recipient by infusion; this technique has been used successfully for many decades, and the lifetime and distribution of some cell populations after infusion are now well known.
- Cells within the circulation can transmigrate through endothelial barriers to reach a local tissue site. The process of transmigration occurs in a series of steps; some of the molecular participants in adhesion and transmigration have been discovered.
- Cells in the circulation can find their way to specific tissue sites; cells rely in part on the molecular composition of the local endothelium to determine their location in the body.
- Cells that are transplanted into a host can persist for long periods of time under the right conditions. The long-term persistence of donor organ cells that are widely distributed in the host is evidence of the capacity of transplanted cells to migrate long distances and to survive.

Acknowledgement

This chapter benefited greatly from editing and suggestions from Dr. Martin S. Kluger.

Exercises

Exercise 10.1

Consider the mathematical model presented in Equations 10-1, which were taken from the paper by Iadocicco *et al.* [7].

a) Compare the equations presented in this chapter with the comparable ones in the paper (Equations 1a to 1d). What variables have been changed? Justify any differences that you find.
b) State and verify the assumptions that were made in reducing the set of four equations (Equation 10-1) to the "compact model" indicated in Equations 2a and 2b in the paper.
c) Verify the equilibrium solution found in the section Methods 1.

Exercise 10.2 (provided by Linda G. Griffith)

Several investigators have proposed that the rate of bone healing in an alloplast device might be increased if a source of progenitor cells were included at the time of implant. Two such sources are possible: (1) whole marrow, which can be readily obtained in the operating room at the time of surgery; (2) stem cells purified from marrow, an approach which likely requires an extra procedure and handling of the cells outside the operating room. In the case of marrow, only a very small fraction ($\ll 1\%$) of the cells are progenitors for bone. Thus, in the case of creating new bone in large alloplasts, it may be useful to purify the progenitors because of mass transfer issues.

a) Compare the maximum number and concentration of cells that can be implanted in a 1 mm thick versus a 1 cm thick device if oxygen is the limiting nutrient. You may assume the cells are homogeneously distributed in a porous matrix (infinite slab geometry), that the minimum allowable concentration of oxygen is 50% of that in the tissue surrounding the implant, that the oxygen concentration in the tissue surrounding the implant is 0.1 mM, and that the purified stem cells and whole marrow consume oxygen at the same rate, 4×10^{-11} mol/million cells-sec.
b) Compare the time required for devices (both the 1 mm and the 1 cm) seeded with either marrow or purified stem cells, seeded at maximum density calculated in part (a), to grow to a tissue-like density of 1×10^8 cells/cm^3. You can assume that the cell growth rate is proportional to the number of cells present, and that the time required for cells to double in number is 2 days. You may assume that only the progenitors grow and that the purified stem cells contain only progenitors while in marrow the fraction of progenitors is 0.00001. You may also assume that the other cells in marrow are "inert" (that is, do not grow) for this calculation. You may also assume that blood vessels grow at a rate that can supply the cells with adequate nutrients.

References

1. Starr, D., *Blood: An Epic History of Medicine and Commerce*. New York: Alfred A. Knopf, 1998.
2. Eadie, G.S., I.W. Brown, and W.G. Curtis, The potential life span and ultimate survival of fresh red blood cells in normal healthy recipients as studied by simultaneous CR-51 tagging and differential hemolysis. *Journal of Clinical Investigation*, 1954, **34**, 629.
3. Hogg, J.C., et al., Erythrocyte and polymorphonuclear cell transit time and concentration in human pulmonary capillaries. *Journal of Applied Physiology*, 1994, **77**(4), 1795–1800.
4. Mollison, P.L., *Blood Transfusion in Clinical Medicine*, 6th ed. Oxford: Blackwell Scientific Publishers, 1979.
5. Koller, M.R. and B.O. Palsson, Tissue engineering: reconstitution of human hematopoiesis *ex vivo*. *Biotechnology and Bioengineering*, 1993, **42**, 909–930.
6. Andrade, W.N., M.G. Johnston, and J.B. Hay, The relationship of blood lymphocytes to the recirculating lymphocyte pool. *Blood*, 1998, **91**(5), 1653–1661.
7. Iadocicco, K., L.H.A. Monteiro, and J.G. Chaui-Berlinck, A theoretical model for estimating the margination constant of leukocytes. *BMC Physiology*, 2002, **2**(3), http://www.biomedcentral.com/1472–6793/2/3.
8. Melder, R.J., et al., Systemic distribution and tumor localization of adoptively transferred lymphocytes in mice: comparison with physiologically based pharmacokinetic model. *Neoplasia*, 2002, **4**(1), 3–8.
9. Abbas, A.K., A.H. Lichtman, and J.S. Pober, *Cellular and Molecular Immunology*, 4th ed. Philadelphia, PA: W.B. Saunders, 2000.
10. von Andrian, U. and C. Mackay, T-cell function and migration—Two sides of the same coin. *New England Journal of Medicine*, 2000, **343**, 1020–1034.
11. Rosenberg, S.A., Progress in the development of immunotherapy for the treatment of patients with cancer. *Journal of Internal Medicine*, 2001, **250**, 462–475.
12. Fisher, B., et al., Tumor localization of adoptively transferred indium-111 labeled tumor infiltrating lymphocytes in patients with metastatic melanoma. *Journal of Clinical Oncology*, 1989, **7**(2), 250–261.
13. Rosenberg, S.A., et al., Gene transfer into humans: immunotherapy of patients with advanced melanoma, using tumor-infiltrating lymphocytes modified by retroviral gene transduction. *New England Journal of Medicine*, 1990, **323**(9), 570–578.
14. Wolfe, J.T., et al., Review of immunomodulation by photophoresis: treatment of cutaneous T-cell lymphoma, autoimmune disease, and allograft rejection. *Artificial Organs*, 1994, **18**(1), 888–897.
15. Melder, R.J., et al., Imaging of activated natural killer cells in mice by positron emission tomography: preferential uptake in tumors. *Cancer Research*, 1993, **53**, 5867–5871.
16. Chambers, A.F., et al., Early steps in hematogenous metastasis of B16F1 melanoma cells in chick embryos studied by high-resolution intravital videomicroscopy. *Journal of National Cancer Institute*, 1992, **84**, 797–803.
17. MacDonald, I.C., et al., Intravital videomicroscopy of the chorioallantoic microcirculation: a model system for studying metastasis. *Microvascular Research*, 1992, **44**, 185–199.
18. Weiss, L., Deformation-driven destruction of cancer cells in the microvasculature [letter]. *Clinical and Experimental Metastasis*, 1993, **11**, 430–436.

19. Humphries, M.J., K. Olden, and K.M. Yamada, A synthetic peptide from fibronectin inhibits experimental metastasis of murine melanoma cells. *Science*, 1986, **233**, 467–470.

20. Starzl, T., et al., Cell migration, chimerism, and graft acceptance. *The Lancet*, 1992, **339**, 1579–1582.

21. Nelson, J.L., Microchimerism: incidental byproduct of pregnancy or active participant in human health. *Trends in Molecular Medicine*, 2002, **8**(3), 109–113.

22. Anderson, C.C. and P. Matzinger, Immunity or tolerance: opposite outcomes of microchimerism from skin grafts. *Nature Medicine*, 2001, **7**, 80–87.

23. Triulzi, D.J. and M.A. Nalesnik, Microchimerism, GVHD, and tolerance in solid organ transplantation. *Transfusion*, 2001, **41**, 419–426.

24. Parkhurst, M.R. and W.M. Saltzman, Quantification of human neutrophil motility in three-dimensional collagen gels: effect of collagen concentration. *Biophysical Journal*, 1992, **61**, 306–315.

25. Parkhurst, M.R. and W.M. Saltzman, Leukocyte migration in three-dimensional gels of midcycle cervical mucus. *Cellular Immunology*, 1994, **156**, 77–94.

26. Lauffenburger, D., C. Rothman, and S. Zigmond, Measurement of leukocyte motility and chemotaxis parameters with a linear under-agarose migration assay. *Journal of Immunology*, 1983, **131**, 940–947.

27. Buettner, H.M., D.A. Lauffenburger, and S.H. Zigmond, Measurement of leukocyte motility and chemotaxis parameters with the Millipore filter assay. *Journal of Immunological Methods*, 1989, **123**, 25–37.

28. Saltzman, W.M., et al., Three-dimensional cell cultures mimic tissues. *Annals of the New York Academy of Science*, 1992, **665**, 259–273.

29. Saltzman, W.M., T.L. Livingston, and M.R. Parkhurst, Antibodies to CD18 influence the migration of neutrophils through collagen gels. *Journal of Leukocyte Biology*, 1999, **65**, 356–363.

30. Mombach, J.C.M. and J.A. Glazier, Single cell motion in aggregates of embryonic cells. *Physical Review*, 1996, **76**(16), 3032–3035.

31. Dunn, E.H., Primary and secondary findings in a series of attempts to transplant cerebral cortex in the albino rat. *Journal of Comparative Neurology*, 1917, **27**, 565–582.

32. Murphy, J.B. and E. Strum, Conditions determining the transplantability of tissues in the brain. *Journal of Experimental Medicine*, 1923, **38**, 183–197.

33. Bjorklund, A., et al., Intracerebral grafting of neuronal cell suspensions I. Introduction and general methods of preparation. *Acta Physiol. Scand. Suppl.*, 1983, **522**, 1–7.

34. Bjorklund, A., et al., Intracerebral grafting of neuronal cell suspensions II. Survival and growth of nigral cell suspensions implanted in different brain sites. *Acta Physiol. Scand. Suppl.*, 1983, **522**, 9–18.

35. Schmidt, R.H., et al., Intracerebral grafting of neuronal cell suspensions III. Activity of intrastriatal nigral suspension implants as assessed by measurements of dopamine synthesis and metabolism. *Acta Physiol. Scand. Suppl.*, 1983, **522**, 19–28.

36. Gage, F.H., et al., Intracerebral grafting of neuronal cell suspensions VIII. Survival and growth of implants of nigral and septal cell suspensions in intact brains of aged rats. *Acta Physiol. Scand. Suppl.*, 1983, **522**, 67–75.

37. Gage, F.H., et al., Intracerebral grafting of embryonic neural cells into the adult host brain: an overview of the cell suspension method and its application. *Developmental Neuroscience*, 1983, **6**, 137–151.

38. Bjorklund, A. and U. Stenevi, eds., *Neural Grafting in the Mammalian CNS*. Amsterdam: Elsevier, 1985.
39. Dunnett, S.B. and A. Bjorklund, eds., *Neural Transplantation: A Practical Approach*. Practical Approach Series, ed. D. Rickwood and B.D. Hames. New York: Oxford University Press, 1992.
40. Lois, C. and A. Alvarez-Buylla, Long-distance neuronal migration in the adult mammalian brain. *Science*, 1994, **264**, 1145–1148.
41. Saltzman, W.M., *Drug Delivery: Engineering Principles for Drug Therapy*. New York: Oxford University Press, 2001.
42. Saltzman, W.M., et al., Fibroblast and hepatocyte behavior on synthetic polymer surfaces. *Journal of Biomedical Materials Research*, 1991, **25**, 741–759.
43. Young, A.L., The physiology of lymphocyte migration through the single lymph node *in vivo*. *Seminars in Immunology*, 1999, **11**, 73–83.
44. Abbas, A.K., A.H. Lichtman, and J.S. Pober, *Cellular and Molecular Immunology*, 2nd ed. Philadelphia, PA: W.B. Saunders, 1994.
45. Edelson, R.L. Transimmunization: the science catches up to the clinical success. *Transfusion and Apheresis Science*, 2002, **26**, 177–180.

11

Delivery of Molecular Agents in Tissue Engineering

All truths wait in all things;
They neither hasten their own delivery, nor resist it...

Walt Whitman, *Leaves of Grass*

The previous chapter provided some examples of tissue engineering, in which cells that were isolated and engineered outside of the body are introduced into a patient by direct injection of a cell suspension, typically into the circulatory system. But the field of tissue engineering also points to treatments that are conceptually different from variations on cell transfusion technology; tissue engineering promises the regrowth of adult tissue structure through application of engineered cells and synthetic materials [2]. In support of this broad claim, the field of tissue engineering can point to some initial successes. For example, synthetic materials are now available that accelerate healing of burns and skin ulcers [3]. In addition, *in vitro* cell culture methods now allow the amplification of a patient's own cells for cartilage repair or bone marrow transplantation.

But major obstacles to the widespread application of tissue engineering remain. Tissue engineers have not yet learned how to reproduce complex tissue architectures, such as vascular networks, which are essential for the normal function of many tissues. In fact, the tissue engineering concepts that have been demonstrated in the laboratory to date involve arrangements of cells and materials into precursor tissues (or neotissues) that develop according to natural processes that are already present within the cells or the materials at the time of implantation (Table 11.1). These methods may be suitable for production of some tissues in which either the structure is relatively homogeneous (such as cartilage, in which a tissue structure can reform after the implantation of chondrocytes into a tissue defect) or the structure develops naturally (such as in some tissue-engineered skin, in which the stratified epithelium develops naturally by culturing at an air–liquid interface [4]).

The engineering of many tissue structures—such as the branching architectures found in many tissues or the intricate network architecture of the nervous system—will probably require methods for introducing and changing molecular signals during the process of neo-tissue development. For example,

318

Table 11.1
Stages of Development in Selected Examples of Tissue Engineering

Tissue	Neotissue	Stages of Development	Agents of Interest	Ref.
Vascular networks	Human dermal microvascular endothelial cells within a degradable PLLA matrix (*in vivo*)	Dispersed cells (day 1) Tubular structures (day 5) Functional microvessels (day 7)		[84]
	Flk1 + cells derived from embryonic stem cells within a 3D collagen matrix (*in vitro* and *in vivo*)	Aggregates (day 0) Process formation (day 3) Organized tubular structures formed of multiple cell lineages (day 5)	VEGF	[85]
	Bcl-2 transduced human umbilical vein endothelial cells within a 3D collagen/fibronectin matrix (*in vitro* and *in vivo*)	Organization into cords (day 1) Formation of vascular structures and complex multicellular walls (31 to 60 days)		[86]
Bone	Bone morphogenetic protein in PLA-DX-PEG copolymer matrix (*in vivo*)	Repair of 2 mm bone defects (time and dose-dependent over 2–4 weeks)	rhBMP-2	[87]
	Osteogenic cells cultured in presence of TGF-β1 (*in vitro*)	Formation of 3D aggregates (1–2 days) Production of bone minerals (3–10 days)	TGF-β1	[88]
Cartilage	Free and liposome-encapsulated TGF-β1 in fibrin matrix (*in vivo*)	Migration of mesenchymal cells into matrix (days) Differentiation of cells into mature chondrocytes (weeks)	TGF-β1	[89]
Peripheral nerve	Fibrin matrices with bioactive peptides (*in vivo*)	Regrowth of axons into gap of severed dorsal root (4 weeks)		[90]
Central nervous tissue	PLGA microspheres dispersed within brain cell aggregates (*in vitro* and *in vivo*)	Release of NGF and accumulation in tissue (hours to days) Differentiation (days)	NGF	[11]
Thymic organ	Thymic stromal cells and progenitors within 3D tantalum-coated carbon matrix (*in vivo*)	Formation of confluent stromal layer on matrix (14 days) Co-culture with hematopoietic progenitors to produce T cells (14 days)		[91]

Abbreviations: transforming growth factor β (TGF-β), vascular endothelial growth factor (VEGF), basic fibroblast growth factor (bFGF), bone morphogenic protein (BMP), nerve growth factor (NGF), epidermal growth factor (EGF).

it is well known that chemical gradients of factors known as morphogens induce the formation of structures during development [5, 6]; some of the attributes of morphogens were introduced in Chapter 3. In addition, changes of agent concentration with time can influence the state of differentiation of cells within tissues; growth factors and transcription factors are two well-known examples of agents that function in this manner. With these examples in mind, it is natural to hypothesize that developing the capability to control the physical placement and lifetime of molecular signals is essential for tissue engineering.

Consider a simple model of a tissue engineering environment—which we call a neotissue—in which a synthetic material is combined with living cellular material; further, assume that the synthetic material is designed to create time- and space-dependent variations in concentration of an agent in the vicinity of the material (Figure 11.1a). Biomaterials science is advancing at a remarkable pace, resulting in a wide selection of technology for implantable synthetic materials [7, 8]. Within the spectrum of tissue engineering applications, this synthetic material could represent a drug delivery system intended to release growth factors into a wound bed (Figure 11.1b), a segment of a polymeric mesh intended to provide agent delivery as well as a physical support for cell attachment and migration in the regenerating tissue (Figure 11.1c), or a micro-fabricated prosthetic element intended to integrate in a stable fashion with cells from the host tissue (Figure 11.1d).

A spectrum of biomaterials technologies is presented in Figure 11.1; the specific requirements for delivery of an agent—that is, the identity of the molecular agent(s), its desired concentration in the tissue, and the rate of change of agent concentration with time and spatial position—will undoubtedly differ for each of these materials and every clinical application. This chapter attempts to put these technologies into perspective with regard to their potential for the delivery of molecular agents. In particular, several general questions are addressed here: What options does modern biomaterials technology offer for the controlled delivery of drugs or agents that influence the formation of tissue structure? What are the limits of agent delivery in cases where the drug must be present in time- or space-varying concentrations in order to produce the desired effect? What are the basic principles of agent transport that must guide the design and development of these delivery systems?

11.1 Technology for Controlled Delivery of Molecular Agents in Tissue Engineering

11.1.1 Controlled Release Methods in Tissue Engineering

Introduction to Controlled Release. Controlled release technology has been studied for many decades and is embodied in devices such as Norplant® and Gliadel®, which are used clinically for prevention of pregnancy and brain

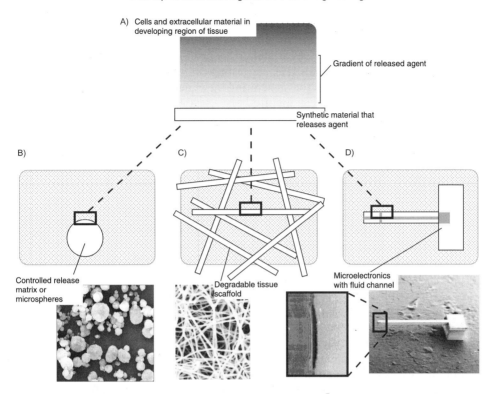

Figure 11.1. Methods for controlled delivery of agents into localized regions of tissue. Panel A shows the general situation in which an agent (indicated by white) is released from a synthetic materials into the tissue (indicated by grey/black), producing a gradient of the agent in the tissue surrounding the material. This general situation can occur with different materials, as illustrated in panels B through D. (B) Controlled release technology can provide continuous agent release from a solid material. The inset shows poly(lactide-co-glycolide) microspheres that release NGF (photograph from [11]). (C) Agent delivery by release from a degradable porous scaffold composed of either synthetic polymers or natural polymers such as collagen (shown in inset) or fibrin. (D) Agent delivery from a system with microfluidic channels. The microelectronic probe (shown in the right inset) has an internal microchannel (shown at higher magnification in the left inset), which is indicated by the grey-shaded region in the schematic illustration. In this final panel, microfabrication and photos were provided by A. Spence, S. Retterer, and M.S. Isaacson (Cornell University).

tumor therapy, respectively [9]. Controlled release has many direct applications to tissue engineering. For example, local delivery of growth factors can be accomplished by encapsulating the agent within a biocompatible polymer matrix or microsphere. The controlled-release polymer system is then implanted at the desired tissue site, where it releases the soluble factor directly into the interstitial space of the tissue (Figure 11.1b). The diffusible agent may influence survival or the function of damaged cells within the local tissue, or provide a signal that elicits cell proliferation or migration within the tissue region. For example, controlled delivery of NGF prevents degeneration of cholinergic neurons in the brain [10, 11]. Similarly, continuous infusions of epidermal growth factor (EGF) stimulate the proliferation of neural precursors in the brains of adult animals [12], suggesting that controlled delivery of EGF may some day be useful for generating new neurons in the adult brain. Signaling molecules that are involved in development and regeneration of various tissues have been identified (some examples are listed in Table 11.1; others are described in the section that follows).

Classes of Molecular Agents that Might be Useful in Tissue Engineering.   Growth factors are one class of agents that might be productively delivered to developing neo-tissues. A variety of protein growth factors that influence cell growth and differentiation have been described, and many of these factors have been tested for safety and effectiveness in human populations (see Section 11.2.1). But other classes of agents may also be good candidates for controlled delivery in tissue engineering, including agents that potentiate the immune response or modify local gene expression.

Transcription factors are transregulatory proteins that bind to specific DNA sequences (called enhancers) and modulate the efficiency and rate of transcription by interaction with the promoter. The expression of certain transcription factors is restricted to specific cell types, where they are responsible for controlling the expression of genes that characterize the state of differentiation of the cell. Transcription factors are well known for their role in patterning in the embryo and cell differentiation. In addition, the activity of some transcription factors can be regulated by hormones, such as retinoic acid and steroid hormones, which bind to the transcription factor and thereby control its biological activity. Local delivery of transcription factors, or drugs that modulate transcription factors, could provide for local control of gene expression in cells within a developing neo-tissue.

Advances in immunosuppression have greatly reduced the problem of immune rejection of transplanted organs. This improvement is primarily due to the introduction of the cyclic peptide cyclosporine, which inhibits the expression of cytokine genes in T cells (through its action on a T cell transcription factor). While cyclosporine has increased the survival of donor organs such as kidney, heart, and liver, it does not work in all cases and side effects, such as renal damage, are possible at high dose. Local delivery of cyclosporine has been successful in special cases, such as topical delivery to transplanted skin [13]. The use of controlled delivery systems for local delivery of agents that modulate the immune response may be particularly valuable in tissue engineering. Other agents that influence immune effector cells, such as antibodies against targeting selected cell populations, cytokines or other concepts that might not be prudent for systemic therapy, may be suitable for local administration. The development of local delivery methods for immunosuppression could reduce concerns regarding immunocompatibility and increase the pool of donor cells, which, in turn, could broaden the range of possibilities for effective design and implementation of tissue engineering concepts.

Controlled Release Methods. Controlled release implants are typically composed of inert, biocompatible polymers such as poly(ethylene-co-vinyl acetate) (EVAc), or biodegradable polymers, such as poly(lactide-co-glycolide) (PLGA). EVAc matrix systems have been used to release protein hormones [14], growth factors [11, 15–17], antibodies [18–21], antigens [22, 23], and DNA [24]. EVAc matrices allow a high degree of control over agent release, versatility in permitting release of a wide range of agents, and good retention of biological activity. Biodegradable polymers have also been used to release growth factors [25–27], protein hormones [28, 29], antibodies [30], antigens [31–33], and DNA [24, 34]. Biodegradable materials disappear from the implant site after protein release, which may be a significant advantage in tissue engineering applications. Polymer gels may also be useful for topical [35] or localized [36] protein delivery. Systems that release multiple protein factors are also possible [37].

Controlled growth factor delivery systems can also be used in conjunction with biocompatible matrices or porous scaffolds that provide morphological guides for assembly of regenerating tissue (Figure 11.1c). On a macroscopic level, the overall shape of the polymer scaffold provides boundaries for regrowth of the tissue. On a microscopic level, the polymeric material provides a solid framework for cell growth and tissue organization at a local site, permitting cell attachment and migration within a controllable microenvironment. This technology is described more completely in Chapter 12. A controlled delivery system can be placed in the vicinity of a polymer scaffold, allowing the creation of gradients of biological activity over the volume of the scaffold. Alternately, the materials that have been used for tissue engineering scaffolds can, in many cases, be modified to allow for controlled release of active molecular agents from the scaffold material itself.

Some of the desired characteristics of polymer scaffolds for tissue engineering have been described [2, 38, 39]. In certain cases, polymer scaffolds are sufficient to produce regeneration; for example, poly(glycolic acid) fiber meshes seeded with cultured chondrocytes produce new cartilage after transplantation [40, 41]. In other cases, tissue regeneration is more difficult to achieve and requires additional biological signals. For example, liver cells transplanted on synthetic polymer supports provide some regeneration of hepatic function, but biological function is improved when cell transplants are supplemented with hepatic growth factors (by enriching growth factors at the transplant site by surgical rearrangement of the vasculature, for example [42]).

In some cases, therefore, it might be useful to produce a polymeric material that serves multiple functions in a tissue engineering application. A multifunctional polymeric system might be designed to provide controlled release of an essential factor as well as structural support for the regenerating tissue. Recently, new approaches for multifunctional polymeric systems have been introduced in tissue engineering, including highly porous materials with embedded agents [34, 43], microparticles that are assembled with tissue progenitor cells [11], and hydrogels that are photopolymerized around cells [44]. This last technique allows cell adhesion signals, as well as linkages that are degradable by cell-secreted enzymes, to be inserted into the polymer structure. Growth factors can be retained for longer periods by chemical immobilization. NGF [45], TGF-β [46], and EGF [47] possess biological activity when chemically immobilized to a surface.

Recently, methods for surface immobilization have been developed that result in gradients of the bound agent (Figure 11.2). Alternatively, the growth factor can be modified by conjugation to a water-soluble carrier, which prolongs its retention at a local site [26, 48–50]. Methods for producing materials that release the immobilized factor in response to a trigger, such as enzymatic activity released by a migrating cell, have also been demonstrated [51, 52].

11.1.2 Microfluidic Systems for Controlled Release and Tissue Assembly

Microfluidics and Microfluidic Devices. Microfluidics is the development of miniaturized devices for handling fluids. Microfluidic devices are composed of networks of interconnected channels, pumps, valves, mixers, separators, and a variety of other components—all on the scale of microns or less. Microfluidic systems have many potential applications including chemical analysis, microchemical reactors, combinatorial chemistry, DNA and protein separations and analysis, and cell sorting. These diverse applications reflect the many advantages in processing fluid systems on small dimensions [53–55]. Precise volumes of fluid can be moved rapidly and efficiently. Chemical analysis is especially accurate owing to the combination of small sample volumes and sensitive detection methods. Diagnostic and delivery methods

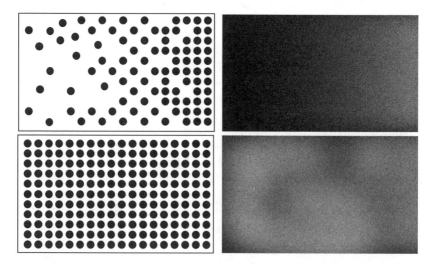

Figure 11.2. Surface gradients of agents: controlled presentation of molecules attached to a surface by immobilization in either uniform (bottom) or right-to-left gradient (top). In these photos, a fluorescently labeled protein was immobilized to a synthetic polymer hydrogel. Images of agent on the hydrogel *in vitro* were collected via epifluorescence microscopy [Gemeinhart and Saltzman, unpublished data].

often can be integrated in a single device. Microfluidic devices have low power requirements, and certain devices can be made suitable for implanting into tissue. Techniques for fabricating microfluidic circuits include reactive-ion etching, lithography, embossing, casting, and molding.

Microfluidic devices require a mechanism for pumping the fluid, in a controlled fashion, through the microscopic mechanical elements. A variety of pumping methods are available, including electro-osmotic pumping for ionic fluids, positive displacement pumps using piezoelectric components, pneumatic pumps, and bubble or surface-tension pumps that rely on moving gas–liquid interfaces to displace fluids. Flow rates up to 100 µL/min have been achieved in an electro-osmotic flow, although a significant voltage must be applied across the channel to achieve high flow rates [55, 56]. In addition, electrokinetic flows can be compromised by contamination on the channel walls and ohmic heating. Some of the same mechanisms that are used to pump fluids can be exploited to construct valves that regulate the flow in microfluidic circuits [57]. Thus, a variety of passive and externally actuated valves, using piezoelectric, electromagnetic, or pneumatic control, have been designed, including valves that rely on controlling the position of a bubble or a gas–liquid interface in a microchannel [53].

Microfluidic Systems for Cell Patterning.   How can microfluidic systems be useful in developing new tools for drug delivery and tissue engineering? One area of application is the induction of pattern formation in cell cultures by microfluidic control of cell positioning. The use of microfabrication techniques to pattern cells on surfaces was demonstrated more than a decade ago [58], and a recent review summarizes developments since then [59]. The underlying idea in many applications is to use microfluidic channels to deliver precise amounts of cell-binding agents, usually proteins, to specific locations on a substrate. The agent is adsorbed or otherwise immobilized only on the part of the substrate that is in contact with the fluid. Subsequently, cells that bind to the immobilized agent can be introduced through the same microchannels that were used to deliver the agents to the substrate, which leads to the formation of specific patterns of cell deposition.

These principles of microfluidics can be used to develop intricate arrangements of multiple cell types on a substrate by introducing agents that differ in cell adhesion selectivity within individual microchannels. Subtle arrangements are possible because of an intrinsic property of microfluidic flows: when fluid streams are combined in microchannels, the combined streams show no inertially induced instabilities that could disrupt the boundary between them. Instead, the combined streams flow in parallel down the microchannel with only diffusional exchange, which is a relatively slow process. This characteristic of low Reynolds number flow can be used to create spatial patterns of agent adsorption—and therefore cell adhesion—within single microchannels. For example, if one of the streams contains an adhesive glycoprotein that adsorbs to the material, the glycoprotein adsorbs nonspecifically on the part of the channel in contact with that particular stream [60]. Multiple fluid streams can be combined into a single channel with the glycoprotein present in every other stream. As a result, the surface of the channel exhibits stripes of glycoprotein adsorption. If cells that bind to the glycoprotein are then introduced into the channel, they will bind along the glycoprotein stripes. By selecting the microchannel geometry and controlling the relative flow rates of various streams, a variety of cell culture patterns can be formed inside a microchannel.

These basic techniques are building blocks that can be used to fabricate more complicated cell culture patterns. For example, by combining several microfluidic layers that contain spatial variations in their surface properties, three-dimensional cell culture patterns composed of multiple types of cells can be formed [61]. These three-dimensional patterning techniques have been used to place cancer cells in close proximity with endothelial cells, resulting in spatial arrangements that could be used to mimic blood vessel formation in tumors. Microfluidic systems may also prove useful in patterning cells that are not attached to a solid substrate. As a first step, a microfluidic system has been used to form intricate, stable, three-dimensional patterns of freely suspended vesicles under controlled conditions [62].

Microfluidic Systems for Local Agent Delivery.   A second application of microfluidics in tissue engineering is even more closely related to drug delivery: the use of microfabricated prostheses to deliver chemical agents to precisely defined regions of tissue or even into the interior of cells. Arrays of silicon microprobes and microneedles have been fabricated using anisotropic etching [63]. The probes have the shape of a pyramid and range in height from a few to several hundred micrometers. The tips of the probes are smaller than $0.1\,\mu m$, which means they can easily penetrate the cell membrane either to deliver an agent through the probe tip or to provide access for intracellular measurements and analysis. The microarrays have been used to deliver a plasmid vector containing a gene for β-glucuronidase to tobacco cells, which soon after showed a transient expression of β-glucuronidase. Similar techniques have been used to fabricate arrays of hollow microcapillaries [64]. Because the lumen diameter of the microcapillaries is known precisely and does not vary along the capillary length, more precise control of the volume of fluid delivered to cells is possible. However, the microcapillaries do not have a sharp tip, and therefore they may not be able to penetrate smaller targets such as bacterial cells or viruses.

Individual microchannel probes have also been developed to deliver precise amounts of an agent to localized regions of tissue. For example, a silicon-based probe for delivery to neural tissue consists of several parallel microchannels that are housed in a flat shank about $70\,\mu m$ wide and $4\,mm$ in length [65]. Some channels can be used to deliver various agents to the tissue, while other channels are used to measure electrical signals from the neurons. The probes have been used to modulate the neuronal activity of guinea pig brain tissue by sequentially injecting solutions of kainic acid, a neural stimulant, and γ-aminobutyric acid, a neural depressant [65].

Similar microfabrication techniques have been used to construct micro-needles and microneedle arrays for intravenous injection [66, 67]. The micro-needles have a rectangular cross-section with typical dimensions of $20 \times 40\,\mu m$ and a wall thickness of about $20\,\mu m$. An array of 25 such microneedles can deliver flow rates ranging from 50 to $650\,\mu L/min$. Microneedles containing multiple outlet ports have also been fabricated. Although it has yet to be demonstrated, the microneedle arrays could provide a means for sustained transdermal drug delivery.

Microfabrication techniques have also been used to construct controlled release microchips [68]. The microchips contain an array of small reservoirs that are filled with various agents to be delivered to the surrounding tissue. The opening of each reservoir is sealed with a material that can be selectively dissolved by an electrochemical reaction. One embodiment of the process uses reservoirs that are sealed with a thin gold membrane that also acts as the anode in an electrochemical reaction. When release of the compound from a specific reservoir is desired, a potential of about $1\,V$ is applied to the membrane to cause it to dissolve, which allows the agent to diffuse out of the reservoir. A variety of drugs, including liquids, solids, and gels, can be delivered from the microchip in a controlled and sustained release. The amount of drug in each reservoir can be adjusted arbitrarily, and the release rate can be programmed or controlled remotely, which could enable precise control of delivery rates to match particular therapeutic requirements.

11.2 Controlled Release of Agents in Time and Space

11.2.1 Tissue Regeneration is a Step-wise Process Involving Timed Introduction of Molecular Agents

Developmental Signals and Tissue Engineering.   Natural processes of development and regeneration occur in a sequence of steps; molecular signals and cellular responses unfold in time through a coordinated sequence of spatial changes. The step-wise nature of development is long known. Recent studies are revealing a complex relationship between secreted signals and cell fate; for example, gradients of FGF-8 influence the cytoarchitectonic map of the cortex [69], and gradients of BDNF and NT-3 change with time to control the spatial pattern of innervation in the cochlea [70]. In adults, the step-wise mechanisms of regeneration are being revealed in studies of angiogenesis [71] and wound healing [3]; carefully orchestrated patterns of soluble bioactive agents are observed in both cases.

In tissue engineering, the transformation of a neotissue into a functional replacement tissue also occurs in a series of steps, in which each step potentially involves different biological signals. The step-wise pattern of transformation from a neotissue into a functioning tissue has been documented in many studies including tissue-engineered skin, nerve, and heart valves (Table 11.1).

Clinical Experience with Molecular Agents of Interest in Tissue Engineering. Although several individual agents that seemed promising—such as VEGF for angiogenesis and PDGF for wound healing enhancement—have been tested in humans, the clinical experience so far is disappointing. Platelet-derived growth factor (PDGF), for example, is a component of an FDA-approved product for healing of diabetic ulcers; the topically applied gel is manufactured by Ortho-McNeil from recombinant PDGF that is produced by Chiron. Many other protein growth factors have been tested for effectiveness in therapy. Fibroblast growth factor (bFGF) has been intravenously administrated to patients in the first 12 hours after thromboembolic stroke; although initial clinical trials were promising, the phase 2/3 trial was halted after 300 patients were tested, because of adverse side effects. NGF has been tested in a variety of clinical applications including systemic administration of the protein and local gene therapy to produce NGF in the brain. Subcutaneous administration of recombinant human NGF, produced by Genentech, reduced the sensory neuropathy associated with HIV infection in some patients [72], but early results were not considered promising enough to earn FDA approval. In a recent preliminary clinical study, topical application of NGF (10 µg/eye, 6 to 10 times daily) led to healing of corneal neurotrophic ulcers with few side effects [73], although this local therapy has not yet been through extensive trials.

Angiogenic factors, or factors that stimulate the formation of new blood vessels, are among the first tissue engineering agents to be tested in humans. Two such agents were championed by two of the most successful biotechnology companies in the U.S.: Genentech (VEGF) and Chiron (FGF-2). Although the production and pre-clinical testing of these compounds represent milestones in the development of protein therapies, and have led to advances in the understanding of angiogenic mechanisms in animals, both agents were unsuccessful in phase 2 clinical trials.

At present, it is difficult to determine whether the failure of these particular agents in clinical trials is due to a problem with the mechanism of action of the agents in humans or a failure to deliver the agent in the correct dose at the target tissue for the appropriate length of time. A definitive test for this new class of therapeutic compounds requires a reliable and controllable technique for the precise control of agent delivery and localization. Providing this level of control over local agent delivery could be the most important initial contribution of controlled release and microfluidics in tissue engineering. In retrospect this failure is easily rationalized, considering the vast difference between administration of single agents (even powerful ones) and the deliberate temporal and spatial coordination of chemical signals that occurs during regeneration.

11.2.2 Controlled Release Materials, Microfluidics, and Temporal Control of Agent Delivery. One major advantage of drug delivery methods in tissue engineering is the potential to control the spatial or temporal pattern of agent delivery. By localizing the source of agent release in the neotissue, gradients of biological activity can be produced within the microenvironment; stable gradients of growth factors and other proteins are maintained near the surface of polymers immersed in unstirred fluids or embedded in collagen gels [74, 75]. It has long been speculated that gradients of soluble factors, called morphogens, can influence pattern formation and tissue development in embryos (see Chapter 3). Interestingly, the gradients produced by controlled release polymers are similar to signaling gradients measured in embryos. Gradients of biological activity can be maintained in animal tissues for several weeks by a single administration of a controlled release polymer [76] (Figure 11.3). By utilizing controlled release, the biological effects of potent signaling molecules are confined to the tissue immediately surrounding (usually within ~1 mm) the implant [77].

Many controlled release systems rely on dissolution of solid material or partitioning from a non-aqueous phase as an element of release. High concentrations of agent can therefore, be delivered to the tissue. In the case of NGF (Figure 11.3), tissue doses of greater than 30,000 ng/mL were achieved; this concentration is ~10,000 times higher than the concentration of NGF that is active in tissue culture. Once the agent is released from the material, transport deeper into the tissue depends on properties of the agent (for example, its size, solubility, and stability) and properties of the local tissue space (for example, its cellular composition, vascularity, rates of interstitial flow). The dynamics of agent release from a controlled delivery device and local transport in the tissue have been most thoroughly studied in the brain [78], although the basic prin-

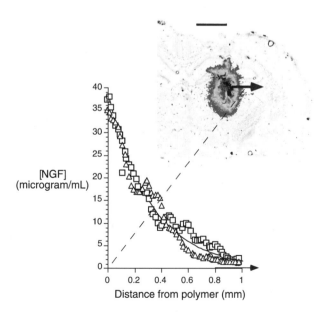

Figure 11.3. Concentration gradients produced by controlled release systems, surrounding a controlled release polymer matrix (photo and graph of gradients adapted from Krewson and Saltzman [92]).

ciples appear to apply to other tissues, even tissues with markedly different architectures such as the reproductive tissue [79].

Controlled release from polymeric materials has some important limitations for sustained delivery to a local site. Because most controlled release systems depend on diffusion of agent through the material during release, the rate of agent release typically decreases with time. When the system is used for local delivery to a tissue, the decreasing rate of agent release is reflected in a decreasing concentration of agent in the tissue adjacent to the material (Figure 11.4). An important advantage of microfluidic delivery systems is the potential to control the rate of agent delivery to the tissue continuously with time, which would allow for temporal control of the peak concentration, that is, the concentration in the tissue immediately adjacent to the delivery system. Provided that only small volumes of fluid are introduced with the agent, the dynamics of agent transport in the tissue are independent of the delivery system; therefore, microfluidic systems will also lead to agent gradients in the local tissue. But, by controlling the rate of agent delivery, a microfluidic device can (in principle) be used to produce patterns of agent concentration that are programmable with time (Figure 11.4).

11.2.3 Control of Spatial Gradients using Controlled Release Materials and Microfluidics.

When agents are delivered by controlled release materials into the brain, the local movement of molecules is determined by the balance between agent diffusion, in which molecules move away from the material by transport down a concentration gradient, and clearance, in which molecules are removed from the transport pathway by degradation, metabolism, binding, or partitioning into capillaries. This balance of diffusion and clearance leads to the development of stable gradients of agent in the tissue near the implanted material (Figures 11.3 and 11.4).

The size of the treated region of tissue (that is, the region that is exposed to concentrations within the biologically active range) is determined by the relative rates of diffusion and clearance. For most agents—including proteins, small drugs, and even virus-sized particulates—the relative rates of diffusion and clearance produce a region of treatment that is approximately 1 mm in size (Figure 11.4). Models of the local transport of molecular agents can be used to examine mechanisms of agent migration and to predict the effect of changes in system variables (such as agent size and clearance rate) on the size of the treated region of tissue. The mathematical and physical principles for modeling agent transport are reviewed in Appendix B. One example of the use of these principles has already been outlined in Chapter 3 (see Equations 3-1 to 3-3 and the related discussion); other examples are provided in the exercises at the end of this chapter.

In many cases this limited range of agent penetration may be beneficial, since highly potent compounds must be confined to specific anatomic regions. However, in other cases it may be desirable to deliver an agent over larger regions; for example, regions of ~1 cm in diameter correspond roughly to the size of neuroanatomical nuclei in the human brain. One simple method for

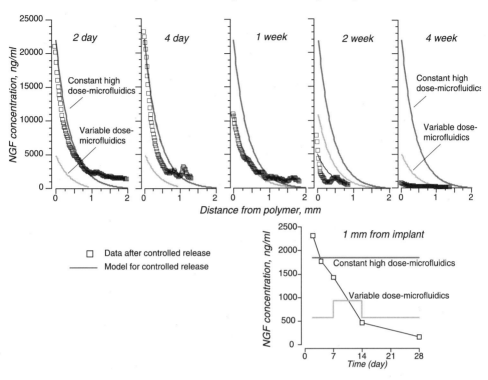

Figure 11.4. Dynamics of NGF delivery to a localized region of tissue. This figure shows NGF concentrations in the tissue surrounding an implanted controlled release matrix (see Figure 11.3). Measured concentrations in the tissue (squares) are dramatically elevated for several weeks after implantation. The fall of concentration with distance from the implant is due to a balance between agent diffusion (down the gradient, into the tissue) and agent disappearance from the tissue (by metabolism or clearance); mathematical models can be used to predict the tissue spatial profiles and their rate of change with time [93], as shown by the thin black lines. In principle, microfluidic drug delivery allows the option of controlling the rate of agent delivery to the tissue over time and therefore could be used to maintain a continuously high concentration or a variable concentration. The graph at the bottom indicates the concentration of agent that would be experienced by a cell 1 mm from the implant surface in each of the delivery scenarios.

dispersing active protein over a larger volume would require controlled placement of a suspension of cells or microspheres into the brain interstitium. Mathematical models of agent transport have been used to predict agent concentrations following delivery from polymer matrices and microspheres (Figure 11.5; details of the calculations have appeared elsewhere [80], but these calculations are similar to the ones presented in Chapter 3). Computer-generated images—in which colors correspond to ranges of concentration—provide a useful means for comparing agent concentration profiles following release from both a polymer matrix and uniformly distributed polymeric microspheres. When small spheres are spaced less than 1 mm apart, larger regions

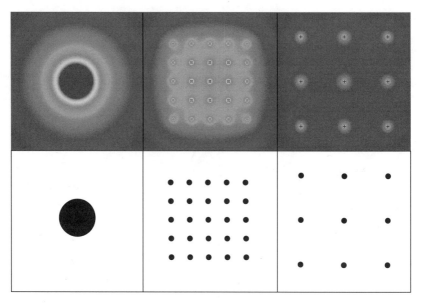

Figure 11.5. Delivery by arrays of controlled release systems. The figure shows concentration gradients surrounding large matrices (~1 mm in diameter) or arrays of smaller microspheres (~10 μm in diameter arranged with close, 1 mm, or distant spacing), adapted from computer-generated predictions as described by Mahoney and Saltzman [80].

of high agent concentration are visible. When microspheres are placed greater than 2.5 mm apart, they essentially behave as isolated point sources distributed throughout the tissue. In this configuration, the volume of tissue exposed to therapeutic agent concentration is small. This method of computer simulation (based on the experimentally measured characteristics of agent transport, as in Figure 11.3 for the case of NGF) can be coupled with radiological studies to guide the placement of ensembles of controlled release systems in a tissue to tailor agent distribution to the anatomy of a tissue region or disease process. In tissue engineering, this pharmacotectonic approach to agent delivery can be used to localize regenerative agents within irregularly shaped regions of tissue or neotissue.

In other cases it may be advantageous to deliver agents to tissue in such a way that they spread over distances that are much larger than the penetration distance shown in Figure 11.5. One possibility is to deliver fluids by pumping them directly into tissue through a microneedle or other prosthetic device. In this case, the transport of the agent in the tissue is enhanced by convection, which may be capable of carrying the agent further than the diffusion penetration distance. The diffusion penetration distance is governed by the rate of diffusion modified by the rate of agent clearance. Diffusion rates are determined by the physicochemical properties of the agent and tissue, and are independent of the delivery scheme. In convection-based delivery, the penetration distance is determined by the relative rates of convection and elimination, and convection rates can be determined by the delivery scheme.

The velocity of fluid in tissue under constant infusion through a microneedle is determined by a variety of factors, including the structure of the tissue and the interstitial matrix and fluid transport across microvascular membranes and into lymphatics, if present. A simple model views convection in the interstitial space as flow through a porous medium governed by Darcy's law, which gives a linear relationship between flow rate and the pressure gradient with coefficients that reflect the extracellular volume fraction and the tissue hydraulic conductivity. If an agent is dissolved in the fluid, its transport is governed by a combination of convection, diffusion, and clearance.

The relative importance of convection in comparison with diffusion is determined by the Peclet number. For example, calculations for the continuous infusion of a 180 kDa protein at a rate of 3.5 µL/min through a needle in the brain yield a Peclet number that exceeds 10 at a distance of almost 2 cm from the injection point [81]. Thus, diffusion is unimportant over this distance, and the injected protein is predicted to advance outward from the injection point in a sharp front. After 12 hr of continuous infusion, the front is located 1.5 cm from the injection point with little loss in protein concentration at the leading edge. The front will continue to advance as long as infusion continues, but the fluid velocity decreases with increasing distance from the injection point. Eventually, the velocity will decrease to the point that diffusion becomes significant.

Delivering compounds continuously and promoting their spread over relatively large distances (~1 cm) is important in delivering anti-cancer agents to brain tumors. However, in tissue engineering applications, it may be important to deliver smaller volumes of potent morphogens or other growth agents at specified locations [82, 83]. Furthermore, since cell behavior in the neotissue can be sensitive to concentration gradients, it may be desirable to control concentration profiles in order to stimulate directional or spatial changes. In this event, it may be possible to combine microfluidic systems with convection-enhanced delivery to control the location and profile of agents at distant locations from the injection point (Figure 11.6). Microfluidic circuits can be designed to deliver flow rates and outlet concentrations of agents that vary in time in prescribed ways. For example, if a discrete bolus of an agent is infused through a microneedle, it will spread through the tissue radially as a spherical shell whose thickness depends on the volume of the bolus and the distance from the injection point (Figure 11.7). The location of the shell can be controlled by adjusting the infusion rate as the shell advances. With only a single infusion point, the spherical symmetry of the shell will be preserved as it advances, at least in homogeneous tissue. However, if the agent is delivered by infusion at a series of spatial locations (as in Figure 11.6), then more complex shapes can be formed by allowing the shells from the delivery points to overlap with each other. Furthermore, if the concentrations of the agent differ among the various infusion points, then concentration gradients can be estab-

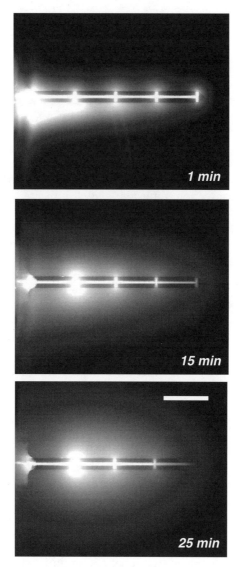

Figure 11.6. Flow in a microfluidic channel. The figures show flow and delivery of 3 kDa dextran through a microfluidic channel at 1, 15, and 25 min after introduction of dextran to the reservoir (left side of photo). The microfluidic device was implanted within an agarose gel; diffusion of dextran from the channel into the surrounding gel can be observed. Scale bar = 500 μm. Figure provided by Scott Retterer.

lished within the overlapping shells far from the injection points. Of course, clearance of the agent and diffusion would eventually degrade the concentration profile that is established at the end of infusion, but the infusion cycle could be repeated to reestablish the desired profile.

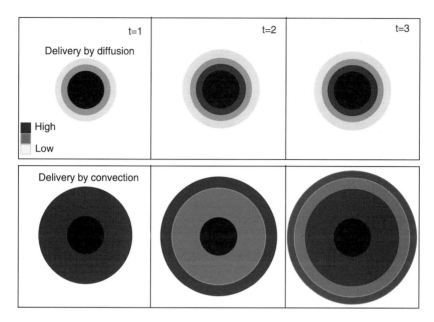

Figure 11.7. Local spread of agents predicted by models of diffusion and convection. Local spread by diffusion is shown in the top three panels. In this case, concentration gradients develop within the tissue near the device and remain stable until the agent is completely released (compare to Figure 11.4). Local spread of agents can be enhanced by convection, as illustrated in the bottom three panels. Convection can enhance the penetration distance, as shown in the left panel, but it can also allow for programmed changes in infusion concentration with time. The change in color of the outermost red region in the panel F reflects degradation of the agent with time. The delivery vehicle is shown in black; concentration ranges are indicated by shades of grey.

11.3 Future Applications of Controlled Delivery in Tissue Engineering

Controlled release is a well-established approach in drug delivery. However, the combination of controlled release technology and microfluidics is likely to produce new delivery methods for a variety of biological agents (including drugs, proteins, and genes) that are essential in tissue engineering. Microfluidics not only provides new tools for fabricating controlled release platforms, but also provides a new method for delivering agents directly to tissue. The essential feature of delivery with microfluidics is that diffusion can be combined with convection to offer greater versatility in design than is available with controlled release alone. In particular, the penetration distance of an agent in tissue can be increased by using convection-based delivery, and if flow rates, concentrations, and release sequences can be controlled using microfluidics, then spatial patterns of agents could be established to direct tissue growth and other cellular responses.

Unlike controlled release, which has been tested extensively both in animals and in humans, microfluidic methods have not been challenged by long-term use in a tissue environment. Furthermore, the materials that are frequently used to fabricate laboratory microfluidic prototypes may not be appropriate for clinical applications. The ultimate clinical impact of microfluidics on tissue engineering may depend not only on our understanding of the physics underlying the delivery method, but also on our ability to develop compatible microfluidic devices. In any event, it is clear that controlled release and microfluidics are key methods in tissue engineering.

Summary

- The engineering of many tissue structures—such as the branching architectures found in many tissues or the intricate network architecture of the nervous system—will require new methods for producing controlled spatial and temporal gradients of agents in developing tissues.
- Controlled release technology has many direct applications to tissue engineering; for example, local delivery of growth factors can be accomplished by encapsulating the agent within a biocompatible polymer matrix or microsphere.
- Controlled growth factor delivery systems can also be used in conjunction with biocompatible matrices or porous scaffolds that provide morphological guides for assembly of regenerating tissue within a controllable microenvironment.
- Microfluidic devices, which are composed of networks of interconnected channels, pumps, valves, mixers, and separators, will be useful in developing new tools for drug delivery and tissue engineering, including microfluidic control of cell positioning and local agent delivery.
- In tissue engineering, the transformation of a neotissue into a functional replacement tissue occurs in a series of steps, in which each step potentially involves different biological signals that can be introduced by controlled delivery methods.
- Modeling of the dynamics of agent diffusion and convection at local tissue sites will be an essential tool for developing new delivery systems that provide spatial and temporal control over agent delivery.

This chapter was revised and expanded from an original manuscript, co-authored by W.M. Saltzman and W.L. Olbricht, that appeared previously [1].

Exercises

Exercise 11.1

Ethylene–vinyl acetate copolymer discs are prepared, containing dispersed particles of BSA and nerve growth factor (particle composition BSA:NGF 2500:1 by weight). The matrices contain 40% particles (by weight) and the particles were sieved to be less than 178 µm in diameter. The matrices contained either (1) unlabeled NGF and were 2 mm in diameter, ~0.5 mm thick, weighing 5.5 mg or (2) ^{125}I-NGF and were 2 mm in diameter, ~0.8 mm thick, weighing ~10 mg.

The discs were incubated in phosphate-buffered saline and the cumulative amount of NGF released was measured as a function of time. Data are provided in the table below.

Day	NGF (ng)	^{125}I-NGF (ng)
0	0	0
1	202.53	148.5
2	290.58	204.3
3	332.46	248.7
4	357	286.2
7	381.9	384.6
11	401.7	459.3

a) Justify the following statement: "NGF is released by diffusion through the polymer matrix." Calculate the diffusion coefficient for NGF in the matrix.
b) Estimate the diffusion coefficient for NGF in buffered saline. Justify your technique.
c) Can you reconcile the answers you obtained in parts a) and b)?
d) Why are labeled and unlabeled NGF released at different rates?

Exercise 11.2

Polymer discs containing ^{125}I-NGF (see Exercise 11.1) were implanted into the brains of adult rats. Local NGF concentrations were measured by quantitative autoradiography. A typical concentration profile, showing NGF concentration as a function of distance from the polymer, is shown in Figure 11.3. The data was obtained from an animal 48 hr after polymer implantation.

a) Develop a mathematical model that will allow you to predict the concentration of NGF in the interstitial space of the brain as a function of distance and time. In the simplest form, this model should contain two parameters: the diffusion coefficient D and an elimination rate constant k. You should relate these parameters to the physiology and anatomy of the tissue.
b) Use the data in Figure 11.3 to estimate D and k.
c) Expand your model to predict NGF concentration profiles in the brain at 1, 6, and 24 hr, as well as 1 week and 1 month (you will need to consider the data and solutions in Exercise 11.1 to address this issue fully).
d) Estimate the rate of NGF permeation through brain capillaries. Describe the procedure you used and justify your estimate.

e) On the basis of the results of parts (c) and (d), estimate concentrations of NGF in the blood at 1, 6, 24, and 48 hr, 1 week, and 1 month. Assume that the half-life for NGF in the plasma is 10 min.

Exercise 11.3 (provided by Linda G. Griffith)

An approach to regenerating bone in a defect is to implant a scaffold which releases a chemotactic factor for bone progenitor cells and draws them into the scaffold from surrounding tissue. One such factor, BMP, is believed to induce both migration and differentiation of bone progenitor cells, and evidence suggests it operates as a chemotactic factor at *low* concentrations ($\leq 50\%$ receptor occupancy) and as a differentiation factor at *high* concentrations ($\sim$ saturation of receptors). Although the goal is to have bone form only inside the scaffold, it is often observed that bone forms out in the tissue adjacent to the scaffold. When this happens, bone formation inside the scaffold is poor—that is, a rim of bone tissue forms around the scaffold and penetrates only part way in.

a) If you assume that the concentration of the BMP at the surface of the scaffold may be $\gg K_d$ in some cases, propose a hypothesis to explain why bone might occur out in the tissue.
b) The K_d for BMP, measured for progenitor cells, is 2 nM. Estimate the concentration of BMP required in the external medium to achieve 50% receptor occupancy (that is, the chemotactic limit) and receptor saturation ($\sim$90% receptor occupancy). You may assume the conditions are steady state, no ligand depletion, and constant receptor number (no receptor turnover).
c) Develop an equation for the concentration profile of BMP, C_{bmp}, being released from a scaffold into tissue, where it is consumed at a first-order rate process $k_c C_{bmp}$ by cellular uptake and by another first-order rate process $k_c C_{bmp}$ due to diffusion into blood. You may assume one-dimensional rectangular coordinates (that is, diffusion in the x direction only away from the scaffold) and that the concentration of BMP at the surface of the scaffold is constant at C_0. You may further consider the tissue to be an "infinite sink", that is, that it stretches to infinity away from the surface of the scaffold (hint—this is necessary for one of the boundary conditions).
d) In one experiment, a set of scaffolds was prepared which contained different amounts of BMP, resulting in concentrations of BMP at the surface of the device of approximately 10, 1 and 0.1 μg/cm^3. The molecular weight of BMP is 20,000. For each device, predict the distance from the surface of the scaffold where bone formation is observed if $k_b = 1.8 \times 10^{-4}\,\text{s}^{-1}$ and $k_c = 0.9 \times 10^{-4}\,\text{s}^{-1}$ on the basis of the criteria you propose in part (a). If you are not confident of your answer to (a), you may assume bone starts to form when the local concentration of BMP is 0.04 μg/cm^3.

Exercise 11.4 (provided by Linda G. Griffith)

Nguyen et al. [94] have proposed a model for studying angiogenesis inhibitors based on the well-accepted chick embryo chorioallantoic membrane or "CAM" assay for studying angiogenesis. In the CAM assay, an angiogenic stimulus is placed in a collagen gel on top of the CAM of a shell-less egg, and the growth of vessels into the gel is quantified. Figure 1 of the research paper depicts the geometry of the assay. The thickness of the gel, which is not stated in the paper, can be estimated as 1.25 mm on the basis of the dimensions given of the mesh (4 mm × 4 mm) and the volume of collagen gel (20 μL). Angiogenesis is induced into the collagen gel from the underlying CAM by including FGF in the gel. FGF binds to heparin, a property which mediates many aspects of its bioactivity. FGF is "stored" in matrix which has high heparan sulfate proteoglycan (HSPG) content, and the diffusion of FGF through matrix is hindered by substantial FGF content.

FGF also binds to a variety of other negatively charged polyionic species. In the research paper, the molecule sucralfate (aluminum sucrose octasulfate, $M_w = 2,086$) was used to maintain FGF in a stable state in the gel and control its release to induce angiogenesis in the CAM. Sucralfate is not soluble in the collagen gel; it is present as small gel-like particles. The objective of this paper is to describe an assay which can be used to screen inhibitors of angiogenesis: the inhibitor is placed on *top* of the collagen gel containing FGF/sucralfate, and the reduction of blood vessel penetration in the gel is compared to controls for a standard dose of FGF.

a) On the basis of the data in the paper and the information given above, calculate the molar concentrations of FGF ($M_w = 18,000$) and sucralfate in the collagen gel at the start of the experiment. If one sucralfate molecule can bind one FGF, which molecule is in excess? If twenty sucralfates are required to bind each FGF? One hundred?

b) Do you expect the transient diffusion of FGF through the collagen gel to be significantly affected by the presence of the sucralfate? You will need to make several assumptions to evaluate the effects: it is likely that the affinity of FGF for sucralfate is significantly less than its affinity for heparin; the K_d for the heparin–FGF interaction is 50–500 nM (depending on who did the measurement, which heparin they used, and how the affinity was measured).

c) Angiogenesis in the CAM assay is typically scored according to the vessel density reaching to the top of the collagen gel after a certain time point. The inhibitors used in the work were placed on top of the gel; that is, distant from the CAM by ~1.25 mm (the thickness of the gel). Results for inhibition of angiogenesis are shown in Figure 2 of [94]. To interpret these results, it is useful to know the physicochemical properties of these materials, which are not given in the paper: (I) beta-cyclodextrin tetradecasulfate (bCTD)/hydrocortisone. Cyclodextrin is a ring-shaped molecule containing seven glucose units; the version used here has 14 sulfates (two on each glucose). Hydrocortisone, a hydrophobic steroid, intercalates in the center of the ring, increasing the effective solubilty of HC. Approximate molecular weight of the complex is 2,000. (II) U24067—an uncharged fluorinated sparingly soluble (hydrophobic) molecule, $M_w \simeq 500$. (III) AGM 1470— properties unavailable. (IV) protamine – protein isolated from fish sperm, $M_w \sim 5,000$; highly positively charged.

Given that the inhibitor must diffuse into the gel to prevent angiogenesis, do you think the assay has a bias for certain types of compounds? Does the data in Figure 2 support any hypothesis regarding a bias based on physicochemical properties?

Exercise 11.5 (provided by Linda G. Griffith)

Consider a skin wound healing situation, for example, a thermal wound on pigs [95], in which epidermal growth factor (EGF) is applied in an attempt to hasten repopulation of the wound by dermal fibroblasts. The specific growth rate μ of the fibroblasts is defined as $\mu = (1/n)(dn/dt)$, where n is the cell number. A design correlation for fibroblast proliferation response to EGF has been found by Knauer et al. [96] in which μ depends on the number of EGF–EGFR complexes per cell, C, according to the relationship $\mu(c) = \mu_{max} C/(K + C)$ where $\mu_{max} = 0.03$ hr-L and $K = 10^4$ #/cell. Recall the simple model for ligand–receptor binding presented in Chapter 4, with parameter values $k_f = 7 \times 10^7 \, \text{M}^{-1}\text{min}^{-1}$, $k_r- = 0.35 \, \text{min}^{-1}$, $k_e = 0.2 \, \text{min}^{-1}$, $k_f = 0.02 \, \text{min}^{-1}$.

a) If the dermal fibroblasts are found to possess 3×10^4 #/cell EGFR in the absence of EGF, determine the EGFR synthesis rate per cell, V_r.
b) Normal dermal tissue is approximately 10% fibroblasts by volume; wounded tissue initially contains no cells. Estimate the number of cells (and corresponding concentration) required to fill a wound bed of dimensions $0.1 \times 1 \times 1$ cm. If the wound bed is initially invaded by migrating fibroblasts to a level of about 0.1% by volume, estimate the cell growth rate required to repopulate the entire bed to normal tissue cell concentration within a week. Is the number you obtain reasonable?
c) Early attempts to provide EGF-enhanced skin wound healing involved inclusion of the peptide growth factor into a cream applied to the wound bed. Loss of EGF occurs by proteolytic degradation and by diffusion into the bloodstream, with a combined rate constant of approximately $0.01 \, \text{min}^{-1}$. It also occurs by EGFR-mediated uptake and degradation. Given the various parameter values above, calculate the transient EGF concentration in the wound bed following application for a series of possible initial doses.
d) On the basis of your findings in part (c), predict the time needed for tissue regeneration as a function of applied EGF dose.

e) As an alternative, one could apply a biomaterial matrix in the wound bed, which might release EGF at a controlled rate. Employing this approach, determine an optimal set of loading and release specifications for such a device, assuming that no mass transfer limitations are present (i.e, all EGF released is instantly uniformly distributed).

f) Consider an alternative technology for enhanced wound healing: delivering the gene for EGF to fibroblasts in the wound bed so that they can stimulate their own proliferation in an autocrine manner. Let the fraction of cells taking up and expressing the gene be ϕ (that is, the delivery efficiency) and the ligand production rate per expressing cell to be V_L, #/cell-time. We need to determine target specifications for ϕ and V_L as are necessary to yield an enchanced tissue regeneration following the situation outlined above. Employ the same receptor–ligand trafficking dynamics model as above, but for the autocrine cells an additional feature must be introduced: the existence of a boundary layer of volume V_{sec} ($\sim$500 μm^3) surrounding each producing cell, into which the autocrine ligand is first secreted; it can either bind to a cell receptor from this layer or diffuse into the bulk medium, where it may then bind to receptors of other cells with rate constant Δ($\sim$1 min^{-1}). Determine the number of EGF–EGFR complexes on the ligand-producing (autocrine) and on nonproducing (paracrine) cell subpopulations for select values of ϕ and V_{sec}. Also, determine the proliferation rates of the cells at the time needed for tissue regeneration. Which is more important: a higher value of ϕ or of V_{sec}? How does this gene therapy approach compare to the controlled-release approach of part (e) above?

Exercise 11.6 (provided by Linda G. Griffith)

Consider the BMP release data reported by Uludag et al. [97]. In this paper, they describe the pharmacokinetics of rhBMP2 and rhBMP4 release from several different types of carrier matrices and attempt to correlate bone formation with retention of BMP at the site. Iodinated BMP formulations were added to the carrier and implanted subcutaneously. At various timepoints, the matrices were removed and the amount of acid-precipitable (that is, protein-linked) ^{125}I was determined. Also, the amount of bone formation was determined by examining the mineralization. Suggestion: use a database program such as Excel for this problem.

a) Refer to the data in Figure 2 of the paper, which shows the percent of BMP retained in the graft site as a function of time for 15 days for four carriers. For rhBMP2 (CHO) and rhBMP4, calculate the total amount released during each time period (moles) and use this amount to calculate a release rate (for example, mol/hr) for each of the four carriers. Use the information provided in the materials and methods section under "Implant Preparation" to convert percent retained to absolute amounts. Plot your data for the release rate as a function of time for each carrier. Do the plots look like what you expected?

b) Use the information provided about the volumes and geometries of the carriers to estimate the flux of **BMP** out of each device for the data you converted in part (a). For lack of any additional information, you may assume the gelatin capsule is a sphere with the volume given. Use the flux to calculate a concentration gradient at the surface of each device. You may assume that the diffusion coefficient of **BMP** in the tissue next to the implanted device is $\sim 10^{-6}\,\text{cm}^2/\text{s}$. Plot the flux for each device as a function of time.

c) In experiments with other growth factors, the penetration distance into tissue (that is, the distance away from the device where the concentration falls to about 1% of the initial concentration) has been observed to be $\sim 500\,\mu\text{m}$ (0.5 mm, see Figure 11.3). If we assume that consumption is first order, show that the concentration profile away from the implant site is $C = C_0 e^{-x\sqrt{k_1/D_{\text{bmp}}}}$ where k_1 is the first-order rate constant and x is the distance from the surface of the release device (recall the analysis of growth factor penetration of tissue in Chapter 4). Estimate a value for the first-order rate constant by setting $C/C_0 = 0.01$ at $x = 500\,\mu\text{m}$. What value do you get if the concentration decrease occurs over a distance of only $200\,\mu\text{m}$?

d) Using the value of the rate constant you derive in part (c) along with the concentration profiles calculated from the data in part (b), estimate values for C_0 for the initial two time points in each plot. This value of C_0 will correspond to the **BMP** in the solution phase. Much of the **BMP**, however, remains bound to the matrix. Compare the values you get for C_0 to the values you get for the total concentration of **BMP** in the device, which is the percentage of the original amount (see materials and methods, as in part (a)) divided by the total volume of the device. Do your values support any of the author's conclusions?

e) If the K_d for **BMP** binding to its receptor is 0.1 nM and an osteoprogenitor cell has a length of $\sim 20\,\mu\text{m}$, are the gradients at the surface of the device physiologically relevant to induce cell migration?

References

1. Saltzman, W.M. and W.O. Olbricht, Building drug delivery into tissue engineering. *Nature Reviews Drug Discovery*, 2002. **1**, 177–186.
2. Langer, R. and J.P. Vacanti, Tissue engineering. *Science*, 1993, **260**, 920–932.
3. Singer, A.J. and R.A.F. Clark, Cutaneous wound healing. *New England Journal of Medicine*, 1999, **341**, 738–746.
4. Black, A.F., et al., In vitro reconstruction of a human capillary-like network in a tissue-engineered skin equivalent. *FASEB Journal*, 1998, **12**, 1331–1340.

5. Wolpert, L., Positional information and pattern formation. *Current Topics in Developmental Biology*, 1971, **6**, 183–224.
6. Gurdon, J.B. and P.-Y. Bourillot, Morphogen gradient interpretation. *Nature*, 2001, **413**, 797–803.
7. Peppas, N.A. and R. Langer, New challenges in biomaterials. *Science*, 1994 **263**, 1715–1720.
8. Ratner, B., et al., eds., *Biomaterials Science: An Introduction to Materials in Medicine*. San Diego: Academic Press, 1996.
9. Saltzman, W.M., *Drug Delivery: Engineering Principles for Drug Therapy*. New York: Oxford University Press, 2001.
10. Hoffman, D., L. Wahlberg, and P. Aebischer, NGF released from a polymer matrix prevents loss of ChAT expression in basal forebrain neurons following a fimbria–fornix lesion. *Experimental Neurology*, 1990, **110**, 39–44.
11. Mahoney, M.J. and W.M. Saltzman, Transplantation of brain cells assembled around a programmable synthetic microenvironment. *Nature Biotechnology*, 2001, **19**, 934–939.
12. Craig, C.G., et al., In vivo growth factor expansion of endogenous subependymal neural precursor cell populations in the adult mouse brain. *Journal of Neuroscience*, 1996, **16**(8), 2649–2658.
13. Hewitt, C.W. and K.S. Black, Overview of a 10-year experience on methods and compositions for inducing site-specific immunosuppression with topical immuno-suppressants. *Transplantation Proceedings*, 1996, **28**(2), 922–923.
14. Brown, L., et al., Controlled release of insulin from polymer matrices: control of diabetes in rats. *Diabetes*, 1986, **35**, 692–697.
15. Edelman, E.R., et al., Controlled and modulated release of basic fibroblast growth factor. *Biomaterials*, 1991, **12**, 619–626.
16. Murray, J., et al., A micro sustained release system for epidermal growth factor. *In Vitro*, 1983, **19**, 743–748.
17. Krewson, C.E., M. Klarman, and W.M. Saltzman, Distribution of nerve growth factor following direct delivery to brain interstitium. *Brain Research*, 1995, **680**, 196–206.
18. Saltzman, W.M. and R. Langer, Transport rates of proteins in porous polymers with known microgeometry. *Biophysical Journal*, 1989, **55**, 163–171.
19. Radomsky, M.L., et al., Controlled vaginal delivery of antibodies in the mouse. *Biology of Reproduction*, 1992, **47**, 133–140.
20. Saltzman, W.M., Antibodies for treating and preventing disease: the potential role of polymeric controlled release. *Critical Reviews in Therapeutic Drug Carrier Systems*, 1993, **10**(2), 111–142.
21. Sherwood, J.K., et al., Controlled release of antibodies for sustained topical passive immunoprotection of female mice against genital herpes. *Nature Biotechnology*, 1996, **14**, 468–471.
22. Pries, I. and R. Langer, A single-step immunization by sustained antigen release. *Journal of Immunological Methods*, 1979, **28**, 193–197.
23. Wyatt, T.L., et al., Antigen-releasing polymer rings and microspheres stimulate mucosal immunity in the vagina. *Journal of Controlled Release*, 1998, **50**, 93–102.
24. Luo, D., et al., Controlled DNA delivery systems. *Pharmaceutical Research*, 1999, **16**(8), 1300–1308.
25. Camarata, P.J., R. Suryanarayanan, and D.A. Turner, Sustained release of nerve growth factor from biodegradable polymer microspheres. *Neurosurgery*, 1992, **30**, 313–319.

26. Krewson, C.E., et al., Stabilization of nerve growth factor in polymers and in tissues. *Journal of Biomaterials Science*, 1996, **8**, 103–117.

27. Gombotz, W.R., et al., Controlled release of TGF-beta 1 from a biodegradable matrix for bone regeneration. *Journal of Biomaterials Science, Polymer Edition*, 1993, **5**(1–2), 49–63.

28. Johnson, O.L., et al., A month-long effect from a single injection of microencapsulated human growth hormone. *Nature Medicine*, 1996, **2**(7), 795–799.

29. Mathiowitz, E., et al., Polyanhydride microspheres as drug carriers. II. Microencapsulation by solvent removal. *Journal of Applied Polymer Science*, 1988, **35**, 755–774.

30. Sherwood, J.K., R.B. Dause, and W.M. Saltzman, Controlled antibody delivery systems. *Bio/Technology*, 1992, **10**, 1446–1449.

31. Cleland, J.L., Design and production of single-immunization vaccines using polylactide polyglycolide microsphere systems, in M.F. Powell and M.J. Newman, eds., *Vaccine Design: The Subunit and Adjuvant Approach*. New York: Plenum Press, 1995, pp. 439–462.

32. Marx, P.A., et al., Protection against vaginal SIV transmission with microencapsulated vaccine. *Science*, 1993, **260**, 1323–1327.

33. Whittum-Hudson, J.A., et al., Oral immunization with an anti-idiotypic antibody to the exolipid antigen protects against experimental *Chlamydia trachomatis* infection. *Nature Medicine*, 1996, **2**(10), 1116–1121.

34. Shea, L.D., et al., Controllable DNA delivery from three-dimensional polymer matrices for tissue engineering. *Nature Biotechnology*, 1999, **17**(6), 551–554.

35. Puolakkainen, P.A., et al., The enhancement in wound healing by transforming growth factor-beta 1 depends on the topical delivery system. *Journal of Surgical Research*, 1995, **58**(3), 321–329.

36. Hill-West, J.L., R.C. Dunn, and J.A. Hubbell, Local release of fibrinolytic agents for adhesion prevention. *Journal of Surgical Research*, 1995, **59**, 759–763.

37. Richardson, T.P., et al., Polymeric system for dual growth factor delivery. *Nature Biotechnology*, 2001, **19**, 1029–1034.

38. Hubbell, J.A., Biomaterials in tissue engineering. *Bio/Technology*, 1995, **13**, 565–576.

39. Baldwin, S.P. and W.M. Saltzman, Polymers for tissue engineering. *Trends in Polymer Science*, 1996, **4**, 177–182.

40. Freed, L., et al., Neocartilage formation *in vitro* and *in vivo* using cells cultured on synthetic biodegradable polymers. *Journal of Biomedical Materials Research*, 1993, **27**, 11–23.

41. Vacanti, C.A., et al., Synthetic polymers seeded with chondrocytes provide a template for new cartilage formation. *Plastic and Reconstructive Surgery*, 1991, **88**, 753–759.

42. Uyama, S., et al., Delivery of whole liver-equivalent hepatocyte mass using polymer devices and hepatotrophic stimulation. *Transplantation*, 1993, **55**, 932–935.

43. Lo, H., M. Ponticello, and K. Leong, Fabrication of controlled release biodegradable foams by phase separation. *Tissue Engineering*, 1995, **1**, 15.

44. Mann, B.K., et al., Smooth muscle cell growth in photopolymerized hydrogels with cell adhesive and proteolytically degradable domains: synthetic ECM analogs for tissue engineering. *Biomaterials*, 2001, **22**, 3045–3051.

45. Carbonetto, S.T., M.M. Gruver, and D.C. Turner, Nerve fiber growth on defined hydrogel substrates. *Science*, 1982, **216**, 897–899.

46. Mann, B.K., R.H. Schmedlen, and J.L. West, Tethered-TGF-beta increases extracellular matrix production of vascular smooth muscle cells. *Biomaterials*, 2001, **22**(5), 439–444.

47. Kuhl, P.R. and L.G. Griffith, Tethered epidermal growth factor as a paradigm of growth factor-induced stimulation from the solid phase. *Nature Medicine*, 1996, **2**, 1022–1027.

48. Belcheva, N.B., et al., Synthesis and characterization of polyethylene glycol–mouse nerve growth factor conjugates. *Bioconjugate Chemistry*, 1999, **6**, 932–937.

49. Knusli, C., et al., Polyethylene-glycol modification of GM-CSF enhances neutrophil priming activity but not colony stimulating activity, *British Journal of Haematology*, 1992, **82**(4), 654.

50. Bentz, H., J.H. Schroeder, and T.D. Estridge, Improved local delivery of TGF-beta2 by binding to injectable fibrillar collagen via difunctional polyethylene glycol. *Journal of Biomedical Materials Research*, 1998, **39**(4), 539–548.

51. Sakiyama-Elbert, S.E. and J.A. Hubbell, Controlled release of nerve growth factor from a heparin-containing fibrin-based cell ingrowth matrix. *Journal of Controlled Release*, 2000, **69**(1), 149–158.

52. Sakiyama-Elbert, S.E., A. Panitch, and J.A. Hubbell, Development of growth factor fusion proteins for cell-triggered drug delivery. *FASEB Journal*, 2001, **15**(7), 1300–1302.

53. Dario, P., et al., Microsystems in biomedical applications. *Journal of Micromechanics and Microengineering*, 2000, **10**, 235–244.

54. Whitesides, G.M. and A.D. Stroock, Flexible methods for microfluidics. *Physics Today*, 2001, **54**, 42–46.

55. Paul, P.H., M.G. Garguilo, and D.J. Rakestraw, Imaging of pressure- and electro-kinetically driven flows through open capillaries. *Analytical Chemistry*, 1998, **70**, 2459–2467.

56. Paul, P.H., et al., Electrokinetic pump application in micro-total analysis systems: mechanical actuation to HPLC, in *Micro Total Analysis Systems 2000*. The Netherlands: Kluwer Academic, 2000, pp. 583–590.

57. Quake, S.R. and A. Scherer, From micro- to nanofabrication with soft materials. *Science*, 2000, **290**, 1536–1540.

58. Hammarback, J.A., et al., Guidance of neurite outgrowth by pathways of substratum-adsorbed laminin. *Journal of Neuroscience Research*, 1985, **13**, 213–220.

59. Folch, A. and M. Toner, Microengineering of cellular interactions. *Annual Review of Biomedical Engineering*, 2000, **2**, 227–256.

60. Takayama, S., et al., Patterning cells and their environments using multiple laminar fluid flows in capillary networks. *Proceedings of the National Academy of Sciences*, 1999, **96**, 5545–5548.

61. Chiu, D.T., et al., Patterned deposition of cells and proteins onto surfaces by using three-dimensional microfluidic systems. *Proceedings of the National Academy of Sciences*, 2000, **97**, 2408–2413.

62. Thorsen, T., et al., Dynamic pattern formation in a vesicle-generating microfluidic device. *Physical Review Letters*, 2001, **86**, 4163–4166.

63. McAllister, D.V., M.G. Allen, and M.R. Prausnitz, Microfabricated microneedles for gene and drug delivery. *Annual Review of Biomedical Engineering*, 2000, **2**, 289–313.

64. Chun, K., et al., Fabrication of array of hollow microcapillaries used for injection of genetic materials into animal/plant cells. *Japan Journal of Applied Physics, Part 2*, 1999, **38**, 279–281.

65. Chen, J. and K.D. Wise, A multichannel neural probe for selection chemical delivery at the cellular level. *IEEE Transactions on Biomedical Engineering*, 1997, **44**, 760–769.
66. Brazzle, J.D., I. Paputsky, and A.B. Frazier, Fluid-coupled hollow metallic micromachined needle arrays. *Proceedings of SPIE Conference on Microfluidic Devices Systems*, 1998, **3515**, 116–124.
67. Brazzle, J.D., S. Mohanty, and A.B. Frazier, Hollow metallic micromachined needles with multiple output ports. *Proceedings of SPIE Conference on Microfluidic Devices and Systems*, 1999, **3877**(35), 257–266.
68. Santini, J.T., et al., Microchips as controlled drug-delivery devices. *Angew. Chem. Int. Ed.*, 2000, **39**, 2396–2407.
69. Fukuchi-Shimogori, T. and E.A. Grove, Neocortex patterning by the secreted signaling molecule FGF8. *Science*, 2001, **294**, 1071–1074.
70. Farinas, I., et al., Spatial shaping of cochlear innervation by temporally regulated neurotrophin expression. *Journal of Neuroscience*, 2001, **21**(16), 6170–6180.
71. Carmeliet, P. and R.K. Jain, Angiogenesis in cancer and other diseases. *Nature*, 2000, **407**, 249–257.
72. McArthur, J.C., et al., A phase II trial of nerve growth factor for sensory neuropathy associated with HIV infection. *Neurology*, 2000, **54**, 1080–1088.
73. Lambiase, A., et al., Topical treatment with nerve growth factor for corneal neurotrophic ulcers. *New England Journal of Medicine*, 1998, **338**(17), 1174–1180.
74. Radomsky, M.L., et al., Macromolecules released from polymers: diffusion into unstirred fluids. *Biomaterials*, 1990, **11**, 619–624.
75. Beaty, C.E. and W.M. Saltzman, Controlled growth factor delivery induces differental neurite outgrowth in three-dimensional cell cultures. *Journal of Controlled Release*, 1993, **24**, 15–23.
76. Krewson, C.E. and W.M. Saltzman, Transport and elimination of recombinant human NGF during long-term delivery to the brain. *Brain Research*, 1996, **727**, 169–181.
77. Mahoney, M.J. and W.M. Saltzman, Millimeter-scale positioning of a nerve-growth-factor source and biological activity in the brain. *Proceedings of the National Academy of Sciences*, 1999, **96**, 4536–4539.
78. Mak, M., et al., Distribution of drugs following controlled delivery to the brain interstitium. *Journal of Neuro-Oncology*, 1995, **26**, 91–102.
79. Kuo, P.Y., J.K. Sherwood, and W.M. Saltzman, Topical antibody delivery systems produce sustained levels in mucosal tissues and blood. *Nature Biotechnology*, 1998, **16**, 163–167.
80. Mahoney, M.J. and W.M. Saltzman, Controlled release of proteins to tissue transplants for the treatment of neurodegenerative disorders. *Journal of Pharmaceutical Sciences*, 1996, **85**(12), 1276–1281.
81. Morrison, P.F., et al., High-flow microinfusion: tissue penetration and pharmacodynamics. *American Journal of Physiology*, 1994, **266**, R292–R305.
82. Lonser, R.R., et al., Direct convection delivery of macromolecules to peripheral nerves. *Journal of Neurosurgery*, 1998, **89**, 610–615.
83. Lonser, R.R., et al., Direct convective delivery of macromolecules to the spinal cord. *Journal of Neurosurgery*, 1998, **89**, 616–622.
84. Nor, J.E., et al., Engineering and characterization of functional microvessels in immunodeficient mice. *Laboratory Investigation*, 2001, **81**(4), 453–463.
85. Yamashita, J., et al., Flk1-positive cells derived from embryonic stem cells serve as vascular progenitors. *Nature*, 2000, **408**, 92–96.

86. Schechner, J.S., et al., *In vivo* formation of complex microvessels lined by human endothelial cells in an immunodeficient mouse. *Proceedings of the National Academy of Sciences*, 2000, **97**(16), 9191–9196.
87. Saito, N., et al., A biodegradable polymer as a cytokine delivery system for inducing bone formation. *Nature Biotechnology*, 2001, **19**, 332–335.
88. Kale, S., et al., Three-dimensional cellular development is essential for *ex vivo* formation of human bone. *Nature Biotechnology*, 2000, **18**, 954–958.
89. Hunziker, E.B., Growth-factor-induced healing of partial-thickness defects in adult articular cartilage. *Osteoarthritis and Cartilage*, 2001, **9**, 22–32.
90. Schense, J.C., et al., Enzymatic incorporation of bioactive peptides into fibrin matrices enhances neurite extension. *Nature Biotechnology*, 2000, **18**, 415–419.
91. Poznansky, M.C., et al., Efficient generation of human T cells from a tissue-engineered thymic organoid. *Nature Biotechnology*, 2000, **18**, 729–734.
92. Krewson, C.E. and W.M. Saltzman, Targeting of proteins in the brain following release from a polymer, in V.H.L. Lee, M. Hashida, and Y. Mizushima, eds., *Trends and Future Perspectives in Peptide and Protein Drug Delivery*. Amsterdam: Harwood Academic Publishers, 1995, pp. 273–291.
93. Saltzman, W.M. and M.L. Radomsky, Drugs released from polymers: diffusion and elimination in brain tissue. *Chemical Engineering Science*, 1991, **46**, 2429–2444.
94. Nguyen, M., Y. Shing, and J. Folkman, Quantitation of angiogenesis and antiangiogenesis in the chick-embryo chorioallantoic membrane. *Macrovascular Research*, 1994, **47**, 31–40.
95. Brown, G.L., et al. Enhancement of epidermal regeneration by biosynthetic epidermal growth factor. *Journal of Experimental Medicine*, 1986, **163**, 1319.
96. Knauer, D.J. et al., Relationship between epidermal growth factor receptor occupancy and mitogenic response. *Journal of Biological Chemistry*, 1984, **259**, 5623.
97. Uludag, H. et al., Implantation of recombinant human bone morphogenetic proteins with biomaterial carriers. *Journal of Biomedical Materials Research*, 2000, **50**, 227–238.

12

Cell Interactions with Polymers

> You look at where you are going and where you are and it never makes any sense, but then you look back at where you've been and a pattern seems to emerge. And if you project forward from that pattern, then sometimes you can come up with something.
>
> Robert M. Pirsig, *Zen and the Art of Motorcycle Maintenance*

Synthetic and natural polymers are an important element in new strategies for producing engineered tissue. Polymers are currently used in a wide range of biomedical applications, including applications in which the polymer remains in intimate contact with cells and tissues for prolonged periods [1, 2]. As discussed in Chapter 1, several classes of polymers have proven to be most useful in biomedical applications and, therefore, might be appropriate for tissue engineering applications. To produce tissue-engineered materials composed of polymers and cells, however, it is first necessary to understand the influence of these polymeric materials on cell viability, growth, and function.

12.1 Characterizing Cell Interactions with Polymers

Cell interactions with polymers are usually studied using cell culture techniques. While *in vitro* studies do not reproduce the wide range of cellular responses observed following implantation of materials, the culture environment provides a level of control and quantification that cannot usually be obtained *in vivo*. Cells in culture are generally plated over a polymer surface and the extent of cell adhesion and spreading on the surface can be measured. By maintaining the culture for longer periods the influence of the substrate on cell viability, function, and motility can also be determined. Since investigators use different techniques to assess cell interactions with polymers, and because the differences between techniques are critically important for interpretation of interactions, some of the most frequently used *in vitro* methods are reviewed in this section.

Before any measurement of cell interaction with a polymer substrate can be attempted, the polymeric material and the cells must come into contact. Preferably, this contact should be controlled (or at least understood) by the experimentalist. This is a critical, and often overlooked, aspect of all of these measurements. Some materials are easily fabricated in a format suitable for study; polystyrene films, for example, are transparent, durable, and strong. Other materials must be coated onto a rigid substrate (such as a glass coverslip) prior to study. Cell function is sensitive to chemical, morphological, and mechanical properties of the surface; therefore, almost every aspect of material preparation can introduce variables that are known to influence cell interactions.

12.1.1 Adhesion and Spreading

Most tissue-derived cells require attachment to a solid surface for viability and growth. For this reason, the initial events that occur when a cell approaches a surface are of fundamental interest. In tissue engineering, cell adhesion to a surface is critical because adhesion precedes other events such as cell spreading, cell migration and, often, differentiated cell function. A number of techniques for quantifying the extent and strength of cell adhesion have been developed. The most important of these techniques (for example, sedimentation-detachment assay, centrifugation assay, fluidflow chambers, micropipette assays) are presented in Chapter 6 (see Figure 6.6). Many different techniques are used, making it difficult to compare studies performed by different investigators. This situation is further complicated by the fact that cell adhesion depends on a large number of experimental parameters [3], many of which are difficult to control.

12.1.2 Migration

The migration of individual cells within a tissue is a critical element in the formation of the architecture of organs and organisms [4]. Similarly, cell migration is likely to be an important phenomenon in tissue engineering since the ability of cells to move, either in association with the surface of a material or through an ensemble of other cells, will be an essential part of new tissue formation or regeneration. Cell migration is also difficult to measure, particularly in complex environments. Fortunately, a number of useful techniques for quantifying cell migration in certain situations have been developed. As in cell adhesion, however, no technique has gained general acceptance, so it is often difficult to correlate results obtained by different techniques or different investigators. These techniques, including under-agarose, filter assaying, and direct visualization, are discussed in Chapter 7 (see Figure 7.2).

12.1.3 Aggregation

Cell aggregates are important tools in the study of tissue development, permitting correlation of cell–cell interactions with cell differentiation, viability, and migration, as well as subsequent tissue formation. The aggregate morphology permits re-establishment of cell–cell contacts normally present in tissues; therefore, cell function and survival are often enhanced in aggregate culture [5–10]. Because of this, cell aggregates may also be useful in tissue engineering, enhancing the function of cell-based hybrid artificial organs [11] or reconstituted tissue transplants [12].

Aggregates are usually formed by incubating cells in suspension, using gentle rotational stirring to disperse the cells [13]. While this method is suitable for aggregation of many cells, serum or serum proteins must be added to promote cell aggregation in many cases [14], thus making it difficult to characterize the aggregation process and to control the size and composition of the aggregate. Specialized techniques can be used to produce aggregates in certain cases, principally by controlling cell detachment from a solid substratum. For example, stationary culture of hepatocytes above a nonadherent surface [5, 7] or attached to a temperature-sensitive polymer substratum [15] have been used to form aggregates. Recently, synthetic polymers produced by linking cell-binding peptides (such as RGD and YIGSR) to both ends of poly(ethylene glycol) (PEG) have been used to promote aggregation of cells in suspension [16].

The kinetics and extent of aggregation can be measured by a variety of techniques. Often, direct visualization of aggregate size is used to determine the extent of aggregation, following the pioneering work of Moscona [13]. The kinetics of aggregation can be monitored in this manner as well, by measuring aggregate size distributions over time. This procedure is facilitated by the use of computer image analysis techniques [16, 17] or electronic particle counters, where sometimes the disappearance of single cells (instead of the growth of aggregates) is followed [18]. Specialized aggregometers have been constructed to provide reproducible and rapid measurements of the rate of aggregation; in one such device, small-angle light scattering through rotating sample cuvettes was used to produce continuous records of aggregate growth [19].

12.1.4 Cell Function

In tissue engineering applications, particularly those in which cell–polymer hybrid materials are prepared, one is usually interested in promotion of some cell-specific function. For example, protein secretion [20] and detoxification [21] are essential functions for hepatocytes used for transplantation or liver support devices; therefore, measurements of protein secretion and intracellular enzyme activity (particularly the hepatic P_{450} enzyme system) are frequently used to assess hepatocyte function. Similarly, the expression and activity of enzymes involved in neurotransmitter metabolism (such as choline acetyltransferase or tyrosine hydroxylase) are often used to assess the function of neurons. Production of extracellular matrix (ECM) proteins is important in the physiology of many cells, and production of collagen and glycosaminoglycan has been used as an indicator of cell function in chondrocytes [22], osteoblasts [23], and fibroblasts [24]. In some cases the important cell function involves the coordinated activity of groups of cells, such as the formation of myotubules in embryonic muscle cell cultures [25] or the contraction of the matrix surrounding the cells [26]. In these cases, cell function is monitored by watching for changes in the morphology of the culture.

12.2 Cell Interactions with Polymer Surfaces

12.2.1 Effect of Polymer Chemistry on Cell Behavior

Synthetic Polymers.   For cells attached to a solid substrate, cell behavior and function depend on the characteristics of the substrate. Consider, for example, experiments described by Folkman and Moscona, in which cells were allowed to settle onto surfaces formed by coating conventional tissue-culture polystyrene (TCPS) with various dilutions of pHEMA [27]. As the amount of pHEMA added to the surface was increased, cell spreading decreased, as refected by the average cell height on the surface. The degree of spreading, or average height, correlated with the rate of cell growth (Figure 12.1), suggesting that cell shape, which was determined by the adhesiveness of the surface, modulated cell proliferation. In these experiments, two simple polymers (TCPS and pHEMA) were used to produce a series of surfaces with graded adhesivity, permitting the identification of an important aspect of cell physiology. These experiments clearly demonstrate, however, that the nature of a polymer surface will have important conquences for cell function, an observation of considerable significance with regard to the use of polymers in tissue engineering.

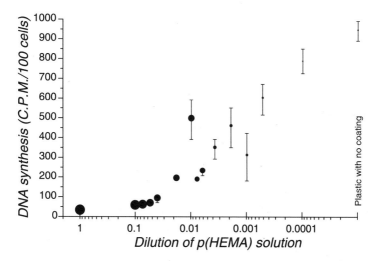

Figure 12.1. Cell shape and growth are modulated by properties of a polymer surface. Cell culture surfaces were produced by evaporating diluted solutions of pHEMA onto TCPS. The uptake of [^{3}H]thymidine was used as a measure of proliferation. The size of the symbol represents the relative cell height: small symbols represent cells with small heights and therefore significant spreading; large symbols represent cells with large heights and therefore negligible spreading. Data replotted from Folkman and Moscona [27].

Following an experimental rationale similar to that employed by Folkman and Moscona, a number of groups have examined the relationship between chemical or physical characteristics of the substrate and behavior or function of attached cells. For example, in a study of cell adhesion, growth, and collagen synthesis on synthetic polymers, fetal fibroblasts from rat skin were seeded onto surfaces of 13 different polymeric materials [24]. The polymer surfaces had a range of surface energies. as determined by static water contact angles, from very hydrophilic to very hydrophobic (Table 12.1). On a few of the surfaces (PVA and cellulose), little cell adhesion and no cell growth was observed. On most of the remaining surfaces, however, a moderate fraction of the cells adhered to the surface and proliferated. The rate of proliferation was relatively insensitive to surface chemistry: the cell doubling time was ~ 24 hr, with slightly slower growth observed for two very hydrophobic surfaces (PTFE and PP, see Table 12.2). Collagen biosynthesis was also correlated with contact angle, with higher rates of collagen synthesis per cell for the most hydrophobic surfaces.

Results from a number of similar studies are summarized in Tables 12.1 and 12.2. Cell adhesion appears to be maximized on surfaces with intermediate wettability (Table 12.1, Table 12.2, and Figure 12.2) [24, 28]. For most surfaces, adhesion requires the presence of serum and, therefore, this optimum is probably related to the ability of proteins to adsorb to the surface. In the absence of serum, adhesion is enhanced on positively charged surfaces [28]. Cell spreading on copolymers of HEMA (hydrophilic) and EMA (hydrophobic) was highest at an intermediate HEMA content, again corresponding to intermediate wettability [29]; spreading correlated with fibronectin adsorption [30]. The rate of fibroblast growth on polymer surfaces appears to be relatively independent of surface chemistry [31–33]. Cell viability may also be related to interactions with the surface [34]. The migration of surface-attached fibroblasts [33], endothelial cells [35], and corneal epithelial cells [36] is also a function of polymer surface chemistry (Table 12.1).

Surface Modification.   Polymers can frequently be made more suitable for cell attachment and growth by surface modification. In fact, polystyrene (PS) substrates used for tissue culture are usually treated by glow-discharge [38] or exposure to sulfuric acid to increase the number of charged groups at the surface, which improves attachment and growth of many types of cells. Other polymers can also be modified in this manner. Treatment of pHEMA with sulfuric acid, for example, improves adhesion of endothelial cells and permits cell proliferation on the surface [39]. Modification of PS or PET by radio-frequency plasma deposition enhances attachment and spreading of fibroblasts and myoblasts [40]. Again, many of the effects of these surface modifications appear to be secondary to increased adsorption of cell attachment proteins, such as fibronectin and vitronectin, to the surface. On the other hand, some reports have identified specific chemical groups at the polymer surface—such as hydroxyl (–OH) [41, 42], or surface C–O functionalities [40]—as important factors in modulating the fate of surface-attached cells.

Table 12.1
Cell Attachment, Growth, and Motility on Commonly Used Biomedical Materials.

Polymer	Water Contact Angle (°)	Cell Adhesion (% Control)	Fibroblast Doubling Time (hr)	Cell Migration (mm)
PTFE	105–116[a,l,m]	28[f] 50[a] 70[m]	60[a]	nm[f] 0.5[j]
PE	94 – 97[a,k,l,m,n]	83[a] 78[m]	25[a]	1.0[j]
PP	92–97[a,m]	67[a] 75[m]	36[a]	
PS	75–90[a,k]	100[a] 85[m]	20[a]	1.2[j]
PET	61–65[a,k]	53[f] 20[g] 100[a] 77[m]	24[a]	nm[f] 1.1[j]
Nylon	61[a]	92[a] 78[m]	27[a]	
TCPS	35–68[a,b,k,l,n]		22[a]	1.8[j]
Poly(vinyl alcohol) (PVA)	42[a]		ng[a]	
Glass	26–45[a,l,n]	75[a] 100[m]	19[a] 21[e]	1.2[j]
Cellulose	18[a]	4[a] 27[m]	ng[a]	
PEU[h]	57–86[h,k,l]			
PMMA	65–80[k,l,n]	85[m]		1.0[j]
PVF	75[l]			0.6[j]
PVDF				0.5[j]
FEP	105–111[l,m,n]	62[m]		0.4[j]
PDMS	100–104[k,l]	67[m]		
pHEMA	60–80[k]			

[a]Fetal rat skin fibroblasts with 10% fetal calf serum; static water contact angles were measured; n.g. = no growth [24].

[b]Human umbilical vein endothelial cells with 20% human serum: receding water contact angles [28].

[c]Bovine aortic endothelial cell with 10% fetal calf serum [156].

[d]Mouse 3T3 fibroblasts with no serum [29].

[e]Mouse 3T3 fibroblasts with 10% calf serum [32].

[f]Human adult endothelial cells with 20% fetal calf serum; n.m. = no motility [35].

[g]Human adult endothelial cells with 20% bovine serum; polymers pretreated with fibronectin [157].

[h]Polyurethane (PEU) based on poly(tetramethylene oxide)methylene diphenylene diisocyanate and 1,4-butanediol; receding water contact angles [72].

[i]Dissociated fetal neurons with 20% serum; cell adhesion relative to poly-L-lysine control; the HEMA preparations contain trace MAA [64].

[j]Cell motility determined as outgrowth area in cm^2; corneal epithelial cells [36].

[k]Water in air contact angles [34].

[l]PBS in air contact angles [44].

[m]L cells with 10% serum [37].

[n]Water contact angles [31].

Tissue Engineering Practice

Table 12.2
Cell Attachment and Growth on Acrylic Copolymers

Polymer	% HEMA	Receding Water Contact Angle (°)	Cell Adhesion (% control)	Fibroblast Doubling Time (hr)
pHEMA		4[b]	0[b]	ng[e]
			5[c]	
			1[d]	
			5[e]	
			20[i]	
p(HEMA-*co*-MMA)				
	75	8[b]	6.6[b]	
	50	26[b]	30[b]	
	25	39[b]	47[b]	
	0	57[b]	41[b]	
p(HEMA-*co*-MAA)				
	90		20[c]	
	80		30[c]	
	70		40[c]	
p(HEMA-*co*-DEAEMA)				
	90		10[c]	
	80		50[c]	
	70		30[c]	
p(HEMA-*co*-EMA)				
	80–83		23[d]	
	70–73		23[d]	ng[e]
			27[e]	
	58–60		31[d]	ng[e]
			42[e]	
	50		55[e]	23[e]
			53[i]	
	40		19[d]	23[e]
			55[e]	
	30–32		60[e]	23[e]
	0		24[d]	24[e]
p(HEMA-*co*-MAA)	85	3	0[b]	
p(HEMA-*co*-TMAEMA-Cl)	85			
p(MMA-*co*-MAA)	85% MMA	4	58[b]	
p(MMA-*co*-TMAEMA-Cl)	85% MMA	1	73[b]	
pGMA			60[i]	
pHPMA			80[i]	

EMA = ethyl methacrylate, MAA = methacrylic acid, MMA = methyl methacrylate,
GMA = glyceryl methacrylate, HPMA = N-(2-hydroxypropyl)methacrylamide, ng = no
growth observed. Lettered footnotes are the same as in Table 12.1.

So far, no general principles that would allow prediction of the extent of attachment, spreading, or growth of cultured cells on different polymer surfaces have been identified. For specific cells, however, interesting correlations have been made with parameters such as the density of surface hydroxyl groups [41], density of surface sulfonic groups [43], surface free energy [31, 44, 45] (Figure

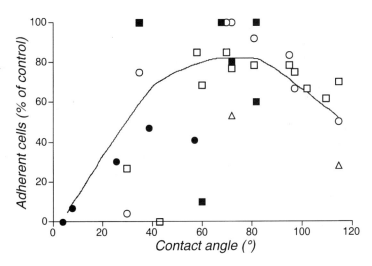

Figure 12.2. Relationship between cell adhesion and water-in-air contact angle. Data replotted from Tamada and Ikada for fibroblasts (open squares) [24], Ikada for L cells (open circles) [37], Hasson et al. for endothelial cells (open triangles) [35], van Wachem et al. for endothelial cells (filled circles) [28], and Saltzman et al. for fibroblasts (filled squares) [33].

12.3), fibronectin adsorption [40], and equilibrium water content [42], but exceptions to these correlations are always found. Complete characterization of the polymer, including both bulk and surface properties, is critical to understanding the nature of the cell–polymer interactions. Many commonly used polymers are complex, containing components which are added to enhance polymerization or to impart desired physical properties, often in trace quantities. Surface characterization is essential and must be performed on the exact material that will be used for cell culture, since lot-to-lot variations in the surface properties of commercially available polymers can be significant [46].

While the interactions of cells with implanted polymers are much more difficult to measure, the surface chemistry of polymers appears to influence cell interactions *in vivo*. For example, the ability of macrophages to form multinucleated giant cells at the material surface correlates with the presence of certain chemical groups at the surface of hydrogels: macrophage fusion decreases in the order $(CH_3)_2N- > -OH = -CO-NH- > -SO_3H > -COOH$ ($-COONa$) [47, 48]. A similar hierarchy has been observed for CHO (Chinese hamster ovary) cell adhesion and growth on surfaces with grafted functional groups: CHO cell attachment and growth decreased in the order $-CH_2NH_2 > -CH_2OH > -CONH_2 > -COOH$ [49].

Biodegradable Polymers. After implantation, biodegradable polymers slowly degrade and then dissolve. This feature may be important for many tissue engineering applications, since the polymer will disappear as functional tissue regenerates [50]. For this reason, interactions of cells with a variety of biode-

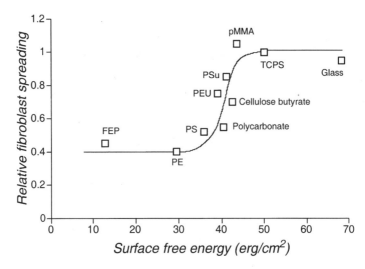

Figure 12.3. Relationship between cell spreading and surface free energy. Data obtained for fibroblasts cultured on a variety of polymer surfaces. Data replotted from van der Valk et al. [31] and Schakenraad et al. [44]. Abbreviations are defined in Table 12.1 or in the text.

gradable polymers have been studied. Biodegradable polymers may provide an additional level of control over cell interactions: during polymer degradation, the surface of the polymer is constantly renewed, providing a dynamic substrate for cell attachment and growth.

Homopolymers and copolymers of lactic and glycolic acid (PLA, PGA, PLGA; see Appendix A) have been frequently examined as cell culture substrates, since they have been used as implanted sutures for several decades [51–54]. Chondrocytes proliferated and secreted glycosaminoglycans within porous meshes of PGA and foams of PLA [55]. Rat hepatocytes attached to blends of biodegradable PLGA polymers and secreted albumin for 5 days in culture [20]. Neonatal rat osteoblasts also attached to PLA, PGA, and PLGA substrates and synthesized collagen [23].

Cell adhesion and function have also been examined on a variety of other biodegradable polymers. When cells from an osteogenic cell line were seeded onto polyphosphazenes produced with a variety of side groups, the rates of both cell growth and polymer degradation depended on side group chemistry [56]. Fibroblasts and hepatocytes attached to poly(phosphoesters) with a variety of side group functionalities [33].

Synthetic Polymers with Adsorbed Proteins.   Cell attachment, migration, and growth on polymer surfaces appear to be mediated by proteins, either adsorbed from the culture medium or secreted by the cultured cells. Since it is difficult to study these effects *in situ* during cell culture, often the polymer surfaces are pretreated with purified protein solutions. In this way, the investigators hope that subsequent cell behavior on the surface will represent cell behavior in the presence of a stable layer of surface-bound protein. A major problem with this approach is the difficulty in determining whether surface conditions, that is, the density of protein on the surface, change during the period of the experiment.

As described earlier, cell spreading, but not attachment, correlates with fibronectin adsorption to a variety of surfaces [30, 36, 40]. Rates of cell migration on a polymer surface are usually sensitive to the concentration of pre-adsorbed adhesive proteins [57, 58], and migration can be modified by addition of soluble inhibitors to cell adhesion [59]. It appears that the rate of migration is optimal at intermediate substrate adhesiveness, as one would expect from mathematical models of cell migration [3]. In fact, a recent study shows a clear correlation between adhesiveness and migration for CHO cells [60].

The outgrowth of corneal epithelial cells from explanted rabbit corneal tissue has been used as an indicator of cell attachment and migration on biomaterial surfaces [61]. When corneal cell outgrowth was measured on ten different materials that were preadsorbed with fibronectin, outgrowth generally increased with the ability of fibronectin to adsorb to the material (Table12.1) [36]. Exceptions to this general trend could be found, suggesting that other factors (perhaps stability of the adsorbed protein layer) are also important.

Hybrid Polymers with Immobilized Functional Groups.   Surface modification techniques have been used to produce polymers with surface properties that are more suitable for cell attachment [37]. For example, chemical groups can be added to change the wettability of the surface, which often influences cell adhesion (Figure 12.2), as described above. Alternatively, whole proteins such as collagen can be immobilized to the surface, providing the cell with a substrate that more closely resembles the ECM found in tissues [24]. Collagen and other ECM molecules have also been incorporated into hydrogels, either by adding the protein to a reaction mixture containing monomers and initiating the radical polymerization [62–64], or by mixing the protein with polymer, such as pHEMA, in an appropriate solvent [25]. To isolate certain features of ECM molecules, and to produce surfaces that are simpler and easier to characterize, smaller biologically active functional groups have been used to modify surfaces. These biologically active groups can be oligopeptides [65], saccharides [66], or glycolipids [67].

Certain short amino acid sequences, identified by analysis of active fragments of ECM molecules, appear to bind to receptors on cell surfaces and mediate cell adhesion. For example, the cell-binding domain of fibronectin contains the tripeptide RGD (Arg–Gly–Asp, see Chapter 6).* Cells attach to surfaces containing adsorbed oligopeptides with the RGD sequence, and solu-

---

* Amino acids are identified by their one-letter abbreviations: A = alanine, R = arginine, N = asparagine, D = aspartic acid, B = asparagine or aspartic acid, C = cysteine, Q = glutamine, E = glutamic acid, Z = glutamine or glutamic acid, G = glycine, H = histidine, I = isoleucine, L = leucine, K = lysine, M = methionine, F = phenylalanine, P = proline, S = serine, T = threonine, W = trypotophan, Y = tyrosine, V = valine.

ble synthetic peptides containing the RGD sequence, reduce the cell binding activity of fibronectin [68], demonstrating the importance of this sequence in adhesion of cultured cells. A large number of ECM proteins (fibronectin, collagen, vitronectin, thrombospondin, tenascin, laminin, and entactin) contain the RGD sequence. The sequences YIGSR and IKVAV on the A chain of laminin also have cell binding activity, and appear to mediate adhesion in certain cells.

Because RGD appears to be critical in cell adhesion to ECM, many investigators have examined the addition of this sequence to synthetic polymer substrates. Synthetic RGD-containing peptides have been immobilized to PTFE [69], PET [69], polyacrylamide [70], PEU [71, 72], poly(carbonate urethane) [73], PEG [74], PVA [75], PLA [76], and poly(N-isopropylacrylamide-co-N-n-butylacrylamide) [77] substrates. The addition of cell-binding peptides to a polymer can induce cell adhesion to otherwise non-adhesive or weakly adhesive surfaces [65, 72]. Cell spreading and focal contact formation are also modulated by the addition of peptide [78, 79] (Figure 12.4). Since cells contain cell adhesion receptors that recognize only certain ECM molecules, use of an appropriate cell-binding sequence can lead to cell-selective surfaces as well, where the population of the cells that adhere to the polymer is determined by the peptide [79].

The presence of serum proteins attenuates the adhesion activity of peptide-grafted PEU surfaces [72], highlighting a difficulty in using these materials *in vivo*. This problem may be overcome, however, through the development of base materials that are biocompatible yet resistant to protein adsorption. One of the most successful approaches for reducing protein adsorption or cell adhesion is to produce a surface rich in PEG. A variety of technqiues have been used including surface grafting of PEG [80], adsorption of PEG-containing copolymers, and semi-interpenetrating networks [81]. It may be possible to immobilize PEG-star polymers to increase the density of PEG chains at the surface [82]. Polymer substrates composed of PEG in highly crosslinked matrices of acrylic acid and trimethyloylpropane triacrylate completely resisted protein adsorption and cell adhesion, but readily supported adhesion after derivatization with cell-binding peptides [83]. Alternatively, matrices formed directly from synthetic polypeptides may also be useful for cell adhesion. Genes coding the β-sheet of silkworm silk have been combined with genes coding fragments of fibronectin to produce proteins that form very stable matrices with cell adhesion domains (Pronectin F, Protein Polymer Technologies, Inc.). Synthetic proteins based on peptide sequences from elastin have been used as cell culture substrates: in the presence of serum, fibroblasts and endothelial cells adhered to the surfaces of matrices formed by γ-irradiation crosslinking of polypeptides containing repeated sequences GGAP, GGVP, GGIP, and GVGVP [84].

Surface adsorption of homopolymers of basic amino acids, such as polylysine and polyornithine, frequently enhance cell adhesion and growth on polymer surfaces. Covalently bound amine groups can also influence cell attachment and growth. Polymerization of styrene with monamine- or diamine-containing monomers produced copolymers with ~8% mono- or diamine side chains, which enhanced spreading and growth: diamine–PS > mono-

a

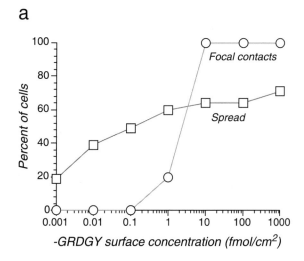

b

Peptide	Human foreskin fibroblasts	Human vascular smooth muscle cells	Platelets	Human umbilical vein endothelial cells
-GRGDY	85	93	0	90
-GYIGSRY	79	88	0	84
-GPDSGRY	56	62	0	66
-GREDVY	9	7	0	89
-None	9	10	0	8

Figure 12.4. Cell adhesion to surfaces with immobilized peptides (data from [78, 79]). (a) Fibroblast spreading on surfaces with immobilized –GRGDY. (b) Cell-selective surfaces: fraction of cells spread for several immobilized peptides.

amine–PS > PS [85]. Similarly, diamines coupled to glass surfaces enhanced the spreading and cytoskeletal organization of human fibroblasts [86].

The immobilization of saccharide units to polymers can also influence cell attachment and function. N-p-vinylbenzyl-o-β-D-galactopyranosyl-(1–4)-D-gluconamide has been polymerized to form a polymer with a polystyrene backbone and pendant lactose functionalities [87, 88]. Rat hepatocytes adhere to surfaces formed from this polymer, via asialoglycoprotein receptors on the cell surface, and remain in a rounded morphology consistent with enhanced function in culture. In the absence of serum, rat heptaocytes will adhere to similar polymers with pendant glucose, maltose, or maltotriose [87]. Similar results

have been obtained with polymer surfaces derivatized with N-acetyl glucosamine, which is recognized by a surface lectin on chicken hepatocytes [89].
Glucosamine has also been incorporated into N-(2-hydroxypropyl)methacryl-
amide hydrogels by radical copolymerization with methacryloylated glucosamine [64], and a variety of carbohydrates have been immobilized on
polyacrylamide discs [66].

12.2.2 Electrically Charged or Electrically Conducting Polymers

A few studies have examined cell growth and function on polymers that are
electrically charged. Piezoelectric polymer films, which were produced by high
intensity corona poling of poly(vinylidene fluoride) or poly(vinylidene fluoride-
co-trifluoroethylene) and should generate transient surface charge in response
to mechanical forces, enhanced the attachment and differentiation of mouse
neuroblastoma cells (Nb2a), as determined by neurite number and mean
neurite length [90, 91]. These observations may also be important *in vivo*.
For example, positively poled poly(vinylidene fluoride-*co*-trifluoroethylene)
nerve guidance channels produced greater numbers of myelinated axons than
either negatively poled or unpoled channels [92].

Electrically conducting polymers might be useful for tissue engineering
applications because their surface properties can be changed by application of
an applied potential. For example, endothelial cells attached and spread on
fibronectin-coated polypyrrole films in the oxidized state, but became rounded
and ceased DNA synthesis when the surface was electrically reduced [93].

12.2.3 Influence of Surface Morphology on Cell Behavior

The microscale texture of an implanted material can have a significant effect on
the behavior of cells in the region of the implant. Fibrosarcomas developed
with high frequency, approaching 50% in certain situations, around implanted
Millipore filters; the tumor incidence increased with decreasing pore size in the
range of 450 to 50 μm [94, 95]. In a recent study, porous polymer membranes
containing certain structural features (nominal pore size > 0.6 μm and fibers/
strands < 5 μm) were associated with enhanced new vessel growth [96].

The behavior of cultured cells on surfaces with edges, grooves, or other
textures is different from behavior on smooth surfaces. In many cases, cells
oriented and migrated along fibers or ridges in the surface, a phenomenon
called contact guidance from early studies on neuronal cell cultures [97, 98].
Fibroblasts have also been observed to orient on grooved surfaces [99], particularly when the texture dimensions are 1 to 8 μm [100]. The degree of cell
orientation depends on both the depth [101] and pitch [100] of the grooves. Not
all cells exhibit the same degree of contact guidance when cultured on identical
surfaces: BHK and MDCK cells oriented on 100 nm-scale grooves in fused
quartz, while cerebral neurons did not [101]. Fibroblasts, monocytes, and
macrophages, but not keratinocytes or neutrophils, spread when cultured on
silicon oxide with grooves with a 1.2 μm depth and 0.9 μm pitch [102]. The

variation in responses to a surface with grooves and edges is shown in Table 12.3.

Substrates with peaks and valleys also influence the function of attached cells. PDMS surfaces with 2 to 5 μm texture maximized macrophage spreading [103]. Similarly, PDMS surfaces with 4 or 25 μm^2 peaks uniformly distributed on the surface provided better fibroblast growth than 100 μm^2 peaks or 4, 25 or 100 μm^2 valleys [103].

The micro-scale structure of a surface has a significant effect on cell migration, at least for the migration of human neutrophils. In one study, microfab-

Table 12.3
Summary of the Effect of Parallel Ridges/Grooves on Cell Behavior

Cells	Material	h/d (μm)	w(μm)	s(μm)	Result
Chick heart fibroblasts [19]	Glass	* *	2 4	2 4–12	Not aligned Aligned
Human gingival fibroblasts [27]	Epon	5 92	36–78 100–162	36–78 101–162	Aligned Not aligned
Teleost fin mesenchymal cells [28]	Quartz	0.8–1.1	1–4	1–4	Aligned with increasing width
BHK, MDCK, and chick embryo neurites [20]	Silicon or ECM protein-coated silicon	0.2–1.9	2–12	2-12	Aligned with increasing depth and alignment depending on depth
Hippocampal neurons [21]	Quartz	0.014 1.1	1 4	1 4	Not aligned Aligned
Xenopus spinal cord neurons [21]	Quartz	0.014–1.1	1–4	1–4	Aligned
Epithelial tissue and cells [18]	Polystyrene	1 or 5	1–10	1–10	Migration was enhanced along the grooves; more significant effect with deeper grooves
Osteoblasts [29]	Ti or Ca–P coated silicon	3, 10, or 30	5	42	Aligned and increased bone-like nodule formation
Murine macrophage P388D1 [30]	Fused silica or ECM protein-coated silica	0.03–0.282	2 or 10	*	Aligned with increasing depth or decreasing width

Abbreviations used: BHK, baby hamster kidney; MDCK, Madin Darby canine kidney; ECM, extracellular matrix; h, height of ridges; d, depth of grooves; w, width of ridges; s, spacing between ridges; *, data not specified. Adapted from [158].

rication technology was used to create regular arrays of micrometer-size holes ($2\,\mu m \times 2\,\mu m \times 210\,nm$) on fused quartz and photosensitive polyimide surfaces [159]. The patterned surfaces, which possessed a basic structural element of a 3-D network (that is, spatially separated mechanical edges), were used as a model system for studying the effect of substrate microgeometry on neutrophil migration. The edge-to-edge spacing between features was systematically varied from $6\,\mu m$ to $14\,\mu m$ with an increment of $2\,\mu m$. The presence of evenly distributed holes at the optimal spacing of $10\,\mu m$ enhanced the random motility coefficient μ (defined in Chapter 7, see Equation 7-2) by a factor of 2 on polyimide, a factor of 2.5 on collagen-coated quartz, and a factor of 10 on uncoated quartz. The biphasic dependence of neutrophil migration on 2-D patterned substrate was strikingly similar to that previously observed during neutrophil migration within 3-D networks (as illustrated in Figure 7.6), suggesting that microfabricated materials provide relevant models of 3-D structures with precisely defined physical characteristics. Perhaps more importantly, these results illustrate that the microgeometry of a substrate, when considered separately from adhesion, can play a significant role in cell migration. This result was confirmed by looking at cell migration on surfaces of fixed geometry, but with different surface treatments [158].

12.2.4 Use of Patterned Surfaces to Control Cell Behavior

A variety of techniques have been used to create patterned surfaces containing cell adhesive and non-adhesive regions. Patterned surfaces are useful for examining fundamental determinants of cell adhesion, growth, and function. For example, individual fibroblasts were attached to adhesive micro-islands of palladium that were patterned onto a non-adhesive pHEMA substrate using microlithographic techniques [104]. By varying the size of the micro-island, the extent of spreading and hence the surface area of the cell was controlled. On small islands ($\sim 500\,\mu m^2$) cells attached, but did not spread. On larger islands ($4,000\,\mu m^2$), cells spread to the same extent as in unconfined monolayer culture. Cells on large islands proliferate at the same rate as cells in conventional culture, and most cells attached to small islands proliferate at the same rate as suspended cells. For 3T3 cells, however, contact with the surface enhanced proliferation, suggesting that anchorage can stimulate cell division by simple contact with the substrate as well as by increases in spreading.

A number of other studies have employed patterned surfaces in cell culture. Micrometer-scale adhesive islands of self-assembled alkanethiols were created on gold surfaces, using a simple stamping procedure [105], which served to confine cell spreading to the islands. When hepatocytes were attached to these surfaces, larger islands ($10,000\,\mu m^2$) promoted growth, while smaller islands ($1,600\,\mu m^2$) promoted albumin secretion. Stripes of a monoamine- derivatized surface were produced on fluorinated ethylene–propylene films by radio-frequency glow discharge [106]. Since proteins adsorbed differently to the monamine-derivatized and the untreated stripes, striped patterns of cell attachment were produced. A similar approach, using photolithography to produce hydrophilic patterns on a hydrophobic surface, produced complex patterns of neuroblastoma attachment and neurite extension [107]. A variety of substrate microgeometries were created by photochemical fixation of hydrophilic polymers onto TCPS or of hydrophobic polymers onto PVA through patterned photomasks: bovine endothelial cells attached and proliferated preferentially on either the TCPS surface (on TCPS/hydrophilic patterns) or the hydrophobic surface (on PVA/hydrophobic patterns) [108]. When chemically patterned substrates were produced on self-assembled monolayer films, using microlithographic techniques, neuroblastoma cells attached to and remained confined within amine-rich patterns on these substrates [109].

Surfaces containing gradients of biological activity have also been useful tools in cell biology, particularly for examining haptotaxis, the directed migration of cells on surfaces with gradients of immobilized factors [110, 111].

12.3 Cell Interactions with Polymers in Suspension

Most of the studies reviewed in the preceding section concerned the growth, migration, and function of cells attached to a solid polymer surface. This is a relevant paradigm for a variety of tissue engineering applications, where polymers will be used as substrates for the transplantation of cells or as scaffolds to guide tissue regeneration *in situ*. Polymers may also be important in other aspects of tissue engineering. For example, polymer microcarriers can serve as substrates for the suspension culture of anchorage-dependent cells, and therefore might be valuable for the *in vitro* expansion of cells or cell transplantation [112]. Immunoprotection of cells suspended within semipermeable polymer membranes is another important approach in tissue engineering, since these encapsulated cells may secrete locally active proteins [113] or function as small endocrine organs [114] within the body.

The idea of using polymer microspheres as particulate carriers for the suspension culture of anchorage-dependent cells was introduced by van Wezel [115, 116]. As described above for planar polymer surfaces, the surface characteristics of microcarriers influence cell attachment, growth, and function. In the earliest studies, microspheres composed of diethylaminoethyl (DEAE)–dextran were used; these spheres have a positively charged surface and are routinely used as anion-exchange resins. DEAE–dextran microcarriers support the attachment and growth of both primary cells and cell lines, particularly when the surface charge is optimized [117]. In addition to dextran-based microcarriers, microspheres that support cell attachment can be produced from PS [89, 118, 119], gelatin [120], and many of the synthetic and naturally occurring polymers described in the preceding sections. The surface of the microcarrier can be modified chemically, or by immobilization of proteins [118], peptides [118], or carbohydrates [89].

Suspension culture techniques can also be used to permit cell interactions with complex three-dimensional polymer formulations. For example, cell seeding onto polymer fiber meshes during suspension culture result in more uniform cell distribution within the mesh than can be obtained by inoculation in static culture [121].

In cell encapsulation techniques, cells are suspended within thin-walled capsules or solid matrices of polymer. Alginate forms a gel with the addition of divalent cations under very gentle conditions and therefore has been frequently used for cell encapsulation [122]. Certain synthetic polymers, such as polyphosphazenes, can also be used to encapsulate cells by cation-induced gelation [123]. Low-melting-temperature agarose has also been studied extensively for cell encapulsation [124]. Methods for the microencapsulation of cells within hydrophilic or hydrophobic polyacrylates by interfacial precipitation have been described [125, 126], although the thickness of the capsule can limit the permeation of compounds, including oxygen, through the semipermeable membrane shell. Interfacial polymerization can be used to produce conformal membranes on cells or cell clusters [127], thereby providing immunoprotection while reducing the diffusional distances.

Hollow fibers are frequently used for macroencapsulation; cells and cell aggregates are suspended within thin fibers composed of a porous, semipermeable polymer. Chromaffin cells suspended within hollow fibers formed from copolymer of vinyl chloride and acrylonitrile, which are commonly used as ultrafiltration membranes, have been studied as potential treatments for cancer patients with pain [128] or Alzheimer's disease [113]. Other materials have been added to the interior of the hollow fibers to provide a matrix that enhances cell function or growth: chitosan [129], alginate [114], and agar [130] have been used as internal matrices.

12.4 Cell Interactions with Three-Dimensional Polymer Scaffolds and Gels

Cells within tissues encounter a complex chemical and physical environment that is quite different from commonly used cell culture conditions. *In vitro* methods for growing cells in tissue-like environments may have direct application in tissue engineering [50, 131]. Previous investigators have used three-dimensional cell culture methods to simulate the chemical and physical environment of tissues [132–140]. White blood cells, fibroblasts, pancreatic cells, epithelial cells and nervous tissue cells have been cultured in gels containing ECM components and the dynamics of cell motility [141, 142], aggregation [143], and force generation [26] within gels have been studied. Often, tissue-derived cells cultured in ECM gels will reform multicellular structures that are reminiscent of tissue architecture.

Gels of agarose have also been used for three-dimensional cell culture. Chondrocytes dedifferentiate when cultured as monolayers, but re-express a differentiated phenotype when cultured in agarose gels [22]. When fetal striatal cells were suspended in three-dimensional gels of hydroxylated agarose, $\sim$50% of the cells extended neurites in gels containing between 0.5 and 1.25% agarose, but no cells extended neurites at concentrations above 1.5%. This inhibition of neurite outgrowth correlated with an average pore radius of greater than 150 nm [144]. Neurites produced by PC12 cells within agarose gels, even under optimal conditions, are much shorter and fewer in number than neurites produced in gels composed of ECM molecules [143].

Macroporous hydrogels can also be produced from pHEMA-based materials, using either freeze–thaw or porosigen techniques [145]. These materials, when seeded with chondrocytes, may be useful for cartilage replacement [146]. Similar structures may be produced from PVA by freeze–thaw crosslinking [147]. Although cells adhere poorly to pHEMA and PVA surfaces, adhesion proteins can be added during the formation to encourage cell attachment and growth. Alternatively, water-soluble polymers containing adhesive peptides, such as RGDS, have been photopolymerized to form a gel matrix around vascular smooth muscle cells: cells remain viable and elongate within the gel during subsequent culture [148].

Fiber meshes [149] and foams [150–152] of PLGA, PLA, and PGA have been used to create three-dimensional environments for cell proliferation and function, and to provide structural scaffolds for tissue regeneration (Figures 12.5 and 12.6). When cultured on three-dimensional PGA fiber meshes, chondrocytes proliferate, produce both glycosaminoglycans and collagen, and form structures that are histologically similar to cartilage [153]. The physical dimensions of the polymer fiber mesh influence cell growth rate, with slower growth in thicker meshes [154]. Changing the fluid mechanical forces on the cells during tissue formation also appears to influence the development of tissue structure [121].

In addition to fiber meshes, porosity can be introduced into polymer films by phase separation, freeze drying, salt leaching, and a variety of other methods (reviewed in [160]). It is now possible to make porous, degradable scaffolds with controlled pore architectures and oriented pores (Figure 12.7). Fabrication methods that provide control over the structure at different length scales may be useful in the production of three-dimensional tissue-like structures (Figure 12.8).

Summary

- Cell adhesion, spreading, migration, and function on a substratum depend on the chemical, physical, and mechanical nature of the substratum.
- Except for a few cases, cell interactions with a polymeric material cannot be predicted.
- Many materials of interest in tissue engineering are hybrids, composed of synthetic polymers and proteins, peptides, or oligosaccharides.
- A variety of methods are now available for the construction of three-dimensional materials (or materials that stimulate formation of three-dimensional tissue structures). These materials are essential for tissue engineering.

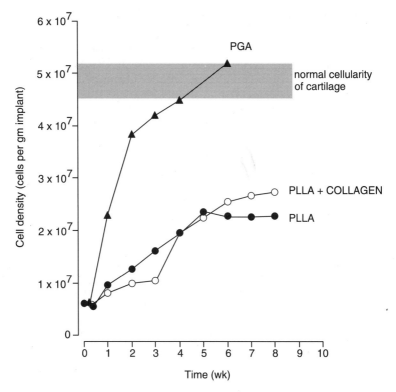

Figure 12.5. Chondrocyte growth on three-dimensional polymer substrata in culture. Freshly isolated bovine chondrocytes, harvested from the femoral patellar grove, were allowed to attach to a PGA fiber mesh (14 μm fibers, 60,000 MW, 91–97% porosity) (closed triangles) or a porous PLLA sponge (104,000 MW, 91% porosity) either uncoated (closed circles) or coated with type I collagen (open circles). Reprinted from [55].

Exercises

Exercise 12.1

Write the chemical structures for all of the polymers listed in Table 1.2. You may use the information in Appendix A.

Exercise 12.2

A polyester fiber used for surgical sutures is poly[oxy(1-oxoethylene)]. Write the structure of this polymer and suggest an alternate name.

Exercise 12.3

a) What is a vinyl polymer?

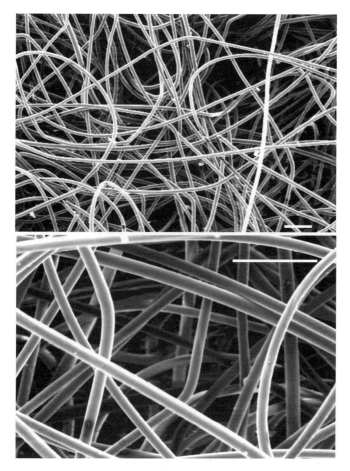

Figure 12.6. Scanning electron micrographs showing low (top) and high (bottom) image fixation views of a PGA fiber mesh. Scale bar is 100 μm in both panels. Photo provided by Peter Fong.

b) What is the difference between a step-reaction polymerization and a chain-reaction polymerization?
c) Write a reaction mechanism for free radical chain polymerization to produce either poly(methyl methacrylate) or polyacrylamide; be sure to include initiation, propagation, and termination steps.

Exercise 12.4

Calculate the number-average molecular weight, M_n, the weight-average molecular weight, M_W, and the polydispersity for a hypothetical polymer sample that contains:

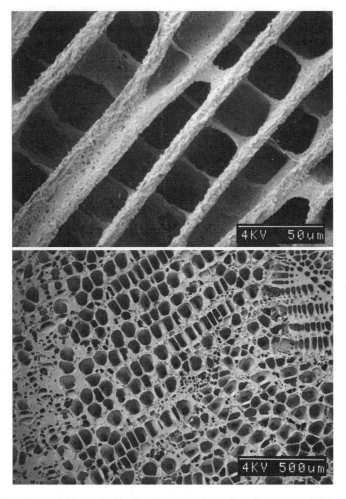

Figure 12.7. Degradable scaffolds for cell transplantation. Porous scaffolds were produced by freeze drying from a 5% solution of PLGA/PLLA in dioxane. Photo provided by Erin Lavik.

a) equimolar amounts of polymer having molecular weights of 20×10^3, 60×10^3, and 100×10^3;

b) equal mass amounts of polymer having molecular weights of 20×10^3, 60×10^3, and 100×10^3.

Exercise 12.5

Develop a model for the degradation of a thin polymer film which is being used as a cell culture substrate. A uniform poly(L-lactic acid) film, of thickness L, is firmly attached to a glass substrate.

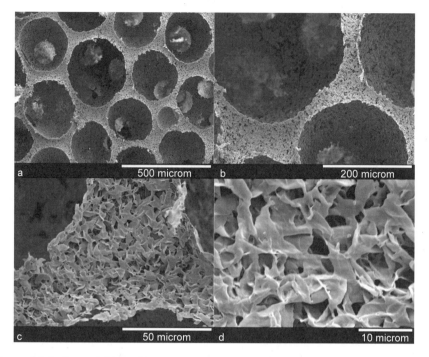

Figure 12.8. Degradable scaffolds with regular spherical pores. These highly porous scaffolds were produced by casting PLLA round an ensemble of paraffin spherical particles and then dissolving the paraffin slowly in hexane. Panels (a) through (d) show increasing magnification of a matrix produced under one set of conditions, revealing the 100 μm scale structure of the material provided by the paraffin spheres and the sub-micrometer-scale structure in the polymer interstitial space. By varying the conditions used to produce the scaffold, both the large-scale and small-scale structure of the material can be adjusted. Reprinted from [164]. Photo provided by Peter Ma.

a) Assuming no degradation, calculate the concentration of water in the film as a function of time. Assume that the diffusion coefficient for water in polymer is 1×10^{-7} cm^2/s and the film thickness is 100 μm.

b) Write a balanced chemical equation for the hydrolysis of poly(L-lactic acid).

c) Assume that the poly(L-lactic acid) has an initial number-average molecular weight of 10,000. Further assume that this polymer sample is in an aqueous solution, so that water is readily available. Write kinetic equations describing the change in molecular weight as a function of time.

d) Write the differential equations for determining poly(L-lactic acid) molecular weight within the film as a function of position and time, given your results for water penetration (part a) and polymer degradation.

Exercise 12.6

Protein molecules can adsorb on a glass surface; in fact, protein adsorption is considered to be a prerequisite for cell attachment to a surface. Prepare a model for accumulation of proteins on the surface.

a) Write a differential equation for diffusion of proteins to the surface from the bulk fluid phase. Include the necessary initial and boundary conditions.
b) Determine the steady-state protein flux to the surface, assuming that protein is not depleted from the fluid, that absorption on the surface is instantaneous, and that the surface can accommodate all of the protein molecules that arrive.
c) Albumin has a hydrodynamic radius of ~3.0 nm; assume that it has the same size when adsorbed onto the surface. How many albumin molecules can fit in a monolayer on the surface (per unit surface area)?
d) Determine the surface concentration of albumin as a function of time. Assume that molecules adsorb and that the rate of adsorption decreases exponentially with surface concentration; that is, when there are no molecules on the surface, adsorption is very rapid, but the rate of adsorption decreases with increasing number of molecules on the surface, becoming equal to zero when a complete monolayer is formed. Use the diffusion coefficient for albumin in water (8.3×10^{-7} cm^2/s at 25°C).

Exercise 12.7

A suspension of cells in a protein-rich medium is placed into a tissue culture dish.

a) Why do proteins reach the surface of the dish first?
b) How does this change if the chemical properties of the surface change?

Exercise 12.8 (provided by Rebecca Kuntz Willits)

Peptide–polymer conjugates are frequently used in tissue-engineered constructs. Why? Discuss the peptide sequences that would be useful for TE constructs and why they would be useful. Would you design these peptide–polymer conjugates as degradable? Why/why not?

Exercise 12.9

In the experiments by Folkman and Moscona (Figure 12.1), surfaces of varying adhesivity were produced by adding dilutions of pHEMA onto a tissue culture polystyrene surface. Describe these surfaces in as much detail as possible. Use a diagram to indicate how the surface changes (chemically and physically) as more pHEMA is added. Make sure that you include all features, particularly those that are in the range of 1–10 µm (that is, cell-sized).

Exercise 12.10 (provided by Christine Schmidt)

Consider the mechanical testing of polymers. When an amorphous polymer is pulled in a tensile test, the polymer becomes thinner at the center as shown below (a phenomenon called necking). However, as the stress increases, the neck does not continue to thin and instead, the remainder of the polymer deforms (that is, the neck disappears). Explain this behavior (why does the neck not continue to deform?) in terms of the polymer properties discussed in Appendix A.

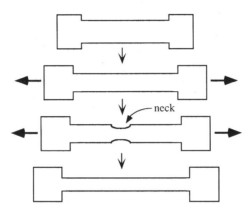

Exercise 12.11 (provided by Christine Schmidt)

To assess the utility of a novel material for use as a nerve guidance channel, you test the material *in vitro*. To analyze how the nerve cells interact with the material, you use phase contrast microscopy to monitor the extension of neurites (axons) from the nerve cell bodies on your material. You analyze 100 axons for each experimental case. The data from your studies are given below:

Control (plastic)	Mean axon length = 20 µm ± 5 µm
Control (plastic + collagen)	Mean axon length = 80 µm ± 8 µm
Novel material	Mean axon length = 50 µm ± 7 µm

a) What can you conclude about the migration velocity of the growth cone on the different materials?
b) What study could you perform, and what technique would you use, to confirm your conclusion above?
c) What *key* cytoskeletal protein is likely to be found in the periphery of the growth cone? Justify.
d) How could you determine which cytoskeleton protein is found in the growth cone?

Exercise 12.12 (provided by Linda G. Griffith)

You have convinced a surgeon that he can use a new scaffold that you designed (called "Mend-a-bone") to transplant marrow cells into a bone defect. The scaffold is a porous, sponge-like scaffold that can be seeded with a marrow cell suspension. The cells then adhere to the scaffold and are stabilized for transplant into a bone defect.

Your surgeon colleague has become convinced to consider the engineering aspects of marrow cell transplantation. He has a patient who was in a motorcycle accident, and she needs multiple bone grafts. He decides he will treat two of the defects with "Mend-a-bone" seeded with the patient's marrow. One of the defects, in a long bone, is ~4 cm thick. The other defect, in a hand bone, is only ~0.5 cm thick. His concern is that if he puts too many marrow cells in the scaffold, diffusion of nutrients might limit cell survival. He emails you to ask what cell concentrations are suitable for each of the grafts.

After getting some more information from him, you decide to model the graft as a slab of thickness $2L$ containing uniformly distributed cells at a concentration of N_c cells/cm^3. You suspect that either oxygen or a growth factor will limit cell survival in the graft, and that it is present at the surface of the device at a concentration of C_{A0}. You further presume that the cells are consuming the rate-limiting substrate at a zero-order rate q_A (mol/cell-s). Finally, you assume that all the cells have the same uniform volume, 10^{-9} cm^3/cell.

a) Draw the coordinate system appropriate for mass transfer in this system. Label the boundary conditions, the dimensions, the direction of transport, and the important variables governing reaction rate.

b) Derive the appropriate term for the zero-order volumetric consumption rate of "component A" in the graft as a function of the cell concentration N_c cells/cm^3.

c) What maximum cell concentrations would you recommend for each graft dimension if oxygen is limiting and is present at the surface at $C_{A0} = 0.1x \times 10^{-6}$ mol/cm^3 and $q_A = 2 \times 10^{-17}$ mol/cell-s? You may presume that the diffusion coefficient of oxygen at 37°C in the scaffold is the same as that in tissue, 2×10^{-5} cm^2/s.

d) You have some data that suggest the soluble peptide signaling molecule epidermal growth factor (EGF) is required as a cell survival signal for the bone progenitor cells present in marrow, and that cells will die if the concentration of EGF in their environment drops below 0.1 nM. (that is, 1×10^{-10} mol/L or 1×10^{-13} mol/cm^3). While the data on consumption rates for EGF are scarce, you find some papers indicating that cells consume roughly 2 molecules of EGF per second. If the concentration of EGF in the fluid at the surface of the device is ~ 1 nM, and you presume that all cells present in marrow consume EGF at the same rate, should you change the suggestions you made in part (c) on the basis of diffusion EGF limitations? You may assume that the diffusion coefficient of EGF in culture medium is 1×10^{-5} cm^2/s.

Exercise 12.13 (provided by Linda G. Griffith)

Despite many studies on the use of EGF in clinical wound healing and significant commerical investment in R&D for use of EGF, there are as yet no viable clinical products using EGF for wound healing. It has been proposed that it might be more efficacious to deliver EGF in a form where it cannot be internalized but can still be bound by its receptor (EGFR); that is, by tethering EGF to a solid (non-internalizable) substrate via a long water-soluble polymer chain which allows EGF to diffuse freely over some volume prescribed by the length of the tether (~70 nm) but which keeps it localized (see [161]). The use of scaffolds to achieve guided tissue regeneration makes this approach appear feasible from a development standpoint. Further, the unique chemical properties of EGF—it has just one primary amine—allow it to be covalently linked to a tether in a single conformation that should presumably be competent to bind the receptor.

a) The molecule of interest for tethering EGF, polyethylene oxide (PEO), is widely used in biomaterials to inhibit protein and cell adhesion to surfaces. Because PEO is a highly swollen random coil in solution, there is concern that EGFR may not be able to bind EGF when it is tethered to PEO because the PEO will sterically prevent access to the EGF molecule. To test whether binding of EGF would be affected by the PEO tether, soluble conjugates comprising one EGF molecule linked to a tether were prepared and the receptor-mediated internalization properties were examined in the following experiment. B82 cells were serum-starved at 37°C for three hours before addition of ^{125}I-labeled EGF–PEO conjugate (16.4 pM). Parallel cultures were incubated for 1–20 minutes at 37°C and then transferred to an ice bath where the medium was removed and the cells washed twice in WHIPS buffer. *Surface radioactivity* was removed by washing the cells twice in acid strip solution, allowing the cells to incubate for 8 minutes in the acid strip during the first wash and 4 minutes during the second wash. *Internalized ligand* was then removed by solubilizing the cells in 1N NaOH. The following data were obtained for the conjugate (error is ± 10% on each measurement for three measurements):

Time (min.)	No. of Surface Complexes	No. of Internal Complexes
2	88	82
4	100	78
6	117	89
8	111	156
10	116	158
12	119	217
14	170	348
16	186	447
18	207	568
20	264	782

The endocytic rate constant for soluble EGF on B82 cells has been reported as $k_e = 0.15 \, \text{min}^{-1}$. Based on these data, does it appear that the PEO tether significantly influences the binding of EGF to EGFR?

b) A more direct way to compare the binding efficiency of EGF and EGF–PEO conjugate to EGFR would be to measure the dissociation constant K_d, which has a value of ~1 nM. Why do you think this was not done?

c) A major concern in using the tethered EGF approach is the possible implications for signaling by the EGFR, as the EGF–EGFR complex remains active and signals in intracellular compartments. Posner and co-workers have hypothesized that the retention of signaling capacity by EGFR, once internalized, is what leads to qualitative differences in signaling by insulin receptor and EGFR in hepatocytes, since both receptors are receptor tyrosine kinases. In liver, under steady-state conditions of administration of soluble EGF, Posner found that there are ~7 times as many active EGF–EGFR complexes inside the cell as at the cell surface. This raises the issue of whether the tethered EGF will be as effective at stimulating cell growth as soluble EGF. To test whether soluble and tethered EGF would signal with equal efficiency, it is desired to carry out a series of dose–response experiments to compare whether soluble and tethered EGF complexes signal with equal efficiency in hepatocytes. It is assumed that the DNA synthesis response is proportional to the number of receptor-ligand complexes as described by Knauer et al. for fibroblasts [165]. Primary rat hepatocytes have ~265,000 EGFR per cell and spread to an area of ~1600 μm^2 on the culture substrate. The K_d for soluble EGF interacting with the hepatocyte EGFR is 1 nM. It is possible to tether the EGF molecules to the substrate using a tether of ~70 nm in length, and it may be assumed that the tethered EGF diffuses freely within the volume circumscribed by the fully extended tether. With this information, estimate the surface density (molecules EGF/μm^2) required to achieve 1%, 10%, 50%, 90%, and 100% occupancy of surface EGFR by tethered EGF. Can you think of ways to experimentally measure the number of complexes in the tethered case? Provided you have antibodies to the EGFR, EGF, and activated EGFR, are there experimental techniques you can suggest that might allow you to assess whether the receptor occupancy you estimate is close to what is actually achieved?

Exercise 12.14 (provided by Erin Lavik)

This exercise introduces some of the concepts involved in the fabrication of three-dimensional tissue engineering scaffolds.

a) *Fabrication by salt leaching.* You've just been hired at Austin Inc., a new tissue engineering company. Your boss comes in on your first day and tells you that the company needs highly porous scaffolds (>95% porous), with pore diameters on the order of 180 μm made from poly(lactic acid), poly(lactic-*co*-glycolic acid), and poly(caprolactone). You do some research and find that salt leaching will allow you to make a large number of scaffolds quickly. Salt leaching is accomplished by pouring a polymer solution over salt, evaporating the solvent, and then leaching the salt in water. You decide to make 100 scaffolds with the dimensions of 1 mm by 1 cm by 2 cm. How much polymer do you need? How much salt?

b) Qualitatively discuss what solvent you would dissolve the polymer in, at what concentration, and why. (All three polymers are soluble in chloroform, methylene chloride, dioxane, and dimethylsulfoxide.) (Hint: you may want to consider such properties as viscosity and evaporation rate in your answer.)

c) Now you want to leach the salt. How much water do you need?

d) *Other scaffold-making methods.* Your boss returns, delighted that you have made such brilliant scaffolds, but it turns out that the scaffolds need to have a pore structure with the pores oriented normal to the plane of the scaffold. How do you make the scaffold?

e) *Mechanical properties and scaffold fabrication.* You've been promoted at Austin Inc. The company has been taking the oriented scaffolds you make and using them to tissue-engineer an artificial artery, but has been having problems with the arterial implants not having the same mechanical properties (compliance) as the native tissue. You are asked to solve the problem. Following a search of the literature as well as data from the company, you decide that you need to fabricate scaffolds with an elastic modulus of 10^6 Pa and a tensile strength greater than 10^5 Pa. You have:

- PLLA with a tensile strength of 10×10^5 psi and a modulus of 5×10^5 psi;
- PLGA with a tensile strength of 7×10^3 psi and a modulus of 3×10^5 psi;
- PCL with a tensile strength of 3×10^3 psi and a modulus of 4×10^4 psi. What do you do?

f) You've now made great scaffolds with the appropriate modulus and you set out to seed them with endothelial cells. What technique might you use to seed the scaffolds? What are the pros and cons of static versus dynamic seeding? What can you do to augment attachment of the cells to the scaffold?

g) Your cells grow very slowly, so you seed the scaffold for three weeks. When you test the mechanical properties of the cell-seeded scaffold what are you likely to find? (Hint, you're using degradable polymers in warm medium for several weeks.) What can you do to deal with the changes you encounter?

Exercise 12.15 (provided by Rebecca Kuntz Willits)

How would you design a chitosan scaffold to increase ECM deposition throughout the scaffold (as opposed to just on the surface)? Why would this be beneficial?

Suppose a tissue-engineered scaffold of collagen and glycosaminoglycan is fabricated. Why is it beneficial to have the protein in the original scaffold if it will be replaced or covered by cell-secreted ECM?

References

1. Peppas, N.A. and R. Langer, New challenges in biomaterials. *Science*, 1994, **263**, 1715–1720.
2. Marchant, R.E. and I. Wang, Physical and chemical aspects of biomaterials used in humans, in R.S. Greco, ed., *Implantation Biology*. Boca Raton, FL: CRC Press, 1994, pp. 13–53.
3. Lauffenburger, D.A. and J.J. Linderman, *Receptors: Models for Binding, Trafficking, and Signaling*. New York: Oxford University Press, 1993, 365 pp.
4. Trinkhaus, J.P., *Cells into Organs. The Forces that Shape the Embryo*, 2nd ed, 1984. Englewood Cliffs, NJ: Prentice-Hall.
5. Koide, N., et al., Continued high albumin production by multicellular spheroids of adult rat hepatocytes formed in the presence of liver-derived proteoglycans. *Biochemical and Biophysical Research Communications*, 1989, **161**, 385–391.
6. Landry, J., et al., Spheroidal aggregate culture of rat liver cells: histotypic reorganization, biomatrix deposition and maintenance of functional activities. *Journal of Cell Biology*, 1985, **101**, 914–923.
7. Parsons-Wingerter, P. and W.M. Saltzman, Growth versus function in three-dimensional culture of single and aggregated hepatocytes within collagen gels. *Biotechnology Progress*, 1993, **9**, 600–607.
8. Cirulli, V., P.A. Halban, and D.G. Rouiller, Tumor necrosis factor-α modifies adhesion properties of rat islet B cells. *Journal of Clinical Investigation*, 1993, **91**, 1868–1876.
9. Matthieu, J., et al., Aggregating brain cell cultures: A model to study brain development, in *Physiological and Biochemical Basis for Perinatal Medicine*. Basel: Karger, 1981, pp. 359–366.
10. Peshwa, M.V., et al., Kinetics of hepatocyte spheroid formation. *Biotechnology Progress*, 1994, **10**, 460–466.
11. Nyberg, S.L., et al., Evaluation of a hepatocyte-entrapment hollow fiber bioreactor: a potential bioartificial liver. *Biotechnology and Bioengineering*, 1993, **41**, 194–203.
12. Langer, R. and J.P. Vacanti, Tissue engineering. *Science*, 1993, **260**, 920–932.
13. Moscona, A.A., Rotation-mediated histogenic aggregation of dissociated cells. A quantifiable approach to cell interactions *in vitro*. *Experimental Cell Research*, 1961, **22**, 455–475.
14. Matsuda, M., Serum proteins enhance aggregate formation of dissociated fetal rat brain cells in an aggregating culture. *In Vitro Cellular & Developmental Biology*, 1988, **24**, 1031–1036.

15. Takezawa, T., et al., Characterization of morphology and cellular metabolism during the spheroid formation by fibroblasts. *Experimental Cell Research*, 1993, **208**, 430–441.
16. Dai, W., J. Belt, and W.M. Saltzman, Cell-binding peptides conjugated to poly(ethylene glycol) promote neural cell aggregation. *Bio/Technology*, 1994, **12**, 797–801.
17. Munn, L.L., et al., Analysis of lymphocyte aggregation using digital image analysis. *Journal of Immunological Methods*, 1993, **166**, 11–25.
18. Orr, C.W. and S. Roseman, Intercellular adhesion. I. A quantitative assay for measuring the rate of adhesion. *Journal of Membrane Biology*, 1969, **1**, 109–124.
19. Thomas, W.A. and M.S. Steinberg, A twelve-channel automatic recording device for continuous recording of cell aggregation by measurement of small-angle light-scattering. *Journal of Cell Science*, 1980, **41**, 1–18.
20. Cima, L., et al., Hepatocyte culture on biodegradable polymeric substrates. *Biotechnology and Bioengineering*, 1991, **38**, 145–158.
21. Gutsche, A.T., et al., Rat hepatocyte morphology and function on lactose-derivatized polystyrene surfaces. *Biotechnology & Bioengineering*, 1996, **49**, 259–265.
22. Benya, P.D. and J.D. Shaffer, Dedifferentiated chondrocytes reexpress the differentiated collagen phenotype when cultured in agarose gels. *Cell*, 1982, **30**, 215–224.
23. Ishaug, S.L., et al., Osteoblast function on synthetic biodegradable polymers. *Journal of Biomedical Materials Research,* 1994, **28**, 1445–1453.
24. Tamada, Y. and Y. Ikada, Fibroblast growth on polymer surfaces and biosynthesis of collagen. *Journal of Biomedical Materials Research*, 1994, **28**, 783–789.
25. Stol, M., M. Tolar, and M. Adam, Poly(2-hydroxyethyl methacrylatea)-collagen composites which promote muscle cell differentiation *in vitro*. *Biomaterials*, 1985, **6**, 193–197.
26. Barocas, V.H., A.G. Moon, and R.T. Tranquillo, The fibroblast-populated collagen microsphere assay of cell traction force. Part 2. Measurement of the cell traction parameter. *Journal of Biomechanical Engineering*, 1995, **117**, 161–170.
27. Folkman, J. and A. Moscona, Role of cell shape in growth control. *Nature*, 1978, **273**, 345–349.
28. van Wachem, P.B., et al., Adhesion of cultured human endothelial cells onto methacrylate polymers with varying surface wettability and charge. *Biomaterials*, 1987, **8**, 323–328.
29. Horbett, T.A., et al., Cell adhesion to a series of hydrophilic–hydrophobic copolymers studied with a spinning disc apparatus. *Journal of Biomedical Materials Research*, 1988, **22**, 383–404.
30. Horbett, T. and M. Schway, Correlations between mouse 3T3 cell spreading and serum fibronectin adsorption on glass and hydroxyethylmethacrylate-ethylmethacrylate copolymers. *Journal of Biomedical Materials Research*, 1988, **22**, 763–793.
31. van der Valk, P., et al., Interaction of fibroblasts and polymer surfaces: relationship between surface free energy and fibroblast spreading. *Journal of Biomedical Materials Research*, 1983, **17**, 807–817.
32. Horbett, T., M. Schway, and B. Ratner, Hydrophilic-hydrophobic copolymers as cell substrates: Effect on 3T3 cell growth rates. *Journal of Colloid and Interface Science*, 1985, **104**, 28–39.
33. Saltzman, W.M., et al., Fibroblast and hepatocyte behavior on synthetic polymer surfaces. *Journal of Biomedical Materials Research*, 1991, **25**, 741–759.

34. Ertel, S.I., et al., *In vitro* study of the intrinsic toxicity of synthetic surfaces to cells. *Journal of Biomedical Materials Research*, 1994, **28**, 667–675.

35. Hasson, J., D. Wiebe, and W. Abbott, Adult human vascular endothelial cell attachment and migration on novel bioabsorbable polymers. *Archives of Surgery*, 1987, **122**, 428–430.

36. Pettit, D.K., A.S. Hoffman, and T.A. Horbett, Correlation between corneal epithelial cell outgrowth and monoclonal antibody binding to the cell binding domain of adsorbed fibronectin. *Journal of Biomedical Materials Science*, 1994, **28**, 685–691.

37. Ikada, Y., Surface modification of polymers for medical applications. Biomaterials, 1994, **15**(10), 725–736.

38. Amstein, C. and P. Hartman, Adaptation of plastic surfaces for tissue culture by glow discharge. *Journal of Clinical Microbiology*, 1975, **2**, 46–54.

39. Hannan, G. and B. McAuslan, Immobilized serotonin: a novel substrate for cell culture. *Experimental Cell Research*, 1987, **171**, 153–163.

40. Chinn, J., et al., Enhancement of serum fibronectin adsorption and the clonal plating efficiencies of Swiss mouse 3T3 fibroblast and MM14 mouse myoblast cells on polymer substrates modified by radiofrequency plasma deposition. *Journal of Colloid and Interface Science*, 1989, **127**, 67–87.

41. Curtis, A., et al., Adhesion of cells to polystyrene surfaces. *Journal of Cell Biology*, 1983, **97**, 1500–1506.

42. Lydon, M., T. Minett, and B. Tighe, Cellular interactions with synthetic polymer surfaces in culture. *Biomaterials*, 1985, **6**, 396–402.

43. Kowalczynska, H.M. and J. Kaminski, Adhesion of L1210 cells to modified styrene copolymer surfaces in the presence of serum. *Journal of Cell Science*, 1991, **99**, 587–593.

44. Schakenraad, J.M., et al., The influence of substratum surface free energy on growth and spreading of human fibroblasts in the presence and absence of serum proteins. *Journal of Biomedical Materials Research*, 1986, **20**, 773–784.

45. Baier, R., et al., Human platelet spreading on substrata of known surface chemistry. *Journal of Biomedical Materials Research*, 1985, **19**, 1157–1167.

46. Tyler, B.J., B.D. Ratner, and D.G. Castner, Variations between Biomer lots. I. Significant differences in the surface chemistry of two lots of a commercial poly (ether urethane). *Journal of Biomedical Materials Research*, 1992, **26**, 273–289.

47. Smetana, K., Cell biology of hydrogels. *Biomaterials*, 1993, **14**(14), 1046–1050.

48. Smetana, K., et al., The influence of hydrogel functional groups on cell behavior. *Journal of Biomedical Materials Research*, 1990, **24**, 463–470.

49. Lee, J.H., et al., Cell behavior on polymer surfaces with different functional groups. *Biomaterials*, 1994, **15**(9), 705–711.

50. Vacanti, J.P., et al., Selective cell transplantation using bioabsorbable artificial polymers as matrices. *Journal of Pediatric Surgery*, 1988, **23**, 3–9.

51. Kulkarni, R.K., et al., Biodegradable poly(lactic acid) polymers. *Journal of Biomedical Materials Research*, 1971, **5**, 169–181.

52. Schmitt, E.E. and R.A. Polistina, *Surgical sutures*. U.S. Patent 3,297,033, January 10, 1967.

53. Wasserman, D. and A.J. Levy, *Nahtmaterials aus weichgemachten Lacttid-Glykolid-Copolymerisaten*. German Patent Offenlegungsschrift 24 06 539, 1975.

54. Schneider, M.A.K., *Elément de suture absorbable et son procédé de fabrication*. French Patent 1,478,694, 1967.

55. Freed, L., et al., Neocartilage formation *in vitro* and *in vivo* using cells cultured on synthetic biodegradable polymers. *Journal of Biomedical Materials Research*, 1993, **27**, 11–23.

56. Laurencin, C.T., et al., Use of polyphosphazenes for skeletal tissue regeneration. *Journal of Biomedical Materials Research*, 1993, **27**, 963–973.

57. DiMilla, P.A., et al., Maximal migration of human smooth muscle cells on fibronectin and type IV collagen occurs at an intermediate attachment strength. *Journal of Cell Biology*, 1993, **122**, 729–737.

58. Calof, A.L. and A.D. Lander, Relationship between neuronal migration and cell–substratum adhesion: laminin and merosin promote olfactory neuronal migration but are anti-adhesive. *Journal of Cell Biology*, 1991, **115**(3), 779–794.

59. Wu, P., et al., Integrin-binding peptide in solution inhibits or enhances endothelial cell migration, predictably from cell adhesion. *Annals of Biomedical Engineering*, 1994, **22**, 144–152.

60. Palecek, S.P., et al., Integrin–ligand binding properties govern cell migration speed through cell-substratum adhesiveness. *Nature*, 1997, **385**, 537–540.

61. Pettit, D.K., *Invest. Ophthalmol. Vis. Sci.*, 1990, **31**, 2269.

62. Civerchia-Perez, L., et al., Use of collagen–hydroxyethylmethacrylate hydrogels for cell growth. *Proceedings of the National Academy of Sciences*, 1980, **77**, 2064–2068.

63. Carbonetto, S.T., M.M. Gruver, and D.C. Turner, Nerve fiber growth on defined hydrogel substrates. *Science*, 1982, **216**, 897–899.

64. Woerly, S., et al., Synthetic polymer derivatives as substrata for neuronal cell adhesion and growth. *Brain Research Bulletin*, 1993, **30**, 423–432.

65. Massia, S.P. and J.A. Hubbell, Covalent surface immobilization of Arg–Gly–Asp– and Tyr–Ile–Gly–Ser–Arg-containing peptides to obtain well-defined cell-adhesive substrates. *Analytical Biochemistry*, 1989, **187**, 292–301.

66. Schnaar, R.L., et al., Adhesion of hepatocytes to polyacrylamide gels derivitized with N-acetylglucosamine. *Journal of Biological Chemistry*, 1978, **253**, 7940–7951.

67. Blackburn, C.C. and R.L. Schnaar, Carbohydrate-specific cell adhesion is mediated by immobilized glycolipids. *Journal of Biological Chemistry*, 1983, **258**(2), 1180–1188.

68. Pierschbacher, M.D. and E. Ruoslahti, Cell attachment activity of fibronectin can be duplicated by small synthetic fragments of the molecule. *Nature*, 1984, **309**, 30–33.

69. Massia, S.P. and J.A. Hubbell, Human endothelial cell interactions with surface-coupled adhesion peptides on a nonadhesive glass substrate and two polymeric biomaterials. *Journal of Biomedical Materials Research*, 1991, **25**, 223–242.

70. Brandley, B. and R. Schnaar, Covalent attachment of an Arg–Gly–Asp sequence peptide to derivatizable polyacrylamide surfaces: support of fibroblast adhesion and long-term growth. *Analytical Biochemistry*, 1988, **172**, 270–278.

71. Lin, H.-B., et al., Synthesis of a novel polyurethane co-polymer containing covalently attached RGD peptide. *Journal of Biomaterials Science, Polymer Edition*, 1992, **3**, 217–227.

72. Lin, H., et al., Synthesis, surface, and cell-adhesion properties of polyurethanes containing covalently grafted RGD-peptides. *Journal of Biomedical Materials Research*, 1994, **28**, 329–342.

73. Breuers, W., et al., Immobilization of a fibronectin fragment at the surface of a polyurethane film. *Journal of Materials Science: Materials in Medicine*, 1991, **2**, 106–109.

74. Drumheller, P.D., D.L. Ebert, and J.A. Hubbell, Multifunctional poly(ethylene glycol) semi-interpenetrating polymer networks as highly selective adhesive substrates for bioadhesive peptide grafting. *Biotechnology and Bioengineering*, 1994, **43**, 772–780.

75. Matsuda, T., et al., Development of a novel artificial matrix with cell adhesion peptide for cell culture and artificial and hybrid organs. *Transactions of the American Society for Artificial Internal Organs*, 1989, **35**, 677–679.

76. Barrera, D.A., et al., Synthesis and RGD peptide modification of a new biodegradable copolymer: poly(lactic acid-*co*-lysine). *Journal of the American Chemical Society*, 1993, **115**, 11010–11011.

77. Miura, M., et al., Application of LCST polymer–cell receptor conjugates for cell culture on hydrophobic surfaces. *Seventeenth Annual Meeting of the Society for Biomaterials*. Scottsdale, Arizona, USA, 1991.

78. Massia, S.P. and J.A. Hubbell, An RGD spacing of 440 nm is sufficient for integrin $\alpha V \beta 3$-mediated fibroblast spreading and 140 nm for focal contact and stress fiber formation. *Journal of Cell Biology*, 1991, **114**, 1089–1100.

79. Hubbell, J.A., et al., Endothelial cell-selective materials for tissue engineering in the vascular graft via a new receptor. *Bio/Technology*, 1991, **9**, 568–572.

80. Desai, N.P. and J.A. Hubbell, Biological responses to polyethylene oxide modified polyethylene terephthalate surfaces. *Journal of Biomedical Materials Research*, 1991, **25**, 829–843.

81. Drumheller, P.D. and J.A. Hubbell, Densely crosslinked polymer networks of poly(ethylene glycol) in trimethylolpropane triacrylate for cell-adhesion-resistant surfaces. *Journal of Biomedical Materials Research*, 1995, **29**, 207–215.

82. Merrill, E.W., Poly(ethylene oxide) star molecules: Synthesis, characterization, and applications in medicine and biology. *Journal of Biomaterials Science, Polymer Edition*, 1993, **5**, 1–11.

83. Drumheller, P.D. and J.A. Hubbell, Polymer networks with grafted cell adhesion peptides for highly biospecific cell adhesive surfaces. *Analytical Biochemistry*, 1994, **222**, 380–388.

84. Nicol, A., et al., Elastomeric polytetrapeptide matrices: Hydrophobicity dependence of cell attachment from adhesive (GGIP)n to nonadhesive (GGAP)n even in serum. *Journal of Biomedical Materials Research*, 1993, **27**, 801–810.

85. Kikuchi, A., K. Kataoka, and T. Tsuruta, Adhesion and proliferation of bovine aortic endothelial cells on monoamine- and diamine-containing polystyrene derivatives. *Journal of Biomaterials Science, Polymer Edition*, 1992, **3**(3), 253–260.

86. Massia, S.P. and J.A. Hubbell, Immobilized amines and basic amino acids as mimetic heparin-binding domains for cell surface proteoglycan-mediated adhesion. *Journal of Biological Chemistry*, 1992, **267**, 10133–10141.

87. Kobayashi, A., et al., Enhanced adhesion and survival efficiency of liver cells in culture dishes coated with a lactose-carrying styrene homopolymer. *Makromolekulare Chemie—Rapid Communications*, 1986, **7**, 645–650.

88. Kobayashi, A., K. Kobayashi, and T. Akaike, Control of adhesion and detachment of parenchymal liver cells using lactose-carrying polystyrene as substratum. *Journal of Biomaterials Science, Polymer Edition*, 1992, **3**(6), 499–508.

89. Gutsche, A.T., et al., N-acetylglucosamine and adenosine derivatized surfaces for cell culture: 3T3 fibroblast and chicken hepatocyte response. *Biotechnology and Bioengineering*, 1994, **43**, 801–809.

90. Valentini, R.F., et al., Electrically charged polymeric substrates enhance nerve fiber outgrowth *in vitro*. *Biomaterials*, 1992, **13**, 183–190.

91. Makohliso, S.A., R.F. Valentini, and P. Aebischer, Magnitude and polarity of a fluoroethylene propylene electret substrate charge influences neurite outgrowth *in vitro*. *Journal of Biomedical Materials Research*, 1993, **27**, 1075–1085.

92. Fine, E.G., et al., Improved nerve regeneration through piezoelectric vinylidene-fluoride–trifluoroethylene copolymer guidance channels. *Biomaterials*, 1991, **12**, 775–780.

93. Wong, J.Y., R. Langer, and D.E. Ingber, Electrically conducting polymers can noninvasively control the shape and growth of mammalian cells. *Proceedings of the National Academy of Sciences, USA*, 1994, **91**, 3201–3204.

94. Goldhaber, P., The influence of pore size on carcinogenicity of subcutaneously implanted Millipore filters. *Proceedings of the American Association for Cancer Research*, 1961, **3**, 228.

95. Goldhaber, P., Further observations concerning the carcinogenicity of Millipore filters. *Proceedings of the American Association for Cancer Research*, 1962, **4**, 323.

96. Brauker, J., et al., Neovascularization of immunoisolation membranes: the effect of membrane architecture and encapsulated tissue. *Transplantation Proceedings*, 1992, **24**, 2924.

97. Weiss, P., Experiments on cell and axon orientation *in vitro*: the role of colloidal exudates in tissue organization. *Journal of Experimental Zoology*, 1945, **100**, 353–386.

98. Weiss, P., *In vitro* experiments on the factors determining the course of the out-growing nerve fiber. *Journal of Experimental Zoology*, 1934, **68**, 393–448.

99. Brunette, D., Fibroblasts on micromachined substrata orient hierarchically to grooves of different dimensions. *Experimental Cell Research*, 1986, **164**, 11–26.

100. Dunn, G.A. and A.F. Brown, Alignment of fibroblasts on grooved surfaces described by a simple geometric transformation. *Journal of Cell Science*, 1986, **83**, 313–340.

101. Clark, P., et al., Cell guidance by ultrafine topography *in vitro*. *Journal of Cell Science*, 1991, **99**, 73–77.

102. Meyle, J., K. Gultig, and W. Nisch, Variation in contact guidance by human cells on a microstructured surface. *Journal of Biomedical Materials Research*, 1995, **29**, 81–88.

103. Schmidt, J.A. and A.F. von Recum, Macrophage response to microtextured silicone. *Biomaterials*, 1992, **12**, 385–389.

104. O'Neill, C., P. Jordan, and G. Ireland, Evidence for two distinct mechanisms of anchorage stimulation in freshly explanted and 3T3 Swiss mouse fibroblasts. *Cell*, 1986, **44**, 489–496.

105. Singhvi, R., et al., Engineering cell shape and function. *Science*, 1994, **264**, 696–698.

106. Ranieri, J.P., et al., Selective neuronal cell adhesion to a covalently patterned monoamine on fluorinated ethylene propylene films. *Journal of Biomedical Materials Research*, 1993, **27**, 917–925.

107. Matsuda, T., T. Sugawara, and K. Inoue, Two-dimensional cell manipulation technology: an artificial neural circuit based on surface microprocessing. *ASAIO Journal*, 1992, **38**, M243–M247.

108. Matsuda, T. and T. Sugawara, Development of surface photochemical modification method for micropatterning of cultured cells. *Journal of Biomedical Materials Research*, 1995, **29**, 749–756.

109. Matsuzawa, M., et al., Containment and growth of neuroblastoma cells on chemically patterned substrates. *Journal of Neuroscience Methods*, 1993, **50**, 253–260.

110. Brandley, B. and R. Schnaar, Tumor cell haptotaxis on covalently immobilized linear and exponential gradients of a cell adhesion peptide. *Developmental Biology*, 1989, **135**, 74–86.

111. Brandley, B.K., J.H. Shaper, and R.L. Schnaar, Tumor cell haptotaxis on immobilized N-acetylglucosamine gradients. *Developmental Biology*, 1990, **140**, 161–171.

112. Demetriou, A., et al., Replacement of liver function in rats by transplantation of microcarrier-attached hepatocytes. *Science*, 1986, **23**, 1190–1192.

113. Emerich, D.F., et al., Implantation of polymer-encapsulated human Nerve Growth Factor-secreting fibroblasts attenuates the behavioral and neuropathological consequences of quinolinic acid injections into rodent striatum. *Experimental Neurology*, 1994, **130**, 141–150.

114. Lacy, P.E., et al., Maintenance of normoglycemia in diabetic mice by subcutaneous xenografts of encapsulated islets. *Science*, 1991, **254**, 1782–1784.

115. van Wezel, A.L., Growth of cell strains and primary cells on microcarriers in homogeneous culture. *Nature*, 1967, **216**, 64–65.

116. van Wezel, A., Monolayer growth systems: homogeneous unit processes. *Animal Cell Biotechnology*, 1985, **1**, 265–282.

117. Levine, D., D. Wang, and W. Thilly, Optimization of growth surface parameters in microcarrier cell culture. *Biotechnology and Bioengineering*, 1979, **21**, 821–845.

118. Jacobson, B. and U. Ryan, Growth of endothelial and HeLa cells on a new multipurpose microcarrier that is positive, negative or collagen coated. *Tissue & Cell*, 1982, **14**, 69–83.

119. Fairman, K. and B. Jacobson, Unique morphology of HeLa cell attachment, spreading and detachment from microcarrier beads covalently coated with a specific and non-specific substratum. *Tissue & Cell*, 1983, **15**, 167–180.

120. Wissemann, K. and B. Jacobson, Pure gelatin microcarriers: synthesis and use in cell attachment and growth of fibroblast and endothelial cells. *In Vitro Cellular & Developmental Biology*, 1985, **21**, 391–401.

121. Freed, L.E. and G. Vunjak-Novakovic, Cultivation of cell–polymer tissue constructs in simulated microgravity. *Biotechnology and Bioengineering*, 1995, **46**, 306–313.

122. Lim, F. and A.M. Sun, Microencapulated islets as bioartificial endocrine pancreas. *Science*, 1980, **210**, 908–910.

123. Bano, M.C., et al., A novel synthetic method for hybridoma cells encapsulation. *Bio/Technology*, 1991, **9**, 468–471.

124. Nilsson, K., et al., Entrapment of animal cells for production of monoclonal antibodies and other biomolecules. *Nature*, 1983, **302**, 629–630.

125. Dawson, R.M., et al., Microencapsulation of CHO cells in a hydroxyethyl methacrylate–methyl methacrylate copolymer. *Biomaterials*, 1987, **8**, 360–366.

126. Sefton, M., et al., Microencapsulation of mammalian cells in a water-insoluble polyacrylate by coextrusion and interfacial precipitation. *Biotechnology and Bioengineering*, 1987, **29**, 1135–1143.

127. Sawhney, A.S., C.P. Pathak, and J.A. Hubbell, Modification of islet of Langerhans surfaces with immunoprotective poly(ethylene glycol) coatings via interfacial polymerization. *Biotechnology and Bioengineering*, 1994, **44**, 383–386.

128. Joseph, J.M., et al., Transplantation of encapsulated bovine chrommafin cells in the sheep subarachnoid space: a preclinical study for the treatment of cancer pain. *Cell Transplantation*, 1994, **3**, 355–364.

129. Zienlinski, B.A. and P. Aebischer, Chitosan as a matrix for mammalian cell encapsulation. *Biomaterials*, 1994, **15**, 1049–1056.

130. Sullivan, S.J., et al., Biohybrid artificial pancreas: long-term implantation studies in diabetic, pancreatectomized dogs. *Science*, 1991, **252**, 718–721.

131. Thompson, J., et al., Heparin-binding growth factor 1 induces the formation of organoid neovascular structures *in vivo*. *Proceedings of the National Academy of the Sciences USA*, 1989, **86**, 7928–7932.

132. Yang, J., et al., Sustained growth and three-dimensional organization of primary mammary tumor epithelial cells embedded in collagen gels. *Proceedings of the National Academy of Sciences USA*, 1979, **76**, 3401–3405.

133. Richards, J., et al., Method for culturing mammary epithelial cells in a rat tail collagen gel matrtix. *Journal of Tissue Culture Methods*, 1983, **8**, 31–36.

134. Bell, E.B., B. Ivarsson, and C. Merrill, Production of a tissue-like structure by contraction of collagen lattices by human fibroblasts with different proliferative potential. *Proceedings of the National Academy of Sciences USA*, 1979, **75**, 1274–1278.

135. Chen, J., E. Stuckey, and C. Berry, Three-dimensional culture of rat exocrine pancreatic cells using collagen gels. *British Journal of Experimental Pathology*, 1985, **66**, 551–559.

136. Schor, S., Cell proliferation and migration on collagen substrata *in vitro*. *Journal of Cell Science*, 1980, **41**, 159–175.

137. Schor, S., A. Schor, and G. Bazill, The effects of fibronectin on the migration of human foreskin fibroblasts and Syrian hamster melanoma cells into three-dimensional gels of native collagen fibres. *Journal of Cell Science*, 1981, **48**, 301–314.

138. Schor, S., T. Allen, and C. Harrison, Cell migration through three-dimensional gels of native collagen fibres: collagenolytic activity is not required for the migration of two permanent cell lines. *Journal of Cell Science*, 1980, **46**, 171–186.

139. Haston, W. and P. Wilkinson, Visual methods for measuring leukocyte locomotion. *Methods in Enzymology*, 1988, **162**, 17–38.

140. Saltzman, W.M., et al., Three-dimensional cell cultures mimic tissues. *Annals of the New York Academy of Science*, 1992, **665**, 259–273.

141. Dickinson, R.B., S. Guido, and R.T. Tranquillo, Biased cell migration of fibroblasts exhibiting contact guidance in oriented collagen gels. *Annals of Biomedical Engineering*, 1994, **22**, 342–356.

142. Parkhurst, M.R. and W.M. Saltzman, Quantification of human neutrophil motility in three-dimensional collagen gels: effect of collagen concentration. *Biophysical Journal*, 1992, **61**, 306–315.

143. Krewson, C.E., et al., Cell aggregation and neurite growth in gels of extracellular matrix molecules. *Biotechnology and Bioengineering*, 1994, **43**, 555–562.

144. Bellamkonda, R., et al., Hydrogel-based three-dimensional matrix for neural cells. *Journal of Biomedical Materials Research*, 1995, **29**, 663–671.

145. Oxley, H.R., et al., Macroporous hydrogels for biomedical application: methodology and morphology. *Biomaterials*, 1993, **14**, 1064–1072.

146. Corkhill, P.H., J.H. Fitton, and B.J. Tighe, Towards a synthetic articular cartilage. *Journal of Biomaterials Science, Polymer Edition*, 1993, **4**, 615–630.

147. Cascone, M.G., et al., Evaluation of poly(vinyl alcohol) hydrogels as a component of hybrid artificial tissues. *Journal of Materials Science: Materials in Medicine*, 1995, **6**, 71–75.

148. Moghaddam, M.J. and T. Matsuda, Development of a 3D artificial extracellular matrix. *Transactions of the American Society of Artificial Internal Organs*, 1991, **37**, M437–M438.

149. Mikos, A.G., et al., Preparation of poly(glycolic acid) bonded fiber structures for cell attachment and transplantation. *Journal of Biomedical Materials Research*, 1993, **27**, 183–189.

150. Lo, H., M. Ponticello, and K. Leong, Fabrication of controlled release biodegradable foams by phase separation. *Tissue Engineering*, 1995, **1**, 15.

151. Lo, H., et al., Poly(L-lactic acid) foams with cell seeding and controlled release capacity. *Journal of Biomedical Materials Research*, 1996, **44**(4), 446–455.

152. Thomson, R.C., et al., Fabrication of biodegradable polymer scaffolds to engineer trabecular bone. *Journal of Biomaterials Science, Polymer Edition*, 1995, **7**(1), 23–38.

153. Puelacher, W.C., et al., Design of nasoseptal cartilage replacements synthesized from biodegradable polymers and chondrocytes. *Biomaterials*, 1994, **15**(10), 774–778.

154. Freed, L.E., G. Vunjak-Novakovic, and R. Langer, Cultivation of cell–polymer cartilage implants in bioreactors. *Journal of Cellular Biochemistry*, 1993, **51**, 257–264.

155. Dai, W. and W.M. Saltzman, Fibroblast aggregation by suspension with conjugates of poly(ethylene glycol) and RGD. *Biotechnology & Bioengineering*, 1996, **50**, 349–356.

156. McAuslan, B. and G. Johnson, Cell responses to biomaterials I: Adhesion and growth of vascular endothelial cells on poly(hydroxyethyl methacrylate) following surface modification by hydrolytic etching. *Journal of Biomedical Materials Research*, 1987, **21**, 921–935.

157. Pratt, K., S. Williams, and B. Jarrell, Enhanced adherence of human adult endothelial cells to plasma discharge modified polyethylene terephthalate. *Journal of Biomedical Materials Research*, 1989, **23**, 1131–1147.

158. Tan, J. and W.M. Saltzman, Topographical control of human neutrophil motility as micropatterned materials with various surface chemistry. *Biomaterials*, 2002, **23**, 3215–3225.

159. Tan, J., H. Shen, and W.M. Saltzman. Micron-scale positioning of features influences the rate of polymorphonuclear leukocyte migration. *Biophysical Journal*, 2001, **81**, 2569–2579.

160. Yang, S., K.F. Leong, Z. Du, and C.R. Chua, The design of scaffolds for use in tissue engineering. Part 1. Traditional factors. *Tissue Engineering*, 2001, **7**(6), 679–689.

161. Kuhl, P.R. and L.G. Griffith. Tethered epidermal growth factor as a paradigm of growth factor-induced stimulation from the solid phase. *Nature Medicine*, 1996, **2**, 1022–1027.

162. Diguglielmo, G., P. Baass, W. Ou, B. Posner, and J. Bergeron, Compartmentalization of SHC, GRB2 and MSOS, and hyperphosphorylation of RAF-1 by EGF but not insulin in liver parenchyma. *Embo Journal*, 1994, **13**(18), 4269–4277.

163. Baass, P., G. Diguglielmo, F. Authier, B. Posner, and J. Bergeron, Compartmentalized signal-transduction by receptor tyrosine kinases. *Trends in Cell Biology*, 1995, **5**(12), 465–470.

164. Ma, P.X. and J.W. Choi. Biodegradable polymer scaffolds with well-defined interconnected spherical pore networks. *Tissue Engineering*, 2001, **7**(1), 23–33.

165. Knauer, D.J., H.S. Wiley, and D.D. Cunningham, Relationship between epidermal growth factor receptor occupancy and mitogenic response. *Journal of Biological Chemistry*, 1984, **259**, 5623–5631.

13

Approaches to Tissue Engineering

"I'm not afraid of failing. It's just that I don't know how to turn myself into the wind."

Paulo Coelho, *The Alchemist*

The first part of this book has proposed that tissue engineering is a modern realization of a practice with ancient origins. Tissue engineering is different because technologies that are now available permit generation of synthetic materials that mimic biological materials as well as clinically useful quantities of biological components (such as proteins and cells). These technologies have emerged from rapid advances in the biological sciences and engineering over the past few decades. Since tissue engineering is new, however, few examples of successful tissue engineering are available. The reader, upon recognizing this early stage of development, might presume that the prospects for a compelling chapter on "Approaches to Tissue Engineering" are bleak. Instead, I am convinced that this is the most exciting of times to write such a chapter, because the precedents are not yet assembled and the field has not yet been reduced to systematic divisions. But there are many challenges.

The challenge begins with organization of information. Written reviews of tissue engineering to date adopt different organizational structures. For example, an early influential review was organized around replacement strategies for different organ or tissue systems [1]. A similar, although more encyclopedic, approach was used in the first two editions of an edited textbook [2]. This is a sensible arrangement, given that tissue engineering is an interdisciplinary area of study that has emerged in response to rather specific clinical needs, such as the shortage of donor livers and the paucity of grafts for skin. But it is a difficult arrangement for the teacher and student, as it does not require reconciliation between approaches used to solve different problems. For example, although regeneration of skin and liver differs in many essential ways, there are important areas of intersection. As a consequence, an organ or tissue-based approach does not easily allow for assimilation of new knowledge that is acquired by successes made on particular problems.

What is tissue engineering and how can the basic principles, which are developed in Part 2 of this book, be integrated into a strategy for the engineering of replacement tissues? The previous three chapters describe important, but focused, elements of tissue engineering practice: cell delivery, agent delivery, and cell interactions with synthetic materials. These are elements of tissue engineering but they do not define the subject, nor do they illustrate boundaries in its application. In defining the topic more completely, the present chapter admits that there is no simple answer to the question, but instead attempts to illuminate the essential elements of tissue engineering by focusing on four unifying, but hopefully not overly restrictive, themes:

1. Tissue engineering involves the replacement of tissue structure and function. This idea was introduced earlier, in Chapter 2. If this is true, then the end result of a tissue engineering procedure must be quantifiable by functional or structural endpoints. For example, the success of a method for replacement of pancreas function can be measured by regulation of glucose concentration or maintenance of insulin secretion. The success of a bone tissue engineering approach can be evaluated by examination of the histological structure and the mechanical properties of the newly formed bone.
2. Tissue engineering usually involves the introduction of a biological product (either cells, genes, or proteins) that initiate or support a process of regeneration. The production and application of cells is, in particular, a unique (but not defining) feature of tissue engineering.
3. Tissue engineering usually involves a synthetic component that serves to organize or constrain the biological product.
4. Tissue engineering represents a logical extension of the well-established practice of artificial organs.

This final theme is the most specific, and represents the easiest place to start.

13.1 Artificial Organs

13.1.1 Artificial Kidney

The kidney provides an essential excretory function by removing water-soluble waste molecules from the blood and concentrating them in a liquid form. Remarkably, it performs this function while maintaining the blood balance of essential ions (such as Na^+ and K^+) and with a minimal loss of total body water ($\sim 1\,L/day$). Our metabolic machinery is diverse, and therefore the kidney is responsible for excretion of thousands of different chemicals. Loss of kidney function results in an accumulation of toxic molecules in the blood. The end-products of nitrogen metabolism are a particularly important subset of these chemicals; for example, blood concentration of urea rises to toxic levels during kidney failure.

Hemodialysis is a life-extending procedure for $\sim 200{,}000$ patients with end-stage renal disease in the United States [3]. The success of hemodialysis is a direct result of engineering analysis; the formulation of a mathematical description of solute movement during hemodialysis, which was based on classical chemical engineering principles [4], produced improvements in artificial kidney design and operation [5].

The technology of dialysis was developed to provide an artificial replacement for kidney function. Most artificial kidneys function by controlling the contact of a patient's blood with a dialysate solution (Figure 13.1). Contact is indirect; solute exchange is regulated by an artificial membrane that serves as a common boundary for the flowing liquid streams. Chemical extraction from the blood is controlled via the permeability characteristics of the membrane and the flowrates of blood and dialysate (Q_B and Q_D, respectively).

The most commonly used artificial kidneys contain an array of hollow fibers (Figure 13.1b). The parallel arrangement of hollow fibers provides convenient flow pathways for both blood and dialysate and an extensive surface area for solute exchange. The total surface area S available for exchange of molecules is given by

$$S = N\pi dL \tag{13-1}$$

where N is the number of hollow fibers in the unit, d is the diameter of each fiber, and L is the length of each fiber. For a 10,000-fiber unit, with fibers of diameter 200 μm and length 20 cm, the total surface area is $\sim 1.3\,\text{m}^2$.

Assuming steady-state operation, and focusing on the movement of one type of molecule (solute A), the overall rate of solute removal from the blood, N_T, must equal the rate of solute appearance in the dialysate:

$$N_T = Q_B(C_B - C_{B_o}) = Q_D(C_{D_o} - C_{D_i}) \tag{13-2}$$

N_T must also be equal to the total number of molecules that cross the dialysis membrane as a result of diffusion of solute through the membrane. The local rate of solute movement from blood to dialysate is given by

$$N_x = K(C_{B_x} - C_{D_x}) \tag{13-3}$$

where N_x is the local flux through the dialysis membrane at position x, and is the product of the concentration difference between blood and dialysate at x and an overall transfer coefficient K. A mass balance on a volume element corresponding to the blood-containing region from x to $x + dx$ gives

$$Q_B(C_{B_x} - C_{B_{x+dx}}) = K(C_{B_x} - C_{D_x})w\,dx \tag{13-4}$$

which can be rearranged to give

$$\frac{dC_B}{(C_B - C_D)} = -\frac{Kw\,dx}{Q_B} \tag{13-5}$$

A similar mass balance can be written on the dialysate-containing region from x to $x + dx$ to give

$$\frac{dC_D}{(C_B - C_D)} = -\frac{Kw\,dx}{Q_D} \tag{13-6}$$

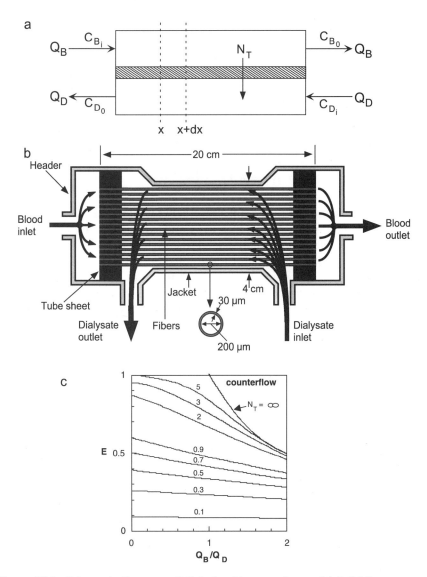

Figure 13.1. Schematic diagrams of dialysis with a membrane. (a) Solid lines indicate passive diffusion, which is driven by a concentration gradient. In counter-current operation, blood flows in one direction (across the top of the membrane) and dialysate flows in the opposite direction. (b) Hollow fiber dialysis device operating in counter-current flow. (c) Extraction ratio as a function of blood flowrate (redrawn from Figure 9.10 in [6]). The extraction ratio is shown for different operating parameters in counter-current operation.

Subtracting Equation 13-6 from 13-5 yields the differential equation

$$\frac{d(C_B - C_D)}{C_B - C_D} = -K\left(\frac{1}{Q_B} - \frac{1}{Q_D}\right)w\,dx \qquad (13\text{-}7)$$

which can be integrated over the length of the dialysis unit to yield:

$$\ln\left(\frac{C_{B_o} - C_{D_i}}{C_{B_i} - C_{D_o}}\right) = -KwL\left(\frac{1}{Q_B} - \frac{1}{Q_D}\right) \qquad (13\text{-}8)$$

Using Equation 13-2 to eliminate the variables Q_B and Q_D leads to the design equation for counter-current flow dialysis

$$N_T = KA\frac{\delta C_1 - \Delta C_2}{\ln(\Delta C_1 - \Delta C_2)} \qquad (13\text{-}9)$$

where ΔC_1 is the concentration difference between blood and dialysate at the left-hand side of Figure 15.1a ($C_{B_i} - C_{D_o}$) and ΔC_2 is the concentration difference between blood and dialysate at the right-hand side of the Figure ($C_{B_o} - C_{D_i}$). Equation 13-9 relates the total rate of solute movement across the dialysis membrane—which is equal to the total rate of solute removal from the blood—to characteristics of the dialyzer (that is, flow pattern, membrane permeability, and membrane area) and operational variables (that is, inlet and outlet concentrations).

The overall performance of a dialysis unit can be expressed in a number of ways: dialysance, clearance, or extraction ratio. Dialysance D^* is expressed in units of flowrate:

$$D^* = \frac{Q_B(C_{B_i} - C_{B_o})}{C_{B_i} - C_{D_i}} \qquad (13\text{-}10)$$

Clearance C^* is an extension of a concept used frequently to describe behavior of the kidneys and is commonly used to describe the overall performance of artificial kidneys. Clearance can be interpreted as the blood flowrate that can be completely cleared of a solute (that is, the volume per unit time of blood that could have all of the solute removed):

$$C^* = \frac{Q_B(C_{B_i} - C_{B_o})}{C_{B_i}} = \frac{N_T}{C_{B_i}} \qquad (13\text{-}11)$$

The extraction ratio E^* is the solute concentration change in the blood compared to the theoretical solute concentration change that would occur if the blood and dialysate came to equilibrium:

$$E^* = \frac{C_{B_i} - C_{B_o}}{C_{B_i} - C_{D_i}} \qquad (13\text{-}12)$$

Equations 13-10 through 13-12 are defined for counter-current flow operation, as illustrated in Figure 13.1.

If the inlet dialysate stream contains no solute ($C_{D_i} = 0$, which is the usual situation for most solutes that are to be removed), the extraction ratio can be written in terms of characteristics of the dialysis unit:

$$E^* = \frac{1 - e^{\gamma(1-z)}}{z - e^{\gamma(1-z)}} \qquad (13\text{-}13)$$

where γ is the relative rate of membrane transfer to blood flow (KA/Q_B) and z is the relative rate of blood flow to dialysate flow (Q_B/Q_D). Equation 13-13, which applies to a unit in counter-current operation, was obtained by calculating concentrations as a function of device design and is shown in Figure 13.1c. A similar analysis can be performed for other configurations (see Figure 9.10 of the book by Cooney [6], or Chapter 6 of Fournier [73]).

The present analysis assumes that diffusion is the only mechanism for molecular exchange across the membrane. This is not always true; hemodialysis units are sometimes operated with a pressure drop across the membrane to provide an additional ultrafiltration flux of water from the blood to the dialysate. Ultrafiltration may serve an important clinical function by allowing for regulation of the fluid volume of the patient. The more advanced operation with ultrafiltration is now possible because materials with good separation characteristics that also permit the convective movement of water are now available. Figure 13.2 shows some of the basic membrane structures that can be used in hemodialysis, ultrafiltration, and other blood purification operations. Asymmetric membranes—which possess a thin layer for size selectivity and a thicker, more porous layer for mechanical strength—are an important development in this area. These membranes also provide a good illustration of an advancement in materials science (that is, methods for the reliable production of asymmetric membrane materials) that has permitted a more sophisticated form of medical therapy.

13.1.2 Artificial Pancreas

The pancreas produces the protein hormone insulin and releases it into the bloodstream as necessary for maintenance of normal blood glucose levels. The physiology of pancreatic function involves a complex network of cellular interactions and molecular signals, but the essential function is conceptually simple (Figure 13.3a). Cells within the pancreas secrete insulin; the rate of insulin secretion depends on the glucose concentration in the blood. Other cells in the body store glucose; the rate of glucose removal from the blood depends on insulin concentration. Because this function is conceptually simple, patients with type II diabetes (that is, patients with abnormal pancreas function who require supplemental insulin) can control their blood glucose levels by periodically injecting doses of insulin; the timing and quantity of the injected dose is based on estimated or measured levels of glucose in the blood. In this manner, one of the functions of the pancreas is replaced by adding appropriate amounts of insulin to the blood as needed to maintain glucose levels.

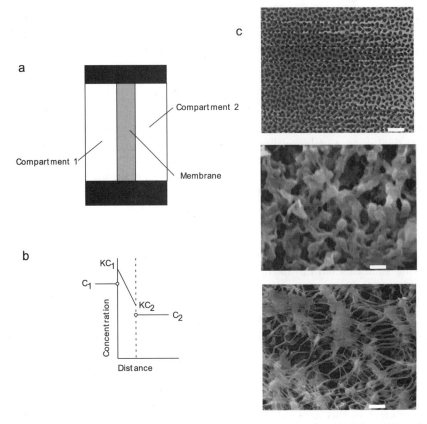

Figure 13.2. Different structures of membrane for size separation. (a) The ability of a membrane to regulate the passage of any given solute is often determined experimentally by holding the membrane between two compartments (usually aqueous compartments in tissue engineering applications) that contain different concentrations of the solute of interest. In this case, compartment 1 initially contains a higher concentration than compartment 2, so the solute diffuses from compartment 1 to 2. (b) Relationship between concentrations in the aqueous compartments and concentrations in the membrane for the situation illustrated in panel (a). (c) Scanning electron micrographs of the membrane morphology for three different types of membrane materials: an anopore ceramic membrane (top); a PVDF membrane (middle); and a PTFE membrane (bottom). In each photo, the white scale bar indicates 1 μm. The photographs in panel (c) were kindly provided by Andrew Zydney.

Insulin injection therapy is effective in many patients, but it is imperfect. The normal pancreas continuously secretes insulin in response to continuous sensing of glucose concentration; the injection of insulin mimics this function without the high level of regulation (that is, without continuous sensing and evaluation of the need for insulin). Patients with diabetes have long-term side effects of their illness that correlate with the precision of glucose control. In addition, the injection of insulin does not provide other functions naturally performed by a normal pancreas.

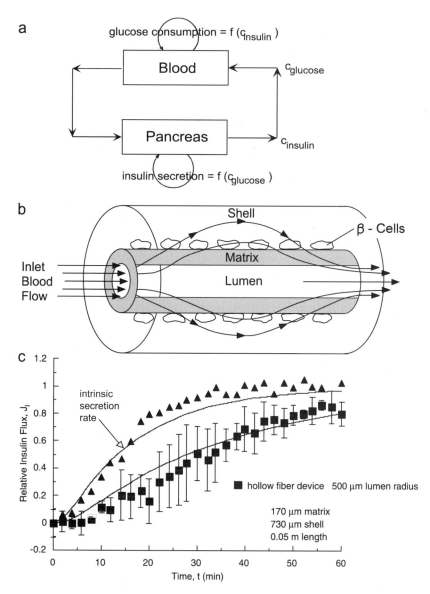

Figure 13.3. Design and operation of an artificial pancreas. (a) Schematic model for the function of the pancreas, in which insulin is secreted in response to glucose concentration in the blood. Both the sensing and the secretion function are present within islet cells in the pancreas. (b) Hollow fiber device for long-term culture of pancreatic islets and contact with blood through a hollow fiber membrane. (c) Mathematical models of solute movement in the hollow fiber device can be used to describe the changes in glucose and insulin concentration that are observed experimentally. Model and data from Pillarella and Zydney [7].

Cells of the pancreas can sense glucose concentration and release insulin in response (see Figure 2.7 in Chapter 2). An artificial pancreas can therefore use normal pancreatic cells as functional units. For example, cells from the pancreatic islets of Langerhans can be added to an artificial device that is conceptually similar to the hollow fiber hemodialyzer (Figure 13.3b). Because of their position within the device, islet cells are exposed to glucose concentrations from the flowing blood, but they are protected from immunological reactions due to blood cells and proteins.

Analysis of the artificial pancreas is similar to that of the artificial kidney, but is complicated by the presence of living cells. The model developed by Pillarella and Zydney [7] analyzes the transport in three separate phases: lumen (L), membrane or matrix (M), and shell (S), as shown in Figure13.3b. A mass conservation equation for insulin (*i*) or glucose (*g*) can be written in each phase:

$$\frac{\partial C_a}{\partial t} + u\frac{\partial C_a}{\partial z} + v\frac{\partial C_a}{\partial r} = \frac{D_a}{r}\frac{\partial}{\partial r}\left[r\frac{\partial C_a}{\partial r}\right] + R_a \tag{13-14}$$

where the subscript *a* represents either *i* or *g*. This model is consistent with experimental information on the release of insulin from hollow fiber-type devices (Figure 13.3c).

There has been considerable progress in the translation of this concept into a working system for clinical use. One design for an implantable biohybrid artificial pancreas employs an annular-shaped acrylic housing 9 cm in diameter, 2 cm high, weighing 50 g, and containing 30–35 cm of coiled tubular membrane with an inner diameter of 5–6 mm and a wall thickness of 120–140 μm [8]. This membrane material was connected to standard 6 mm PTFE graft for connection to the vasculature. This design provides a total membrane surface area of 60 cm^2 and a total cell compartment volume of 5–6 mL; islets are seeded within the device as a suspension in agar. Ability of these devices to produce insulin was tested *in vitro* when seeded with 1–2 × 10^5 canine islets; islets within the device produced insulin for many months in response to changes in glucose concentration, with a time lag of ~ 21 min. When implanted into pancreatectomized dogs, the need for insulin in these animals was decreased to ~ 0 while the fasting blood glucose level was decreased from ~ 250 mg/dL to 150 mg/dL. It has, however, been difficult to develop similar devices of an adequate size to use in humans, because of problems with coagulation within the fiber lumen and surgical connection of the synthetic device to the patient's vessels, as well as difficulty in identifying the appropriate source for islets.

13.1.3 Artificial Liver

Fulminant liver failure presents a dramatic and life-threatening situation. Patients experience rapid progression of jaundice, clotting disorders, and encephalopathy, which leads to death in 50 to 80% of cases. The liver can recover from pathological changes, and frequently does. Unfortunately, in many cases, the progression of disease is more rapid than the process of regeneration; the patient therefore succumbs. Because of the diverse functions of the liver (Table 2.2), the loss of metabolic, synthetic, and regulatory functions of the liver creates multisystem failures. The only current therapy is orthotopic liver transplantation, with one-year survivals now exceeding 70%. But donors are severely limited and many patients die awaiting a donor liver. Artificial measures to support the patients with rapidly progressive disease would be extremely useful.

Extraordinary efforts are frequently enlisted to provide temporary support for patients awaiting liver transplants, including *ex vivo* perfusion through animal livers. Xenoperfusion was first used to support patients in liver failure in 1965. Studies of pig-liver perfusion suggest that this treatment can reduce serum bilirubin and ammonia levels while reducing the symptoms of hepatic encephalopathy. This approach is limited, however, since each perfused liver only retains essential functions for a few hours. Other approaches to liver support include charcoal hemoperfusion, plasmapheresis, hemodialysis, and cross-circulation with humans and animals (see [9]).

At least four different artificial liver assist devices have been tested clinically using hepatocytes from either a well-differentiated human hepatoblastoma [10] or hepatocytes from pigs [11]. In one system, HepatAssist, porcine hepatocytes are used in a hollow fiber bioreactor, two charcoal columns, a membrane oxygenator, and a pump (see Figure 13.4). Blood is first separated by plasmapheresis prior to HepatAssist treatment of the plasma fraction. A review article compares the technologies that are currently available [12].

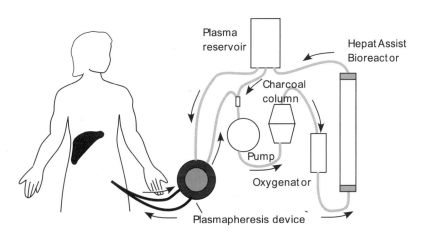

Figure 13.4. Design of an extracorporeal liver assist device; schematic diagram of the components of the HepatAssist device developed by Circe Biomedical. According to the manufacturer's website: "The HepatAssist System includes a hollow fiber bioreactor containing hepatocytes, two charcoal columns, a membrane oxygenator, and a pump (as shown in figure). The HepatAssist System is used in combination with a commercially available plasma separation machine, which diffuses plasma through the HepatAssist circuit before it is reconstituted with the blood cells and returned to the patient."

13.2 Roles of the Synthetic Component

As suggested by the examples of the previous section, synthetic materials—such as membranes with size-dependent permeability—are essential ingredients in the construction of artificial organs. Similarly, synthetic components are a fundamental part of most tissue engineering approaches. The synthetic component may serve one or more of several functions: selective permeability for compartmentalization; support of mechanical structure as a substitute for ECM; controlled release; or controlled presentation of signaling molecules. Some of these elements have been described in previous chapters (controlled release in Chapter 11, support of mechanical structure in Chapter 12, controlled presentation of signaling molecules in both). In this section, therefore, the focus is on materials with selective permeability, and on uses of these materials to create isolated compartments, which allow for regulated molecular interaction between the compartments.

13.2.1 Membranes for Isolation (Selective Permeability of the Material)

Membrane Materials Used in Hemodialysis and Hollow Fiber Bioreactors. Many of the membrane materials that are used for hemodialysis are composed of cellulose or cellulose derivatives. Although several synthetic materials have been developed that have greater strength, support higher solute fluxes, and interact less with flowing blood (Table 13.1, Figure 13.2), the cellulose-based materials are useful in dialysis as well as in other biomedical applications that require a material to keep two aqueous phases separate while allowing for the exchange of selected molecules.

The materials that have been used for hollow fiber bioreactors (such as those described above for the artificial pancreas and liver) are similar to the materials used in dialysis. Cellulose, and derivatives of cellulose, polysulphone, poly(acrylonitrile-*co*-vinyl chloride), and PMMA are commonly used.

Table 13.1
Polymeric Materials Used as Dialysis Membranes

Material	Flux	Biocompatibility
Cellulose	Low	Low
Cellulose diacetate	High/Low	Moderate
Cellulose triacetate	High	High
Diethylaminoethyl-substituted cellulose	High	Moderate
Polyacrylonitrile–methallyl sulfonate copolymer	High	High
Polyacrylonitrile–methacrylate copolymer	High	High
Polymethylmethacrylate	High/Low	High
Polysulfone	High	High

Information from [3].

Selective Permeation Properties of Materials. Many dialysis membranes that are designed to separate small molecules (less than 1,000 dalton) from the blood appear to function by a solution–diffusion mechanism (Figures 13.2a and 13.2b). Recall the expression used to evaluate fluxes through biological membranes in Chapter 9:

$$P = k_s = \frac{KD_m}{L} \tag{9-1}$$

in which the permeability of the material P is related to the equilibrium partition coefficient K, the diffusion coefficient of the solute in the membrane D_m, and the thickness of the membrane L. Equation 9-1 demonstrates that the overall permeability for a solute in a membrane depends on properties of the membrane/solute pair. For small molecules that can dissolve into the membrane material, the equilibrium partition coefficient is a measure of the relative solubility of the solute in the membrane compared to the solubility of the same solute in water ($K = C_{membrane}/C_{water}$). The overall flux of solute through the membrane material (given by Equation 9-2) depends on the magnitude of the solubility of the solute in the membrane, K, and the rate of diffusion of the solute through the membrane material, D_m. Therefore, according to the solution–diffusion mechanism, a dialysis membrane can function to exclude penetration of a solute because of either the low solubility in the membrane material or the slow rate of diffusion within the material.

For larger molecules, especially molecules that are soluble in water, penetration through the membrane requires physical openings, or pores, that are larger than the molecule (Figure 13.5). Recall the discussion of permeation

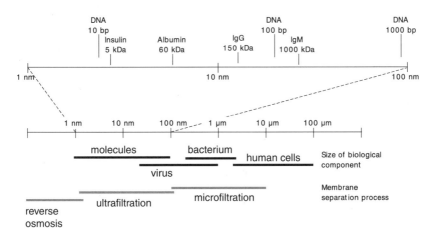

Figure 13.5. Molecular size and molecular weight cutoffs for membranes. The length scale shows the range of dimensions of interest for membrane-based separations. Many biological molecules are in the size range (1–100 nm) that is separable by ultrafiltration membranes. Real membrane materials have pores with a distribution of sizes, so molecular weight "cutoffs" are not sharply defined.

through porous materials in Chapter 9 (Section 9.2.2). Here we are considering synthetic membranes in which the natural equilibrium partition coefficient for the solute/material pair is near zero, because of the limited ability of the solute to dissolve in the membrane material (for example, most proteins do not dissolve appreciably in non-porous synthetic polymers). To allow for permeation, water-filled pores must be present in the membrane material; the physical size of the aqueous pores then determines the size selectivity of the overall membrane. The apparent solubility of the solute in the membrane is determined by the volume fraction of aqueous pores in the material, as well as by the partition coefficient between the pore fluid and the bulk fluid (Φ, defined in Chapter 9). Figure 13.5 provides a rough estimate of the physical size of the biological molecules that are of interest in tissue engineering. A membrane that regulates the transport of any particular solute (insulin, for example) but excludes another solute (antibody class IgG, for example) must have pores that are large enough to permit passage of the smaller molecule (insulin) but not the passage of the larger molecule (IgG).

Porous membranes rarely contain a uniform population of pores. The pores within the material have a distribution of sizes and shapes and, therefore, no membrane is perfect in its ability to transport solutes selectively based on size. Imagine a porous membrane that contains a distribution of pores of different sizes, ranging from 10 to 1000 nm in size: molecules that are smaller than 10 nm ($\sim$ 100 kDa proteins) will pass through any of the pores, whereas molecules that are between 10 and 100 nm $\sim$ 100 kDa protein to 1,000 kbase DNA) will only pass through a fraction of total pores and hence will be transported at a lower flux. When membranes are characterized by their "molecular weight cutoff," it is important to realize that this means the membrane allows for passage of *most* of the molecules smaller than the cutoff (for example, 90% of molecules smaller than the cutoff number) and prohibits passage of *most* of the molecules larger than the cutoff (for example, 95% of the molecules larger than the cutoff value). The percentage of molecules that escape the desired cutoff value depends on properties of the material—such as the narrowness of the size distribution in the physical pores in the membrane—as well as properties of the solute such as the flexibility of the solute and, therefore, its ability to squeeze through pores that are comparable to the solute in size. This characteristic of porous polymer materials is important in tissue engineering; it is difficult to design a membrane that totally excludes the passage of IgG, for example, while still permitting passage of a substantial flux of insulin.

Hydrogel Materials.   Many promising materials for tissue engineering are hydrogels (Figure 13.6). Hydrogel materials are constructed from water-soluble polymers that are crosslinked into three-dimensional networks so that the resulting network is insoluble. Water can penetrate into these materials because the individual polymer chains are water-soluble, but crosslinking prevents their complete dissolution. The internal structure of the hydrogel resembles that of extracellular matrix; crosslinked polymer chains are surrounded

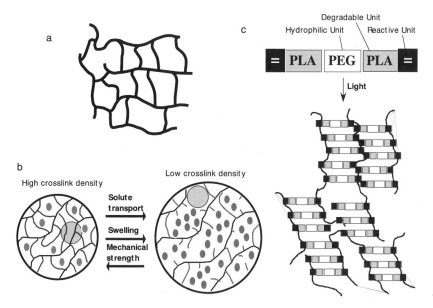

Figure 13.6. Structure and function in hydrogels. (a) Hydrogel materials are crosslinked polymer networks that swell in water. (b) Crosslink density in the network influences the properties of the material. Higher crosslinking densities produce increased mechanical properties. Lower crosslinking densities allow more absorption of water into the network (small grey ovals). Lower crosslink densities—and more swollen hydrogels—permit the transport of large solutes (for example, the large grey circle represents a solute that would diffuse through the less crosslinked network but not through the more highly crosslinked network). (c) Schematic diagram of a biodegradable hydrogel network, synthesized from a water-swellable polymer (PEG) that is crosslinked with degradable linkages. The crosslinking, in this case, is accomplished by light, using photoactive crosslinkers. Diagrams provided by Kristi Anseth.

by a water-rich interstitial fluid. The characteristics of the material can be engineered to suit the application by varying the chemistry (and therefore the water solubility) of individual chains and the degree of crosslinking.

Some of the properties of hydrogels with regard to cellular interactions were discussed in Chapter 12. But hydrogels are also of great interest in tissue engineering because of their solute permeation characteristics. Because they are swollen with water, even large molecules such as proteins can dissolve into the membrane structure. Diffusion of solutes through the material can be manipulated by changing the chemistry and the crosslink density within the gel phase [13, 14].

Lack of mechanical strength is a problem for hydrogels in many tissue engineering applications. Hydrogels have a low compressive modulus, for example, when compared to other polymeric materials and to natural tissues (Table 13.2 compare these values to the properties tabulated for other materials in Table 5.1).

Table 13.2
Some Polymeric Materials Used for Cell Encapsulation

Material	Compressive Modulus (kPa)	Tensile Modulus (MPa)	Reference
Photocrosslinked PLA/PEG hydrogel (wet)	100–1500		[69]
HEMA hydrogel (wet)		0.2–0.3	[70]
Crosslinked hyaluronic acid (wet)		1	[71]
95% porosity PGA, scaffold coated with PLA (wet)	1–20		[72]

Polymer Membranes for Immunoprotection. Immune rejection leads to the rapid destruction of transplants of non-autologous cells; for example, notice the rapid loss of hepatocyte function after transplantation in animals without immunosuppression, illustrated in Figure 2.5. To prevent this undesired response, transplanted cells are often isolated from the host's immune system with semipermeable membranes or semipermeable polymer coatings. In the artificial organs discussed above, the role of the polymeric membrane was to isolate components of the patient's blood from cells within the device (illustrated in Figures 13.3 and 13.4 for pancreatic cells and hepatocytes, respectively). In encapsulated cell applications, the polymer material is used to separate transplanted cells from the rest of the host in a format that still allows for transplantation of the encapsulated cell device (Figure 13.7). In contrast to the artificial organ-type systems described earlier in the chapter, encapsulated cell systems are not usually connected to the circulatory system.

An important recent development in encapsulated cell design, however, involves intentionally selecting membrane materials that recruit a microvascular network, allowing for more ready adsorption of released products into the blood [15, 16]. This is part of an overall effort in the biomaterials community to understand the response of tissues to materials, and to design materials that produce a tissue response that is optimized for the purpose of the material [17, 18].

To provide functional separation of the transplanted cells from the host, it is generally assumed that the polymeric material surrounding the cells must prohibit the entry of components of the immune system while allowing for free exchange of nutrients and oxygen. The molecular weight cutoff of the immunoisolation membrane or filter is less than 50 kDa, which is sufficient to allow for diffusion of low molecular weight secretory factors and to permit exchange of nutrients and wastes, but prevents the permeation of lymphocytes, antibodies, and other immune proteins. The presence of these polymers, however, limits the application of protective membranes to situations that do not require vascularization or innervation of the transplanted cells. Immunoisolation by polymers potentially allows for the long-term implantation of secretory cells without the use of immunosuppressive drugs that would normally be required to prevent rejection of foreign tissue.

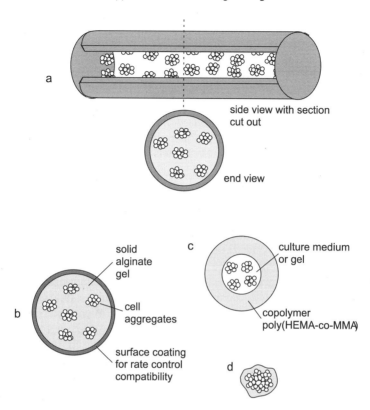

a — side view with section cut out

end view

b — solid alginate gel / cell aggregates / surface coating for rate control compatibility

c — culture medium or gel / copolymer poly(HEMA-co-MMA)

d

Figure 13.7. Methods for encapsulation of living cells: (a) encapsulation of cells within a hollow fiber; (b) suspension in alginate microspheres; (c) entrapment within hollow spheres of synthetic polymers; or (d) formation of a conformal layer of polymer on the cell surface.

Methods for Cell Encapsulation. Alginate has been used extensively as a material for cell encapsulation. Pancreatic cells were first encapsulated in alginate microspheres in 1980 [19]. After encapsulation in alginate droplets, the spheres are coated with poly(L-lysine) (PLL) for stabilization. In general, alginate microspheres are not stable unless coated with PLL, which reduces their biocompatibility. The poor compatibility of PLL surfaces can be reduced by adding an additional thin layer of alginate over the PLL; the additional alginate layer serves to reduce the overgrowth of the surface by fibroblast-like and macrophage-like cells. These three-layered microencapsulated islets can survive in rodents for many months [20].

The procedures for forming the outer layer can be modified to change its chemical properties or to alter the permeability. For example, PEG-graft-poly(L-lysine) polymers improve biocompatibility and can be added to the outer layer by coacervation [21]. The PEG-graft-PLL coacervates with the alginate, but more poorly than PLL alone, presumably because of its larger molecular weight which prevents efficient diffusion to the alginate surface. The

PEG-graft-PLL-coated alginate spheres therefore have good biocompatibility, but also good permeability to moderate-sized proteins such as albumin. To reduce the permeability, pentalayered microcapsules were fabricated as alginate/PLL/alginate/PLL-g-MPEG/alginate, so that the last layer of alginate could seal the areas of permeability defect in the alginate/PLL-g-MPEG spheres.

Synthetic polymers can also be used for microencapsulation of cells. For example, Eudragit RL, a water-insoluble polyacrylate, has been used to microencapsulate red blood cells [22]. Hydrogels of 2-hydroxyethyl methacrylate (HEMA) and methyl methacrylate (MMA) have also been used to encapsulate living cells [23]. These materials have excellent biocompatibility and a long history of use in medical devices; HEMA is used in contact lenses and MMA is the main ingredient in bone cement. To encapsulate cells, the monomers of HEMA and MMA are copolymerized to produce poly(HEMA-*co*-MMA) by solution polymerization. A cell suspension in culture medium is pumped through a coaxial needle with polymer solution (10% w/v in PEG-200). Capsules are formed by shearing at a hexadecane/air interface (30 capsules/min) and captured in a bath containing buffered saline solution. The procedure produces capsules that are several hundred micrometers in diameter.

The synthetic polymer layer can be a substantial barrier to diffusion of nutrients and cell products; this may be a problem, as in the situation for encapsulated islets where the polymer layer creates a lag time in cell performance (recall discussion in Chapter 2). One method for increasing the rate of diffusion, without sacrificing the size-selectivity of the material, is to deposit very thin polymer layers on the surface of cells or cell aggregates (Figure 13.7d). A thin biocompatible layer can be formed by photopolymerization, which depends on the use of a photoactivated macromer [24]. To form the surface layer, the cells are suspended in a solution containing a biocompatible photoactivator (such as eosin Y) and then washed extensively so that all but the surface-adsorbed activator is removed. When the treated cells are exposed to pre-polymer solutions and then exposed to light, a thin layer of polymerized gel forms around the surface of the cells. An alternate method for reducing diffusional limitations is to create microvessels as close as possible to the outer surface of the membrane, or even within the membrane material.

Models of Solute Transport within Encapsulated Systems. The effect of an additional diffusional barrier on the performance of encapsulated cells can be predicted by mathematical models. Consider an encapsulated tissue mass that is implanted into the body and therefore surrounded by tissues of the host (Figure 13.8). Solutes can diffuse within the interior of the encapsulated tissue. In addition, the solute may be generated (for example, a protein secreted by the cells) or consumed (for example, a nutrient required for cell metabolism):

$$D_i^{\text{cell}} \frac{1}{r^2} \frac{\partial}{\partial r} \left[r^2 \frac{\partial C_i^{\text{cell}}}{\partial r} \right] + R_i^{\text{cell}} = 0 \qquad (13\text{-}15)$$

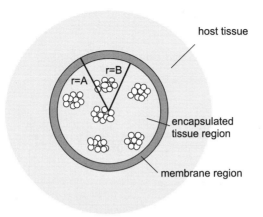

Figure 13.8. Movement of nutrients and secreted proteins in encapsulated tissues. The basic model describes a single implanted device which contains uniformly distributed cells and is surrounded by tissue.

which is valid in the region $0 < r < B$. The solute can also diffuse, but perhaps at a different rate, within the membrane material; however, the solute is not generated or consumed in this region:

$$D_i^{mem} \frac{1}{r^2} \frac{\partial}{\partial r}\left[r^2 \frac{\partial C_i^{mem}}{\partial r} \right] = 0 \qquad (13\text{-}16)$$

which is generally thinner than the cell-rich region $(B < r < A)$. Finally, the solutes diffuse to the surface of the capsule within the interstitial space, which may also contain sources for production or consumption of the solute:

$$D_i^{body} \frac{1}{r^2} \frac{\partial}{\partial r}\left[r^2 \frac{\partial C_i^{body}}{\partial r} \right] + R_i^{body} = 0 \qquad (13\text{-}17)$$

which applies in the region $A < r$. These three differential equations are accompanied by a set of boundary conditions:

$$
\left.
\begin{aligned}
&\partial C_i^{cell} = 0; && r = 0 \\[1em]
&C_i^{mem} = K_{m:c} C_i^{cell}; && -D_i^{mem}\left[\frac{\partial C_i^{mem}}{\partial r} \right] = -D_i^{cell}\left[\frac{\partial C_i^{cell}}{\partial r} \right]; && r = B \\[1em]
&C_i^{body} = K_{b:m} C_i^{mem}; && -D_i^{body}\left[\frac{\partial C_i^{body}}{\partial r} \right] = -D_i^{mem}\left[\frac{\partial C_i^{mem}}{\partial r} \right]; && r = A \\[1em]
&C_i^{body} = C_o; && r \to \infty
\end{aligned}
\right\}
$$

$$(13\text{-}18)$$

The rates of solute production and generation in the cellular region $(r < B)$ and in the body $(r > A)$ will vary, depending on the species of interest. Consider the situation in which the cells inside the device are producing insulin at a constant rate ($R_i^{cell} = S$) and the insulin is not produced or consumed outside of the device ($R_i^{body} = 0$). In this case, Equations 13-5 through 13-18 can be solved to yield

$$C_{insulin} =$$

$$\begin{cases} \dfrac{SB^2}{6D_{insulin}^{cell}} + \dfrac{SB^2}{3D_{insulin}^{body}} + \dfrac{SB^2}{3A}\left(\dfrac{1}{D_{insulin}^{body}} - \dfrac{1}{D_{insulin}^{mem}}\right) - \dfrac{S}{6D_{insulin}^{cell}}r^2; & 0 < r < B \\[2em] \dfrac{SB^3}{3D_{insulin}^{mem}}\dfrac{1}{r} + \dfrac{SB^3}{3A}\left(\dfrac{1}{D_{insulin}^{body}} - \dfrac{1}{D_{insulin}^{mem}}\right); & B < r < A \\[2em] \dfrac{SB^3}{3D_{insulin}^{body}}\dfrac{1}{r}; & A < r \end{cases}$$

$$(13\text{-}19)$$

Figure 13.9 shows the concentration profiles predicted from Equation 13-19.

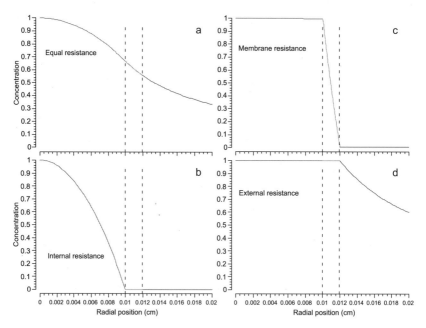

Figure 13.9. Secretion of insulin by encapsulated cells. Equation 13-19 is plotted for a microencapsulated islet tissue with $B = 100\,\mu m$ and $A - B = 20\,\mu m$. Concentration is normalized by the rate of secretion S. The relative rate of diffusion was changed in each panel: (a) D^{cell}, D^{mem}, $D^{body} = 10^{-6}\ cm^2/s$; (b) $D^{cell} = 10^{-9}\ cm^2/s$, D^{mem}, $D^{body} = 10^{-6}\ cm^2/s$; (c) $D^{mem} = 10^{-9}\ cm^2/s$, D^{cell}, $D^{body} = 10^{-6}\ cm^2/s$; and (d) $D^{body} = 10^{-9}\ cm^2/s$, D^{mem}, $D^{cell} = 10^{-6}\ cm^2/s$.

Applications of Encapsulated Cells.   Encapsulated cell systems have been used in a variety of biomedical applications, but mostly in the replacement of islet cell function. A few of these applications are illustrated in this section; many more examples have been reported. A review of the historical development of these encapsulated cell systems, including early clinical testing, is available [25].

To replace islet cell function—Alginate-encapsulated islets can be maintained for many weeks in culture; they retain their responsiveness to glucose, demonstrating a short time lag to insulin secretion following glucose stimulation. The microencapsulated islets are typically several hundred micrometers in diameter. In the first animal studies, the microencapsulated cells maintained normoglycemia in rats for ~ 3 weeks, compared to maintenance for ~ 1 week for unencapsulated cells [19].

Islets have also been encapsulated in poly(acrylonitrile-*co*-vinyl chloride) hollow fibers [26]. In initial studies, when fibers (600 μm inner diameter, 730 μm outer diameter) were filled with 100 rat islets and implanted intraperitoneally in mice, normoglycemia was maintained for only 7 days, presumably because the islets aggregated within the center of the hollow fiber. Later studies employed 2 cm long fibers containing 500 or 1,000 islets that were suspended in alginate within the acrylic hollow fibers and implanted subcutaneously or intraperitoneally in mice. Normoglycemia was maintained in the majority of mice for > 60 days following a single implant. The structure of the outer wall of the hollow fiber was important in maintaining normoglycemia for subcutaneously implanted fibers, but not for intraperitoneally implanted fibers, indicating that the site of implantation—as well as the properties of the material—is an important variable in the effectiveness of the device.

To provide controlled release of bioactive molecules—Encapsulated cell systems have also been used in the nervous system. In this case, the goal was generally to provide for controlled release of a molecule that is secreted by the encapsulated cells. For example, PC12 cells have been used to provide a controlled release of dopamine; dopamine release was detectable for 6 months [27]. Encapsulated cell systems have been used to deliver ciliary neurotrophic factor to the spinal cord [28] and the retina [29].

Encapsulated cell systems that provide controlled release may be useful in cancer treatment. For example, encapsulated cell systems can release molecules that treat cancer pain [30]. In another example, encapsulated cells that produced an angiogenesis inhibitor, endostatin, were effective in the treatment of animals with intracranial and extracranial tumors [31, 32].

13.2.2 Materials as Scaffolds (Structural Support Properties of the Material)

Most mammalian cells require a solid surface for attachment in order to proliferate and maintain their differentiated state (see Chapter 4). Cells attach with varying affinity to synthetic and natural polymer surfaces, as described in Chapter 12. One of the most important roles for a synthetic material in tissue engineering is to serve as a substrate for the attachment, migration, growth, and function of cells. Our ability to engineer tissues will depend on our ability to manufacture materials (based on synthetic, natural, or hybrid components) which will interact with cells in predictable ways. Cell interactions with polymers were reviewed in Chapter 12; this section presents some approaches for exploiting these interactions in tissue engineering.

Selective Cell Adhesion—Tissue-Engineered Blood Vessels.   Some aspects of tissue engineering involve the preferential attachment and growth of specific cell populations. For example, vascular grafts frequently fail because they are not biocompatible; that is, they cause unwanted reactions such as thrombosis (clot formation within the vessel) after prolonged contact with flowing blood (see [33] for a review of historical development and references). Natural blood vessels have a living cell layer—the endothelium—that provides a compatible interface between the flowing blood and the stationary vessel matrix. Therefore, it is reasonable to speculate that synthetic vessels could be made more compatible by attaching a uniform layer of endothelial cells on the surface.

In the early 1950s a number of materials for replacement vessels were tested. Many materials (nylon, orlon, polyethylene, polyurethane) had insufficient stability for long-term use; PTFE and Dacron (PET) emerged as the most acceptable. Dacron and expanded PTFE, produced by a special stretching process at high temperature, are now preferred and widely used as a synthetic vessel replacement material. But synthetic grafts of these materials are only useful for the replacement of large vessels; even the best totally synthetic grafts have a failure rate of $\sim 50\%$ for vessels that are 6–10 mm in diameter, and they are not used in vessels 3–5 mm in diameter. The problem with synthetic grafts is the reactivity of components of flowing blood to the surface of the vessel; eventually, platelets and proteins will adhere to even the most inert synthetic materials, initiating a biological process that leads to blockage of the vessel lumen and failure of the graft. This problem is most severe for smaller vessels.

Natural vessels remain patent because the surface of the vessel—a confluent layer of endothelial cells—is non-reactive. Perhaps, then, the synthetic grafts can be made to be more biocompatible by growing a surface layer of endothelial cells on the internal surface of the vessel. It is now known that synthetic materials can be made to promote the adhesion and growth of specific types of cells, sometimes by modifying the surface chemistry (see Section 12.2.1). For example, by covalent coupling of cell adhesion peptides to polymer surfaces, the surface can be made to selectively attach only endothelial cells, not smooth muscle cells or platelets or fibroblasts [34–37]. But, to function as a biocompatible lining, the interior of the vessel must be covered with a confluent layer of endothelial cells.

The goal of this tissue engineering problem is to provide a replacement blood vessel that has a biocompatible endothelial cell layer on the lumenal surface. One can imagine several different approaches to solving this problem; other tissue engineering situations present a similar range of choices [38]. Functional tissue could be achieved by: (1) *in situ* regeneration, in which the synthetic material is implanted in the body with the intention of recruiting endothelial cells from the adjacent host tissue; or (2) *in vitro* tissue formation, in which the material is seeded with cells outside of the body and then implanted at some later point; or (3) *in vitro* tissue production, which is the same as (2), except that the tissue is allowed to develop to maturity before implantation.

Each approach presents slightly different problems. In all cases, attachment, migration, and growth on the adhesive material is important. But, in each different case, what are the possible patterns of cell growth and migration that lead to a full monolayer of cell coverage? What are the optimal patterns of growth and migration? What is the source of the cells that are used to line the synthetic vessel? With cell source in mind, perhaps the best approach would involve *in situ* tissue regeneration, which should result in a vessel that is composed of cells from the host. But tissue development will take time after transplantation, which may not be acceptable. Alternately, the graft could be preloaded with cells from another donor, but an immune reaction to the transplanted cells may develop. For *in vitro* tissue development, questions beyond cell source quickly emerge. Is *in vitro* production even possible? That is, can all of the correct biological factors be identified and provided to the vessel *in vitro*? The answer to this question appears to be yes (see [39, 40]), but the best strategy for achieving a tissue-engineered blood vessel—of several promising strategies that have been reported—is not yet known; several different strategies look promising. Exercise 13-9 encourages you to think quantitatively about some of these issues.

Three-Dimensional Structures Formed from Cells and Particles. A three-dimensional structure can be created by attaching cells to the surface of particulates, as in the use of microcarriers for liver cell transplantation [41]. In this case, hepatocytes are allowed to attach to the surface of microcarrier beads and then transplanted, by localized injection, into rats. In one realization of this approach, the hepatocytes remained viable after transplantation and were able to conjugate bilirubin and secrete albumin for many days (Figure 2.5).

The goal of cell transplantation is this situation will depend on the clinical application, and the properties of the particles can be selected to match the goals. In some applications, it may be sufficient for the particles to be stable (that is, they do not degrade or change with time after implantation) and for the properties of the cells to remain static (that is, they continue to function for a prolonged period, preferably without substantial changes in function during the period). In these situations, it might be possible to model the function of these implanted tissues using the same approach that was developed in Equations 13-15 through 13-18. Some parts of the mathematical description would have to be changed: there is no immunoisolation barrier and it may not be appropriate to assume that the cell/particle mass is homogeneous with respect to transport and functional properties.

In other clinical applications, it might be desirable for the transplanted cell/particle system to evolve and transform after implantation. The cell/particle system that is formed outside of the body is sometimes called a "neotissue."

The neotissue can be assembled *in vitro* to mimic some of the functions of the *in vivo* environment that are known to be important for development of differentiated cells or tissue structures (Figure 13.10). After this neotissue is transplanted, the intent is for it to change and develop into a new, stable, functional tissue in the host. One can then imagine that the properties of the particles should change after transplantation: perhaps they disappear slowly because they are formed from a degradable material. One can also imagine that the cellular components evolve: perhaps the cells proliferate to form a larger cell mass, or rearrange to form more complicated tissue structures, or differentiate from a proliferative to a functional phenotype, or intermingle with cells from the host.

What is the optimal size and composition for particles that are used as supports for transplanted cells or neotissues? The answer to this question is not known and probably depends on the specifics of the transplanted cells and the clinical application. But it is possible to imagine this same approach using particles that are much smaller than individual cells (see [42]), or even using soluble molecules instead of cells (see [43]).

Porous Scaffolds for Attachment and Transplantation of Cells. Methods for producing three-dimensional matrices or fiber meshes from biocompatible polymers are discussed in Chapter 12. These meshes may be useful for a variety of cell delivery or tissue regeneration applications, as discussed in this section. The earliest example of this approach used degradable polymeric materials that were intended to serve as physical scaffolds for cell growth after implantation [44]. Since that time, a wide variety of materials and methods have been developed in an effort to translate this basic concept into clinical applications.

The addition of bioactive molecules can influence the development of tissue structure around the scaffold material. For example, when fiber meshes of expanded PTFE were coated with collagen type I or IV and allowed to equilibrate with heparin binding growth factor 1 (HBGF-1) [45] and then implanted into the peritoneal cavity of rats, a freshly vascularized tissue— called "organoid neovascular structures" by the authors—was formed around the mesh. The vessels of this organoid appeared to be continuous with the preexisting vasculature of the rat. When hepatocytes were transplanted into this newly vascularized space, the cells were able to maintain bilirubin conjugation for several months. More recent applications of this approach use synthetic degradable materials (such as PLA and PLGA); biological function on the surface of the material is often added by chemical coupling of peptide sequences, as described in Section 12.2.1.

Some other published examples illustrate some of the potential power of this approach. Figure 12.5 illustrated the growth of cartilage cells on PLA and PLGA polymer scaffolds; the characteristics of the scaffold influence the rate of cell growth in the material. A second example is shown in Figure 13.11. Alginate hydrogels have been used for cell encapsulation (see above) and more recently as scaffolds for tissue engineering. The suitability of alginate as a tissue engineering scaffold can be enhanced substantially by tailoring its

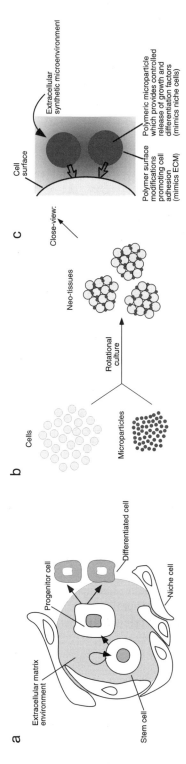

Figure 13.10. Formation of neotissues. (a) Stem cell niche (adapted from [67]). (b) Assembly of cells and controlled-release polymeric microparticles together to create transplantable neotissues. (c) Neotissues contain programmable, synthetic extracellular microenvironments which mimic aspects of the *in vivo* stem cell environment. Reprinted from [42].

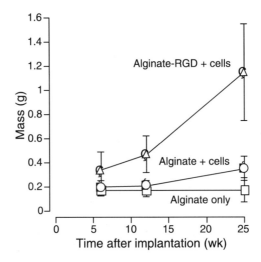

Figure 13.11. Growth of cartilage cells in an alginate matrix (data obtained from [46]). Bovine articular cartilage cells were embedded in an alginate matrix and implanted into mice. The rate of cell growth was influenced by the chemistry of the alginate matrix. When cell adhesive RGD peptides were coupled to the alginate, the greatest increase in cell mass (and size of the resulting implant) was observed.

adhesion properties—by adding covalently bound cell adhesive peptides, for example [46].

For further information on the state of the art in polymer scaffold design and engineering, a review article is recommended [47].

13.3 Control of the Biological Component

In most cases, tissue engineering will require a source of cells for transplantation.* The source of the cells may be from the patient (autograft), from another person (allograft), or from another species (xenograft). The cell source is frequently limited and the number of cells needed to treat a single patient is usually substantial. In some cases, the growth of cells is the most important barrier to therapy; with hematopoietic stem cells, which can be introduced into the blood for repopulation of peripheral tissues, isolation and amplification of the stem cells is the biggest engineering challenge.

---

*Some strategies of tissue engineering do not involve new cells, but instead attempt to reorganize or redirect the growth of cells within a patient. For example, nerve guides to facilitate the repair of damaged nerve (Figure 2.4) do not necessarily require transplantation of new cells, although the presence of cells may enhance the therapy (as we will see in the next chapter). More generally, materials for repair of a tissue defect may operate without cells in situations where the material enhances the ingrowth of host cells (Figure 2.3).

How do we obtain sufficient numbers of cells for a tissue engineering treatment? Cells are a characteristic part of many tissue engineering products, and the success of tissue engineering depends on our ability to harvest cells, to select for desired properties or engineer new ones, and to grow cells outside of the body. This section considers two different examples of *in vitro* cell growth in tissue engineering. One example involves amplification of specific cells within a harvested tissue population, such as the production of hematopoietic stem cells. The other example illustrates the special challenges involved with the development of bioreactors for the growth of cells on tissue engineering constructs.

Some of the methods for analyzing cell growth in culture were introduced in Chapter 4. Here, we extend that discussion to consider the development of bioreactors for tissue engineering by first considering the basic elements of bioreactor design.

13.3.1 Models for Ideal Bioreactors

Engineers use two different ideal reactor models. The ideal stirred tank model assumes that molecules entering a compartment are instantaneously and uniformly distributed throughout the compartment (Figure 13.12a). Reactor per-

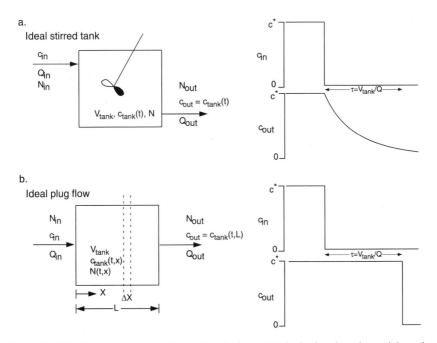

Figure 13.12. Ideal models for bioreactor design. (a) Ideal stirred-tank model, and response of the stirred tank to a step change in concentration of an inert tracer at the inlet. (b) Ideal plug flow model and its response to a step change in concentration of tracer at the inlet.

formance is often characterized by considering the behavior of a non-reactive dye that is introduced into the reactor under controlled conditions. Assume that an ideal stirred tank is operating with an inlet stream containing a dye molecule that does not react within the tank; if the tank has been operating for a long enough time, the concentration of the dye within the tank, the concentration of dye in the outlet stream, and the concentration in the inlet stream are all equal (c^*). If the inlet stream is suddenly changed, so that it now contains no dye molecules ($c_{in} = 0$), the concentration of dye in the tank and in the outlet stream will slowly decrease. Our basic assumption regarding the ideal stirred tank leads to several predictions: (1) the dye concentration throughout the tank is always uniform but changes with time, $c_{tank}(t)$; (2) the outlet concentration is equal to the concentration in the tank ($c_{tank} = c_{out}$); and (3) the tank/outlet concentration changes in a predictable way in response to the step-change in inlet concentration:

$$c_{out} = c^* e^{-t/\tau} \tag{13-20}$$

where t is the time after initiation of the step-change in inlet concentration and τ is a characteristic time for the compartment ($= V_{tank}/Q$). For this example, the characteristic time is equal to the time required for the outlet concentration to decrease from c^* to $0.37\, c^*$.

The second model is ideal plug flow (Figure 13.12b), in which molecules moving through the region do not mix, but rather travel in an orderly fashion from inlet to outlet. The simplest physical model of ideal plug flow is slow fluid flow through a long tube: each "packet" of fluid enters the tube just after some other packet, and remains behind its neighbor from inlet to outlet. Each packet emerges from the tube in the order that it entered. The time required for a packet to move from inlet to outlet is $\tau(= V_{tank}/Q)$; a step change in inlet concentration produces a step change in outlet concentration that is offset by τ (Figure 13.12b).

These two ideal models display different behaviors in response to a step change in inlet concentration of a tracer. In principle, then, one can determine whether a bioreactor of unknown performance is more like a stirred or plug flow model by examining the response of that box to a step change in the inlet concentration of an inert tracer molecule.

13.3.2 Cell Growth and Differentiation in Culture

How do these ideal reaction vessels function when used as bioreactors for the growth of cells? Consider the stirred tank reactor (Figure 13.12a); in this case, N indicates cell number per volume, c indicates concentration of some substrate or nutrient, and Q represents the flowrate of total fluid. A mass balance on cell number can be obtained (IN $-$ OUT $+$ GEN $=$ ACC):

$$Q_{in} N_{in} - Q_{out} N_{out} + V r_N = \frac{d(VN)}{dt} \tag{13-21}$$

where r_N is the rate of production of cells within the reactor. The rate of cell production can be found from the Monod model (Equation 4-30):

$$r_N = \frac{k_{p,\max} c}{K_M + c} N \qquad (13\text{-}22)$$

Using a similar mass balance approach on the substrate molecules yields

$$Q_{in} c_{in} - Q_{out} c_{out} + V r_c = \frac{d(Vc)}{dt} \qquad (13\text{-}23)$$

in which the consumption rate of the substrate molecules, r_c, is given by

$$r_c = -\frac{1}{Y_{N/c}} r_N = -\frac{1}{Y_{N/c}} \left(\frac{k_{p,\max} c N}{K_m + c} \right) \qquad (13\text{-}24)$$

where $Y_{N/c}$ is the yield coefficient for the production of cells on the substrate of interest:

$$Y_{N/c} = \frac{N - N_0}{c_0 - c} \qquad (13\text{-}25)$$

which provides a relationship between the amount of substrate consumed and the number of cells produced. Equations 13-21 to 13-24 can be used to calculate the expected change in cell number as a function of time when the inlet conditions and the parameters ($k_{p,\max}$, K_m, $Y_{N/c}$) are known.

Batch Bioreactor. Consider first the simplest case of a batch reactor, in which a certain number of cells and a certain concentration of substrate are introduced into the reactor at time $t = 0$, when the substrate concentration and cell concentration are c_0 and N_0, but there is no inlet or outlet flow at any time during growth of the cells. In this situation, the cell mass balance equation (Equation 13-21) can be solved (using the definitions of the cell production rate, Equation 13-22, and the yield coefficient, Equation 13-25) to give

$$k_{p,\max} t = \left(\frac{Y_{N/c} K_m}{N_0 + Y_{N/c} c_0} + 1 \right) \ln \left(\frac{N}{N_0} \right) + \left(\frac{Y_{N/c} K_m}{N_0 + Y_{N/c} c_0} \right) \ln \left(\frac{c_0}{c} \right) \qquad (13\text{-}26)$$

In most cases K_m will be small, so that Equation 13-26 can be written in a reduced, approximate form:

$$k_{p,\max} t = \ln \left(\frac{N}{N_0} \right) \qquad (13\text{-}27)$$

Note that this expression is equivalent to Equation 4-28 for proliferation of cells in a uniform environment with no restraints on growth (that is, no limitation of substrate).

Continuous Well-Stirred Bioreactor. The simplest reactor that provides for continuous operation (and therefore continuous production of cells) is the well-stirred reactor shown in Figure 13.12a. If the reactor is operated at steady-state and the contents of the reactor are well mixed, the cell balance equation reduces to

$$QN_{in} - QN_{out} + Vr_N = 0 \qquad (13\text{-}28)$$

where the rates of flow for the inlet and outlet streams are equal (Q), the contents of the vessel are constant with time (accumulation $= 0$), the concentration of cells in the outlet stream is equal to the concentration in the reactor ($N_{out} = N$), and the rate of cell production is constant (r_N). If the inlet stream contains no cells ($N_{in} = 0$), then Equation 13-21 implies that the rate of cell removal from the reactor is equal to the rate of cell production in the reactor:

$$QN = Vr_N \qquad (13\text{-}29)$$

The dilution rate D for the reactor is defined as the ratio of the rate of flow through the system to the volume of the reactor ($D = Q/V$), and the Monod equation is used for the rate of cell production:

$$DN = \frac{k_{p,max}c}{K_M + c}N \qquad (13\text{-}30)$$

Since the substrate concentration is constant within the reactor, an effective cell production rate constant μ can be defined:

$$DN = \mu N \qquad (13\text{-}31)$$

which suggests that the overall growth rate for cells in the reactor, μ, and the dilution rate, D, must be equal for steady-state operation of the bioreactor ($\mu = D$). An operator can adjust the rate of growth by increasing the dilution rate (that is, by increasing the inlet flow rate Q for a reactor of fixed volume V). If the dilution rate is increased above the maximum growth rate of the cells ($k_{p,max}$), however, cell growth will not keep pace with cell removal via the outlet stream and the cells will be washed out of the bioreactor (that is, $N = 0$). Notice that this state satisfies Equation 13-31, but this is not a satisfactory solution since the goal of the bioreactor was to produce cells (that is, have $N > 0$).

Plug Flow Bioreactor.   In the plug flow reactor, continuous cell production can also be achieved with steady-state operation. But in this situation the concentration of cells is a function of location in the reactor. This situation is most readily analyzed by considering a cell or substrate balance within a small cross-section of the reactor (Figure 13.12b):

$$QN|_x - QN|_{x+\Delta x} + A\Delta x r_N = 0 \qquad (13\text{-}32)$$

where A is the cross-sectional area of the bioreactor. Rearrangement of this equation yields, in the limit as Δx goes to zero,

$$\frac{Q}{A}\frac{dN}{dx} = r_N \qquad (13\text{-}33)$$

If it is noticed that the velocity of flow through the reactor (Q/A) is equal to the first derivative of the spatial variable x with time,

$$\frac{\mathrm{d}x}{\mathrm{d}t} = \text{velocity} = \frac{Q}{A} \tag{13-34}$$

then the design equation for the plug flow reactor (Equation 13-33) can be written in a form that is equivalent to the expression for a simple batch reactor:

$$\frac{\mathrm{d}N}{\mathrm{d}t} = r_N \tag{13-35}$$

13.3.3 Bioreactors for Tissue Engineering Products

Hematopoietic Cell Bioreactors. Bioreactors that are similar to the ideal reactors described above have been used for tissue engineering applications. For example, the cultivation of hematopoietic cells has been studied actively for many decades and, most recently, the focus of this effort has been on the growth of stem cells and progenitor cells from hematopoietic populations [48]. Several variables are known to be important for control of both the rate of growth and the state of cell differentiation; some of these variables are common for mammalian cell bioreactors (oxygen concentration, pH, substrate and waste concentrations) and others are specific to these particular cell cultures (cytokines and growth factors, recall Figure 4.5). Design of a bioreactor attempts to account for all of these variables.

For hematopoietic cell culture, three basic approaches are used. Batch culture can be accomplished in tissue culture flasks or other vessels, but usually gas-permeable culture bags are used for culture on a scale that is useful clinically. There are many advantages to this approach, but the technique does not permit control of the culture conditions during the growth period and it is not easy to add feed mixtures (such as cytokines) during the culture process. Therefore, conditions within batch or static bioreactors are constantly changing with time. Stirred reactors are also used, usually by modification of the kinds of stirred vessels or spinner flasks that have been developed for mammalian cell culture (see [49] for a review). Immobilized cell bioreactors are also employed, in an attempt to mimic the three-dimensional structure normally present in bone marrow spaces. In this case, cells are often grown after attachment to porous polymer microcarriers (described in Chapter 12), although detachment of cells for harvesting at the end of the reaction is often difficult. Hollow fiber reactors—which could potentially be used to create plug flow reactors for control of conditions inside the reaction vessel—have been attempted with hematopoietic cells, but with limited success due to difficulty in harvesting them. A variation on this approach, using grooved culture surfaces which retain cells as a nutrient-rich medium is continuously perfused over the surface, is now commonly used for stem cell expansion in clinical practice [50].

In all of these culture systems described above, cytokines are added to the culture medium in order to create a suitable culture environment. In the bone marrow, stem cells are surrounded by stromal cells that release cytokines and create a microenvironment that is specialized for cell growth and differentiation (Figure 4.8). It might be possible to mimic some of these conditions by co-culture of hematopoietic cells with stromal cells, although development of systems that are safe and efficient on a clinical scale is a challenge for the future [48]. New concepts in culture dynamics may be useful for designing hematopoietic cell expansion bioprocesses, by also accounting for the responses of mature and maturing cells within the population in order to produce optimized transplants that contain not only amplified stem cell populations but also cells that support and enhance engraftment [51]. An important emerging concept suggests that the maintenance of self-renewal in stem cell populations requires that ligand–receptor (that is, cytokine–cytokine receptor) complexes be maintained above a critical threshold level [52].

Other Tissue Engineering Bioreactors.   Many tissue engineering systems benefit from the design of bioreactors that offer control of cell growth and differentiation, as described above, but that also provide environmental conditions that influence the development of tissue structure. For example, bioreactors for cartilage tissue engineering replicate the mechanical forces that maintain cell phenotype (such as high hydrostatic pressure) [53]. Similar bioreactors and bioprocesses have been developed for tissue engineering of heart valves [54] and vessels [39, 40].

A common problem in most bioreactors is the presence of high mixing forces, which can disrupt the formation of the cell–cell interactions that lead to tissue development. For that reason, bioreactors that provide mixing under low shear conditions may be particularly well suited to tissue engineering. One such reactor was developed by scientists at NASA, and involves a bioreactor vessel that rotates slowly on its central axis [55–57]. Dynamic imaging studies of microcarriers and cells within this bioreactor demonstrate that properties of the microcarrier (such as size and density) and the operation of the reactor can be manipulated to promote tissue formation [58]. These bioreactors can also be modified to accommodate porous polymer scaffolds and can facilitate some manipulations that are difficult to accomplish under conventional culture conditions, such as seeding of a millimeter-scale porous polymer with cells [59], assembly of large cell aggregates [60], or assembly of microcarriers and cells [61]. When cartilage cells were cultivated on polymeric scaffolds in this bioreactor, both the properties of the reactor and the properties of the scaffold were significant variables in the final composition and mechanical properties of the engineered cartilage [62]; cell/scaffold systems that developed in the rotating wall bioreactor had properties that were closer to those of native cartilage.

13.3.4 Control of Vascularization within Tissue-Engineered Materials

The microcirculation of tissues in the bodies plays a critical role in the supply of nutrients and removal of waste products. As we have seen at several different points in the previous chapters, the development of vascularization within tissue-engineered products remains one of the most difficult and central problems. There has been some progress in the development of model systems for obtaining vasculature in constructs (see Table 11.1, for example), but lack of vascularization remains one of the most troubling problems in current clinical products such as tissue-engineered skin (as we will see in Chapter 14). It is interesting that tissue-engineering of cartilage has advanced more rapidly than tissue engineering of many other tissues; cartilage is avascular, making it easier to approach as a tissue engineering product.

Much is known about the process of vessel and vessel network development in embryos and during tissue remodeling; imaging methods and computer modeling are being used to expand and assimilate this information and apply it in tissue engineering contexts [63]. A review paper that outlines the current state of the art and presents some of the practical problems with control of vascularization in tissue engineering is also recommended for further reading [64].

13.4 Replacement of Tissue Structure or Function

How do we evaluate the success of a tissue engineering approach in replacement of function or structure? There is no simple answer to this question, but there are approaches to the answer that can be outlined. The success of the approach must be evaluated by different methods depending on whether one is replacing a metabolic function or a structural function of the tissue (see Figure 2.1 and related discussion). First, the replacement of metabolic function in an organism is considered. In the following sections, the replacement of structural function is outlined.

13.4.1 Metabolic Function of Tissue-Engineered Constructs

Pharmacokinetic studies in drug development usually involve the development of compartmental analogs of physiological systems and mathematics to describe the accumulation, movement, and elimination of molecules within the body. The goal of pharmacokinetic modeling is to describe the fate of the drug molecules in the body, so that one can determine the duration of effectiveness, optimal dose, and potential for toxicity. Development of pharmacokinetic models has impacted drug development, discovery, and approval for use at many levels (see Chapter 7 of [65] for an introduction). Although the objective of tissue engineering may involve more than the delivery and migration of a single molecular agent, pharmacokinetic models can still be tremendously important in evaluating the success of tissue engineering approaches.

Consider a simple model of a patient receiving dialysis (Figure 13.13). In this model, the patient is represented by a single compartment, which contains a solute that is normally eliminated by the kidneys. In the absence of normal kidney function, the concentration of the solute in the body, C_B, is elevated. The goal of dialysis is to remove solute and reduce the concentration in the

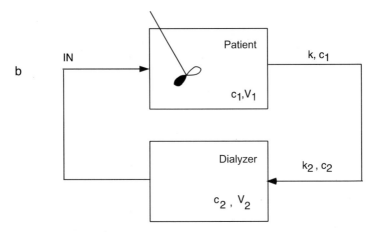

Figure 13.13. A simple model for the effectiveness of dialysis at removal of a single solute, which assumes that the solute distribution in the body can be approximated with one compartment.

blood. Therefore, the effectiveness of an artificial kidney can be quantified by examining its impact on the circulating blood concentration of the solute.

During the dialysis procedure, blood is removed from the patient, circulated through the dialysis unit, and returned to the patient (Figure 13.13). An overall mass balance can be used to calculate the change in solute concentration in the blood:

$$V_B \frac{dC_B}{dt} = N_T \tag{13-36}$$

where V_B is the volume of distribution of the solute in the patient and N_T is the total rate of solute removal due to the dialysis operation. (Some solutes will distribute throughout the blood volume of the patient ($\sim 5\,L$); other solutes may have a more extensive or limited distribution, due to the physical and biological properties of the solute.) The rate of solute removal depends on the blood concentration, as described in Equation 13-2, which can be substituted into Equation 13-36:

$$V_B \frac{dC_B}{dt} = Q_B(C_{B_o} - C_{B_i}) \tag{13-37}$$

The inlet and outlet concentrations in the blood are related by the performance equation for the dialyzer (see Section 13.1.1) If we assume counter-current operation and a dialysate stream that is initially free of solute, the expressions for extraction ratio (Equations 13-12 and 13-13) can be combined to yield

$$\frac{C_{B_i} - C_{B_o}}{C_{B_i}} = \frac{1 - e^{\gamma(1-z)}}{z - e^{\gamma(1-z)}} \tag{13-38}$$

which can be approximated by

$$\frac{C_{B_i} - C_{B_o}}{C_{B_i}} = 1 - e^{-\gamma} \tag{13-39}$$

when the blood flowrate is significantly slower than the dialysate flowrate ($\gamma \simeq 0$). This simplification leads to an expression for the outlet blood concentration as a function of the inlet blood concentration:

$$C_{B_o} = C_{B_i} e^{-KA/Q_B} \tag{13-40}$$

which can be substituted into the mass balance, Equation 13-6, to yield a first-order differential equation:

$$\frac{dC_{B_i}}{dt} = \frac{Q_B}{V_B} C_{B_i} \left(d^{-KA/Q_B} - 1 \right) \tag{13-41}$$

In this final differential equation, the concentration of solute in the blood at the inlet to the dialyzer is assumed to be equal to the uniform concentration in the body ($C_B = C_{B_i}$). If the initial concentration at the start of dialysis ($t = 0$) is C_{init}, then the solute concentration in the body should decrease during dialysis according to

$$C_{B_i} = C_{init} \exp\left[\frac{Q_B}{V_B} \left(e^{-KA/Q_B} - 1 \right) t \right] \tag{13-42}$$

which is illustrated in Figure 13.14.

When a patient receives dialysis, it can be quantified in terms of a "dose." The usual means for quantifying the dose that a patient receives is based on the clearance, defined in Equation 13-11:

$$\text{Dose} = \frac{C^* T}{V_B} \tag{13-43}$$

where V_B is the volume of the patient's total body water and T is the time of the dialysis treatment. The clearance, C^*, is determined by the properties of the dialysis operation (that is, the value of the clearance could be determined for any one of the curves shown in Figure 13.14). The total body water is estimated for the particular patient. For a particular patient on a specific dialysis machine, therefore, the dose of dialysis is a function of the time of treatment, as indicated in Equation 13-43.

While the formula for calculating dose is simple, there are many potential problems in determining each of the values in a clinical setting [66]. But this approach, in which the effectiveness of therapy is linked quantitatively to the change in a metabolic parameter (change in concentration of some key solute, such as urea, indicated by C in Figure 13.14), can be extended to other artificial organs (such as extracorporeal liver support systems) and tissue engineering organ replacements (such as encapsulated cells).

The problem of quantification of function becomes more difficult as the complexity of the metabolic organ's function increases. For example, the liver performs thousands of metabolic functions simultaneously (see Table 2.2); any of these could potentially used as the basis for quantifying the "effectiveness"

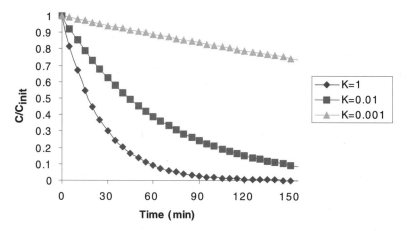

Figure 13.14. Effectiveness of dialysis for the one-compartment model. Equation 13-42 is plotted for typical dialysis parameters: $Q_B = 200 \, \text{mL/min}$, $A = 1 \, \text{m}^2$, $V_B = 5 \, \text{L}$, and $0.001 < K < 1$.

of a tissue-engineered liver. But a particular tissue engineering device may be much more effective at replacing one function (for example, albumin secretion) than it is at replacing another function (for example, metabolism of acetaminophen). For a complex organ, therefore, an analysis that shows quantitative measures of performance for an ensemble of important functions is preferred; this might require assigning priorities to metabolic functions for tissues with multiple functions.

As tissue engineering products, such as encapsulated cells and cell-loaded polymer scaffolds, enter the clinical setting, tissue engineers will increasingly face this challenge: quantification of the effectiveness of their tissue engineering approach. In the case of metabolic tissues we can rely on the strong foundation provided by pharmacokinetic analysis, but there is still much to be done in translating these methods for appropriate use in tissue engineering.

13.4.2 Mechanical Function of Tissue-Engineered Constructs

It might appear, at first glance, that the evaluation of success for an engineered tissue with largely structural function—such as bone or cartilage—would be more straightforward than the pharmacokinetic analysis that was just described for metabolic function. A tissue-engineered bone or cartilage should be similar, from a mechanical standpoint, to the bone or cartilage it is intended to replace [68].

In some situations, the relationship between structure and mechanical function may be straightforward (but not exactly simple). For example, the primary mechanical function of articular cartilage is to withstand a compressive load; therefore, the compressive modulus of tissue-engineered cartilage should be an important indicator of its effectiveness. The compressive modulus of native articular cartilage is over 1 MPa (1,000 kPa, Table 5.1).The materials that are most often used as scaffolds for tissue-engineered cartilage are PLA/ PGA scaffolds (which have a modulus of 1 to 20 kPa without cells) or hydrogels (which have a modulus of 1 to 1,500 kPa without cells) (see Table 13.2). If a high-modulus hydrogel (that is, one that is highly crosslinked) is used as the scaffold, then appropriate mechanical function will be available immediately. But if any of the other materials are used, the cells must grow and secrete ECM components that provide the additional mechanical properties in order for the tissue-engineered material to function in its normal role. For polymer scaffolds (composed of PGA or benzylated hyaluronan), which have been seeded with chondrocytes, the compressive modulus obtained after 1 month of cultivation in a bioreactor is 100 to 500 kPa, still lower than the modulus of native cartilage.

How would this technology be applied in a clinical setting? What would a patient experience? The answer to that question depends on choices made during the design of the tissue engineering product. For example, a mismatch in the mechanical properties between the seeded transplant and native tissue will influence the application of this technology. If an implant with mechanical properties that are inferior to native tissue is used, then function of that tissue will be compromised in the patient. Implanted cartilage tissue with a low compressive modulus may not withstand the forces encountered in normal activity, so the patient will not regain full function until additional tissue regeneration occurs *in situ*. How long will this regeneration take? The speed of tissue regeneration and functional recovery will depend on the design of the material (composition of polymer, growth rate of cells, functional activity of the cells, etc.) and on the properties of the implant site. Some of these issues are explored—in cartilage and in other tissue engineering applications—in Chapter 14.

Summary

- Tissue engineering is difficult to define, but involves several definable elements: replacement of tissue structure and function; introduction of biological products that facilitate regeneration; use of a synthetic component that organizes the regeneration process; and extension of concepts that have long been used in the design of artificial organs.
- Many design elements of modern renal dialysis—which is now well developed and accepted as medical therapy—can be used in tissue engineering design.
- Synthetic materials are used in tissue engineering for isolation of tissue compartments, support of mechanical structure, controlled release, and controlled presentation of surface molecules.
- Immunoisolation techniques allow the transplantation of foreign cells into an immunocompetent host, but the material properties that are necessary for long-term immunoisolation are difficult to achieve.

- A variety of biological and mechanical signals can be incorporated into scaffolds for tissue engineering; the current challenge is to translate these advances in scaffold design into functional tissues, which will require a more detailed understanding of the interactions between cells and engineered materials.
- Bioreactor design has been critical in the development of modern tissue engineering practice and is likely to become more important as tissue engineering constructs enter more widespread clinical use.
- The function of tissue-engineered products can be evaluated in terms of metabolic and/or mechanical parameters, but there remain major challenges in determining which, of the many possible parameters that could be measured, will be the most important in gauging the success of any particular tissue replacement.

Exercises

Exercise 13.1

Urea is being filtered from blood using a shell-in-tube exchanger operating in counter-current mode. The mass transfer coefficient for the exchanger is $K = 0.1\,\text{cm/min}$.

a) Assuming flow rates of blood ($Q_B = 200\,\text{mL/min}$) and dialysate ($Q_D = 500\,\text{mL/min}$), calculate the surface area required to achieve a single-pass clearance of 90%.

b) Is this design feasible? What is the necessary "priming" volume for blood in the device?

Exercise 13.2

Consider the bioartificial pancreas that was used to collect the insulin flux data shown in Figure 13.3 (also Figure 2 of Pillarella and Zydney [7]).

a) What is the total amount of insulin that is produced in both hollow fiber devices (shown in panels (a) and (b))? For this answer, you will need to estimate the intrinsic flux from the islets. Justify your estimate.

b) How does this compare with the daily insulin demands of a diabetic?

c) What are the key factors necessary to improve performance?

Exercise 13.3

Consider the model for secretion of insulin by encapsulated islets (Figure 13.9).

a) Solve the set of differential equations, 13–15 through 13–17, with the appropriate boundary conditions, Equation 13–18, and the assumptions given in the text, to obtain Equation 13–19.

b) How would you calculate the rate of insulin release from the encapsulated islet tissue?

c) Calculate the rate of insulin release for each of the devices shown in Figure 13.9.

d) Calculate the internal concentration of insulin at radial position $r = 0$ for each of the devices. Why is it different for each case? What are the consequences of this for performance of the encapsulated cells?

Exercise 13.4

Consider the cells that were analyzed in Exercise 7.2.

a) If you have not done so already, determine the random motility coefficient (μ) and persistence time (P) for these cells, as described in Exercise 7.2, part (a).

b) A polymeric material, similar to the gel matrix used in (a), is implanted into a wound site. The geometry of the site is indicated schematically below. The total length of the matrix is 1.0 cm and its cross-section is 2 cm $\times$ 2 cm. Assume that cell migration is possible only through the interface between normal tissue and gel matrix that is indicated (that is, only migration in the x-direction must be considered). Assume that the normal tissue contains $\sim 5 \times 10^7$ motile cells/mL. If cells attempt to crawl into the matrix, and if the population of cells has the same motile characteristics as the population of cells studied in (a), predict the concentration density of cells within the matrix as a function of time. Plot the cell concentration within the gel matrix as a function of position at 6 hr, 1 day, and 1 week.

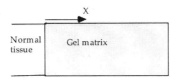

Exercise 13.5

You are designing a porous scaffold that will be seeded with isolated hepatocytes, maintained under culture conditions for some period of time, and then implanted into the abdominal cavity. Describe—as briefly and clearly as possible—the design issues that you would consider with respect to:

a) materials of construction;

b) overall (macroscopic) geometry of the scaffold;

c) microscopic structure of the scaffold;

d) source of cells.

Exercise 13.6 (provided by Michael V. Sefton)

PC12 cells produce dopamine; they may therefore be useful in treating
Parkinson's disease (when dopamine is missing). One approach would be to
encapsulate PC12 cells inside a spherical capsule (400 μm outer diameter (OD);
25 μm wall thickness) and then implant these capsules inside the brain. The
capsules serve to protect the cells from the brain of the recipient. Under one set
of circumstances, the cell density in the capsules is initially 1×10^6 cells /mL
and the capsules are incubated *in vitro* until enough cells grow to fill the entire
capsule.

Doubling time of PC12 cells	8 h
Mass of the mouse	250 g
Ratio of mouse head mass to overall mass	1/10
Ratio of mouse brain mass to head mass	1/5
Dopamine secretion *in vitro*	1 g/107 cells per day
Initial encapsulation cell density	1×10^6 PC12 cells/mL
Dopamine requirement	0.1 g/kg brain mass per day

a) Calculate the necessary incubation time for 50 capsules to produce
   enough dopamine for a mouse.
b) Part (a) assumes exponential growth for PC12 cells within the
   capsules. However, because of oxygen limitations, the growth kinetics
   of PC12 cells is modeled using Monod kinetics (recall Equation 4.23).
   What is the new incubation time based on this modified assumption?
   Relevant data: $K = 2\,\text{g/L}$, $\mu_{max} = 0.15\,\text{hr}$, and $dS/dt = -0.002\,\text{mol/L}$
   per hour (where S is the substrate concentration).
c) How many microcapsules are required to treat a human? State your
   assumptions.

Exercise 13.7 (provided by Linda G. Griffith)

Consider the nutrient limitations for islets encapsulated in microspheres (as
in Figure 13.7) and implanted subcutaneously. Data for the nutrients oxygen,
glucose, and transferrin ($M_w = 88{,}000$) are considered below. You may
assume the fluid surrounding the capsule is equivalent to extracellular fluid
in composition and that the capsule (whatever its size) is completely filled
with islet tissue. You may also assume zero-order nutrient consumption
rates.

a) For *free* (unencapsulated) islets, which nutrient is limiting? If the
   nutrient concentration at the center of the tissue mass is at least 20%
   of that in the external fluid, what is the dimension of the largest tissue
   mass that can be used?
b) If the membrane capsule surrounding the islets is 20 μm thick and
   inhibits oxygen and glucose diffusion by 15% (that is, $D_{membrane}/D_{tissue}$
   $= 0.85$) and transferrin diffusion by 95% (that is, $D_{membrane}/D_{tissue} =$

0.05), what is the maximum diameter of islet which can be used if the nutrient concentration in the center of the islet is at least 20% of that in the surrounding fluid?

c) The characteristic transient diffusion time (time for a solute to penetrate a distance L from the source) is calculated as $\tau = L^2/D$, where D is the diffusion coefficient. Estimate the response time for glucose stimulation of the whole islet and for insulin release.

Nutrient Data

Nutrient	$D_{tissue}(cm^2/s)$	$C_{externalfluid}$	$Q(mol/cm^3\text{-}s)$
Oxygen	1.5×10^{-5}	0.08 mM	2.5×10^{-8}
Glucose	0.4×10^{-5}	2.0 mM	3×10^{-9}
Transferrin	3.0×10^{-7}	100 mg/dL	0.8×10^{-12}
Insulin	0.1×10^{-5}		

Exercise 13.8 (provided by Linda G. Griffith)

It has been suggested that oxygen delivery to cells could be enhanced by increasing the solubility of oxygen in the membrane. Several approaches are available for increasing this solubility—for example, filling the pores in the membrane with perfluorocarbon and using a polymer such as polydimethyl-siloxane (silcone rubber).

a) Derive an equation that relates the steady-state flux of oxygen across a planar "oxygen transport enhancing" membrane of thickness Δx to K, the solubility of oxygen in the membrane relative to that in water; to the concentration driving force, using the water phase as a basis; and to D_m, the diffusion coefficient of oxygen in the membrane. Use your expression to develop a ratio of the steady-state flux across an oxygen transport enhancing membrane to that of a membrane with the properties of water. Under what conditions is oxygen transport enhanced?

b) In general, approaches aimed at increasing the solubility of oxygen in the immunoisolation membrane also inhibit diffusion of other nutrients. Thus, one idea is to make a membrane which has "plugs" of oxygen-permeable material embedded within the membrane to provide an additional conduit for oxygen to the cells. If the oxygen-permeable material has a permeability twice that of the standard immunoisolation membrane, where permeability P is defined as the proportionality between flux and driving force, $J_{oxygen} = P\Delta c_{oxygen}$, what enhancement of oxygen transfer can be expected if the oxygen-permeable material makes up 10% of the total membrane surface area? If it makes up 50% of the surface area?

Exercise 13.9

For all of the parts of this exercise, consider a synthetic replacement vessel that is 1 cm in length. For each of the questions below, you will need to make some assumptions; state them clearly.

a) How many endothelial cells will it take to form a confluent monolayer on the surface of the vessel lumen? Plot the number of cells as a function of vessel diameter.

b) Estimate the proliferation rate of endothelial cells (use information from Chapter 4). How long will it take to produce the number of cells that are needed to cover the surface of the vessels studied in part (a)? Solve this problem for each tissue engineering scenario outlined in the chapter (*in situ* regeneration, *in vitro* tissue development, and *in vitro* tissue production), stating the cell source and assumptions for each.

c) Assume that there is an abundant source of endothelial cells at each end of the vessel. Further assume that cells can migrate into the vessel along the surface of the lumen, but do not divide while migrating. Estimate the migration rate of endothelial cells (use information from Chapter 7). How long will it take to cover the vessel wall with migrating cells?

d) How are your answers different if the vessel is 10 cm long?

Exercise 13.10 (provided by Rebecca Kuntz Willits)

a) Discuss possible rejection pathways of immunoisolated cells. What are the benefits associated with encapsulating xenogenic cells?

b) List at least three parameters that are important to consider when constructing an immunoisolation device.

Exercise 13.11 (provided by Rebecca Kuntz Willits)

Develop an expression, beginning with a mass balance, to investigate the movement of a growth factor through newly implanted tissue. Describe your system, including assumptions and boundary conditions, and include diffusion, convection and binding (mol/vol-t) in your model. How (mathematically) would this model change if the new tissue were immunoisolated from the body?

Exercise 13.12 (provided by Linda G. Griffith)

Islet cells are maintained in a sandwich membrane configuration (Figure 13.15) with flat semipermeable membranes of thickness x_m on each side of a layer of cells of thickness x_c. The membrane is 100 μm thick. The cells consume oxygen at a zero-order rate of 5×10^{-8} mol/cm^3-s. The diffusion coefficient of oxygen in the membrane at 37°C is 1.5×10^{-5} cm^2/s. The diffusion coefficient of oxygen in culture medium at 37°C is 2.3×10^{-5} cm^2/s. Consider the "ends" (edges of the sandwich, on the left and right in the figure) to be oxygen-impermeable.

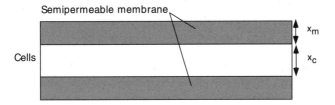

Figure 13.15. Diagram for Exercise 13.12.

a) An experiment is conducted in which the "sandwich" is maintained under well-stirred conditions in equilibrium with air. You may assume that, in this case, the oxygen concentration at the outer surface of each membrane is in equilibrium with air and is equal to 0.27 mM. If $x_c = 40$ mm (about 3–4 cell layers thick), what is the oxygen concentration at the interface between the membrane and the cells?

b) An experiment is conducted in which the "sandwich" lies flat on the bottom of the petri dish under 1 mm of culture medium. In this arrangement, oxygen can diffuse in only from one side. The culture medium is stagnant. What is the oxygen concentration at the outer surface of the membrane through which oxygen is diffusing? At the interface between the cells and the membrane (inner surface)? How do these concentrations change if the medium depth is increased to 1 cm? Do you think a zero-order reaction rate is appropriate in the latter case, and can you suggest an alternative?

Exercise 13.13

a) Show how Equation 13-26 is obtained from Equations 13-21 to 13-25.
b) Under what conditions is Equation 13-27 a good approximation for Equation 13-26 (that is, how small does K_m need to be to make the approximation valid)?

Exercise 13.14

Operation of a continuous, well-stirred bioreactor can sometimes be enhanced by addition of a recycle stream. Assume that a recycle stream is added to the reactor shown in Figure 13.12a by taking a fraction of the outlet stream flow and mixing it with the inlet stream flow (Figure 13.16a). If the fraction of the outlet flow stream that is recycled is equal to α ($Q_{recycle} = \alpha Q$), and the fraction of cells that are recycled is f ($N_{recycle} = f N_{out}$), show that the overall growth rate for the reactor is now given by

$$\mu = D(1 + \alpha(1 - f))$$

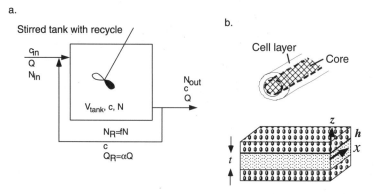

Figure 13.16. Diagrams for Exercises 13.14 and 13.15.

Exercise 13.15 (provided by Linda G. Griffith)

It has been suggested that oxygen transport to immunoisolated cells could be improved by using a hollow fiber design with an oxygen-permeable core (see Figure 13.16b; the encapsulating membrane is not shown). In this design, it is presumed that some advantage is derived by choosing the core such that $KD_c > D_t$, where K is the relative solubility of oxygen in the core material relative to the extracellular fluid, and D_c and D_t are the diffusion coefficients in the core region and the tissue layer, respectively. In the typical construction of hollow fiber encapsulated cell systems, the length L of the hollow fiber is much greater than the inner diameter D in which cells are contained; typical dimensions are $L \simeq 2\,\text{cm}$ and $D \simeq 0.05\,\text{cm}$.

Analyze the potential for such a core to increase the oxygen transport by providing an *estimate* of the oxgen profile along the axis of the core, and comparing the length scale for oxygen transport along the core (that is, the distance required for the oxgen concentration to fall to $\sim 10\%$ of that in the bulk medium) to the length scale of diffusion into the cell mass. For simplicity, neglect the transport resistance of the encapsulation membrane.

Further assumptions which will reduce the complexity of the problem: Use rectangular coordinates—assume a semi-infinite slab arrangement as shown in Figure 13.16b (bottom), with a core of thickness t and a cell layer thickness of h. Oxygen diffuses into the slab of tissue from two opposite directions, $z = 0$ and $z = h$, where $z = h$ corresponds to the cell–fluid interface where the bulk oxygen concentration is c_b. Oxygen enters the core region only at $x = 0$ and diffuses down the core in the x-direction and into the tissue in the z-direction (assume the tissue itself is closed off from the surrounding fluid at $x = 0$, that is, no axial flux in the tissue). It is reasonable to assume that the problem is analogous to finned heat transfer in that transport in the core region is essentially 1-D (in the x-direction) with no significant gradient in the z-direction in the core, and that, as the total length L of the diffusion path in the core increases, the oxygen concentration ultimately falls to approximately zero in the core and that, for long L, the oxygen flux in the x-direction at L is negligibly small. Since only an estimate of the scale of the diffusion path length in the core is needed, you can use zero-order kinetics and make an approximation regarding diffusion into the tissue mass from the core rather than calculating the full 2-D diffusion expression; for example, at what value of x must the maximum value of the flux occur? What does the profile look like if one assumes that this value of the flux prevails along the entire path length? You may also suggest other ways to put bounds on the flux into the tissue mass, for example, by assuming a certain thickness of influence, etc. You should ultimately develop a relationship in which you relate the ratio of diffusion paths L/h to K, and to the diffusion coefficients in each region.

Can you recommend a design that would be superior to the standard hollow fiber?

Exercise 13.16 (provided by Linda Griffith)

A bioreactor has been developed to culture primary hepatocytes in a tissue-like configuration. Hepatocytes maintained in conventional culture (for example, in a tissue culture dish) flatten out on the culture surface, lose their traditional cuboidal morphology, and simultaneously lose the majority of their hepatocyte functions. Within the bioreactor, the cells are cultured in channels on an etched silicon scaffold in a three-dimensional manner. This provides an environment for the hepatocytes to retain, to a greater extent, their cuboidal morphology and hepatocyte function. Channels are 300 μm long × 300 μm wide × 230 μm deep. A top and side view of four of the channels is shown in Figure 13.17a.

Usually, the silicon scaffold is placed in a bioreactor, so that each chamber of the scaffold is continuously perfused with culture medium. The perfusion allows convective mass transfer of oxygen and nutrients to the cells. Assume, however, that an experiment is performed in which the device is used in a simpler mode in which the scaffold (loaded with cells) is maintained within a well-stirred fluid on a flat dish. The flat dish is filled with medium, which you can assume is well mixed everywhere except inside the channels, where the hepatocytes reside (Figure 13.17b).

Within the channels, the void fraction of tissue is 50% (that is, the channels are half-full of tissue) and the tissue is homogeneous within each channel. The oxygen consumption rate for hepatocytes is 9×10^{-8} mol/(cm^3 tissue-s). The diffusion coefficient of oxygen in the culture medium and in the tissue is 2.3×10^{-5} cm^2/s. The medium at the top of the channel ($x = 0$) is in equilibrium with humidified incubator air containing 5% CO_2.

a) Estimate the oxygen concentration at the lowest part of the channel, $x = 230$ μm. If you find that the concentration is zero at the bottom of the channel, then answer this: for what values of x is the concentration greater than zero? In other words, how far does the oxygen penetrate into the channel?

a)

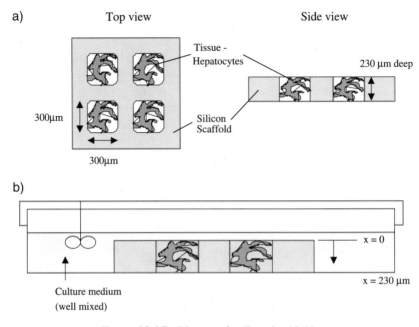

Figure 13.17. Diagram for Exercise 13.16.

b) How is the experiment going to work out? (A fact that may complicate your answer somewhat is our assumption of zero-order oxygen consumption rate.)

c) Why is this apparatus normally used in the presence of a perfusion flow? What will the hepatocytes experience that is different in the normal situation of continuous perfusion?

What is the purpose of using microscale chambers for the hepatocytes? that is, how would the device perform in a perfusion setting, but with chambers that were 2 × larger in each dimension? 10 × larger in each dimension?

References

1. Langer, R. and J.P. Vacanti, Tissue engineering. *Science*, 1993 **260**, 920–932.
2. Lanza, R., R. Langer, and J. Vacanti, eds. *Textbook of Tissue Engineering*, 2nd ed. New York: Academic Press, 2000.
3. Pastan, S. and J. Bailey, Medical progress: dialysis therapy. *New England Journal of Medicine*, 1998, **338**, 1428–1437.
4. Michaels, A.S., Operating parameters and performance criteria for hemodializers and other membrane-separation devices. *Transactions of the American Society for Artificial Internal Organs*, 1966, **12**, 387–392.
5. Colton, C. and E. Lowrie, Hemodialysis: physical principles and technical considerations. *The Kidney*, 1981, **II**, 2nd ed., 2425–2489.

6. Cooney, D.O., *Biomedical Engineering Principles: An Introduction to Fluid, Heat and Mass Transport Processes*. New York: Marcel Dekker, 1976.
7. Pillarella, M.R. and A.L. Zydney, Theoretical analysis of the effect of convective flow on solute transport and insulin release in a hollow fiber bioartificial pancreas. *Journal of Biomechanical Engineering*, 1990, **112**(2), 220–228.
8. Sullivan, S.J., et al., Biohybrid artificial pancreas: long-term implantation studies in diabetic, pancreatectomized dogs. *Science*, 1991, **252**, 718–721.
9. Munoz, S.J., Difficult management problems in fulminant hepatic failure. *Seminars in Liver Disease*, 1993, **13**(4), 395–413.
10. Sussman, N.L., et al., Reversal of fulminant hepatic failure using an extracorporeal liver assist device. *Hepatology*, 1992, **16**, 60–65.
11. Rozga, J., et al., A bioartificial liver to treat severe acute liver failure. *Annals of Surgery*, 1994, **219**, 538–546.
12. Patzer, J.F., Advances in bioartificial liver assisst devices. *Annals of the New York Academy of Sciences*, 2001, **94**, 320–333.
13. Mason, M.N., et al., Predicting controlled-release behavior of degradable PLA-b-PEG-b-PLA hydrogels. *Macromolecules*, 2001, **34**, 4630–4635.
14. Lu, S. and K.S. Anseth, Release behavior of high molecular weight solutes from poly(ethylene glycol)-based degradable networks. *Macromolecules*, 2000, **33**(7), 2509–2515.
15. Sanders, J.E., A.B. Baker, and S.L. Golledge, Control of *in vivo* microvessel ingrowth by modulation of biomaterial local architecture and chemistry. *Journal of Biomedical Materials Research*, 2002, **60**, 36–43.
16. Brauker, J., et al., Neovascularization of synthetic membranes directed by membrane microarchitecture. *Journal of Biomedical Materials Research*, 1995, **29**(12), 1527–1524.
17. Ratner, B.D., Reducing capsular thickness and enhancing angiogenesis around implant drug release systems. *Journal of Controlled Release*, 2002, **78**, 211–218.
18. Sharkawy, A.A., et al., Engineering the tissue which encapsulates subcutaneous implants. I. Diffusion properties. *Journal of Biomedical Materials Research*, 1997, **37**, 401–412.
19. Lim, F. and A.M. Sun, Microencapulated islets as bioartificial endocrine pancreas. *Science*, 1980, **210**, 908–910.
20. O'Shea, G.M. and A.M. Sun, Encapsulation of rat islets of Langerhans prolongs xenograft survival in diabetic mice. *Diabetes*, 1986, **35**, 943–946.
21. Sawhney, A.S. and J.A. Hubbell, Poly(ethylene oxide)-graft–poly(L-lysine) copolymers to enhance the biocompatibility of poly(L-lysine)-alginate microcapsule membranes. *Biomaterials*, 1992, **13**, 863–870.
22. Sefton, M., et al., Microencapsulation of mammalian cells in a water-insoluble polyacrylate by coextrustion and interfacial precipitation. *Biotechnology and Bioengineering*, 1987, **29**, 1135–1143.
23. Dawson, R.M., et al., Microencapulation of CHO cells in a hydroxyethyl methacrylate-methyl methacrylate copolymer. *Biomaterials*, 1987, **8**, 360–366.
24. Pathak, C.P., A.S. Sawhney, and J.A. Hubbell, Rapid photopolymerization of immunoprotective gels in contact with cells and tissue. *Journal of American Chemical Society*, 1992, **114**, 8311–8312.
25. Zielinski, B.A. and M.J. Lysaght, Immunoisolation, in R. Lanza, R. Langer, and J. Vacanti, eds., *Textbook of Tissue Engineering*. New York: Academic Press, 2000, pp. 321–330.

26. Lacy, P.E., et al., Maintenance of normoglycemia in diabetic mice by subcutaneous xenografts of encapsulated islets. *Science*, 1991, **254**, 1782–1784.

27. Winn, S., et al., An encapsulated dopamine-releasing polymer alleviates experimental Parkinsonism in rats. *Experimental Neurology*, 1989, **105**, 244–250.

28. Aebischer, P., et al., Gene therapy for amyotrophic lateral sclerosis (ALS) using a polymer encapsulated xenogenic cell line engineered to secrete hCNTF. *Human Gene Therapy*, 1996, **7**, 851–860.

29. Tao, W., et al., Encapsulated cell-based delivery of CNTF reduces photoreceptor degeneration in animal models of retinitis pigmentosa. *Investigative Ophthalmology & Visual Science*, 2002, **43**(10), 3292–3298.

30. Joseph, J.M., et al., Transplantation of encapsulated bovine chrommafin cells in the sheep subarachnoid space: a preclinical study for the treatment of cancer pain. *Cell Transplantation*, 1994, **3**, 355–364.

31. Read, T., et al., Local endostatin treatment of gliomas administered by micro-encapsulated producer cells. *Nature Biotechnology*, 2001, **19**, 29–34.

32. Joki, T., et al., Continuous release of endostatin from microencapsulated engineering cells for tumor therapy. *Nature Biotechnology*, 2001, **19**, 35–39.

33. Paris, E., et al., Innovations and deviations in therapeutic vascular devices, in S. Dumitriu, ed., *Polymeric Biomaterials*. New York: Marcel Dekker, 1994, pp. 245–275.

34. Massia, S.P. and J.A. Hubbell, An RGD spacing of 440 nm is sufficient for integrin aVβ3-mediated fibroblast spreading and 140 nm for focal contact and stress fiber formation. *Journal of Cell Biology*, 1991, **114**, 1089–1100.

35. Hubbell, J.A., et al., Endothelial cell-selective materials for tissue engineering in the vascular graft via a new receptor. *Bio/Technology*, 1991, **9**, 568–572.

36. Massia, S.P. and J.A. Hubbell, Vascular endothelial cell adhesion and spreading promoted by the peptide REDV of the IIICS region of plasma fibronectin is mediated by integrin α4β1. *Journal of Biological Chemistry*, 1992, **267**, 14019–14026.

37. Massia, S.P. and J.A. Hubbell, Immobilized amines and basic amino acids as mimetic heparin-binding domains for cell surface proteoglycan-mediated adhesion. *Journal of Biological Chemistry*, 1992, **267**, 10133–10141.

38. Griffith, L.G. and G. Naughton, Tissue engineering–Current challenges and expanding opportunities. *Science*, 2002, **295**, 1009.

39. L'Heureux, N., et al., A completely biological tissue-engineered human blood vessel. *FASEB Journal*, 1998, **12**, 47–56.

40. Niklason, L., et al., Functional arteries grown *in vitro*. *Science*, 1999, **284**, 489–493.

41. Demetriou, A., et al., Replacement of liver function in rats by transplantation of microcarrier-attached hepatocytes. *Science*, 1986, **23**, 1190–1192.

42. Mahoney, M.J. and W.M. Saltzman, Transplantation of brain cells assembled around a programmable synthetic microenvironment. *Nature Biotechnology*, 2001, **19**, 934–939.

43. Dai, W., J. Belt, and W.M. Saltzman, Cell-binding peptides conjugated to poly (ethylene glycol) promote neural cell aggregation. *Bio/Technology*, 1994, **12**, 797–801.

44. Vacanti, J.P., et al., Selective cell transplantation using bioabsorbable artificial polymers as matrices. *Journal of Pediatric Surgery*, 1988, **23**, 3–9.

45. Thompson, J., et al., Heparin-binding growth factor 1 induces the formation of organoid neovascular structures *in vivo*. *Proceedings of the National Academy of Sciences USA*, 1989, **86**, 7928–7932.

46. Alsberg, E., et al., Engineering growing tissues. *Proceedings of the National Academy of Sciences*, 2002, **99**(19), 12025–12030.

47. Griffith, L.G., Emerging design principles in biomaterials and scaffolds for tissue engineering. *Annals of the New York Academy of Sciences*, 2002, **961**, 83–95.

48. Noll, T., et al., Cultivation of hematopoietic stem and progenitor cells: biochemical engineering aspects. *Advances in Biochemical Engineering/Biotechnology*, 2002, **74**, 111–128.

49. Shuler, M.L. and F. Kargi, *Bioprocess Engineering: Basic Concepts*, 2nd ed. New York: Prentice Hall, 2002.

50. Koller, M.R. and B.O. Palsson, Tissue engineering of bone marrow, in J.D. Bronzino, ed., *Biomedical Engineering Handbook*. Boca Raton, FL: CRC Press, 1995, pp. 1728–1744.

51. Madlambayan, G.J., et al., Controlling culture dynamics for the expansion of hematopoietic stem cells. *Journal of Hematotherapy & Stem Cell Research*, 2001, **10**, 481–492.

52. Zandstra, P.W., D.A. Lauffenburger, and C.J. Eaves, A ligand–receptor signaling threshold model of stem cell differentiation control: a biologically conserved mechanism applicable to hematopoiesis. *Blood*, 2000, **96**(4), 1215–1222.

53. Darling, E.M. and K.A. Athanasiou, Articular cartilage bioreactors and bioprocesses. *Tissue Engineering*, 2003, **9**(1), 9–26.

54. Hoerstrup, S.P., et al., New pulsatile bioreactor for *in vitro* formation of tissue engineered heart valves. *Tissue Engineering*, 2000, **6**(1), 75–79.

55. Begley, C.M. and S.M. Kleis, The fluid dynamic and shear environment in the NASA/JSC rotating-wall perfused-vessel bioreactor. *Biotechnology and Bioengineering*, 2000, **70**, 32–40.

56. Goodwin, T.J., J.M. Jessup, and D.A. Wolf, Morphologic differentiation of colon carcinoma cell lines HT-29 and HT-29KM in rotating-wall vessels. *In Vitro Cell Developmental Biology*, 1992, **28A**, 47–60.

57. Schwarz, R.P., T.J. Goodwin, and D.A. Wolf, Cell culture for three-dimensional modeling in rotating-wall vessels: applications of simulated microgravity. *Journal of Tissue Culture Methods*, 1992, **14**, 51–58.

58. Pollack, S.R., et al., Numerical model and experimental validation of microcarrier motion in a rotating bioreactor. *Tissue Engineering*, 2000, **6**(5), 519–530.

59. Freed, L.E., G. Vunjak-Novakovic, and R. Langer, Cultivation of cell–polymer cartilage implants in bioreactors. *Journal of Cellular Biochemistry*, 1993, **51**, 257–264.

60. Baldwin, S.P. and W.M. Saltzman, Aggregation enhances catecholamine synthesis in cultured cells. *Tissue Engineering*, 2001, **7**, 179–190.

61. Unsworth, B.R. and P.I. Lelkes, Growing tissues in microgravity. *Nature Medicine*, 1998, **4**(8), 901–907.

62. Pei, M., et al., Bioreactors mediate the effectiveness of tissue engineering scaffolds. *FASEB Journal*, express article 10.1096/fj.oz-0083fje. Published on-line, August 7, 2002.

63. Hirschi, K.K., et al., Vascular assembly in natural and engineered tissues. *Annals of the New York Academy of Sciences*, 2002, **961**, 223–242.

64. Cassell, O.C.S., et al., Vascularization of tissue-engineered grafts: the regulation of angiogenesis in reconstructive surgery and in disease states. *British Journal of Plastic Surgery*, 2002, **55**, 603–610.

65. Saltzman, W.M., *Drug Delivery: Engineering Principles for Drug Therapy*. New York: Oxford University Press, 2001.

66. DePalma, J.R. and J.D. Pittard, Dialysis dose (part I). *Dialysis & Transplantation*, 2001, April, 252–261, 266.
67. Watt, F.M. and B.L.M. Hogan, Out of Eden: stem cells and their niches. *Science*, 2000, **287**, 1427–1430.
68. Butler, D.L., S.A. Goldstein, and F. Guilak, Functional tissue engineering: the role of biomechanics. *Journal of Biomechanical Engineering*, 2000, **122**, 570–575.
69. Bryant, S.J. and K.S. Anseth, Hydrogel properties influence ECM production by chondrocytes photoencapsulated in poly(ethylene glycol) hydrogels. *Journal of Biomedical Materials Research*, 2002, **59**(1), 63–72.
70. Johns, B., et al., Mechanical properties of a pH sensitive hydrogel., *SEM Annual Conference Proceedings*, Society for Experimental Mechanics, 2002.
71. Kirker, K.R., et al., Glycosaminoglycan hydrogel films for wound healing. BED volume, *2001 Bioengineering Conference*, ASME, 50.
72. Moran, J.H., D. Pazzano, and L.J. Bonassar, Characterization of polylactic acid–polyglycolic acid composites for cartilage tissue engineering. *Tissue Engineering*, 2003, **9**(1), 63–70.
73. Fournier, R.L., *Basic Transport Phenomena in Biomedical Engineering*. New York: Taylor & Francis, 1998.

14

Case Studies in Tissue Engineering

O harp and altar, of the fury fused,
(How could mere toil align thy choiring strings!)

Hart Crane, *To Brooklyn Bridge*

This final chapter introduces a few tissue engineering systems that either have been used clinically or are rapidly approaching clinical use for cartilage, skin, and nerve repair. Some of the elements of each tissue engineering system are presented, together with references to the primary literature.

The first example involves engineering of a tissue with an important mechanical function: cartilage. The general approach described for cartilage has been attempted in other structural tissues such as bone, tendon, and skin; there are important common elements among these tissue engineering systems. One common underlying theme, which is emphasized in the first example, is the use of a material as a scaffold for the ingrowth, proliferation, and function of cells, which differentiate into mature functional cells.

After being introduced to this first example and provided with an outline of some experimental results, the reader is then presented with a series of questions: some are intended to stimulate discussion in the classroom, while others can be used as homework assignments or as the basis for independent projects. The main objective of these exercises is to assimilate information from previous chapters and apply it in a situation with clinical application: cartilage tissue engineering.

The second and third examples involve tissue-engineered skin and repair of nerves lost to disease or trauma. No questions are provided with these examples, but the reader is encouraged to identify the connections to material in the preceding chapters.

14.1 Tissue-Engineered Cartilage

14.1.1 Carticel Procedure for Cartilage Repair

One of the first tissue engineering products available to patients is Carticel®, which uses autologous cultured chondrocytes for the repair of cartilage defects in the femoral condyle (spirally curved prominences on the end of the femur that is involved in the knee joint). The procedure has several phases: first, a pea-sized biopsy of healthy knee cartilage is obtained. This tissue is expanded *in vitro* to obtain a large number of cultured cells that are all derived from the patient. In a second procedure, a surgeon prepares the transplant site by removing diseased tissue and preparing the defect (in the clinical trials of this product, the defect had a cross-sectional area of <1 to $20\,cm^2$, with 90% of the defects $<10\,cm^2$). The amplified cell population ($\sim 12 \times 10^6$ cells) is then reintroduced into the prepared defect site, and retained at the site by suturing of a patch of periosteum over the defect.

Cell Amplification and Packaging.   The process of autologous cell amplification takes 5 to 6 weeks; this is the time from removal of the biopsy tissue from the patient to receipt of the ampule of transplantable cells by the surgeon.

1. How many chondrocytes are present in the initial pea-sized biopsy tissue?
2. How long should it take to obtain the 12×10^6 cells from the biopsy tissue, using cell culture techniques? What features of the culture conditions can you control in order to minimize this time? How would you expect this time to vary if you used a similar procedure for cells from other biopsy tissues—that is, from skin, or liver, or muscle, or bone marrow, or lymph node, or intestinal epithelium?
3. What elements do you expect to be added to the cell population during amplification (that is, what things might be in the ampule that is received by the surgeon that were not present in the biopsy specimen)? Which of these things might you be concerned about, if you were a surgeon or patient?

Clinical Outcome.   The product brochure for Carticel reports the following clinical outcome:

> Twenty-two of the initial 23 patients in the Swedish series had histological evaluation of biopsies from the transplant site. Fifteen of those patients had defects of the femoral condyle and 7 had defects of the patella. Six of the 15 femoral condyle patients showed only hyaline cartilage on their biopsy, 5 had a mixture of hyaline and fibrocartilage, and 4 had only fibrocartilage. Of the 6 patients with only hyaline cartilage on biopsy, 2 had minimal to no defects and 4 had more extensive defects (for example, fissures, fibrillations, etc.).

a) Describe the differences between hyaline cartilage and fibrocartilage. Histologically, what do these two types of tissue look like (that is, describe the cellular and extracellular features of each)?
b) What features of the local site of repair would you expect to influence the outcome toward either of these endpoints?
c) Are there any elements that you could add to the cell suspension that is injected into the defect site, or to the surgical procedure used to

deploy the cells, to increase the probability of the most desirable clinical outcome?

14.1.2 Cartilage Repair Using a Cell-Free Matrix with Controlled-Release Differentiation Factor

There is some evidence that defects in cartilage can be repaired, without the introduction of any new cells, by stimulating the process of tissue regeneration at the local site. For this exercise, consider two papers published by Hunziker, in which synovial cells are recruited into the defect site by using two elements: a fibrin matrix to support cell migration [1], and local delivery of transforming growth factor-β1 (TGF-β1) to stimulate differentiation of the cells into chondrocytes [2].

Three-Dimensional Scaffold for Cell Migration to Fill a Defect. Both papers used an animal model in which a defect of controlled size was made in either the rabbit (in which the defects were 1 mm wide, 0.2–0.25 mm deep, and 4-6 mm long) or the Yucatan mini-pig (in which the defects were 0.5 mm wide, 0.6 mm deep, 7–9 mm long). The results are illustrated schematically in Figure 14.1:

- when the defect was untreated (panel A) a few scattered clusters of mesenchymal cells were found in the defect after 2 or 4 weeks;
- when the defect was pre-treated with an enzyme (chondroitanase ABC, panel B), a greater number of cells were found in the defect;
- when the enzyme pre-treatment was used together with a topical application of TGF-β1 (panel C), an even greater number of cells were found, but not enough to fill the defect;
- when the defect was pre-treated with enzyme and filled with a fibrin matrix (panel D), the defect was found to be filled with a low number of cells;
- when the defect was pre-treated with enzyme and filled with a fibrin matrix containing TGF-β1 (panels E, F), the defect was found to be filled with a large number of cells.

The experimental data are consistent with the following model. Enzyme treatment creates a defect surface over which local cells can migrate. TGF-β1 enhances cell accumulation and/or proliferation within the defect site. Presence of a fibrin matrix provides a three-dimensional, space-filling scaffold through which the cells can migrate to fill the defect volume. Again, in the presence of a fibrin matrix, TGF-β1 enhances cell accumulation within the defect site, but now the cells can migrate throughout the three-dimensional volume of the defect.

Now consider the following questions:

a) Why do cells migrate over the enzyme-treated defect surface better than they migrate over the non-treated surface? If you measured the adhesiveness of the defect surface to the migrating cells, do you think

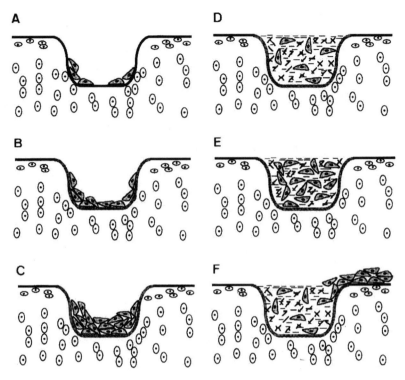

Figure 14.1. Results for repair of a cartilage defect (reproduced from [1]). Schematic illustration of the result of different experimental interventions in the healing of a regular defect in cartilage. See text for details. The different panels represent the outcome with (a) no treatment; (b) enzyme pre-treatment; (c) enzyme pre-treatment plus topical TGF-β1; (d) enzyme pre-treatment and fibrin matrix; (e) and (f) enzyme pre-treatment plus fibrin matrix containing TGF-β1.

that it would be higher in the non-treated or the enzyme-treated case? Use information from Chapter 7 in formulating your answer.

b) Describe the physical structure of the fibrin matrix (or clot), which was created with a solution of 1 mg/mL of fibrinogen and 100 units/mL of thrombin. Can you estimate its physical properties (pore size, porosity, mechanical strength)?

c) The half-life of TGF-β1 is ~5 min when it is *injected intravenously* [3]. If the initial concentration of TGF-β1 in the fibrin clot is 6 ng/mL of fibrinogen solution, what do you expect the concentration of TGF-β1 to be in the defect at 1 d, 1 wk, 2 wk, and 4 wk after treatment? Explain why you should not make this estimate by using a 5 min half-life at the local site. (Hint: This problem is similar to the one described in exercises 11.1 and 11.2.)

d) How do cells fill the defect in the animals that received fibrin matrices? How long should this process take? Recall the model of cell migration through a three-dimensional hydrogel that was introduced in Chapter 7 (exercises 7.2 and 7.5). Using this model, what is the rate of cell migration through the polymer matrix? How is the rate of migration influenced by TGF-β1? The paper suggests that the cells within the defect are recruited from adjacent synovial membrane, and that the cells "stream" across the uninjured cartilage surface to fill the defect. This process potentially involves proliferation of cells, migration across the cartilage surface, and migration through the fibrin matrix. What is the rate-limiting step for this process?

e) Assume that, instead of the small defect used by Hunziker, a defect of the size used in the Carticel procedure was used (1–$20 \, \text{cm}^2$ cross-sectional area, length × width). What would you expect to be the result?

Differentiation of Cells Using Local Delivery of a Protein.   In the experiments described in the first paper [1], no cartilage tissue was formed within any of the experimental animals. Remodeling of the fibrin matrix did occur: a fibrous connective tissue was formed within the joints, even after application of TGF-β1, which is known to induce cartilage formation. Speculating that the source of TGF-β1 used in the previous experiment was short-lived (see question (c) in the previous section), Hunziker repeated these experiments using a liposome/TGF-β1 preparation [2]; with the improved TGF-β1 delivery system, tissue with many of the histological features of cartilage was formed in the defect site.

a) Hunziker used a liposome delivery system in these experiments. Using the information from Chapter 11 as a guide, consider three alternate delivery systems for the TGF-β1 that could be used for this application: a non-degradable matrix system, degradable polymer microparticles, and degradable fibrous mesh (see Figure 11.1). What are the advantages and disadvantages of each?

b) Hunziker describes two possible mechanisms for activity of the liposome/TGF-β1 delivery system: (a) phagocytosis of liposomes by cells in the matrix and subsequent intracellular action, and (b) release of TGF-β1 in the extracellular space and activation of cells via receptors on the cell surface. Which mechanism do you think is the most important, and how would you design an experiment to test each hypothesis?

Scaffold Materials: Three-Dimensional Hydrogel Matrix.   Fibrin matrix is an excellent model matrix and it was employed with great success by Hunziker, but it might not be the best system for clinical use. A variety of other matrix materials is available; some are described in Chapters 12 and 13. Of particular potential interest are hydrogels, which can be engineered to possess many desirable properties including degradability, gel formation under gentle conditions, controlled pore sizes, and controlled mechanical properties. In fact, recalling the discussion at the end of Chapter 13, it is possible to produce hydrogels that have a compressive modulus similar to that of articular cartilage.

In a paper by Bryant and Anseth [4], PEG-based hydrogels are used for the encapsulation of chondrocytes. Consider the properties of these materials, which are summarized in Table 14.1.

a) Recalling the discussion of molecular weight cut-off from Chapter 13, describe the resistance of these materials to the diffusion of the following proteins: insulin, albumin, laminin, collagen type I, and collagen type II. It might be useful to refer to Figure 13.6 and the related discussion. Information on rates of diffusion of macromolecules in hydrogels is available from a variety of sources, including Chapter 4 of [5].

b) Assume that a single viable chondrocyte was encapsulated in each of the four materials listed in Table 14.1. Assume further that this cell is continuously secreting a proteoglycan with a molecular diameter of 90 Å. Plot the proteoglycan concentration as a function of distance from the cell surface for each material. How do your results compare with Figure 3 of the paper [4], which is reproduced in Figure 14.2?

c) In addition to its barrier properties for molecular transport, in what other ways will the hydrogel system influence cell behavior and tissue formation at the defect site? Compare the mechanical environment experienced by the cell in a fibrin matrix and a hydrogel matrix. How will the mechanical properties of the material influence cell function?

d) Can the materials listed in Table 14.1 be used as a matrix for synovial cell ingrowth; that is, could these materials be used in place of fibrin matrix in the papers by Hunziker? If yes, what differences would you expect to observe in the results? If no, how could you change their properties to make them useful in that mode?

14.1.3 Extension to Other Tissue Engineering Applications

It should be obvious that variations on this approach can be used to engineer bone and other structural tissues. The approach would involve formation of a

Table 14.1
Properties of Hydrogels

% PEGDM	Compressive Modulus (kPa)	Mesh size (Å)
10	34	140
20	360	60
30	940	50
40	1400	40

From [4].

4 weeks *in vitro*

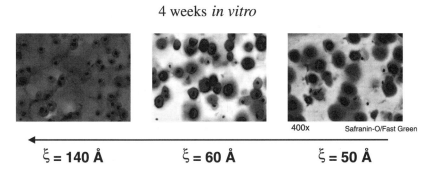

400x   Safranin-O/Fast Green

$\xi = 140$ Å $\xi = 60$ Å $\xi = 50$ Å

Figure 14.2. Proteoglycan distribution in hydrogel encapsulated chondrocytes (reproduced from [4]). Three of the hydrogel materials that are listed in Table 14.1 were used to encapsulate chondrocytes. Each gel was stained to show the presence of proteoglycans after 4 weeks of culture *in vitro*.

fibrous matrix, either cell-free or with transplanted cells, that would occupy the space of the defect initially and guide the transformation into a mature tissue over time; many variables in the matrix and in the procedure can be adjusted to suit the application. (As a thought experiment, make a list of the variables that could be changed in the experiments done by Hunziker and how you would expect them to differ if the goal were to repair damaged bone or skin.) The success of the transformation can be assessed experimentally by observing the histological structure and chemical components of the tissue that forms over time in the defect site. In addition, one could use mechanical tests to verify that the tissue has the desired mechanical properties.

This is a straightforward approach, but is complicated by at least two additional observations. First, the mechanical functions of bone, cartilage, skin, tendon, muscle, and other tissues are complex and it is often not clear which—of the many mechanical metrics one might use to test a material (Table 14.2)—is the most critical for the application under consideration [6]. Second, the mechanical function of a tissue depends on interactions between elements over many length scales, from the geometry of the whole organ to the subcellular components of the resident cells (Figure 14.3). Because of this hierarchy of structure, the tissue engineer must approach the design of a structural tissue with a similar hierarchical perspective [7].

14.2 Tissue-Engineered Skin

A wide variety of materials have been proposed and tested as skin grafts, to prevent dehydration and infection of large open wound areas and to aid healing (Figure 14.4, see review of clinical products [8]) . Some systems are acellular; one of the earliest systems, for example, employs silicone membranes (to retain fluid) together with a collagen/chondroitan sulfate layer to induce blood vessel and connective tissue integration [9–14]. These first systems, which

Table 14.2
Some of the Mechanical Properties
of a Tissue that Might be
Important for Tissue Function

Anisotropy
    Tensile, compressive, shear moduli
    Permeability
    Failure stress and strain
    Fatigue life
Geometry
Inhomogeneity
Nonlinearity
Physicochemical-mechanical coupling
    Residual stresses
    Swelling
    Electrokinetic effects
Tribological properties
    Frictional coefficient
    Wear properties
    Hardness
Viscoelasticity
    Multiphase or poroelastic
    Energy dissipation
    Intrinsic viscoelasticity
    Fluid viscosity

This list was adapted from Table 1
of [6].

evolved into the clinical product Integra®, now the most widely used synthetic skin substitute for burn patients, involved only non-living components: a silicone upper layer and an extracellular matrix lower layer. In clinical use, the silicone layer is replaced after 3 weeks with a thin epidermal graft. Subsequent developments have included autografted cells (from a small graft) in the lower layer prior to use in the patient [14].

Another approach is to take a small biopsy from the patient and expand the autologous epidermal cells *in vitro*, as in the cartilage therapy described earlier in the chapter. But epidermal cells are more difficult to grow than chondrocytes. Using optimized cell culture techniques (for example, by culture with a feeder layer of irradiated 3T3 cells and medium with growth factors), it is possible to achieve a 10,000-fold amplification in cell number by the end of 3 to 4 weeks, which is too slow for many clinical situations.

This time delay can be avoided by using allogeneic cells, which can be prepared in advance and stored frozen. This approach is used by two biological skin substitutes (Figure 14.4): Apligraf®, a collagen-based system containing both allogeneic endothelial cells and fibroblasts, and Dermagraft®, a system based on PLGA fiber meshes containing cultured fibroblasts. The fate of the allogeneic cells used in these products after transplantation is not clear and—while they represent important milestones in tissue engineering with potential

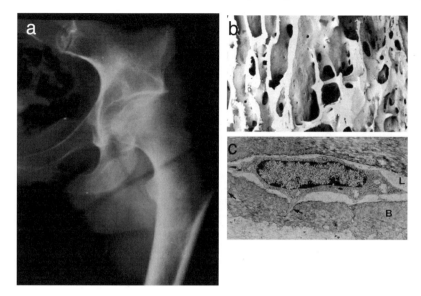

Figure 14.3. Structure property relations occur over a range of length scales. To evaluate the functional properties of a tissue-engineered bone, one must consider the interactions between structure and function at a variety of length scales from the whole organ (a), to the microarchitecture of the tissue (b), to the interaction between cells and extracellular matrix, and even within the cytoplasm of the cell (c). From [7].

benefits to patients—the role of these tissue-engineered materials in clinical practice is still uncertain.

A common problem, which is encountered to varying degrees with all of the current tissue engineered skin products, is the lack of formation of a stable vasculature that is connected to—and perfused by—the blood system of the host. Lack of a robust system of perfused vessels greatly reduces the likelihood of successful engraftment. Indeed, lack of development of an adequate vascular system is a major problem in most tissue engineering products (recall the brief discussion in Section 13.3.2). For skin, this may be an even more important problem to solve, since many patients who would benefit from tissue-engineered skin have damaged vessels in the adjacent host tissue (due to the effect of burns or diabetes, two of the most common indications for skin substitutes) or have limited capacity for angiogenesis (due to advanced age).

One approach for enhancing vascularization, which may be applicable to many tissue engineering products including skin, involves the culture of human endothelial cells within a transplantable matrix; matrices of type I collagen and fibronectin have been used successfully [15]. Under the appropriate culture conditions, human umbilical vein endothelial cells (HUVEC) will form tubular structures after a brief period of culture. When these constructs are transplanted under the skin of a mouse, a HUVEC-lined blood vessel system—that is, perfused by mouse blood—forms within the construct. Genetic

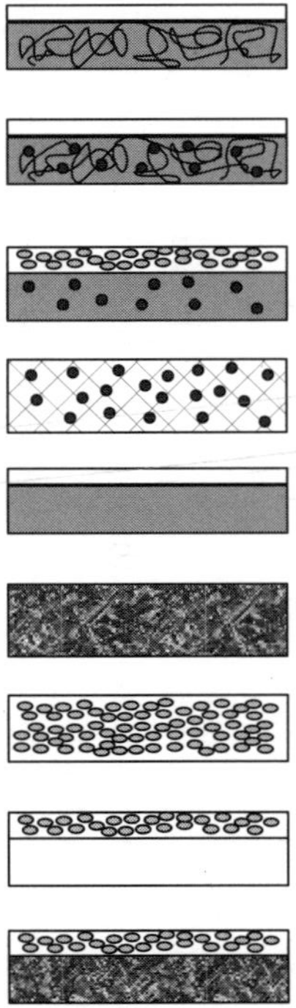

TRADE NAME		COMPOSITION	APPROXIMATE COST per square cm
Biobrane ™ (Dow Hickam/Bertek Pharmaceuticals, Sugar Land, TX)		1.Silicone 2.Nylon Mesh 3.Collagen	$0.82
Transcyte® (Advanced Tissue Sciences Inc., La Jolla, CA)		1.Silicone 2.Nylon Mesh 3.Collagen seeded with neonatal fibroblasts	$9.16
Apligraf® (Organogenesis Inc., Canton, MA and Novartis Pharmaceuticals, East Hanover, NJ)		1.Neonatal keratinocytes 2.Collagen seeded with neonatal fibroblasts	$16.52
Dermagraft® (Advanced Tissue Sciences Inc., La Jolla, CA)		1.Polyglycolic acid or polyglactin-910 seeded with neonatal fibroblasts	$8.31
Integra® (Integra Life Sciences Corporation, Plainsboro, NJ)		1.Silicone 2.Collagen and glycosaminoglycan	$3.86
Alloderm® (Life Cell, Woodlands, TX)		1.Acellular de-epithelialised cadaver dermis	$6.86
Epicel™ (Genzyme, Cambridge, MA)		1.Cultured autologous keratinocytes	$16.28
Laserskin™ (Fidia Advanced Biopolymers, Italy; Vivoderm™ by ER Squibb & Sons Ltd., United Kingdom)		1.Cultured autologous keratinocytes 2.Hyaluronic acid with laser perforations	n/a
Cadaveric allograft (from non-profit skin banks)		1.Cryopreserved in order to retain viability 2.Lyophilized 3.Glycerolized	$0.70

Figure 14.4. Approaches to tissue-engineered skin (from [8]).

engineering of HUVECs, by overexpression of the survival gene Bcl-2, led to an increased vessel density in the construct as well as evidence of vascular remodeling to form arteries and veins. There are many attractive features to this approach, which involves commonly available cells and materials such as collagen that are common in tissue engineering practice. But there are other approaches as well (see Table 11.1 for a few selected examples).

14.3 Tissue Engineering Approaches for Nerve Regeneration

14.3.1 Early Work and Clinical Experience

Several different strategies have been developed for enhancing the regeneration of damaged peripheral nerves [16, 17]. In general, when a nerve is severed, the proximal and distal ends of the severed nerve will reconnect only if the gap between the two severed ends is short. In current clinical practice, the nerve can be repaired only if the gap is short enough (< 1 mm) to permit surgical re-approximation of the distal and proximal ends. For larger defects, the most effective current treatment for bridging defects in peripheral nerves is replace-ment with an autologous nerve; autografts can be used for defects up to 15 cm in length (although some surgeons would limit the autograft to defects under 2 cm). These approaches have serious limitations—the availability of auto-grafts, loss of function at the donor nerve site, fibrosis at the two sites of suturing for the autograft—so new approaches are needed.

Nerve guides of different origin have been used to enhance the natural process of regeneration between proximal and distal ends of a damaged nerve. Figure 2.4 illustrates the use of a tube or conduit that is placed around the proximal and distal ends of the damaged nerve in order to isolate the region through which repair is desired. The conduit provides a number of potential functions including isolation of the region of repair, mechanical guidance of growing nerves from the proximal to the distal end, and protection and accu-mulation of molecular factors (both tropic and trophic) produced by tissue in the distal stump. Conduits from a variety of sources have been examined in animals and in humans, including vein autografts, denatured muscle tissue (sometimes within a nerve guide), and synthetic polymers [17].

Synthetic polymers have been used to facilitate peripheral nerve regenera-tion [18]. In many cases, polymer tubes provide an environment that reorients proximal and distal nerve stumps and isolates the regenerating nerve region (recall Figure 2.4). In most studies, guidance channels composed of hydro-phobic, nondegradable polymers—such as silicone elastomer [18], poly(vinyl chloride) [19], polytetrafluoroethylene (PTFE), poly(acrylonitrile-*co*-vinyl chloride), or polyethylene [20]—were used to separate the regrowth region from the surrounding tissue environment. Biodegradable polymers, such as poly(d,l-lactic acid) or poly(glycolic acid) [21], have also been used.

Early studies, using air-filled silicone tubes as nerve guides, suggest the following sequence of events during nerve regeneration [22]. (1) During the first day after implantation of an air-filled nerve guide, the tube becomes filled with a fluid that possesses neurotrophic activity. (2) During the first week, an asymmetric fibrin matrix appears within the silicone chamber. (3) After the first week, Schwann cells, fibroblasts, and endothelial cells migrate into the chamber along the condensed fibrin matrix. These cells appear first in peripheral regions of the tube, and then more centrally. (4) During the second week, axons appear in the chamber, suggesting that axon growth requires the presence of support- ing cells. The rate of axon elongation is ~ 1 mm/day, faster than the rate of elongation through scar tissue (~ 0.25 mm/day [23]), but slower than the rate of elongation through autografts (~ 3–4 mm/day [24]). (5) Myelination occurs, first proximally then distally, approximately 3 to 5 days following axon growth.

In clinical studies, many silicone-based nerve guides have had to be removed after some period of regeneration, as the device creates irritation within the tissue which is apparent to the patient. In some cases the tube became compressed, halting the regeneration process and causing loss of func- tion. In clinical studies, the PTFE nerve guides perform better than silicone, since there is a reduction in the irritation and hence the need for removal. In all cases, non-degradable guides appear to be limited to the repair of defects that are less than 4 mm in size.

14.3.2 Design of Materials for Use in Nerve Guides

How can the design of materials for use as nerve guides be improved? The time sequence of regeneration within the silicone tube provides a basis for introduc- tion of improved designs. For example, the development of an internal scaf- folding (that is, fibrin matrix) and supporting cells (Schwann cells and fibroblasts) appears to precede the regeneration of axons. Therefore, modifica- tions that speed this process of "organization" within the tube lumen might be expected to enhance regeneration.

The physical and chemical characteristics of material used to construct the guidance channel influence the outcome of peripheral nerve regeneration. For example, the microstructure of the surface in the lumen of the guidance channel also influences regeneration, but it is unclear whether this effect is significant enough to impact the clinical response. Consider the following information, for studies in animal models: poly(ACN-*co*-VC) tubes with smooth and rough surfaces were used to span a 4 mm gap in severed rat sciatic nerve [25]. Smooth tubes enhanced regeneration, producing distinct nerve cables with numerous myelinated neurons and a thin epineural-like layer that did not contact the channel wall, in sharp contrast to rough tubes, which produced a channel-spanning, disorganized matrix containing primarily inflammatory cells and fibroblasts. Presumably the smooth tube wall, which had fewer interac- tions with migrating cells and structural proteins, encouraged the formation of an organized cable-like matrix throughout the tube; this oriented matrix then served as a template for the regenerating neural elements.

In general, most studies have found that nerve regeneration is enhanced when both the proximal and distal ends of the severed nerve are secured within the opposite ends of a polymeric guidance channel. When nondegradable poly(vinyl chloride) tubes and the severed nerve ends were inserted in a variety of orientations, only specific orientations—when both ends of the nerve were within the tube and facing each other—produced successful regeneration [19]. When hollow fibers with selective permeability were used as guidance channels, enhanced regeneration was observed. Even when the distal end of the channel was capped, inhibiting interactions with the distal nerve stump, significant regeneration occurred [26], suggesting that the channel with walls of selective permeability permits exchange of critical nutrients and concentration of essential factors released by the proximal end.

The outcome of regeneration can also be effected by altering the environment within the channel prior to implantation. The influence of extracellular matrix (ECM) molecules on nerve regeneration within the channels is complex, and has not been clearly defined by any of the existing studies. Biodegradable channels filled with Type I collagen permitted nerve regeneration, but were inferior to autografts [21] or saline-filled channels [27] in the rat sciatic nerve, whereas other Type I collagen preparations were superior to autografts [21]. Laminin promotes the attachment and growth of neurites *in vitro* [28], and so is a logical choice for enhancing nerve regeneration *in vivo*. A laminin-rich gel (Matrigel) enhanced sciatic nerve regeneration through biodegradable nerve guidance channels [29] and silicone tubes [30]; empty biodegradable nerve guides were significantly better than laminin-filled guides after 6 weeks in the sciatic nerve of mice [20]. When the silicone tubes were filled with collagen gel ($\sim 1.5\,mg/mL$) or laminin gel (Matrigel) and then used to span a 4 mm gap in mouse sciatic nerves, the laminin-containing gels enhanced regeneration, apparently secondary to rapid infiltration by non-neuronal cells [30]. In permselective guidance channels composed of poly(ACN-*co*-VC), laminin- and collagen-containing gels impeded the regeneration process [27]. Treatment of collagen nerve conduits with laminin had no effect on reinnervation of severed sciatic nerves in the mouse [31]. Amnion membranes appear to influence the pattern of axon regrowth through silicone chambers [32]. In summary, it is clear that the environment within the nerve guide is important, but it is difficult to reconcile all of the available information.

Non-neuronal cells within the channel also influence the extent of regeneration. Permselective guidance channels composed of poly(acrylonitrile-*co*-vinyl chloride), with a molecular weight cut-off of 50,000 dalton, were filled with diluted Matrigel (70:30 DMEM:Matrigel) and either syngeneic or heterologous Schwann cells [33]. The extent of nerve regeneration, as determined by the number of myelinated axons, was inhibited by Matrigel alone (as described in the paragraph above) and by Matrigel with heterologous Schwann cells. Regeneration was enhanced by the addition of syngeneic cells; greater initial cell density led to greater numbers of myelinated axons. In all cases, however, the extent of regeneration was significantly less than that produced by sciatic nerve autografts. Although the mechanism of enhancement by Schwann cells is not known, several factors may contribute: (1) expression of neurotrophic factors by the Schwann cells; (2) expression of cell attachment factors; (3)

enhanced guidance of growing neurons due to the physical orientation of the Schwann cell cable, which forms in the first day following initiation of the culture in the tube; and (4) secretion of proteases or protease inhibitors that are essential for growth cone advancement.

14.3.3 Potential Extensions to Repair in Other Parts of the Nervous System

The previous sections illustrate the complexity of regeneration in the nervous system; the repair of structurally simple nervous tissue—such as a peripheral nerve—has proven to be difficult. It seems clear that biomaterials and tissue engineering will play a role in future treatments for repair in the nervous system. Even more sophisticated strategies will likely be needed for regeneration in other areas of the nervous system. But there are signs of progress in the use of materials for spinal cord repair [34] and for the use of stem cells for repair in the brain [35, 36].

References

1. Hunziker, E.B. and L.C. Rosenberg, Repair of partial-thickness defects in articular cartilage: cell recruitment from the synovial membrane. *Journal of Bone and Joint Surgery*, 1996, **78-A**(5), 721–733.
2. Hunziker, E.B., Growth-factor-induced healing of partial-thickness defects in adult articular cartilage. *Osteoarthritis and Cartilage*, 2001, **9**, 22–32.
3. Coffey, R.J., et al., Hepatic processing of transforming growth factor beta in the rat. *Journal of Clinical Investigation*, 1987, **80**, 750–757.
4. Bryant, S.J. and K.S. Anseth, Hydrogel properties influence ECM production by chondrocytes photoencapsulated in poly(ethylene glycol) hydrogels. *Journal of Biomedical Materials Research*, 2002, **59**(1), 63–72.
5. Saltzman, W.M., *Drug Delivery: Engineering Principles for Drug Therapy*. New York: Oxford University Press, 2001.
6. Butler, D.L., S.A. Goldstein, and F. Guilak, Functional tissue engineering: the role of biomechanics. *Journal of Biomechanical Engineering*, 2000, **122**, 570–575.
7. Goldstein, S.A., Tissue engineering: functional assessment and clinical outcome. *Annals of the New York Academy of Sciences*, 2002, **963**, 183–192.
8. Jones, I., L. Currie, and R. Martin, A guide to biological skin substitutes. *British Journal of Plastic Surgery*, 2002, **55**, 185–193.
9. Yannas, I. and J. Burke, Design of an artificial skin. I. Basic design principles. *Journal of Biomedical Materials Research*, 1980, **14**, 65–81.
10. Yannas, I., et al., Design of an artificial skin. II. Control of chemical composition. *Journal of Biomedical Materials Research*, 1980, **14**, 107–131.
11. Yannas, I., Use of artificial skin in wound management. *The Surgical Wound*, 1981, 171–190.
12. Yannas, I., et al., Wound tissue can utilize a polymeric template to synthesize a functional extension of skin. *Science*, 1982, **215**, 174–176.
13. Yannas, I., et al., Synthesis and characterization of a model extracellular matrix that induces partial regeneration of adult mammalian skin. *Proceedings of the National Academy of Sciences USA*, 1989, **86**, 933–937.

14. Murphy, G., D. Orgill, and I. Yannas, Partial dermal regeneration is induced by biodegradable collagen–glycosaminoglycan grafts. *Laboratory Investigation*, 1990, **63**, 305–313.

15. Schechner, J.S., et al., *In vivo* formation of complex microvessels lined by human endothelial cells in an immunodeficient mouse. *Proceedings of the National Academy of Sciences*, 2000, **97**(16), 9191–9196.

16. Hall, S.M., Regeneration in the peripheral nervous system. *Neuropathology and Applied Neurobiology*, 1989, **15**, 513–529.

17. Meek, M.F. and J.H. Coert, Clinical use of nerve conduits in peripheral-nerve repair: review of the literature. *Journal of Reconstructive Microsurgery*, 2002, **18**(2), 97–109.

18. Lundborg, G., et al., *In vivo* regeneration of cut nerves encased in silicone tubes. *Journal of Neuropathology and Experimental Neurology*, 1982, **41**(4), 412–422.

19. Scaravilli, F., The influence of distal environment on peripheral nerve regeneration across a gap. *Journal of Neurocytology*, 1984, **13**, 1027–1041.

20. Madison, R.D., et al., Peripheral nerve regeneration with entubulation repair: comparison of biodegradable nerve guides versus polyethylene tubes and the effects of a laminin-containing gel. *Experimental Neurology*, 1987, **95**, 378–390.

21. Rosen, J.M., et al., Artificial nerve graft using collagen as an extracellular matrix for nerve repair compared with sutured autograft in a rat model. *Annals of Plastic Surgery*, 1990, **25**, 375–387.

22. Williams, L.R., et al., Spatial-temporal progress of peripheral nerve regeneration within a silicone chamber: parameters for a bioassay. *Journal of Comparative Neurology*, 1983, **218**, 460–470.

23. Ramon y Cajal, S., *Degeneration and Regeneration of the Nervous System*. London: Oxford University Press, 1928.

24. Gutmann, E.L., et al., The rate of regeneration of nerve. *Journal of Experimental Biology*, 1942, **19**, 14–44.

25. Aebischer, P., V. Guenard, and R.F. Valentini, The morphology of regenerating peripheral nerves is modulated by the surface microgeometry of polymeric guidance channels. *Brain Research*, 1990, **531**, 211–218.

26. Aebischer, P., et al., Blind-ended semipermeable guidance channels support peripheral nerve regeneration in the absence of a distal nerve stump. *Brain Research*, 1988, **454**, 179–187.

27. Valentini, R., et al., Collagen- and laminin-containing gels impede peripheral nerve regeneration through semipermeable nerve guidance channels. *Experimental Neurology*, 1987, **98**, 350–356.

28. Sephel, G.C., B.A. Burrous, and H.K. Kleinman, Laminin neural activity and binding proteins. *Developmental Neuroscience*, 1989, **11**, 313–331.

29. Madison, R., et al., Increased rate of peripheral nerve regeneration using bioresorbable nerve guides and a laminin-containing gel. *Experimental Neurology*, 1985, **88**, 767–772.

30. Kjavin, I.J. and R.D. Madison, Peripheral nerve regeneration within tubular prostheses: effects of laminin and collagen matrices on cellular ingrowth. *Cells & Materials*, 1991, **1**, 17–28.

31. Navarro, X., et al., Effects of laminin on functional reinnervation of target organs by regenerating axons. *NeuroReport*, 1991, **2**, 37–40.

32. Danielson, N., et al., Rat amnion membrane matrix as a substratum for regenerating axons from peripheral and central neurons: effects in a silicone chamber model. *Developmental Brain Research*, 1988, **39**, 39–50.

33. Guenard, V., et al., Syngeneic Schwann cells derived from adult nerves seeded in semipermeable guidance channels enhance peripheral nerve regeneration. *Journal of Neuroscience*, 1992, **12**(9), 3310–3320.

34. Teng, Y.D., et al., Functional recovery following traumatic spinal cord injury mediated by a unique polymer scaffold seeded with neural stem cells. *Proceedings of the National Academy of Sciences*, 2002, **99**(5), 3024–3029.

35. Bjorklund, L.M., et al., Embryonic stem cells develop into functional dopaminergic neurons after transplantation in a Parkinson rat model. *Proceedings of the National Academy of Sciences*, 2002, **99**(4), 2344–2349.

36. Freed, C.R., Will embryonic stem cells be a useful source of dopamine neurons for transplant into patient with Parkinson's disease? *Proceedings of the National Academy of Sciences*, 2002, **99**(4), 1755–1757.

APPENDICES

Appendix A

Introduction to Polymers

> These arts open great gates of a future, promising to make the world plastic
> and to lift human life out of its beggary to a god-like ease and power.
>
> Ralph Waldo Emerson, "Works and Days," in *Society and Solitude* (1870).

Polymers are a class of chemicals that are distinguished by repetition. Polymer molecules are formed by bonding several (usually five or more) identical units into a common molecule. The individual unit of a polymer is called a monomer and an individual polymer molecule can contain many thousands of repeated monomer units. Some polymers occur naturally and occupy privileged positions within the described chemical universe: DNA, proteins such as collagen or immunoglobulin, and carbohydrates such as chitin are examples of naturally occurring polymers. Other polymers are produced synthetically and accordingly have lower stature but often higher value. Nylon, polyethylene, and polystyrene have become among the most common materials on earth.

A.1 Polymer Properties

Many of the useful characteristics of polymers arise from this repetitive structure. Polymers can be very large molecules, with molecular weights often exceeding 10^6 daltons, yet their chemical structure is frequently simple and monotonous. Consider a polymer formed by linkage of X units of monomer m:

$$m + m + m + \cdots \rightarrow m_x \qquad \text{(A-1)}$$

The overall chemical structure of this complex molecule can be written by reference to the structure of its monomer, signified here as m. This shortcut nomenclature works for some polymers but it cannot account for the complexity of most polymeric materials, which is enhanced by branching (because monomer units may be connected to each other through multiple sites, rather than just head-to-tail linear), by the presence of multiple monomers (because co-polymers contain more than one monomer unit linked in various combinations), by stereochemistry (because of chirality that exists in the polymer bonds that are formed), and by side-chain complexity (because some of the monomer units may be subsequently modified while others remain unchanged).

Likewise, the properties of polymers can sometimes by summarized simply, even though a complex mixture of properties is embodied in the material. Some of the basic methods for describing the characteristics of polymers are outlined in this section. Excellent books are available on the physics, chemistry, and properties of polymeric systems [1–3].

A.1.1 Molecular Weight Distributions

A polymeric material contains an uncountable number of individual polymer molecules. For simplicity, assume that the material contains only one type of polymer, P. Within the population of molecules are individuals that vary in length: that is, the number of monomers x that are bonded together (Equation A-1) to produce that individual molecule. If the molecular weight of the monomer m is M_1, the molecular weight of a individual molecule with x units is xM_1, or M_x.

The properties of a polymeric material often depend on the size of the individual molecules that comprise the material. Since most polymers are mixtures of individuals with different degrees of polymerization (x in Equation A-1), it is awkward (and difficult) to provide a complete description of the weights of all of the individual molecules. Instead, average molecular weights are defined. The average can be defined in several different ways. The number-average molecular weight $\overline{M}_n$ is based on the number of individuals that have a certain weight:

$$\overline{M}_n = \frac{\sum_x M_x N_x}{\sum_x N_x} \tag{A-2}$$

where N_x is the molar concentration of individual molecules that have x units. The weight-average molecular weight is based on the mass concentration of individuals that have a certain weight:

$$\overline{M}_w = \frac{\sum_x M_x c_x}{\sum_x c_x} = \frac{\sum_x M_x N_x N_x}{\sum_x M_x N_x} \tag{A-3}$$

where c_x is the concentration of the individual molecules that have x units (since $c_x = M_x N_x$).

A.2 Non-degradable Polymers

Among the many classes of polymeric materials now available for biomaterials, non-degradable, hydrophobic polymers are the most widely used. Silicone, polyethylene, polyurethanes, poly(methylmethacrylate), and poly(ethylene-*co*-vinyl acetate) account for the majority of polymeric materials currently used in clinical applications. Consider, for example, the tissue engineering applications listed in Table 1.2 of Chapter 1; many of these applications require a polymer that does not change substantially during the period of use. This section describes some of the most commonly used non-degradable polymers that are used as biomaterials.

A.2.1 Silicone Elastomers

Background. Elastomers of silicone are widely used as biomaterials. In general, silicone elastomers have excellent biocompatibility, inducing only a limited inflammatory response following implantation. In fact, until very recently, it was assumed that silicones were almost completely inert in biological systems. It is now known, however, that certain silicone polymers can provoke inflammatory and immune responses. The biological response to implanted silicone, and the variability of that response among individuals, continues to be the subject of debate.

Silicones, more correctly referred to as poly(siloxanes), are partially inorganic polymers with the general structure

$$\left[\begin{array}{c} R_1 \\ | \\ Si-O \\ | \\ R_2 \end{array} \right]_N \qquad (A\text{-}4)$$

They are usually prepared by hydrolysis of alkylsilicon or arylsilicone halides. Because of their chemical inertness, stability, and excellent mechanical properties, polysiloxanes are used in industrial applications as elastomers, sealants, coatings, lubricating oils, and hydraulic fluids. These polymers are characterized by high chain flexibility and unusually high oxygen permeability. Polysiloxanes are very stable toward hydrolysis, probably as a result of their hydrophobicity. The physical characteristics of polysiloxanes can be modified by varying the polymer molecular weight, degree of crosslinking, and chemical modification. Chemical modification commonly involves introducing substituents in place of one or both of the pendant methyl groups in the structure shown in Equation A-4.

Many of the silicone elastomers that are used in biomedical applications are produced by Dow Chemical Corporation under the trade name Silastic®. For example, a typical medical grade silicone (like Silastic MDX4–4210 medical grade elastomer) contains, after curing, crosslinked dimethylsiloxane polymer and silica for reinforcement. Silcones are also reinforced with PET (Dacron) fiber meshes for certain biomedical applications. For implantable medical devices, it is important to realize that the cured polymer contains residual catalysts and silicone crosslinkers, which are necessary for the polymerization.

Interesting polymers have been produced by copolymerization of siloxanes with other polymers. For example, dimethylsiloxane was copolymerized with ethylene oxide and methyl methacrylate to create a series of polymers with controlled permeability to hydrophilic or hydrophobic steroids, enhanced mechanical properties, and improved adhesion to tissues [4–6].

   Silicone matrix systems have good biocompatibility when implanted subcutaneously [7] or intercranially. Silicone has received FDA approval for many
biomedical applications, including breast prostheses and heart valve prostheses.

Biomedical applications.   *Drug delivery systems*—Silicone elastomers were first
used as the basis for controlled drug delivery systems in 1962, when Folkman
and Long discovered that low molecular weight compounds could diffuse, at a
controlled rate, through the walls of silicone tubing [7–9]. That observation led
to the development of several clinical products for controlled delivery of pharmaceutical agents. Most notably, the Population Council developed tubes of
Silastic (in this case, copolymers of dimethylsiloxane and methylvinylsiloxane)
for the controlled release of the contraceptive hormone levonorgestrel [10, 11].
Norplant devices, which provide reliable contraception for five years after
implantion into the forearm, have been extensively tested in women throughout the world and were approved for use in the United States in late 1990. By
December of 1992 over 600,000 Norplant systems had been implanted in
women in the United States [12]. Early surveys of a fraction of these users
suggested wide enthusiasm for the product [13].
   Silicone can also be formulated into a matrix with dispersed drug. These
matrices can provide a controlled release of small organic molecules, such as
steroids.
   Breast implants—Silicone elastomers are an important element in breast
prostheses. For example, a common type of breast implant is a silicone device
filled with a silicone gel. A possible problem with these devices is the rupture of
the outer layer of silicone, with subsequent leakage of the gel. This gel has been
associated with a variety of diseases. Breast implants based on silicone were
approved for use in humans over 30 years ago, but in a period before the FDA
had clear jurisdication over the approval of medical devices (that jursidication
was provided by the 1976 Medical Device Amendments to the Food, Drug,
and Cosmetic Act). Since that time, and following implantation in over 1
million women, there have been no definitive studies regarding the safety of
these devices. Based on the best information regarding risks and benefits, the
FDA announced in April of 1992 that breast implants filled with silicone gel
would be available only to women who agreed to participate in clinical studies
to evaluate the safety of the product [14]. The best scientific evidence provided
to date provides no link between breast implants and the development of
connective tissue diseases (such as rheumatoid arthritis and systemic lupus
erythematosus) [15], but the question of links between disease and long-term
exposure to implanted silicone remains unanswered [16].

A.2.2 Poly(ethylene-*co*-vinyl acetate)

Background.   Certain copolymers of ethylene and vinyl acetate, poly(ethylene-
co-vinyl acetate) (EVAc, Elvax®, Dupont Corporation), have exceptionally
good biocompatibility and are therefore widely used in implanted and topical

devices. The most commonly used copolymer contains 40% vinyl acetate and has the general structure

$$
\left[\begin{array}{cc} C - C \\ | \quad | \\ H_2 \quad H_2 \end{array} \right]_x \left[\begin{array}{cc} C - C \\ | \quad | \\ H_2 \quad O \\ \qquad | \\ \qquad C = O \\ \qquad | \\ \qquad CH_3 \end{array} \right]_y
\tag{A-5}
$$

The copolymer is synthesized by free radical polymerization from ethylene and vinyl acetate. The most commonly used EVAc (Elvax-40, DuPont) consists of approximately 40% vinyl acetate with a low degree of crystallinity (5–20%). EVAc is hydrophobic; it swells less than 0.8% in water [17].

Biomedical Applications. *Drug delivery systems*—Matrices of EVAc are among the most well-studied drug delivery systems for low molecular weight substances as well as macromolecules. Matrices composed of EVAc and protein can be fabricated by solvent evaporation or compression molding [18]. In solvent evaporation, EVAc, which has been extensively washed to remove low molecular weight oligomers and impurities, is dissolved in methylene choride. The protein of interest is lyophilized, ground, and sieved to a desired particle size range, and suspended in the polymer solution. The suspension is poured into a chilled mold and allowed to solidify. The matrix is then removed from the mold and dried at atmospheric pressure and $-4°C$ for 48 hr and then dried under vacuum at $20°C$ for 48 hr.

The biocompatibility of EVAc matrices has been studied quite extensively. When implanted in the cornea of rabbits—which is sensitive to edema, white-cell infiltration, and neovascularization associated with inflammation—washed EVAc caused no inflammation, whereas unwashed EVAc caused mild inflammation [19]. After seven months of subcutaneous implantion, only a thin capsule of connective tissue surrounded EVAc implants; no inflammation was present and the adjacent loose connective tissue was normal [20]. When implanted in the brains of rats, EVAc matrices produced only mild gliosis [21]. EVAc has shown good biocompatibility in humans over the years and has been approved by the FDA for use in a variety of implanted and topically applied devices.

EVAc has been used in the fabrication of a variety of devices for drug delivery. For example, EVAc was used by Alza in devices to deliver pilocarpine to the surface of the eye for glaucoma treatment (Ocusert®). Currently, EVAc is used in the Progestasert® intrauterine device for the delivery of contraceptive hormones to the female reproductive tract and as a rate-controlling membrane in a number of transdermal devices. Since EVAc is one of the most biocompatible of the polymers that have been tested as implant materials [22], it has been widely studied as a matrix for controlled drug delivery (see [23, 24] for reviews).

A.2.3 Polyurethanes

Polyurethanes were first suggested for use as biomaterials in 1967 [25]. Polyurethane materials have excellent mechanical properties, making them suitable for many different biomedical applications. Currently, a variety of polyurethanes are used in biomedical devices such as coatings for catheters and pacemaker leads (see Table A.1). Because of the long experience with implanted polyurethane devices, there is some interest in using polyurethane matrices to release peptide and protein drugs. The biocompatibility of biomedical polyurethanes appears to be determined by their purity, that is, the effectiveness of the removal from the polymer of catalyst residues and low molecular weight oligomers [26]. The surface properties of commercially available polyurethanes, which are critically important in determining biocompatibility, can vary considerably even among lots of the same commercially available preparation [27]. In some cases, most famously the breast prostheses coated with polyurethane foam, implanted polyurethanes have been reported to degrade into carcinogenic compounds such as toluenediamines [28, 29].

Synthesis.   Polyurethanes can be formed by reacting a bischloroformate with a diamine, for example:

$$Cl - \overset{\overset{\displaystyle O}{\|}}{C} - O - (CH_2)_2 - O - \overset{\overset{\displaystyle O}{\|}}{C} - Cl \; + \; H_2N - (CH_2)_6 - NH_2 \longrightarrow$$

$$\left[\overset{\overset{\displaystyle O}{\|}}{C} - O - (CH_2)_2 - O - \overset{\overset{\displaystyle O}{\|}}{C} - \underset{\underset{\displaystyle H}{|}}{N} - (CH_2)_6 - \underset{\underset{\displaystyle H}{|}}{N} \right]_n$$

$$(A\text{-}6)$$

or by reacting a diisocyanate with a dihydroxy compound, for example ethanediol and hexanediisocyanate:

$$HO - (CH_2)_2 - OH \; + \; O{=}C{=}N - (CH_2)_6 - N{=}C{=}O \longrightarrow$$

$$\left[\overset{\overset{\displaystyle O}{\|}}{C} - \underset{\underset{\displaystyle H}{|}}{N} - (CH_2)_6 - \underset{\underset{\displaystyle H}{|}}{N} - \overset{\overset{\displaystyle O}{\|}}{C} - O - (CH_2)_2 - O \right]_n$$

$$(A\text{-}7)$$

One of the most interesting and useful characteristics of polyurethanes involves block copolymers containing "hard" and "soft" segments to produce an elastomeric material. The production of these polyurethanes is a two-step process, where first an aromatic isocyanate-terminated polymer, in large excess, is reacted with a polyether or polyester containing terminal hydroxyl groups. The product of this reaction is chain extended with a diamine, producing a polymer with urea bonds, $-N-(C=O)-N-$, in addition to the urethane linkages, $-N-(C=O)-O-$. For example:

$$HO \sim\!\!\sim OH + O=C=N-Ar-N=C=O$$

Polyether or polyester

$$+ O=C=N-Ar-N=C=O + H_2N-R'-NH_2$$

"Hard" segment   "Soft" segment

(A-8)

For chain-extended polyurethane elastomers such as the one shown in Equation A-8, the "hard" segments tend to associate into crystalline domains while the soft segments, which form a continuous phase surrounding the discrete crystalline regions, remain amorphous. The utility of segmented polyurethanes like Lycra for biomedical applications such as the total artificial heart, catheters, heart valves, and pacemaker leads was first proposed by Boretos and Pierce [25]. Lycra, a linear segmented polyurethane, was developed by DuPont and is used to make the fiber Spandex. Ethicon manufactures a modified version of this polymer as Biomer. Biomer was used as the basis for the Jarvik-7 artificial heart, but Ethicon has removed Biomer from the general market because of concerns for legal liability [30].

Of the commonly used diisocyanates, 4,4′-diphenylmethane diisocyanate (MDI) forms a semicrystalline hard segment domain which apparently contributes to the excellent mechanical properties of the resulting polyurethane. Other diisocyanates such as 4,4′-dicyclohexylmethane diisocyanate do not crystallize, but still produce polyurethanes with good mechanical properties, probably because these hard segments produce more numerous and smaller microdomains than an MDI polyurethane with the same composition, leading to a more stabilized microstructure [31]. The chemistry of the chain extender can also affect the properties of the polymer. Diamines produce stronger polyurethanes than diols, because the resulting urea linkages within the hard segment participate in hydrogen bonding more readily than the urethane linkages (see Equation A-5). Unfortunately, polyurethanes chain-extended with diamines are more difficult to prepare because they do not dissolve easily in common solvents and, when the temperature is increased, they tend to decompose before they melt. The urea linkages in the diamine-extended polymers may be more susceptible to enzymatic degradation than urethane linkages, which would lead to unwanted degradation in the body [31]. When polyurethane polymer films were implanted subcutaneously in rats, polymers that were chain-extended with butanediol retained mechanical properties better than polymers chain-extended with ethylenediamine. In addition, polymers with MDI in the hard segment were more resistant to cracking and molecular weight changes than polymers with 4,4'-dicyclohexylmethane diisocyanate.

Polyurethanes can be surface-modified to produce materials that are resistant to thrombosis or that interact with cells and tissues in specific ways. Goodman et al. [32] used several different polyurethaneureas composed of hard segments of 4,4-methylene *bis*-phenyl diisocyanate and ethylene diamine with one of four different soft segments ($M_w \sim 1,000$, except PDMS $\sim 2,000$): hydroxybutyl-terminated poly(dimethyl siloxane) (PDMS), poly(ethylene oxide) (PEO), poly(tetramethylene oxide) (PTMO), and poly(propylene oxide) (PPO). The ratio of MDI/ED/soft segment was 2:1:1 for all of the polymers. Polyurethanes such as these can be modified (1) to add sulfonate groups by treating dissolved polymer (usually in DMF) with sodium hydride (NaH) to remove urethane hydrogen and propane sulfone producing $(CH_2)_3SO_3^-$ (this change makes the polymer more polar and it now swells considerably in water); (2) to add C_{18} alkyl groups by treating with NaH and octadecyl iodide ($C_{18}H_{37}I$) (this change makes the surface more hydrophobic [33, 34]; and (3) to add covalently bound RGD-containing peptides to the surface by treating with NaH and β-propiolactone to replace urethane hydrogen with ethyl carboxylate groups followed by coupling of a protected peptide by the N terminus, using the coupling reagent EDCI [32, 35–37].

Biomedical Applications.   Many polyurethenes for biomedical applications are available from commercial manufacturers (see Table A.1): Biomer (Ethicon) is composed primarily of methylene diphenylenediisocyanate, ethylene diamine, and polytetramethylene oxide (2:1:1), see [33]; Biomer and Pellethane were used in the artificial heart program at the University of Utah. Medtronics produces polyurethanes Biostable C-19 and Biostable C-36 using cyclohexane 1,4-diisocyanate, 1,6-hexanediol, and soft segments with 18 or 36 carbons.

Polyurethanes are considered non-degradable, but a recent and well-documented failure of a commonly used breast implant material was due to degradation of the polyurethane coating on the silicone prosthesis. The polyurethane coating on the Meme® implant (Surgitel, Racine, WI) degrades after several years of implantation, releasing small quantities of carcinogenic material (toluenediamine, TDA) [28]. In fact, reasonably high concentrations of TDA have been found in the urine and tissues of women undergoing removal of failing implants [29]. The ester bonds within the polyurethane are subject to hydrolysis within the body, eventually leading to breakdown of the polyurethane chains and physical degradation of the material.

The microscopic events that eventually lead to breakdown and degradation of implanted polyurethanes have been studied [38]. Following implantation, the polymer surface becomes coated with a layer of protein, which

Table A.1
Commercially Available Polyurethanes where the Chemical Structures are Known

Name	Supplier	Description	Structure	Advantage	Disadvantage
Angioflex	Abiomed (Danvers, MA)	Silicone–urethane copolymer	MDI–PTMEG BD–Sil	Good blood compatibility	Difficult to make
Biomer[a]	Ethicon (Somerville, NJ)	Aromatic co(polyetherurea)	MDI–PTMEG EDA	Outstanding flex endurance	Research use only
Bionate	Polymer Technology Group (Berkeley, CA)	Polycarbonate–urethane	Hydroxyl-terminated polycarbonate, aromatic diisocyanate, glycol	Oxidative stability	
BioSpan	Polymer Technology Group (Berkeley, CA)	Segmented polyurethane (replacement for Biomer)	MDI–PTMO mixed diamines	Excellent flex life	
Cardiothane	Kontron, Inc. (Everett, MA)	Silicone–urethane copolymer	MDI–PTMEG-BD–Sil	Good blood compatibility	Difficult to fabricate
Chronoflex	CardioTech International (Woburn, MA)	Aliphatic non-ether	HMDI–???–BD	Biostable	
Elasthane	Polymer Technology Group (Berkeley, CA)	Aromatic ether based	MDI–PTMO–BD	Replacement for Pellethane	
Hemothane	Sarns, Division of 3M (Ann Arbor, MI)	Similar to Biomer	Similar to Biomer	Similar to Biomer	Internal use only
Mitrathane	PolyMedica	Similar to Biomer	Similar to Biomer	Similar to Biomer	Internal use only
Pellethane[a]	Dow Chemical (La Porte, TX)	Aromatic ether-based	MDI–PTMEG BD	Thermoplastic elastomer	Microcracks
Surethane	Cardiac Control (Palm Coast, FL)	Purified Lycra	MDI–PTMEG EDA	Similar to Biomer	Microcracks
Tecoflex	Thermedics (Woburn, MA)	Aliphatic ether-based	HMDI–PTMEG BD	Thermoplastic elastomer	Microcracks

Some of the information revised from [30].

[a]Withdrawn from market.

MDI (methylenebisphenyldiisocyanate (aromatic); PTMEG (polyoxytetramethylenether glycol); PTMO (polyoxytetramethyleneoxide); BD (butanediol); HMD (hydrogenated MDI (cycloaliphatic)); EDA (ethylenediamine). Other commercially available polymers have been investigated for possible use: Lykra Spandex and Tecoflex. Structure and composition of these polymers are discussed in [86].

enhances the adhesion of macrophages. The activated macrophages release oxidative factors, such as peroxide and superoxide anion, which accelerate chemical degradation of the polymer. The complement protein C3bi appears to be critical in the adhesion and activation of phagocytic cells [39].

A.2.4 Others

Polyethylene, Polypropylene, and Polystyrene. Several other common industrial polymers are also used in biomedical applications [40]. Because of its low cost and easy processibility, polyethylene is frequently used in the production of catheters. High-density polyethylene is used to produce hip prostheses, where durability of the polymer is critical. Polypropylene, which has a low density and high chemical resistance, is frequently employed in syringe bodies, external prostheses, and other non-implanted medical applications. Polystyrene is used routinely in the production of tissue culture dishes, where dimensional stability and transparency are important. Styrene–butadiene copolymers or acrylonitrile–butadiene–styrene copolymers are used to produce opaque, molded items for perfusion, dialysis, syringe connections, and catheters.

Poly(tetrafluoroethylene). Poly(tetrafluoroethylene) (PTFE), more commonly known as Teflon$^{®}$ (DuPont) and expanded PTFE (Goretex$^{®}$), is found in vascular grafts. The polymer (Equation A-9) has exceptionally good resistance to chemicals.

$$\left[\begin{array}{cc} F & F \\ | & | \\ -C-C- \\ | & | \\ F & F \end{array}\right]_n \tag{A-9}$$

Poly(vinyl chloride) and Poly[acrylonitrile-*co*-(vinyl chloride)]. Poly(vinyl chloride) has excellent resistance to abrasion, good dimensional stability, and chemical resistance; therefore it is often used in medical tubing and catheter tubes. Poly[acrylonitrile-*co*-(vinyl chloride)]

$$\left[\begin{array}{cc} H & H \\ | & | \\ -C-C- \\ | & | \\ H & Cl \end{array}\right]_x \left[\begin{array}{cc} H & H \\ | & | \\ -C-C- \\ | & | \\ H & C\equiv N \end{array}\right]_y \tag{A-10}$$

has been used to make semipermeable membranes, and is often used in the construction of hollow fibers.

Poly(ethylene terephthalate). A commonly used linear polyester is poly(ethylene terephthlate) (PET), which is synthesized by condensation of terephthalic acid and ethylene glycol and produced under the tradename Dacron.

$$
\left[\begin{array}{c} \overset{O}{\underset{\|}{C}}-\hspace{-4pt}\left\langle\text{benzene ring}\right\rangle\hspace{-4pt}-\overset{O}{\underset{\|}{C}}-O-\overset{H}{\underset{H}{C}}-\overset{H}{\underset{H}{C}}-O \end{array}\right] \qquad \text{(A-11)}
$$

Woven PET fibers are used as vascular grafts and as a reinforcement for a variety of other materials, including laryngeal and esophogeal prostheses.

Poly(methyl methacrylate). Poly(methyl methacrylate) (PMMA) is another vinyl polymer, prepared in large quantities commercially using free radical polymerization:

$$
\left[\begin{array}{cc} H & CH_3 \\ | & | \\ C & C \\ | & | \\ H & C=O \end{array}\right]^{N} \\ \begin{array}{c} | \\ O \\ | \\ CH_3 \end{array} \qquad \text{(A-12)}
$$

PMMA has exceptionally good optical properties; its transparency have made it a popular substitute for glass in applications where breakage must be avoided (Plexiglass). It has a variety of industrial uses including automotive parts and glazings. PMMA was the first implanted synthetic polymeric biomaterial, since it was used as a hip prosthesis in 1947 (see USP XVIII, *The Pharmacopia of the USA* (18th revision), U.S. Pharmacopoeial Convention, Rockville, MD, September 1, 1980). Poly(methyl methacrylate) is currently used in orthopedic applications as bone cement, and in intraocular lenses. More recently, PMMA has been suggested for use as a drug delivery vehicle.

A.3 Biodegradable Polymers

Polymers that slowly dissolve following implantation into the body have many potential uses. A variety of biodegradable polymers have therefore been synthesized and characterized. The physical process of dissolution of a polymer matrix or microsphere, in which a solid material slowly losses mass and eventually disappears, is called *bioerosion*. The mechanism of bioerosion may be simple: for example, the solid polymer may erode by dissolution of the individual polymer chains within the matrix. On the other hand, in many cases the polymer chains within the matrix must change to permit bioerosion. For example, the molecular weight of the polymer may decrease within the matrix following placement within the biological environment. This process, called *biodegradation*, may occur enzymatically, relying on catalysts present within the environment or embedded within the polymer itself, or hydrolytically, if polymers that are susceptible to hydrolytic breakdown are used. As biodegradation proceeds, the molecular weight of the polymer decreases. When the constituent polymer molecules become sufficiently small, they dissolve and the polymer matrix erodes. This process is described in more detail in [41].

This section reviews the characteristics of several families of biodegradable polymers. Readers interested in more details on the synthesis and chemistry of these classes of materials should consult the references provided, or general texts on biodegradable polymers [42].

A.3.1 Polyesters

Polylactide, polyglycolide, and copolymers of lactide/glycolide are among the most commonly used biomaterials for drug delivery and tissue engineering. The interest in these materials has resulted from several characteristics: (1) they break down to naturally occurring metabolites; (2) materials with a variety of useful properties can be obtained by copolymerization of the two monomers; (3) degradation requires only water; and (4) early development of successful suture materials based on these polymers has led to a great deal of experience with these materials in humans, so that their safety is now well documented.

The first synthetic absorbable suture was made from a homopolymer of glycolic acid by Davis & Geek Co. and manufactured under the tradename Dexon (1970). This suture was followed by a second material produced by Ethicon Inc. in 1974, a copolymer of lactide and glycolide known as polyglactine 910 or Vicryl. Both Vicryl and Dexon are made from polymer fibers which are braided to produce a suture. In addition, Vicryl is Teflon-coated for increased smoothness. When used as a suture, Vicryl maintains 50% of its tensile strength for 30 d, compared to 25 d for Dexon, 5–6 d for catgut, and 20 d for chromic catgut. Since their introduction as suture materials these polymers have been used extensively in biomaterials, particularly as drug delivery devices.

Synthesis and Characterization. The polyesters of lactic acid and glycolic acid have the chemical structures

$$\left[\begin{array}{c} O\ \ H \\ \| \ \ \ | \\ -C-C-O- \\ | \\ H \end{array}\right] \qquad \left[\begin{array}{c} O\ \ H \\ \| \ \ \ | \\ -C-C-O- \\ | \\ CH_3 \end{array}\right] \qquad (A-13)$$

Poly(glycolic acid)   Poly(lactic acid)

These biodegradable polyesters can be synthesized by direct polycondensation of lactic and glycolic acid, in which case only low molecular weight polymers are produced which are called poly(lactic acid) (PLA) and poly(glycolic acid) (PGA). Higher molecular weight polymers can be obtained by ring-opening melt polycondensation of cyclic diesters:

$$(A\text{-}14)$$

In that case, the following homopolymers are produced

Poly(L-lactide), PLLA   Poly(D, L-lactide), PDLA   Poly(glycolide), PGA

$$(A\text{-}15)$$

in addition to the copolymer indicated in Equation A-14. Properties of PLA/PGA polymers and copolymers are the subject of several recent reviews [43, 44]. Several groups have studied the synthesis and physical characteristics of this family of polymers in detail [55].

Polymers of ε-caprolactone, a biodegradable polyester with many similarities to the PLA/PGA family, are also useful in drug delivery [45]. The general structure of poly(ε-caprolactone) is

$$(A\text{-}16)$$

This polymer can be produced by a variety of mechanisms, including anionic, cationic, coordination, and radical polymerization [45].

While the copolymers of lactide and glycolide are extremely useful, they are difficult to derivatize. To overcome this limitation, copolymers of

L-lactide and L-lysine have also been produced [46]. These polymers have the structure

$$(A\text{-}17)$$

and might be useful because other functional groups, like peptides, can be coupled to the polymer through the primary amine on the lysine.

When implanted into the bones or soft tissues of rats, pellets of PLA, PLG, and copolymers degrade at different rates [47]. The homopolymers PLA and PGA degrade slowly in tissue, taking many months to disappear (Table A.2). Copolymers degrade more rapidly, probably due to their decreased crystallinity. This characteristic of LA/GA copolymers, that the physical properties can be adjusted by altering the copolymerization ratio, is important in the design of biomaterials. Amorphous polymers may be more suitable for applications where more rapid mass loss is important, or where ease of dispersion and diffusion through the polymer is essential, as in drug delivery. More crystalline polymers, on the other hand, may be more suitable for applications where the polymer must have increased physical strength.

In general, polymers of ε-caprolactone degrade more slowly than comparable lactide or glycolide polymers, making them particularly well suited for long-term drug delivery applications. Alternatively, copolymerization of ε-caprolactone with other monomers or polymers, including lactide and glycolide, results in more rapidly degrading materials.

Biomedical Applications. The first reported biomedical applications of poly(lactic acid) polymers involved use as sutures and prosthetics [48]. In the 1960s American Cyanamid developed synthetic, degradable sutures composed of PGA [49], while Ethicon developed similar materials involving PGA and PLA [50, 51].

In the early 1970s, patents for polylactide/drug mixtures were awarded to DuPont [52, 53]. The first applications for controlled drug delivery involved the release of narcotic antagonists from poly(lactic acid) films [54]. Poly(L(+)-lactic acid) was used to deliver contraceptive steroids [56], and particles of poly(d,l-lactide-*co*-glycolide) (25:75) were used to deliver an antimalarial drug to mice, providing 14 weeks of protection against malarial challenge [57]. Microspheres of poly(d,l-lactic acid) were used to deliver the contraceptive steroid norethisterone to baboons, inhibiting ovulation for six months [58]. In the last 25 years, many different groups have evaluated the use of copolymers of lactide and glycolide for the release of small and large molecules. A product based on this technology is currently available in the United States: Lupron

Table A.2
Characteristics of Biodegradable Polyesters

Material	Molecular weight	$T_g(°C)$	$T_m(°C)$	Crystallinity (%)	Approximate degradation time (month) [Half-life for degradation, from [47]]
Poly(L-lactic acid)	2,000	40	140		
Poly(L-lactide)	50,000 or 100,000	60–67	170–180	37	18–24 [6.5]
Poly(L-lactide-*co*-glycolide) 90:10	N.R.*	~65	~170	22	
Poly(L-lactide-*co*-glycolide) 80:20	N.R.	~65	~120	8	
Poly(L-lactide-*co*-glycolide) 70:30	N.R.	58	None	0	[0.6]
Poly(L-lactide-*co*-glycolide) 50:50	N.R.	~65	None	0	[0.2]
Poly(L-lactide-*co*-glycolide) 30:70	N.R.	~65	None	0	[0.6]
Poly(L-lactide-*co*-glycolide) 20:80	N.R.	~60	~170	20	
Poly(L-lactide-*co*-glycolide) 10:90	N.R.	~60	~205	40	
Poly(glycolide)	50,000	36	210–220	50	2–4 [5]
Poly(D,L-lactide)	N.R.	52–59	None		12–16
Poly(D,L-lactide-*co*-glycolide) 85:15	232,000	45–49	None		5
Poly(D,L-lactide-*co*-glycolide) 75:25	63,000	48	None		
Poly(D,L-lactide-*co*-glycolide) 50:50	12,000–98,000	40–47	None		2
Poly(D,L-lactide-*co*-glycolide) 25:75	N.R.	60	None		
Poly(glycolide)	50,000	36	210–220	50	
Poly(ε-caprolactone)	5,000–100,000	−60	59–64	40–80**	30

Data collected from recent reviews [43–45].

*N.R. = Not reported.

**Crystallinity varies with molecular weight, with higher molecular weights exhibiting the lowest crystallinity.

Depot for endometriosis and prostate cancer. Many other products are under development.

Since PLA and PGA degrade to molecules that are environmentally safe, they were proposed for agricultural applications such as the sustained release of pesticides [59].

A.3.2 Copolymers of Methyl Vinyl Ether and Maleic Anhydride

To control the release of drugs from an eroding or degrading matrix, the erosion or degradation process must occur in an orderly, reproducible manner. Most materials, such as the biodegradable polyesters discussed in the previous section, erode in a disorderly pattern: defects, cracks, and holes that initially appear throughout the material increase in size with time, permitting penetration of water into the matrix and, eventually, loss of mechanical integrity.

To provide better control of polymer matrix erosion, a more orderly degradation and erosion process is needed. In an effort to achieve this goal, materials that erode heterogeneously have been produced. In particular, for materials that erode from the surface only, the kinetics of dissolution and the release of incorporated drugs can be precisely controlled. The first surface-eroding bioerodible polymer formulation was produced at Alza Corporation in the 1970s; it was a copolymer of methyl vinyl ether and maleic anhydride [60]

$$\text{H}_2\text{C}=\text{C}-\text{O}-\text{CH}_3 + \quad \cdots \quad \rightarrow \quad \cdots \quad \text{(A-18)}$$

where the reaction product on the right was obtained after partial esterification. When placed in an aqueous environment, the carboxylic acid groups on the polymer become ionized and the polymer becomes water-soluble. When a matrix of this polymer is placed in water, only the carboxylic acids at the polymer–water interface become ionized. Erosion of the polymer is therefore confined to the polymer surface. The rate of erosion of devices fabricated from these copolymers depends strongly on pH, with the rate increasing as the pH drops. Unfortunately, the erosion products from devices composed of this polymer are macromolecules and are therefore not easily metabolized or excreted by the body.

A.3.3 Poly(ortho esters)

The first poly(ortho ester) for biomedical applications was produced by Choi and Heller at Alza Corporation in the 1970s, and was given the tradename Alzamer®. When placed in an aqueous environment, the polymer degrades to produce a diol and a lactone, which is rapidly converted to γ-hydroxybutyric acid:

$$(A-19)$$

This degradation process is autocatalytic, since the γ-hydroxybutyric acid that is produced catalyzes the hydrolysis reaction. To prevent abrupt degradation and erosion, a basic compound must be incorporated into the polymer. For example, sodium bicarbonate can be incorporated into a polymeric device composed of Alzamer to control the rate of polymer degradation and erosion. Although the polymer has been used for a number of drug delivery applications, it is difficult to produce and requires addition of significant amounts of a basic chemical to prevent uncontrolled degradation [61].

Several improvements on the design and synthesis of poly(ortho esters) have been reported over the last twenty years. One of the most useful of these polymers is shown in Equation (3–7).

$$(A-20)$$

The poly(ortho ester) shown on the left-hand side of Equation A-20 can be synthesized under milder conditions than those required for Alzamer. Since crosslinked polymeric drug delivery devices are usually fabricated by mixing a prepolymer and a diol under mild curing ($\sim 40°C$), care must be taken when using drugs with reactive hydroxyl groups. Most recently, another group of poly(ortho ester) materials was synthesized [62]:

$$
\left[\begin{array}{c} R \quad O{-}CH_2 \\ \diagdown C \diagup \quad | \\ O \diagup \diagdown O{-}CH{-}(CH_2)_4 \end{array}\right]_n \xrightarrow{H_2O}
$$

$$
\begin{array}{c}
O \qquad H_2 \ OH \qquad\qquad OH \\
\| \qquad | \quad | \qquad\qquad | \\
R{-}C{-}O{-}C{-}C{-}(CH_2)_3{-}CH_2 \\
+ \\
OH \ OH \qquad\qquad OH \qquad\qquad O \\
| \quad | \qquad\qquad | \qquad\qquad \| \\
H_2C{-}C{-}(CH_2)_3{-}CH_2 + R{-}C{-}OH \\
+ \\
\qquad\qquad\qquad O \\
\qquad\qquad\qquad \| \\
OH \ OH \qquad\qquad O{-}C{-}R \\
| \quad | \qquad\qquad | \\
H_2C{-}C{-}(CH_2)_3{-}CH_2
\end{array}
$$

$$\text{(A-21)}$$

This polymer is an ointment at room temperature, which may make it appropriate for a variety of topical and peridontal applications. Since the polymer is a viscous liquid at room temperature, proteins and other labile molecules can be mixed into the polymer without using solvents or high temperatures.

A.3.4 Poly-anhydrides

Hydrolysis is the most common mechanism of polymer degradation in biomaterials. Of the linkages that commonly occur in polymers, the anhydride linkage is one of the least stable in the presence of water. In fact, polyanhydride polymers are so senstive to water that they are unsuitable for many potential applications. However, the potential for rapid hydrolysis of the polymer backbone makes anhydride-based polymers attractive candidates for biodegradable materials.

Because of the instability of the anhydride bond in the presence of water, special properties are required for stable polyanhydride devices. A critical element in the development of polyanhydride biomaterials is the need to control hydrolysis within a polymeric device. To obtain implants where hydrolysis is confined to the surface of the polymer, hydrophobic monomers can be polymerized, via anhydride linkages, to produce a polymer that resists water penetration yet degrades into low molecular weight oligomers at the polymer/water interface. By modulating the relative hydrophobicity of the matrix, which can be achieved by appropriate selection of monomers, the rate of degradation can then be adjusted. For example, copolymers of sebacic acid, a hydrophilic monomer, with carboxyphenoxypropane, a hydrophobic monomer, yield

(A-22)

Polymers prepared with different copolymerization ratios can be used to produce implants that degrade in controlled fashion. For more information, recent reviews describe the development, characterization, and applications of polyanhydride polymers [63, 64].

A.3.5 Poly(amino acids)

A common strategy in the design of biodegradable polymers for medical applications has been to use naturally occuring monomers, with the hope that these polymers will degrade into non-toxic components. For example, poly(lactide-*co*-glycolide) degrades into lactic and glycolic acid, which are commonly occurring metabolites. Amino acids are an obvious choice as monomers for the production of new polymeric biomaterials; the large number of structurally related amino acids should lead to a correspondingly wide variety of new materials. Unfortunately, amino acids polymerized by conventional methods usually yield materials that are extremely antigenic and exhibit poor mechanical properties, making it difficult to engineer suitable medical devices.

Several approaches have been developed for producing biodegradable materials using amino acids as starting materials. A few amino acids, such as glutamic acid and lysine, can be modified through their side chains to produce polymers with different mechanical properties. Copolymers of L-glutamic acid and γ-ethyl L-glutamate have been used to release a variety of drugs; variation of the ratio of monomers in the polypeptide influences the rate of degradation of the resulting polymer [65]. Because of the stability of the peptide bond in water, the biodegradation of these implants occurs by dissolution of intact polymer chains and subsequent enzymatic hydrolysis in the liver.

Alternatively, amino acids can be polymerized by linkages other than the conventional peptide bond, yielding pseudopoly(amino acids) [66]. For example, the amino acid serine can be used to produce poly(serine ester), poly(serine imine), or conventional polyserine:

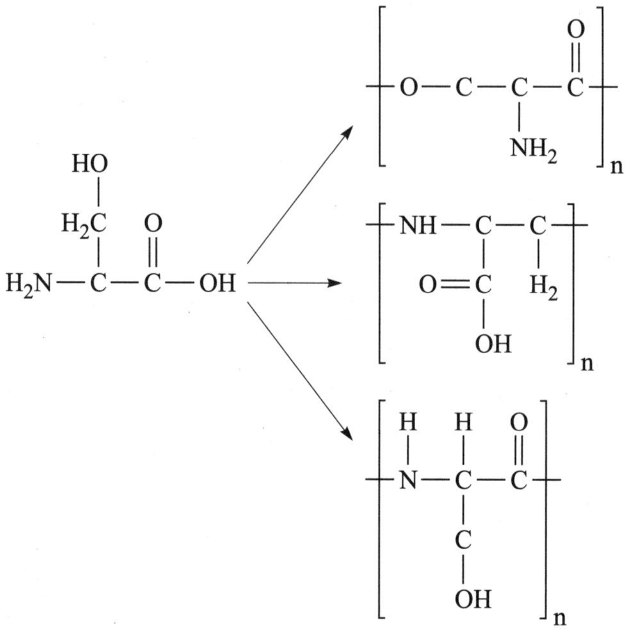

$$
\begin{array}{ccc}
\text{HO} & & \\
| & & \\
\text{H}_2\text{C} & \text{O} & \\
| & || & \\
\text{H}_2\text{N}-\text{C}-\text{C}-\text{OH} & \longrightarrow &
\end{array}
\quad
\left[\begin{array}{c}
\qquad\qquad \text{O} \\
\qquad\qquad || \\
-\text{O}-\text{C}-\text{C}-\text{C}- \\
\qquad | \\
\qquad \text{NH}_2
\end{array}\right]_n
$$

(A-23)

$$
\left[\begin{array}{c}
-\text{NH}-\text{C}-\text{C}- \\
\quad | \quad | \\
\quad \text{O}=\text{C} \quad \text{H}_2 \\
\quad | \\
\quad \text{OH}
\end{array}\right]_n
$$

$$
\left[\begin{array}{c}
\text{H} \quad \text{H} \quad \text{O} \\
| \quad\; | \quad\; || \\
-\text{N}-\text{C}-\text{C}- \\
\quad\; | \\
\quad\; \text{C} \\
\quad\; | \\
\quad\; \text{OH}
\end{array}\right]_n
$$

A.3.6 Phosphorus-Containing Polymers

Polyphosphates and Polyphosphonates, Polyphosphazenes.   Polyphosphazenes have the general structure

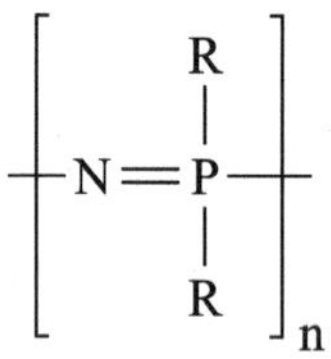

$$
\left[\begin{array}{c}
\text{R} \\
| \\
-\text{N}=\text{P}- \\
| \\
\text{R}
\end{array}\right]_n
$$

(A-24)

Polymers with a variety of chemical, physical, and biological properties can be produced by varying the side groups attached to the phosphorus in the polymer backbone. Different polymers are usually produced by performing substitution reactions on the base polymer, poly(dichlorophosphazene), for example:

$$(A-25)$$

This basic structure provides for considerable flexibility in the design of biomaterials, as described in a recent review [67]. By selection of the side groups on the polymer chain, both hydrophobic and hydrophilic polymers can be produced. Hydrophobic polyphosphazenes may be useful as the basis of implantable biomaterials such as heart valves. The hydrophilic polymers can be used to produce materials with a hydrophilc surface or, when the polymer is so hydrophilic that it dissolves in water, crosslinked to produce hydrogels or solid implants. In addition, a variety of bioactive compounds can be linked to polyphosphazene molecules, allowing the creation of bio-active water-soluble macromolecules or polymer surfaces with biological activity.

A.3.7 Polycarbonates and Polyiminocarbonates

Many of the materials with good biocompatibility have poor processibility or poor mechanical strength. In an effort to design new classes of biodegradable materials with improved physical properties, it was observed that polycarbonates have excellent mechanical strength and are easily processed, but do not degrade under physiological conditions [68]. To prepare polymers with the good mechanical properties of polycarbonates, investigators produced polyiminocarbonates based on bisphenol A:

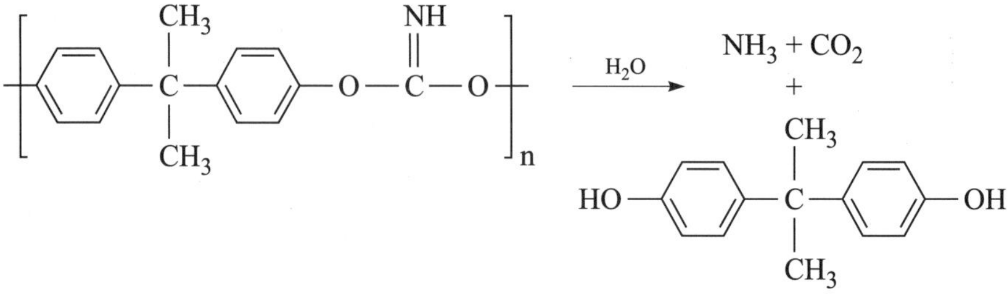

(A-26)

which differ from the comparable bisphenol A-based polycarbonate only in the replacement of the carbonyl oxygen in the polycarbonate by an imino group. The presence of this imino group decreases the stability of the polymer in water, with hydrolytic biodegradation producing ammonia, carbon dioxide, and the biphenol.

Several other structurally similar polymers have been prepared from biphenols with less toxicity than bisphenol A. For example, derivatives of the amino acid tyrosine have been used to produce polyiminocarbonates that have good mechanical properties, such as poly(desaminotyrosyl-tyrosine hexyl ester iminocarbonate) [69]:

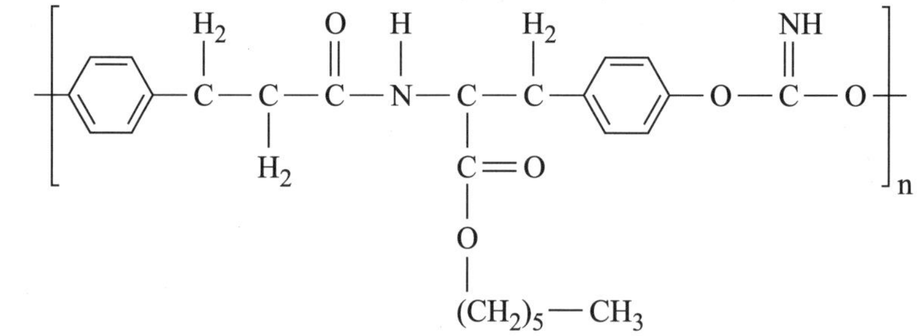

(A-27)

A similar approach can also be used to produce a polycarbonate from derivatives of the dipeptide of tyrosine [70]:

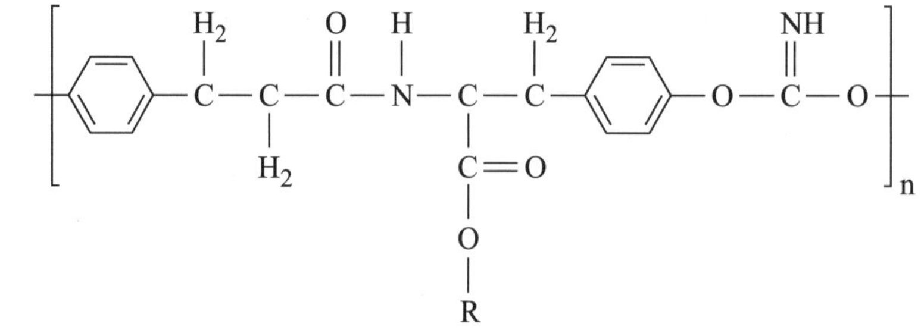

(A-28)

where the properties of the final polymer can be modified by changing the pendant R group in Equation A-28. For example, the length of the pendant chain influences the rate of hydrolysis, with shorter chains permitting more rapid hydrolysis. The hexyl ester is indicated in Equation A-27, but other polymers can also be obtained in the polyiminocarbonate form.

When disks produced from the hexyl esters of the polymers indicated in Equations A-27 and A-28 were implanted subcutaneously in rats, mild tissue responses were observed, comparable to the response produced by implantation of PLA or polyethylene disks [71]. These materials are being evaluated for orthopedic applications [72].

A.3.8 Polydioxanone

Polydioxanone (PDS) was produced in the early 1980s as an absorbable suture material [73]:

$$\left[\begin{array}{c} \quad\ \text{H}\ \ \ \text{H} \quad\quad\ \text{H}\ \ \ \text{O} \\ \quad\ |\ \ \ \ | \quad\quad\ \ |\ \ \ \ \| \\ \text{--O--C--C--O--C--C--} \\ \quad\ |\ \ \ \ | \quad\quad\ \ | \\ \quad\ \text{H}\ \ \ \text{H} \quad\quad\ \text{H} \end{array} \right]_n \qquad (\text{A-29})$$

PDS is produced by polymerization of para-dioxanone. The polymer has unusally high flexibility and, unlike copolymers of lactic and glycolic acid, can be used to produce a variety of monofilament sutures. Since PDS is a polyester, like PLA and PGA, the polymer chains break down by hydrolysis. Currently, PDS is also used in orthopedic applications (Orthosorb®) as a fixation element for bone repair.

A.4 Water-Soluble Polymers

The previous two sections reviewed some of the characteristics of polymers that, in general, are not soluble in water and therefore are typically used as solid materials: fibers, matrices, microspheres, or foams. Water-soluble polymers also are useful as biomaterials. They can be used in their molecular, water-soluble form as agents to modify other materials or as solid, dissolvable matrices (as in the example of copolymers of methyl vinyl ether and maleic anhydride). Alternatively, water-soluble polymers may be crosslinked, by chemical or physical means, into solid materials that swell in water but do not dissolve.

A.4.1 Naturally Occurring Polymers

Sacharrides. Because of their structural diversity, and the opportunity to create a variety of linkages between monomer units, polysaccharides are among the most diverse and important polymers in nature. Consider, for example, the structural similarities and differences in the disaccharides sucrose and lactose:

Sucrose (glucose-α (1, 2)-fructose) Lactose (galactose-β (1, 4)-glucose)

$$(A\text{-}30)$$

Even these disaccharides, with similar molecular composition, have significant chemical differences: here, the fructose unit of sucrose is an example of a five-carbon sugar (pentose); the linkages of the monosaccharides occur between different carbons in sucrose and lactose; and the stereochemistry of the linkage between the sugar units is different. Branched polymers are also common among polysaccharides because of the potential reactivity of all of the carbons within the saccharide ring. Because of this inherent flexibility in polysaccharide chemistry, it is possible to assemble a diverse group of macromolecules; these polymers have diverse functions in nature, serving as structural elements in cells, as energy storage, and as cell–cell recognition molecules. This range of structure and function also provides the opportunity to use polysaccharides as natural and versatile components of biomaterials.

Cellulose is the most abundant organic compound on earth; half of all the organic carbon is in cellulose [74]. Cellulose is a polymer of glucose, with all of the glucose residues connected by β-(1,4) linkages:

$$(A\text{-}31)$$

Because this structural unit is stabilized by hydrogen bonds between the adjacent hexoses, cellulose forms a long straight polymer. Fibrils with high tensile strength can be formed by hydrogen binding between chains that are aligned together.

Chitin, the second most abundant organic compound, is similar to cellulose, except that it is composed of N-acetylglucosamine in a β-(1,4) linkage. (The chitin structure can be recovered from Equation 4-2 by replacing the —OH at carbon 2 with an —NH—CO—CH$_3$.) Because chitin is readily available and occurs naturally in many insects and marine organisms, it is a popular component of cosmetic and health care products. The Japanese Ministry of Health and Welfare approved chitosan as an ingredient for hair care products in 1986, carboxymethyl chitosan as a skin care product in 1987, and chitin nonwoven fabric as a skin substitute in 1988 [75].

Dextran is composed entirely of glucose residues; it is used as a storage polysaccharide in yeasts and bacteria. The linkages in dextran are almost exclusively α-1,6, with an occasional α-1,2, α-1,3, and α-1,4 for branching. The α-1,6 arrangement leads to an open helix confirmation:

$$ \text{(A-32)} $$

Ficoll is a synthetic polymer of sucrose. *Alginate* is a linear polysaccharide from marine organisms, consisting of D-mannuronic and L-guluronic acid residues. Alginate has the important property that it forms a gel in the presence of bivalent cations such as Ca^{++}.

Proteins.   *Collagen*—The chemistry and physical structure of the extracellular matrix protein collagen are discussed in Chapter 6.

A.4.2 Polylysine and Poly(glutamic acid)

$$ \text{(A-33)} $$

Lysine   Glutamic acid

A.4.3 Acrylates and Acrylamides

Background.   Synthetic hydrogels have been frequently used in biomedical applications because of the similarity of their physical properties to those of living tissues [76]. The most widely used synthetic hydrogels are polymers of acrylic acid, acrylamide, and 2-hydroxyethyl methacrylate (HEMA):

Poly(acrylic acid)   Polyacrylamide   Poly(HEMA)

$$
\left[\begin{array}{c} \text{H} \ \ \text{H} \\ |\ \ \ \ | \\ \text{C}-\text{C} \\ |\ \ \ \ | \\ \text{H} \ \ \text{C}=\text{O} \\ | \\ \text{OH} \end{array}\right]_N
\ \ \
\left[\begin{array}{c} \text{H} \ \ \text{H} \\ |\ \ \ \ | \\ \text{C}-\text{C} \\ |\ \ \ \ | \\ \text{H} \ \ \text{C}=\text{O} \\ | \\ \text{NH}_2 \end{array}\right]_N
\ \ \
\left[\begin{array}{c} \text{H} \ \ \text{CH}_3 \\ |\ \ \ \ | \\ \text{C}-\text{C} \\ |\ \ \ \ | \\ \text{H} \ \ \text{C}=\text{O} \\ | \\ \text{O} \\ | \\ \text{CH}_2 \\ | \\ \text{CH}_2 \\ | \\ \text{HO} \end{array}\right]_N
$$

(A-34)

For biomedical applications, the most frequently encountered synthetic hydrogel is poly(2-hydroxyethyl methacrylate) (pHEMA). The characterization and applications of pHEMA have been recently reviewed [77]. Both HEMA and pHEMA are easy and inexpensive to produce. Because of the primary alcohol, the monomer or polymer can be functionalized. In addition, HEMA can be copolymerized with other acrylic or methacrylic derivatives, as well as with other vinyl monomers, resulting in hydrogels with a variety of chemical and physical properties. HEMA has low toxicity in animals, but some preparations can produce local irritation, probably due to the presence of contaminants. PHEMA is among the most biocompatible of the synthetic polymers; implants of pHEMA produce minimal local reaction, and the polymer resists degradation in tissues.

Copolymerization of HEMA with small amounts of methacrylic acid (MAA) (1 to 2 mol %) increases its ability to swell in aqueous urea solutions [78].

Biomedical Applications.   PHEMA has been used extensively in ophthalmic applications as a material for contact or intraocular lenses. In general, cells cannot attach or spread on a pure pHEMA surface. This observation has been used to examine the role of attachment and spreading on cell growth [79, 80] and cell motility. This resistance to cell attachment may underlie pHEMA's excellent biocompatibility, and has led to many studies on the use of hydrogels like pHEMA for the reduction of thrombosis at the surface of blood-contacting biomaterials. Since pHEMA has rather poor mechanical properties and is not suitable for use as a vascular graft material, many hybrid materials have been produced by grafting pHEMA to the surface of polymeric materials with good mechanical properties such as polyurethanes, styrene–butadiene copolymers [81], or polysiloxanes [82].

Photoregulatable polymers—Copolymerization of 2-ethylacrylic acid or methacrylic acid with N-[4-(phenylazo)-phenyl]methacrylamide, a photo-sensitive monomer, results in polymers in which the interaction with lipid biolayers can be photoregulated [83, 84].

Thermally reversible polymers—Poly(n-isopropylacrylamide) is a water-soluble polymer at room temperature, with a lower critical solution temperature (LCST) of 32°C and reversible phase separation; this LCST can be raised or lowered by copolymerization with more or less hydrophilic monomers.

A.4.4 Poly(ethylene glycol)

Poly(ethylene glycol) (PEG) is a simple linear polyether:

$$\mathrm{HO} \left[\begin{array}{cccc} \overset{\displaystyle H}{\underset{\displaystyle H}{|}} & \overset{\displaystyle H}{\underset{\displaystyle H}{|}} \\ C & C & O \end{array} \right]_{n} \begin{array}{cc} \overset{\displaystyle H}{\underset{\displaystyle H}{|}} & \overset{\displaystyle H}{\underset{\displaystyle H}{|}} \\ C & C \end{array} OH \tag{A-35}$$

yet is one of the most frequently used water-soluble polymers in biomedical applications. PEG is useful in biomedical applications because of its high solubility in water, where it behaves as a highly mobile molecule. In addition, it has a large exclusion volume, occupying a larger volume in aqueous solution than other polymers of comparable molecular weight. Because of these properties, PEG molecules in aqueous solution tend to exclude or reject other polymers. It is unusual among the group of water-soluble polymers in that it is also soluble in a variety of organic solvents including methylene chloride, ethanol, and acetone. These properties lead to a number of useful applications: (1) addition of PEG to aqueous solutions of proteins and nucleic acids frequently induces crystallization; (2) addition of high concentrations of PEG to cell suspensions induces cell fusion; (3) immobilization of PEG to polymer surfaces greatly reduces protein adhesion; and (4) covalent coupling of PEG to proteins decreases their immunogenicity and increases their half-life in plasma. PEG is non-toxic and biocompatible.

Low molecular weight PEG (< 1000 Da) is a liquid at room temperature. Higher molecular weight preparations are solids and, when the molecular weight is above 20,000, PEG is frequently referred to as poly(ethylene oxide) (PEO) or polyoxyethylene. In some cases this is a useful distinction, since PEG generally refers to molecules with terminal hydroxyl groups on each end of the molecule (as in Equation 4-6) while PEO generally refers to units of sufficient molecular weight that the end groups are unimportant. PEG has been studied in great detail and its properties and applications are summarized in several books, including a useful summary of the characteristics and applications of PEG [85].

References

1. Flory, P.J., *Principles of Polymer Chemistry*. Ithaca: Cornell University, 1953.
2. Odian, G.G., *Principles of Polymerization*, 3rd ed. New York: Wiley-Interscience, 1991.
3. Rodrigeuz, F., *Principles of Polymer Systems*. 4th ed. London: Taylor & Francis, 1996.
4. Ulman, K., et al., Drug permeability of modified silicone polymers. I. Silicone–organic block copolymers. *Journal of Controlled Release*, 1989, **10**, 251–260.
5. Ulman, K., et al., Drug permeability of modified silicone polymers. II. Silicone–organic grafte copolymers. *Journal of Controlled Release*, 1989, **10**, 261–272.
6. Ulman, K. and C. Lee, Drug permeability of modified silicone polymers. III. Hydrophilic pressure-sensitive adhesives for transdermal controlled drug release applications. *Journal of Controlled Release*, 1989, **10**, 273–281.
7. Folkman, J. and D. Long, The use of silicone rubber as a carrier for prolonged drug therapy. *Journal of Surgical Research*, 1964, **4**, 139–142.
8. Folkman, J. and D. Long, Drug pacemakers in the treatment of heart block. *Annals of the New York Academy of Sciences*, 1964, **11**, 857–868.
9. Folkman, J., D.M. Long, and R. Rosenbaum, Silicone rubber: a new diffusion property useful for general anesthesia. *Science*, 1966, **154**, 148–149.
10. Segal, S., A new delivery system for contraceptive steroids. *American Journal of Obstetrics and Gynecology*, 1987, **157**, 1090–1092.
11. Segal, S.J., The development of Norplant implants. *Studies in Family Planning*, 1983, **14**(6/7), 159.
12. Huggins, G.R. and A.C. Wentz, Obstetrics and gynecology contempo. *JAMA*, 1993, **270**(2), 234–236.
13. Frank, M.L., et al., Characteristics and attitudes of early contraceptive implant acceptors. *Family Planning Perspectives*, 1992, **24**, 208.
14. Kessler, D.A., The basis of the FDA's decision on breast implants. *The New England Journal of Medicine*, 1992, **326**(25), 1713–1715.
15. Gabriel, S.E., et al., Risk of connective-tissue disease and other disorders after breast implantation. *The New England Journal of Medicine*, 1994, **330**, 1697–1702.
16. Angell, M., *Science on Trial: the Clash of Medical Evidence and the Law in the Breast Implant Case*. London: W.W. Norton, 1997, 268 pp.
17. Hsu, T. and R. Langer, Polymers for the controlled release of macromolecules: Effect of molecular weight of ethylene–vinyl acetate copolymer. *Journal of Biomedical Materials Research*, 1985, **19**, 445–460.
18. Siegel, R. and R. Langer, Controlled release of polypeptides and other macro-molecules. *Pharmaceutical Research*, 1984, 2–10.
19. Langer, R. and J. Folkman, Polymers for the sustained release of proteins and other macromolecules. *Nature*, 1976, **263**, 797–800.
20. Brown, L.R., C.L. Wei, and R. Langer, *In vivo* and *in vitro* release of macromole-cules from polymeric drug delivery system. *Journal of Pharmaceutical Research*, 1983, **72**, 1181–1185.
21. During, M.J., et al., Controlled release of dopamine from a polymeric brain implant: *in vivo* characterization. *Annals of Neurology*, 1989, **25**, 351–356.
22. Langer, R., H. Brem, and D. Tapper, Biocompatibility of polymeric delivery systems for macromolecules. *Journal of Biomedical Materials Research*, 1981, **15**, 267–277.
23. Langer, R., New methods of drug delivery. *Science*, 1990, **249**, 1527–1533.

24. Saltzman, W.M., Antibodies for treating and preventing disease: the potential role of polymeric controlled release. *Critical Reviews in Therapeutic Drug Carrier Systems,* 1993, **10**(2), 111–142.

25. Boretos, J.W. and W.S. Pierce, Segmented polyurethane: a new elastomer for biomedical applications. *Science,* 1967, **158**, 1481–1482.

26. Gogolewski, S., Selected topics in biomedical polyurethanes: a review. *Colloid and Polymer Science,* 1989, **267**, 757–785.

27. Tyler, B.J., B.D. Ratner, and D.G. Castner, Variations between Biomer lots. I. Significant differences in the surface chemistry of two lots of a commercial poly (ether urethane). *Journal of Biomedical Materials Research,* 1992, **26**, 273–289.

28. Batich, C. and J. Williams, Toxic hydrolysis product from a biodegradable foam implant. *Journal of Biomedical Materials Research: Applied Biomaterials,* 1989, **23**, 311–319.

29. Chan, S.C., D.C. Birdsell, and C.Y. Gradeen, Detection of toluenediamines in the urine of a patient with polyurethane-covered breast implants. *Clinical Chemistry,* 1991, **37**, 756–758.

30. Szycher, M., A.A. Siciliano, and A.M. Reed, Polyurethane elastomers in medicine, in S. Dimitriu, ed., *Polymeric Biomaterials.* New York: Marcel Dekker, 1994, pp. 233–244.

31. Hergenrother, R.W., H.D. Wabers, and S.L. Cooper, Effect of hard segment chemistry and strain on the stability of polyurethanes: *in vivo* biostability. *Biomaterials,* 1993, **14**, 449–458.

32. Goodman, S.L., S.L. Cooper, and R.M. Albrecht, Integrin receptors and platelet adhesion to synthetic surfaces. *Journal of Biomedical Materials Research,* 1993, **27**, 683–695.

33. Wabers, H.D., et al., Biostability and blood-contacting properties of sulfonate grafted polyurethane and Biomer. *Journal of Biomaterials Science, Polymer Edition,* 1992, **4**, 107–133.

34. Pitt, W.G. and S.L. Cooper, Albumin adsorption on alkyl chain derivatized polyurethanes: I. The effect of C-18 alkylation. *Journal of Biomedical Materials Research,* 1988, **22**, 359–382.

35. Lin, H.-B., et al., Synthesis of a novel polyurethane co-polymer containing covalently attached RGD peptide. *Journal of Biomaterials Science, Polymer Edition,* 1992, **3**, 217–227.

36. Lin, H.-B., et al., Surface properties of RGD-peptide grafted polyurethane block copolymers: variable take-off angle and cold-stage ESCA studies. *Journal of Biomaterials Science, Polymer Edition,* 1993, **4**, 183–198.

37. Lin, H., et al., Synthesis, surface, and cell-adhesion properties of polyurethanes containing covalently grafted RGD-peptides. *Journal of Biomedical Materials Research,* 1994, **28**, 329–342.

38. Anderson, J.M., et al., Cell/polymer interactions in the biodegradation of polyurethanes. *Biodegradable Polymers and Plastics,* 1992, 122–136.

39. McNally, A.K. and J.M. Anderson, Complement C3 participation in monocyte adhesion to different surfaces. *Proceedings of the National Academy of Sciences USA,* 1994, **91**, 10119–10123.

40. Dumitriu, S. and C. Dumitriu-Medvichi, Hydrogel and general properties of biomaterials, in S. Dumitriu, ed., *Polymeric Biomaterials.* New York: Marcel Dekker, 1994, pp. 3–97.

41. Saltzman, W.M., *Drug Delivery: Engineering Principles for Drug Therapy.* New York: Oxford University Press, 2001.

42. Chasin, M. and R. Langer, eds., *Biodegradable Polymers as Drug Delivery Systems.* New York: Marcel Dekker, 1990.
43. DeLuca, P.P., et al., Biodegradable polyesters for drug and polypeptide delivery, in M.A. El-Nokaly, D.M. Piatt, and B.A. Charpentier, eds., *Polymeric Delivery Systems: Properties and Applications.* Washington, DC: American Chemical Society, 1993, pp. 53–79.
44. Lewis, D.H., Controlled release of bioactive agents from lactide/glycolide polymers, in M. Chasin and R. Langer, eds., *Biodegradable Polymers as Drug Delivery Systems.* New York: Marcel Dekker, 1990, pp. 1–42.
45. Pitt, C.G., Poly-ε-caprolactone and its copolymers, in M. Chasin and R. Langer, eds., *Biodegradable Polymers as Drug Delivery Systems,* New York: Marcel Dekker, 1990, pp. 71–120.
46. Barrera, D.A., et al., Synthesis and RGD peptide modification of a new biodegradable copolymer: poly(lactic acid-*co*-lysine). *Journal of the American Chemical Society,* 1993, **115**, 11010–11011.
47. Miller, R.A., J.M. Brady, and D.E. Cutright, Degradation rates of oral resorbable implants (polylactates and polyglycolates): rate modification with changes in PLA/PGA copolymer ratios. *Journal of Biomedical Materials Research,* 1977, **11**, 711–719.
48. Kulkarni, R.K., et al., Biodegradable poly(lactic acid) polymers. *Journal of Biomedical Materials Research,* 1971, **5**, 169–181.
49. Schmitt, E.E. and R.A. Polistina, *Surgical sutures.* U.S. Patent 3,297,033 (Jan. 10, 1967).
50. Wasserman, D. and A.J. Levy, *Nahtmaterials aus weichgemachten Lacttid-Glykolid-Copolymerisaten.* German Patent Offenlegungsschrift 24 06 539, 1975.
51. Schneider, M.A.K., *Elément de suture absorbable et son procédé de fabrication.* French Patent 1,478,694, 1967.
52. Boswell, G.A. and R.M. Scribner, *Polylactid-Arzneimittel-Mischungen.* German Patent Offenlegungsschrift 2 051 580, 1971.
53. Boswell, G.A. and R.M. Scribner, *Polylactide–drug mixtures.* U.S. Patent 3,773,919, 1973.
54. Woodland, J.H., et al., Long-acting delivery systems for narcotic antagonists. *Journal of Medicinal Chemistry,* 1973, **16**(8), 897–901.
55. Gilding, D.K. and A.M. Reed, Biodegradable polymers for use in surgery— polyglycolic/poly(lactic acid) homo- and copolymers. *Polymer,* 1979, **20**, 1459–1464.
56. Jacknicz, T.M., et al., Polylactic acid as a biodegradable carrier for contraceptive steroids. *Contraception,* 1973, **8**, 227–234.
57. Wise, D.L., et al., Sustained release of an antimalarial drug using a copolymer of glycolic/lactic acid. *Life Sciences,* 1976, **19**, 867–874.
58. Beck, L.R., et al., New long-acting injectable microcapsule contraceptive system. *American Journal of Obstetrics and Gynecology,* 1979, **135**, 419–426.
59. Sinclair, R.G., Polymers of lactic and glycolic acids as ecologically beneficial, cost-effective encapsulating materials. *Environmental Science and Technology,* 1976, **7**(10), 955–956.
60. Heller, J., et al., Controlled drug release by polymer dissolution. I. Partial esters of maleic anhydride copolymers, properties and theory. *Journal of Applied Polymer Science,* 1978, **22**, 1991–2009.
61. Heller, J., Development of poly(ortho esters): a historical overview. *Biomaterials,* 1990, **11**, 659–665.

62. Heller, J., et al., Controlled drug release from bioerodible hydrophobic ointments. *Biomaterials*, 1990, **11**, 235–237.

63. Tamada, J. and R. Langer, Review: the development of polyanhydrides for drug delivery. *Journal of Biomaterials Science, Polymer Edition*, 1992, **3**(4), 315–353.

64. Chasin, M., et al., Polyanhydrides as drug delivery systems, in M. Chasin and R. Langer, eds., *Biodegradable Polymers as Drug Delivery Systems*. New York: Marcel Dekker, 1990.

65. Sidman, K.R., et al., Biodegradable, implantable sustained release systems based on glutamtic acid copolymers. *Journal of Membrane Science*, 1980, **7**, 277–291.

66. Kohn, J., Pseudopoly(amino acids), in M. Chasin and R. Langer, eds., *Biodegradable Polymers as Drug Delivery Systems*. New York: Marcel Dekker, 1990, pp. 195–229.

67. Allcock, H.R., Polyphosphazenes as new biomedical and bioactive materials, in M. Chasin and R. Langer, eds., *Biodegradable Polymers as Drug Delivery Systems*. New York: Marcel Dekker, 1990, pp. 163–193.

68. Kohn, J. and R. Langer, Poly(iminocarbonates) as potential biomaterials. *Biomaterials*, 1986, **7**, 176–181.

69. Pulapura, S., C. Li, and J. Kohn, Structure–property relationships for the design of polyiminocarbonates. *Biomaterials*, 1990, **11**, 666–678.

70. Ertel, S.I. and J. Kohn, Evaluation of a series of tyrosine-derived polycarbonates as degradable biomaterials. *Journal of Biomedical Materials Research*, 1994, **28**, 919–930.

71. Silver, F.H., et al., Tissue compatibility of tyrosine-derived polycarbonates and polyiminocarbonates: an initial evaluation. *Journal of Long-term Effects of Medical Implants*, 1992, **1**(4), 329–346.

72. Ertel, S.I. and J. Kohn, Evaluation of poly(DTH carbonate), a tyrosine-derived degradable polymer, for orthopedic applications. *Journal of Biomedical Materials Research*, 1995, **29**, 1337–1348.

73. Ray, J.A., et al., Polydioxanone (PDS), a novel monofilament synthetic absorbable suture. *Surgery, Gynecology & Obstetrics*, 1981, **153**, 497–507.

74. Stryer, L., *Biochemistry*, 2nd ed. New York: W.H. Freeman, 1988.

75. Muzzarelli, R., *In vivo* biochemical significance of chitin-based medical items, in S. Dumitriu, ed., *Polymeric Biomaterials*. New York: Marcel Dekker, 1994, pp. 179–197.

76. Peppas, N.A., *Hydrogels in Medicine and Pharmacy*. Boca Raton, FL: CRC Press, 1987.

77. Montheard, J.-P., M. Chatzopoulos, and D. Chappard, 2-Hydroxyethyl methacrylate (HEMA): chemical properties and applications in biomedical fields. *Journal of Macromolecular Science—Reviews in Macromolecular Chemistry and Physics*, 1992, **C32**(1), 1–34.

78. Pinchuk, L., E.C. Eckstein, and M.R. Van De Mark, The interaction of urea with the generic class of poly(2-hydroxyethyl methacrylate) hydrogels. *Journal of Biomedical Materials Research*, 1984, **18**, 671–684.

79. Folkman, J. and A. Moscona, Role of cell shape in growth control. *Nature*, 1978, **273**, 345–349.

80. Horbett, T., M. Schway, and B. Ratner, Hydrophilic–hydrophobic copolymers as cell substrates: Effect on 3T3 cell growth rates. *Journal of Colloid and Interface Science*, 1985, **104**, 28–39.

81. Hsiue, G.-H., J.-M. Yang, and R.-L. Wu, Preparation and properties of a bio-material: HEMA grafted SBS by gamma-ray irradiation. *Journal of Biomedical Materials Research*, 1988, **22**, 405–415.

82. Seifert, L.M. and R.T. Greer, Evaluation of *in vivo* adsorption of blood elements onto hydrogel-coated silicone rubber by scanning electron microscopy and Fourier transform infrared spectroscopy. *Journal of Biomedical Materials Research*, 1985, **19**, 1043–1071.

83. Ferritto, M.S. and D.A. Tirrell, Photoregulation of the binding of a synthetic polyelectrolyte to phosphatidylcholine bilayer membranes. *Macromolecules*, 1988, **21**, 3117–3119.

84. Ferritto, M.S. and D.A. Tirrell, Photoregulation of the binding of an azobenzene-modified poly(methacrylic acid) to phosphatidylcholine bilayer membranes. *Biomaterials*, 1990, **11**, 645–651.

85. Harris, J.M., ed., *Poly(Ethylene Glycol) Chemistry: Biotechnical and Biomedical Applications*. New York: Plenum Press, 1992.

86. Richards, J.M., et al., Determination of the structure and composition of clinically important polyurethanes by mass spectrometric techniques. *Journal of Applied Polymer Science*, 1987, **34**, 1967–1975.

Appendix B

Analysis of Molecular Transport

You air that serves me with breath to speak!
You objects that call from diffusion my meanings, and give them shape!

Walt Whitman, *Song of the Open Road* (1856)

Most biological processes occur in an environment that is predominantly water: a typical cell contains 70-85% water and the extracellular space of most tissues is 99% water. Even the brain, with its complex arrangement of cells and myelinated processes, is ~80% water. Since water serves as the primary milieu for life processes, it is essential to understand the factors that determine rates of molecular movement in aqueous environments. As we shall see, rates of diffusive transport of molecules vary among biological tissues within an organism, even though the bulk composition of the tissues (that is, their water content) may be similar.

This review of molecular transport analysis is a condensed version of a chapter published earlier [1]. The review begins with the random walk, a useful model from statistical physics that provides insight into the kinetics of molecular diffusion. From this starting point, the fundamental relationship between diffusive flux and solute concentration, Fick's law, is described and used to develop general mass conservation equations. These conservation equations are the starting point for analysis of rates of solute transport in tissues.

B.1 Random Walks

Molecules that are initially localized within an unstirred vessel will spread throughout the vessel, eventually becoming uniformly dispersed. This process, called diffusion, occurs by the random movement of individual molecules; molecular motion is generated by thermal energy. Einstein demonstrated that the average kinetic energy of particles in a system depends on the absolute temperature T [2]:

$$\left\langle \frac{mv_x^2}{2} \right\rangle = \frac{k_B T}{2} \tag{B-1}$$

where v_x is the velocity of a particle on one axis, m is the mass of the particle, and k_B is Boltzmann's constant ($k_B T = 4.14 \times 10^{-14}$ g-cm^2/s^2 at 300 K). The root-mean-square (r.m.s.) velocity can be found from the relationship:

$$v_{\text{rms}} = \sqrt{\langle v_x^2 \rangle} = \sqrt{\frac{k_B T}{m}} \qquad (B\text{-}2)$$

Albumin, a protein of 68,000 M_w, has a predicted r.m.s. velocity of 600 cm/s at 300 K. A molecule moving at this speed should travel 2 m (the height of a very tall person) in about 0.33 s, if it moved in a straight line. Experience teaches us that molecules do not move this rapidly. In fact, rates of diffusive transport are much slower than v_{rms} would suggest. Diffusion is slow because molecules do not travel in a straight path; individual molecules collide with other molecules and change direction frequently, producing a pattern of migration known as a random walk. Since air and water have different molecular densities, the number of collisions per second—and hence the rate of overall dispersion—differs for these fluids.

   These patterns of migration can be simulated by examining particles that follow simple rules for movement: random walkers. Many of the important characteristics of diffusive processes can be understood by considering the dynamics of particles executing simple random walks. The excellent book by Berg [3] provides a useful introduction to the random walk and its relevance in biological systems, which is followed here. Whitney provides a complete, tutorial introduction to a variety of random processes, including the random walk [4].

   Consider, for example, a particle constrained to move on a one-dimensional axis. During a small time interval τ the particle can move a distance δ which depends on the particle's velocity v_x: $\delta = v_x \tau$. Further assume that at the end of each period τ the particle changes its direction of movement, randomly moving to the right or the left with equal probability. At each step in the walk, the decision to move left or right is completely random and does not depend on the particle's previous history of movement. If N identical particles, each moving according to these simple rules, begin at the origin of the coordinate system at $t = 0$, one-half of the particles will be at position $-\delta$ and the other half will be at $+\delta$ at the end of the first interval τ. If the location of one particular particle, indicated by the index i, after $n-1$ such intervals is designated $x_i(n-1)$, then the position of that same particle after n intervals is easily determined:

$$x_i(n) = x_i(n-1) \pm \delta \qquad (B\text{-}3)$$

The mean particle position can be predicted by averaging Equation B-3 over the ensemble of particles, which becomes

$$\langle x(n) \rangle = \frac{1}{N} \sum_{i=1}^{N} x_i(n) = \frac{1}{N} \sum_{i=1}^{N} (x_i(n-1) \pm \delta) = \frac{1}{N} \sum_{i=1}^{N} x_i(n-1) + \frac{1}{N} \sum_{i=1}^{N} (\pm \delta)$$

$$(B\text{-}4)$$

upon substitution of Equation B-3. The averaging operation, designated $\langle \cdot \rangle$, is a conventional arithmetic average: $(1/N)(\sum_{i=1}^{N} \cdot_i)$. The second term on the right-hand side of Equation B-4 is zero, since an equal number of particles will move to the right $(+\delta)$ and to the left $(-\delta)$, which produces

$$\langle x(n) \rangle = \langle x(n-1) \rangle \tag{B-5}$$

Therefore, the average position of the randomly migrating particles in this ensemble does not change with time. For a group of particles that begin at the origin, $x = 0$, the average position will always be at the origin.

Although this random migration does not change the average position of the particle ensemble, it does tend to spread the particles over the axis. The extent of spread can be determined by examining the mean-square displacement of the particle ensemble, $\langle x^2(n) \rangle$:

$$\langle x^2(n) \rangle = \frac{1}{N} \sum_{i=1}^{N} (x_i(n-1) \pm \delta)^2 = \frac{1}{N} \sum_{i=1}^{N} (x_i^2(n-1) \pm 2\delta x_i(n-1) + \delta^2) \tag{B-6}$$

When the summation is expanded, the sum resulting from the middle term on the right-hand side is 0, because an equal number of particles move to the left and right. The first and last terms can be reduced, to yield

$$\langle x^2(n) \rangle = \langle x^2(n-1) \rangle + \delta^2 \tag{B-7}$$

Since the mean-square displacement is initially 0, Equation B-7 indicates that the mean-square displacement increases linearly with the number of steps in the random walk:

$$\left. \begin{aligned} \langle x^2(0) \rangle &= 0 \\ \langle x^2(1) \rangle &= \delta^2 \\ \langle x^2(2) \rangle &= 2\delta^2 \\ &\vdots \\ \langle x^2(n) \rangle &= n\delta^2 \end{aligned} \right\} \tag{B-8}$$

Since the total elapsed time t is equal to $n\tau$, the mean-square displacement also increases linearly with time:

$$\langle x^2(t) \rangle = \left(\frac{\delta^2}{\tau} \right) t \tag{B-9}$$

and the root-mean-square (r.m.s.) displacement, x_{rms}, increases with the square root of time:

$$x_{\text{rms}} \equiv \langle x^2(t) \rangle^{1/2} = \sqrt{2Dt} \tag{B-10}$$

where the diffusion coefficient D is defined thus:

$$D = \delta^2/2\tau \tag{B-11}$$

Experimental measurements, obtained by measuring the rate of spreading of protein molecules in solution, suggest that D for albumin at 300 K is $\sim 8 \times 10^{-7}$ cm^2/s. Since v_x is the particle velocity between changes of direction, which is equal to δ/τ, the distance between direction changes δ can be estimated as $2D/v_x$. For albumin, with $v_x = v_{rms} = 600$ cm/s, this yields a value for δ of 3 $\times 10^{-9}$ cm (or 0.3 Å, small compared to the diameter of albumin which is ~ 60 Å) and a time between direction changes τ of 4×10^{-12} s. This model suggests a different view of albumin movement from that obtained by considering only the r.m.s. velocity of individual particles. The random walk of albumin will require 2.5×10^{10} s or 800 years to travel 2 m (from Equation B-10), a significantly longer time than the r.m.s. velocity would suggest. This simple calculation illustrates the slow progress of diffusing molecules over meter-scale distances (and explains why humans have a circulatory system).

Note that these calculations suggest several important characteristics for diffusion processes:

- since the r.m.s. displacement increases with the square root of time, a diffusing particle that takes T min to diffuse L mm will take $4T$ to diffuse $2L$;
- the diffusion velocity, which might be defined as x_{rms}/t, is inversely proportional to the square root of time and therefore not a useful measure of molecular speed.

This analysis can be extended to two- and three-dimensional random walks by assuming that particle motion in each dimension is independent. The mean-square displacement and r.m.s. displacement for higher dimension random walks become

$$\left.\begin{array}{ll} \langle r^2 \rangle_{2D} = \langle x^2 \rangle + \langle y^2 \rangle = 4Dt & \text{or} \quad \langle r^2 \rangle_{2D}^{1/2} = \sqrt{4Dt} \\ \langle r^2 \rangle_{3D} = \langle x^2 \rangle + \langle y^2 \rangle + \langle z^2 \rangle = 6Dt & \text{or} \quad \langle r^2 \rangle_{3D}^{1/2} = \sqrt{6Dt} \end{array}\right\} \quad \text{(B-12)}$$

For particles executing a random walk, like albumin molecules in buffered water, the calculations above suggest that individual steps in the random walk occur very quickly, over a short time interval. As a consequence, during a typical observation time, each particle takes many steps. The probability that a random walking particle took a total of k steps to the right after a sequence of n steps in the random walk is provided by the binomial distribution:

$$P\left\{\begin{array}{c} \text{particle took } k \\ \text{steps to the right} \\ \text{after } n \text{ steps} \end{array}\right\} = P(k; n, q) = \frac{n!}{k!(n-k)!}(q)^k(1-q)^{n-k} \quad \text{(B-13)}$$

where q is the probability of moving to the right at each step; $q = 1/2$ for an unbiased random walk. For example, after four steps in an unbiased random walk, the binomial distribution can be used to determine the probabilities of finding particles at any location on the axis, as shown in Table B.1.

By using the binomial distribution it is possible to determine $p(x)$, the probability of finding a particle at position between x and $x + dx$, as a function

Table B.1
Characterization of Random Walks with the Binomial Distribution

k	0	1	2	3	4
$n - k$	4	3	2	1	0
x	-4δ	-2δ	0	$+2\delta$	$+4\delta$
$P(k; n, 1/2)$	0.0625	0.25	0.375	0.25	0.0625

The binomial distribution, Equation B-13, was used to calculate the probability of finding a random walker at position x after 4 steps in an unbiased random walk. The position on a coordinate axis x was determined from the number of steps to the right, k, and the number of steps to the left, $n - k : x = \delta(k - (n - k))$.

of time after a large number of individual steps in the random walk have occurred [3]:

$$p(x) = \frac{1}{\sqrt{4\pi Dt}} e^{-x^2/4Dt} dx \tag{B-14}$$

Equation B-14 describes a Gaussian distribution; the random walk model predicts that a group of diffusing particles, initially placed at the origin, will spread over time so that the mean position is unchanged but the variance in the distribution increases as $2Dt$. In the section below, we will see this same distribution emerge from the solution to the macroscopic equations for molecular diffusion.

The rate of movement of particles at any particular location can be estimated by considering the net rate of particle movement at any specific position during the random walk. During a single step in the random walk, which occurs over the time interval τ, the net rate of particle movement between two adjacent positions x and $x + \delta$ is $N(x)/2 - N(x + \delta)/2$, where $N(\cdot)$ gives the number of particles at a given location, because half of the particles at position x will move to the right (ending at $x + \delta$) and half the particles at $x + \delta$ will move to the left (ending at x). The particle flux j_x is defined as the net rate of particle movement per unit area, so that

$$j_x = -\frac{1}{2A\tau}[N(x + \delta) - N(x)] \tag{B-15}$$

Rearranging slightly gives

$$j_x = -\frac{\delta^2}{2\tau}\left[\frac{C(x + \delta) - C(x)}{\delta}\right] \tag{B-16}$$

where $C(x, N(x)/A\delta)$ is the concentration of particles at a given location x. Taking the limit of Equation B-14 as the distance between the adjacent points becomes small yields

$$j_x = -D\frac{\partial C}{\partial x} \tag{B-17}$$

where the diffusion coefficient D is defined as in Equation B-11. Thus, this random walk model also provides a relationship between the spatial concentration distribution and the particle flux. Particles move towards locations with lower concentration; the flux of particles is directly proportional to the concentration gradient and the diffusion coefficient is the constant of proportionality. This expression, often called Fick's law [5], will be of considerable practical value in predicting rates of molecular transport through cells and tissues.

B.2 Equations for the Diffusive Flux (Fick's Law)

This expression for the diffusive flux can be obtained more rigorously by considering the velocities of individual species in a multi-component system. The mass average flux of component A in a mixture, $\bar{j}_A$, is defined on the basis of the velocity of the species of interest, $\bar{v}_A$, relative to the mass average velocity of the system, $\bar{v}$

$$\bar{j}_A = \rho_A(\bar{v}_A - \bar{v}) \tag{B-18}$$

where $\bar{j}_A$, $\bar{v}_A$, and $\bar{v}$ are now vector quantities and the mass average velocity is defined by weighting the velocities of each component by the mass density of that component in the system. For more complete definitions, the derivation of conservation of mass equations, and application of these equations in conventional chemical engineering analysis, the reader is referred to the classical textbook on transport phenomena [6]. The notation used in the present text follows the notation by Bird et al. The flux defined in this manner is due to the presence of concentration gradients in the system, and depends on the diffusion coefficient D_A:

$$\bar{j}_A = -\rho D_A \nabla \omega_A \tag{B-19}$$

where ρ is the total mass density of the system and ω_A is the mass fraction of component A. There are many equivalent ways to express Fick's law for molar or mass fluxes with respect to molar or mass average velocities (see a text on transport phenomena, such as [6] or [7], for examples). In all cases, however, the diffusion coefficient, D_A, is identical. Strictly speaking, this definition of D_A applies to binary mixtures where D_A is the diffusion coefficient of A in a mixture of A and B. In this book, which is primarily concerned with the diffusion of dilute species in an aqueous system containing many additional dilute components, we will use D_A to denote the diffusion coefficient of the species of interest in a multi-component complex system. When used in this manner, D_A is an effective binary diffusion coefficient for A in a multi-component system [6].

Equation B-19 defines the diffusion coefficient D_A, but is inconvenient for many calculations since the flux $\bar{j}_A$ is defined with respect to a moving coordinate system. For binary systems, $\bar{j}_A$ is simply related to the mass flux of A with respect to a stationary coordinate system, $\bar{n}_A$:

$$\bar{n}_A = \omega_A(\bar{n}_A + \bar{n}_B) + \bar{j}_A = \omega_A(\bar{n}_A + \bar{n}_B) - \rho D_A \nabla \omega_A \qquad \text{(B-20)}$$

The mass flux $\bar{n}_A$ is the sum of the diffusive flux $\bar{j}_A$, which accounts for the movement of A due to concentration gradients, and the quantity $\omega_A(\bar{n}_A + \bar{n}_B)$, which accounts for the movement of A due to bulk motion of the fluid. Equation B-20 is the appropriate form of the diffusive flux equation to use for most engineering problems, since quantities are usually measured with respect to some fixed frame of reference. For many of the problems considered here, A is a dilute species in water, in which case $\omega_A \simeq 0$ and the bulk motion term can be neglected.

B.3 Equations of Mass Conservation (Fick's Second Law)

Consider the migration of species A through a homogeneous region of space, such as a small volume of tissue (Figure B.1). General differential equations can be developed to describe the variation of concentration of compound A, C_A, with time and position in the tissue by first considering the conservation of mass within this small volume. Molecules of A can enter through any face of the volume element; they can be generated or consumed within the volume by chemical reaction; they can accumulate within the volume. A general balance equation (in−out + generation = accumulation) yields

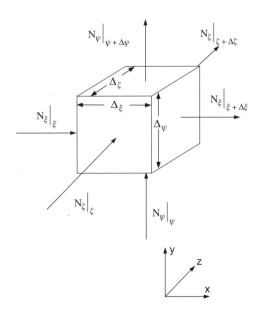

Figure B.1. Differential mass balance on a characteristic element. This diagram shows a simple mass balance in a rectangular coordinate system. Consider the possible sources of consumption or generation of mass within the volume element, say if the element is a small section of tissue.

$$\left[n_x\big|_x \Delta y \Delta z - n_x\big|_{x+\Delta x} \Delta y \Delta z \right] + \left[n_y\big|_y \Delta x \Delta z - n_y\big|_{y+\Delta y} \Delta x \Delta z \right]$$
$$+ \left[n_z\big|_z \Delta x \Delta y - n_z\big|_{z+\Delta z} \Delta x \Delta y \right] + \psi_A \Delta x \Delta y \Delta z = \frac{\partial \rho_A}{\partial t} \Delta x \Delta y \Delta z \tag{B-21}$$

where the first three bracketed terms account for the movement of A through the faces of the volume element, ψ_A is the rate of generation (or negative the rate of consumption) of A per unit volume, and ρ_A is the mass density of A in the volume ($\rho_A = \omega_A \rho$). Dividing each term by the volume ($\Delta x \Delta y \Delta z$) and taking the limit of the resulting expression as the differential volume becomes very small yields

$$-\frac{\partial n_x}{\partial x} - \frac{\partial n_y}{\partial y} - \frac{\partial n_z}{\partial z} + \frac{\partial n_z}{\partial z} + \psi_A = \frac{\partial \rho_A}{\partial t} \tag{B-22}$$

which can be written more simply as

$$-\nabla \cdot \overline{n_A} + \psi_A = \frac{\partial \rho_A}{\partial t} \tag{B-23}$$

which was derived by considering a volume element in rectangular coordinates; identical expressions could be obtained in cylindrical or spherical coordinates.

The mass balance procedure produced a partial differential equation with two dependent variables, solute flux and concentration. To complete this analysis, an appropriate form of Fick's law must be substituted into Equation B-23. Substituting Equation B-20 yields

$$-\nabla \cdot (\omega_A(\overline{n_A} + \overline{n_B}) - \rho D_A \nabla \omega_A) + \psi_A = \frac{\partial \rho_A}{\partial t} \tag{B-24}$$

By recognizing that the sum of the fluxes $\overline{n_A} + \overline{n_B}$ is equal to the density times the mass average velocity, $\rho \overline{v}$, we can reduce this equation to

$$-\nabla \cdot (\rho_A \overline{v}) + \nabla \cdot (\rho D_A \nabla \omega_A) + \psi_A = \frac{\partial \rho_A}{\partial t} \tag{B-25}$$

which is a general expression of the conservation of mass of solute A. Expressions equivalent to Equations B-23 to B-25 could also be written for component B of a binary system; the sum of these individual mass balance equations produces the total mass conservation, or continuity, equation:

$$-\nabla \cdot \rho \overline{v} = \frac{\partial \rho}{\partial t} \tag{B-26}$$

The aqueous systems considered in this text are incompressible (that is, the total density ρ is constant) and Equations B-25 and B-26 can be written as:

$$\nabla \cdot D_A \nabla \rho_A + \psi_A = \frac{D\rho_A}{Dt} \tag{B-27}$$

$$\nabla \cdot \overline{v} = 0 \tag{B-28}$$

where Equation B-28 has been used to eliminate the term involving the velocity gradient in Equation B-27 and the substantial derivative is defined as

$$\frac{D}{Dt}(\,\cdot\,) = \frac{\partial}{\partial t}(\,\cdot\,) + \bar{v}\cdot\nabla(\,\cdot\,) \qquad (B\text{-}29)$$

Equations B-27 and B-28 provide the most compact and general form of the equation of conservation of mass. These expressions are limited only by the assumption that the fluid is incompressible; this assumption is reasonable for all of the problems discussed in this text.

Equations B-20 to B-28 can also be written in terms of molar concentrations and molar fluxes. A summary of the most important equations, expressed in both molar and mass units, is provided in Table B.2. These equations assume that diffusion is isotropic: that is, that the flux of diffusing molecules through some particular plane within a system is proportional to the concentration gradient measured orthogonal to the plane. This assumption is not true for anisotropic media, in which the diffusion characteristics depend on the direction of diffusion. Anisotropic media usually have oriented physical structures, such as crystals or polymers, that provide varying resistances to diffusion in different directions. Anisotropic diffusion may be important for diffusion in biological systems, since the cytoplasm of cells or the extracellular space of tissues can contain highly organized and oriented structures. Consider, for example, the diffusion of compounds in the extracellular space of the brain,

Table B.2
The Basic Equations for Mass Transfer, Derived on a Mass and Molar Basis for Isotropic Diffusion

	Mass	Molar
Average velocity	$\bar{v} = \dfrac{1}{\rho\sum_{i=1}^{n}p_i\bar{v}_i}$	$\overline{V} = \dfrac{1}{c}\sum_{i=1}^{n}c_i\bar{v}_i$
Flux with respect to coordinate system moving at average velocity	$\overline{j_A} = \rho_A(\overline{V_A} - v) = -\rho D_A\nabla\omega_A$	$\overline{J_A} = c_A(\overline{V_A} - \overline{V}) = -cD_A\nabla x_A$
Flux with respect to stationary coordinate system (binary system)	$\overline{n_A} = -\rho D_A\nabla\omega_A + \omega_A(\overline{n_A} + \overline{n_B})$	$\overline{N_A} = -cD_A\nabla x_A + x_A(\overline{N_A} + \overline{N_B})$
General form of conservation of mass for component A (binary system)	$-\nabla\cdot(\rho_A\bar{v} - \rho D_A\nabla\omega_A) + \psi_A = \dfrac{\partial\rho_A}{\partial t}$	$-\nabla\cdot(c_A\overline{V} - cD_A\nabla x_A) + \psi_A^{\mathrm{m}} = \dfrac{\partial c_A}{\partial t}$
Conservation of mass for component A (binary system, incompressible fluid, constant D_A)	$D_A\nabla^2\rho_A + \psi_A = \dfrac{D\rho_A}{Dt}$	$D_A\nabla^2 c_A + \psi_A^{\mathrm{m}} = \dfrac{Dc_A}{Dt}$

The symbols are defined in the text: ψ_A^{m} indicates molar rate of generation of A (mol/cm^3-s).

which may be anisotropic in regions where emanated fibers run in a particular direction.

In the case of anisotropic diffusion, Fick's law, Equation B-19, must be written:

$$
\left.
\begin{aligned}
j_{A_x} &= -\rho \left[D_{11} \frac{\partial \omega_A}{\partial x} + D_{12} \frac{\partial \omega_A}{\partial y} + D_{13} \frac{\partial \omega_A}{\partial z} \right] \\
j_{A_y} &= -\rho \left[D_{21} \frac{\partial \omega_A}{\partial x} + D_{22} \frac{\partial \omega_A}{\partial y} + D_{23} \frac{\partial \omega_A}{\partial z} \right] \\
j_{A_z} &= -\rho \left[D_{31} \frac{\partial \omega_A}{\partial x} + D_{32} \frac{\partial \omega_A}{\partial y} + D_{33} \frac{\partial \omega_A}{\partial z} \right]
\end{aligned}
\right\}
\qquad \text{(B-30)}
$$

where fluxes not only depend on the concentration gradient in the orthogonal direction, but may depend on gradients in the other directions as well. The diffusion coefficients in Equation B-30, D_{nm}, indicate the significance of diffusion in the n-direction due to a gradient in the m-direction. Equation B-30 reduces to Fick's law for isotropic diffusion when the off-diagonal terms are 0—that is, $D_{nm} = 0$ for $n \neq m$—and the diagonal terms are all equal—that is, $D_{nm} = D_A$ for $n = m$. In some cases, appropriate coordinate transformations can be used to reduce the equations describing diffusion in anisotropic media to analogous equations in isotropic media; these techniques are discussed by Crank [8].

The conservation of mass equations listed in the final row of Table B.2 are frequently used to describe the movement of solutes through tissues and cells. These equations were developed by assuming that the tissue is homogeneous throughout the region of interest. Diffusing solute molecules must have equal access to every possible position within the volume of interest and D_A must be constant with respect to both space and time. This assumption is not valid for the diffusion of certain molecules in tissues; for example, consider a molecule that diffuses through the extracellular space of the tissue and does not readily enter cells.

B.4 Solutions to the Diffusion Equation with No Solute Elimination or Generation

When appropriately applied, the equations derived in the section above can be used to predict variations in drug concentration within a tissue following administration. For the description of molecular transport in cells or tissues, the mass conservation equations must be simplified by making appropriate assumptions that are specialized for the geometry of interest. For example, the mass conservation equation in terms of molar fluxes, assuming no bulk flow and no chemical reaction, is

$$
D_A \nabla^2 c_A = \frac{\partial c_A}{\partial t}
\qquad \text{(B-31)}
$$

a commonly used form that is frequently referred to as Fick's second law. When solved subject to the appropriate boundary and initial conditions, this differential equation yields the concentration c_A as a function of time and position within the volume of interest. Since equations equivalent to Equation B-31 arise in a variety of physical settings, detailed solutions for many situations already exist (see the excellent books by Crank [8] and Carslaw and Jaeger [9]).

B.4.1 Rectangular Coordinates

Consider a solute A that is neither consumed nor generated but diffuses with a constant diffusion coefficient D_A. Assume that a bolus of N molecules is injected into a long cylinder, so that all of the molecules are present within an infinitesimal volume at the origin of the coordinate system at $t = 0$. After injection, the molecules will diffuse along the axis of the cylinder, where bulk flow is negligible. This situation will not occur frequently in physiological systems, although it may be a reasonable model for the micro-injection of inert tracers into the axon or dendrite of a neuron [10]. On the other hand, *in vitro* experimental systems are often intentionally arranged into this geometry, which greatly simplifies the subsequent analysis [11, 12].

The concentration of A as a function of time and distance from the site of initial injection can be predicted by solving Equation B-31, expressed in a one-dimensional rectangular coordinate system:

$$D_A \frac{\partial^2 c_A}{\partial x^2} = \frac{\partial c_A}{\partial t} \tag{B-32}$$

subject to the following initial and boundary conditions:

$$\left. \begin{array}{lll} c(x, t) = N\delta(x) & -\infty < x < \infty & t = 0 \\ c(x, t) = 0 & x \to \infty & t > 0 \\ c(x, t) = 0 & x \to -\infty & t > 0 \end{array} \right\} \tag{B-33}$$

where $\delta(x)$ is the unit impulse or Dirac delta function centered at $x = 0$. This equation can be solved by Laplace transform techniques to produce the solution

$$c_A(x, t) = \frac{A}{\sqrt{t}} e^{-x^2/4D_A t} \tag{B-34}$$

where A is a constant of integration. The constant A can be determined by integrating Equation B-34 with respect to x to obtain the total number of diffusing molecules:

$$\int_{-\infty}^{\infty} c_A(x, t) \cdot \pi R^2 dx = \pi R^2 \frac{A}{\sqrt{t}} \int_{-\infty}^{\infty} e^{-x^2/4D_A t} dx = 2\pi R^2 A \sqrt{\pi D_A} = \frac{N}{N_{Av}} \tag{B-35}$$

where R is the radius of the cylinder cross-section and N_{Av} is Avogadro's number. This definite integral reduces to $\sqrt{4D_A t\pi}$. Since the value of the constant A can be determined from Equation B-35, the complete solution is

$$c_A(x, t) = \frac{N}{N_{Av}} \frac{1}{2\sqrt{\pi D_A t}} \frac{1}{2\pi R^2} e^{-x^2/4D_A t} \tag{B-36}$$

This expression is plotted in Figure B.2. The similarity of Equation B-36, which is a solution to the conservation of mass equations, and the Gaussian distribution obtained from random walk calculations (see Equation B-14) is obvious.

A similar analysis can be used to predict concentration profiles in the region on one side of a planar boundary after the concentration is suddenly raised on the opposite side. In this case, the differential equation is still Equation B-32, but the boundary conditions must be modified slightly:

$$\left.\begin{array}{lll} c(x, t) = 0; & \text{for } 0 < x < \infty; & t = 0 \\ c(x, t) = c_0; & \text{for } x = 0; & t > 0 \\ c(x, t) = 0; & \text{for } x \to \infty; & t > 0 \end{array}\right\} \tag{B-33'}$$

Solution of Equation B-32 in this situation yield

$$\frac{c_A}{c_0} = \text{erfc}\left(\frac{x}{2\sqrt{D_A t}}\right) \tag{B-37}$$

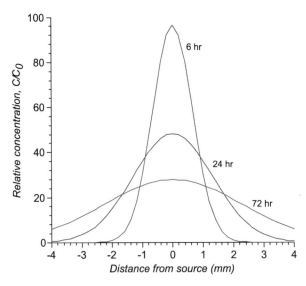

Figure B.2. Concentration profiles for diffusion from a point source. When a concentrated bolus of solute is deposited within a small region of an infinitely long cylinder, the molecules slowly disperse along the axis of the cylinder. The curves shown here are realizations of Equation B-34 for a solute with $D_A = 10^{-7}\,\text{cm}^2/\text{s}$, $R = 0.1\,\text{cm}$, $N = N_{Av}$, and $t = 6, 24, 72$, and $720\,\text{hr}$.

where erfc($\cdot$) is the error function complement, which is simply related to the error function erf($\cdot$):

$$\text{erf}(z) = 1 - \text{erfc}(z) = \frac{2}{\sqrt{\pi}} \int_0^z \exp(-\eta^2) d\eta \tag{B-38}$$

The error function occurs frequently in solutions to the diffusion equation: extensive tables of error functions are available as well as series expansions for approximation [13]. Some values are tabulated in Appendix C. Equation B-37 can be used to examine the penetration of drug molecules into a tissue when suddenly presented at a surface (Figure B.3).

Similarly, if the drug is initially confined to a linear band of width $2w$ and concentration c_0, drug molecules will spread in both directions with time:

$$\frac{c_A}{c_0} = \frac{1}{2}\left[\text{erf}\left(\frac{w+x}{2\sqrt{D_A t}}\right) + \text{erf}\left(\frac{w-x}{2\sqrt{D_A t}}\right)\right] \tag{B-39}$$

3.4.2 Cylindrical Coordinates

Consider the diffusion of solute A from the surface of a cylinder of radius R into a homogeneous tissue. For example, the cylinder might represent the external surface of a capillary that contains a high concentration of a drug.

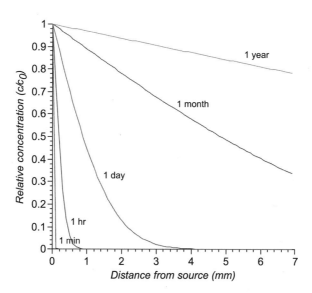

Figure B.3. Concentration profiles for diffusion in a semi-infinite medium. When the concentration of solute is increased within one region of an unbounded space, the molecules slowly penetrate into the adjacent region. The curves shown here are realizations of Equation B-37 for a solute with $D_A = 10^{-7}\,\text{cm}^2/\text{s}$, $R = 0.1\,\text{cm}$, $N = N_{\text{Av}}$, and $t = 6, 24, 72,$ and $720\,\text{hr}$.

The concentration within the tissue in the region $r > R$ can be determined by solving Equation B-31 in cylindrical coordinates:

$$D_A \frac{1}{r} \frac{\partial}{\partial r}\left[r \frac{\partial c_A}{\partial r}\right] = \frac{\partial c_A}{\partial t} \tag{B-40}$$

If the concentration of A in the tissue outside the cylinder is initially 0, and the concentration at the outer surface of the cylinder is maintained at c_0, the initial and boundary conditions can be written as

$$\left. \begin{array}{lll} c(r, t) = 0; & \text{for } R \le r; & t = 0 \\ c(r, t) = c_0; & \text{for } r = R; & t > 0 \\ c(r, t) = 0; & \text{for } r \to \infty & t > 0 \end{array} \right\} \tag{B-41}$$

Solving Equation B-40 subject to Equation B-41 yields

$$\frac{c_A}{c_0} = 1 + \frac{2}{\pi} \int\limits_0^{\infty} e^{-D_A u^2 t} \frac{J_0(ur)\,Y_0(ua) - J_0(ua)\,Y_0(ur)}{J_0^2(ua) - Y_0^2(ua)} \frac{du}{u} \tag{B-42}$$

where J_0 and Y_0 are Bessel functions of the first and second kind of order 0. Equation B-42 is shown graphically in Figure B.4. When the concentration of the solute is maintained at c_0, solute will continue to penetrate into the adjacent medium. For a solute with $D_A = 10^{-7}\,\text{cm}^2/\text{s}$ and a cylinder with $R = 0.1\,\text{cm}$, the solute will penetrate $\sim 0.2\,\text{mm}$ in the first 6 hr, $\sim 0.4\,\text{mm}$ in the first 24 hr, and $\sim 0.6\,\text{mm}$ in the first 100 hr.

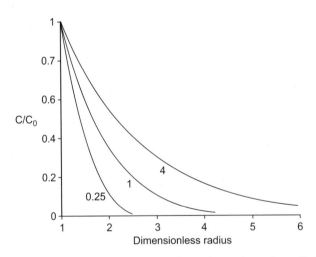

Figure B.4. Concentration of solute diffusing from the surface of a cylinder (reproduced from [7], p. 87). Each curve represents the concentration profile at a different dimensionless time $(D_A t/a^2)$. Dimensionless concentration is shown as a function of distance from the surface of the cylinder. For $D_A = 1 \times 10^{-7}\,\text{cm}^2/\text{s}$ and $R = 0.1\,\text{cm}$, the dimensionless times correspond to 7, 28, and 110 hr.

3.4.3 Spherical Coordinates

Biological systems often exhibit spherical symmetry, or something near it. For example, certain cells are assumed to be spherical, as are vesicles within cells and synthetic vesicles. Therefore, it is frequently convenient to examine the transport of solutes in a spherical coordinate system. Equation B-31 can be expressed in spherical coordinates:

$$D_A \frac{1}{r^2} \frac{\partial}{\partial r} \left[r^2 \frac{\partial c_A}{\partial r} \right] = \frac{\partial c_A}{\partial t} \tag{B-43}$$

where gradients in the θ and ϕ directions are neglected due to symmetry, so that diffusion occurs only in the radial direction. This differential equation can be simplified by making the substitution $u = r c_A$, which produces

$$D_A \frac{\partial^2 u}{\partial r^2} = \frac{\partial u}{\partial t} \tag{B-44}$$

an equation identical to the one obtained for one-dimensional diffusion in a rectangular coordinate system, Equation B-32.

Consider the flux of solute A towards a spherical cell in suspension. If solute is consumed at the surface of the cell, and the rate of consumption is rapid, solute concentrations in the vicinity of the cell can be predicted by solving Equation B-43 subject to the following conditions:

$$\left. \begin{array}{lll} c_A(r, t) = c_0; & \text{for } r \geq R; & t = 0 \\ c_A(r, t) = 0; & \text{for } r = R; & t > 0 \\ c_A(r, t) = c_0; & \text{for } r \to \infty; & t > 0 \end{array} \right\} \tag{B-45}$$

where the initial concentration of solute in the medium surrounding the cell is c_0. The solution to these equations is closely related to the solution of the equations for one-dimensional diffusion in a semi-infinite medium (see Chapter 3 of [8]):

$$\frac{c_A}{c_0} = 1 - \left(\frac{R}{r} \right) \text{erfc} \left[\frac{r - R}{2\sqrt{Dt}} \right] \tag{B-46}$$

For long observation times, Equation B-46 reduces to the steady-state solution:

$$\frac{c_A}{c_0} = 1 - \frac{R}{r} \tag{B-47}$$

Solute concentration in the vicinity of a sphere is shown in Figure B.5. Again, D_A is assumed to be 10^{-7} cm^2/s and R to be 1 mm. The change in concentration penetrates ~0.5 mm in the first 1 hr of absorption by the sphere; as time increases, the decrease in concentration moves progressively deeper into the medium. For the conditions specified in Figure B.5, the approach to steady-state is slow; even after 720 hr (30 days) the concentration profile is still significantly different from the steady-state profile.

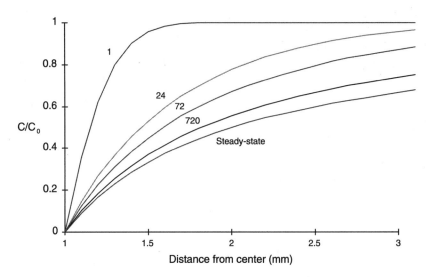

Figure B.5. Concentration profiles in the vicinity of an absorbing sphere. When a perfectly absorbing sphere is placed within an infinite medium, the concentration varies near the surface of the sphere. Concentration profiles are indicated at 1, 24, 72, and 720 hr for a diffusing solute with $D_A = 10^{-7}$ cm^2/s for a sphere of radius 1 mm.

The rate of solute diffusion to the surface of the cell can be calculated from the flux:

$$\text{Rate of disappearance} = -D(4\pi R^2)\frac{dc_A}{dr}\bigg|_{r=R} = 4\pi D R c_0 \qquad \text{(B-48)}$$

Equation B-48 permits the definition of a rate constant for diffusion-limited reaction at a cell surface, k_+. The rate constant, defined as (rate of disappearance) $= k + c_0$, is

$$k_+ = 4\pi D R \qquad \text{(B-49)}$$

This expression for the rate constant, first described by Smoluchowski [14], will be useful in the analysis of rates of diffusion and reaction during ligand–receptor binding (see Chapter 4).

References

1. Saltzman, W.M., *Drug Delivery: Engineering Principles for Drug Therapy*. New York: Oxford University Press, 2001.
2. Einstein, A., A new determination of molecular dimensions. *Annalen der Physik*, 1906, **19**, 289-306.
3. Berg, H.C., *Random Walks in Biology*. Princeton, NJ: Princeton University Press, 1983.

4. Whitney, C.A., *Random Processes in Physical Systems*. New York: John Wiley & Sons, 1990.

5. Fick, A., Ueber Diffusion. *Annalen der Physik*, 1855, **94**, 59–86.

6. Bird, R.B., W.E. Stewart, and E.N. Lightfoot, *Transport Phenomena*. New York: John Wiley & Sons, 1960.

7. Welty, J.R., C.E. Wicks, and R.E. Wilson, *Fundamentals of Momentum, Heat, and Mass Transfer*, 3rd ed. New York: John Wiley & Sons, 1984.

8. Crank, J., *The Mathematics of Diffusion*. 2nd ed. Oxford: Oxford University Press, 1975.

9. Carslaw, H.S. and J.C. Jaeger, *Conduction of Heat in Solids*, 2nd ed. Oxford: Oxford University Press, 1959.

10. Popov, S. and M.M. Poo, Diffusional transport of macromolecules in developing nerve processes. *Journal of Neuroscience*, 1992, **12**(1), 77–85.

11. Radomsky, M.L., et al., Macromolecules released from polymers: diffusion into unstirred fluids. *Biomaterials*, 1990, **11**, 619–624.

12. Lauffenburger, D., C. Rothman, and S. Zigmond, Measurement of leukocyte motility and chemotaxis parameters with a linear under-agarose migration assay. *The Journal of Immunology*, 1983, **131**, 940–947.

13. Abramowitz, M. and I.A. Stegun, *Handbook of Mathematical Functions with Formulas, Graphs, and Mathematical Tables*. Washington, DC: National Bureau of Standards, 1964.

14. Smoluchowski, M., Versuch einer mathematischen Theorie der Koaguationskinetik kolloider Lösungen. *Z. Physik Chem.*, 1917, **92**(9), 129–168.

Appendix C

Useful Data

C.1 Protein Properties

Table C.1
Properties of Some Polypeptides and Proteins

	M_w	N_{aa}	N_c	D_w (10^{-7} cm^2/s)	$t_{1/2}$ (min)
Polypeptide	1,200		1	21±5	
GRGDS synthetic peptide		5	1		$\alpha = 1$; $\beta = 8$ [2]
YRGDS		5	1		$\alpha = 0.5$; $\beta = 160$ [3]
Insulin (bovine)	5,733	51	2		
Ribonuclease (bovine pancreas)	12,640	124	1		
Lysozyme (egg white)	13,930	129	1		
Lactalbumin	14,500			13±3	
Interleukin 2 (recombinant, nonglycosylated, rIL-2)	~15,000				~30 [4]
Myoglobin (horse heart)	16,890	153	1		
Chymotrypsin (bovine pancreas)	22,600	241	3		
Nerve growth factor (mouse)					
F_c fragment from IgG (human)	50,000		2	8.4±0.4	
F_{ab} fragment from IgG (human)	50,000		2	8.3±1.0	
Hemoglobin (human)	64,500	574	4		
Serum albumin (human)	68,500	~550	1		
Serum albumin (cow)	68,000	~550	1	8.3±1.7 [5]	
Hexokinase (yeast)	96,000	~800	4		
F(ab$'$)$_2$ fragment from IgG (human)	100,000		4	6.7±0.24	
Tryptophan synthetase (E. coli)	117,000	~975	4		
γ-globulin (horse)	149,900	~1,250	4		
IgA (human)	150,000	~1,250	4	5.2±0.3	
IgG (human)	150,000	~1,250	4	4.4±1.3	
Glycogen phosphorylase (rabbit muscle)	495,000	~4,100	4		
IgM (human)	970,000		~20	3.2±1.4	
Laminin (EHS sarcoma)	820,000	6477	3		
Glutamate dehydrogenase (bovine liver)	1,000,000	~8,300	~40		
Fatty acid synthetase (yeast)	2,300,000	~20,000	~21		
Tobacco mosaic virus	~40,000,000	~336,500	2,130		

M_w = molecular weight (Da), N_{aa} = number of amino acids, N_c = number of polypeptide chains, D_w = diffusion coefficient in water at 25°C. Protein diffusion coefficients from [1], unless otherwise indicated. $t_{1/2}$ = half-life in the plasma following i.v. injection.

Table C.2
Protein Composition of Human Blood

	M_w	c_p (mg/100 mL)
Albumin	69,000	3,500–4,500
Prealbumin	61,000	28–35
Insulin	5,000	0–29 units/mL
Fibrinogen	341,000	200–600
Erythropoetin	34,000	0.1–0.5 ng/mL
α_1–*globulins*:		
α_1-lipoprotein		
HDL$_2$	435,000	37–117
HDL3	195,000	217–270
α_1-acid glycoprotein (orosomucoid)	44,100	75–100
α_1-antitrypsin (α_1-glycoprotein)	45,000	210–500
Transcortin		7
α_{1x}-glycoprotein		14–35
Haptoglobin	100,000	30–190
α_2–*globulins*:		
Ceruloplasmin	160,000	27–39
α_2-macroglobulin	820,000	220–380
α_2-lipoprotein (low density)	5,000,000–20,000,000	150–230
α_{2HS}-glycoprotein	49,000	8(6)
Zn-α_2-glycoprotein	41,000	4(6)
Prothrombin	62,700	9(6)
β–*globulins*:		
β-lipoprotein	3,200,000	280–440
transferrin	90,000	200–320
β_{1C}-globulin		35
hemoplexin (β_{1B}-globulin)	80,000	80–100
β_2-glycoprotein		20–25
γ–*globulins*:		
γG-immunoglobulin	160,000	1,200–1,800
γM-immunoglobulin	1,000,000	75
γA-immunoglobulin	350,000	100
Enzymes:		
Aldolase		0–7 U/mL
Amylase		4–25 U/mL
Cholinesterase		0.5 pH U or more/hr
Creatinine kinase		40–150 U/L
Lactate dehydrogenase		110–210 U/L
Lipase		<2 U/mL
Nucleotidase		1–11 U/L
Phosphatase (acid)		0.1–0.63 sigma U/mL
Phosphatase (alkaline)		13–39 U/L
Transaminase (SGOT)		9–40 U/mL
TOTAL		**6,726–9,819**

Adapted from [6].

Table C.3
Diffusion Coefficients in Biological Fluids at 37°C

	M_w	D_{saline} or D_{water}	D_{plasma}
Urea		184 [6]	146 [6]
Creatinine		121.5 [6]	87.1 [6]
Glucose	180	90	
Uric acid		121 [6]	74.5 [6]
Sucrose		71.1 [6]	59.0 [6]
Fluorescein	332	74 [7]	—
Inulin		24.0 [6]	21.7 [6]
Dextran	4,000	15	
	16,000	29.3 [6]	24.1 [6]
	9,300	15.4 [5]	
	73,000	7 [5]	
	526,000	5 [5]	
	2,000,000	4.9 [5]	
Bovine serum albumin	68,000	11	
Human IgG	150,000	5.9	

All diffusion coefficients are expressed as 10^{-7} cm^2/s, and corrected to 37°C by assuming $D\mu/T$ is constant. $D_1 = D_2(\mu_2/\mu_1)(T_1/T_2)$. Correction factors from 25°C:
$D^{37} = (37 + 273)/(25 + 273) \times (892/695) = 1.335$; from 20°C
$= (37 + 273)/(20 + 273) \times (1001/695) = 1.524$.

Table C.4
Plasma Half-lives for Proteins

Protein	Plasma Half-life ($t_{1/2}$, min)	Source of Material and Species (Ref.)
Basic fibroblast growth factor (bFGF)	1.5	Recombinant bFGF in rats [8]
γ interferon	11 to 32	Partially purified protein in humans [9]
Nerve growth factor (NGF)	2.4	Purified mouse NGF in rats [10]
Interleukin-2 (IL-2)	30	Recombinant human IL-2 in humans [11]
Erythropoietin (EPO)	300 to 360	Recombinant human EPO in humans [12]
Ciliary neurotrophic factor (CNTF)	3	Recombinant human CNTF in humans

C.2 Blood and Tissue Cell Properties

Table C.5
Cellular Composition of Human Blood

Cell Type	Cell count (10^3 cells/mm^3)	Percentage of WBC	Percentage of Lymphocytes Blood	Lymph	Spleen
Red cells	5,000 ± 350				
Platelets	248 ± 50				
White blood cells	7.25 ± 1.7				
Neutrophils		55			
Eosinophils		3			
Basophils		0.5			
Monocytes		6.5			
Lymphocytes		35			
B cells (class II MHC)			10–15	20–25	40–45
T cells (CD3+)			50–60	50–60	50–60
Helper (CD4+,CD8–)					
Cytolytic (CD4–,CD8+)			20–25	15–20	10–15
Natural killer cells (CD16)			~10	rare	~10

From [13].

Table C.6
Estimated Rates of Blood Cell Production in Humans

Cell Type	Cell Concentration (cells/mL)	Lifespan (days)	Production Rate (10^9 cells/day)
Red cells	5×10^9	120	208
Platelets	2×10^8	8	125
White cells	5×10^6	0.5	50
TOTAL			**383**

Reproduced from [14].

C.3 Mathematical Tables and Functions

Table C.7
Values of the Error Function, erf, and
Error Function Complement, erfc

x	$\mathrm{erf}(x)$	$\mathrm{erfc}(x)$
0	0	1
0.05	0.056372	0.943628
0.1	0.112463	0.887537
0.15	0.167996	0.832004
0.2	0.222703	0.777297
0.25	0.276326	0.723674
0.3	0.328627	0.671373
0.35	0.379382	0.620618
0.4	0.428392	0.571608
0.45	0.475482	0.524518
0.5	0.5205	0.4795
0.55	0.563323	0.436677
0.6	0.603856	0.396144
0.65	0.642029	0.357971
0.7	0.677801	0.322199
0.75	0.711155	0.288845
0.8	0.742101	0.257899
0.85	0.770668	0.229332
0.9	0.796908	0.203092
0.95	0.820891	0.179109
1	0.842701	0.157299
1.05	0.862436	0.137564
1.1	0.880205	0.119795
1.15	0.896124	0.103876
1.2	0.910314	0.089686
1.25	0.9229	0.0771
1.3	0.934008	0.065992
1.35	0.943762	0.056238
1.4	0.952285	0.047715
1.45	0.959695	0.040305
1.5	0.966105	0.033895
1.6	0.976348	0.023652
1.7	0.98379	0.01621
1.8	0.989091	0.010909
1.9	0.99279	0.00721
2	0.995322	0.004678
2.5	0.999593	0.000407
3	0.999978	2.21×10^{-5}
3.5	0.999999	7.43×10^{-7}
4	1	1.54×10^{-8}

Values obtained from [15], pp. 310–311.

References

1. Saltzman, W.M., et al., Antibody diffusion in human cervical mucus. *Biophysical Journal*, 1994, **66**, 508–515.
2. Humphries, M.J., K. Olden, and K.M. Yamada, A synthetic peptide from fibronectin inhibits experimental metastasis of murine melanoma cells. *Science*, 1986, **233**, 467–470.
3. Braatz, J.A., et al., Functional peptide–polyurethane conjugates with extended circulatory half-lives. *Bioconjugate Chemistry*, 1993, **4**, 262–267.
4. Katre, N.V., M.J. Knauf, and W.J. Laird, Chemical modification of recombinant interleukin 2 by polyethylene glycol increases its potency in the murine Meth A sarcoma model. *Proceedings of the National Academy of Sciences*, 1987, **84**, 1487–1491.
5. Kosar, T.F. and R.J. Phillips, Measurement of protein diffusion in dextran solutions by holographic interferometry. *AIChE Journal*, 1995, **41**(3), 701–711.
6. Colton, C., et al., Diffusion of organic solutes in stagnant plasma and red cell suspensions. *Chemical Engineering, Progress Symposium Series*, 1970, **66**, 85–99.
7. Radomsky, M.L., et al., Macromolecules released from polymers: diffusion into unstirred fluids. *Biomaterials*, 1990, **11**, 619–624.
8. Whalen, G.F., Y. Shing, and J. Folkman, The fate of intravenously administered bFGF and the effect of heparin. *Growth Factors*, 1989, **1**, 157–164.
9. Gutterman, J.U., et al., *Cancer Research*, 1984, **44**, 4164–4171.
10. Poduslo, J.F., G.L. Curran, and C.T. Berg, Macromolecular permeability across the blood–nerve and blood–brain barriers. *Proceedings of the National Academy of Sciences USA*, 1994, **91**, 5705–5709.
11. Konrad, M.W., et al., *Cancer Research*, 1990, **50**, 2009–2017.
12. Cohen, A.M., Erythropoietin and G-CSF, in A.H.C. Kung, R.A. Baughman, and J.W. Larrick, eds., *Therapeutic Proteins: Pharmacokinetics and Pharmacodynamics*. New York: W.H. Freeman, 1993, pp. 165–186.
13. Abbas, A.K., A.H. Lichtman, and J.S. Pober, *Cellular and Molecular Immunology*. 2nd ed. Philadelphia, PA: W.B. Saunders, 1994, 457 pp.
14. Koller, M.R. and B.O. Palsson, Tissue engineering: Reconstitution of human hematopoiesis *ex vivo*. *Biotechnology and Bioengineering*, 1993, **42**, 909–930.
15. Abramowitz, M. and I.A. Stegun, *Handbook of Mathematical Functions with Formulas, Graphs, and Mathematical Tables*. Washington, DC: National Bureau of Standards, 1964.

Appendix D

Nomenclature and Abbreviations

D.1 Nomenclature

I attempted to use a nomenclature that was consistent between chapters, but I was not completely successful. Therefore, this table of nomenclature was assembled. In a few cases, the same symbol was used for different purposes in different chapters, and therefore the chapter in which the symbol was used is also included here. In cases where no chapter is indicated, the symbol is used for this purpose throughout.

a	Solute concentration (mg/cm^3), Chapter 7
A	Radius of spherical cell (cm), Chapter 4
A	Cross-sectional area (cm^2)
A	Outer radius (cm), Chapter 13
B	Inner radius (cm), Chapter 13
$c(\ )$	Creep function, Chapter 5
c_A	Concentration of solute A (mg/mL)
C, c	Concentration (mg/mL)
C^*	Clearance (mL/min), Chapter 13
C_B	Concentration of solute in the blood (mg/mL)
C_D	Concentration of solute in the dialysate (mg/mL)
CI	Chemotactic index, Chapter 7
d	Diameter of hollow fiber (cm), Chapter 13
d	Mean displacement (cm), Chapter 7
D	Diffusion coefficient of solute in a system of interest (cm^2-s)
D	Dilution rate (1/s), Chapter 13
D^*	Dialysance (mL/min), Chapter 13
E	Elastic modulus (N/cm^2)
E^*	Extraction ratio, Chapter 13
E_{ion}	Equilibrium membrane potential, Chapter 9
f	Frictional drag coefficient, Chapter 9
f	Fraction of cells moving towards source, Chapter 7
f_c	Fraction of circulating cells, Chapter 10
f_m	Fraction of marginated cells, Chapter 10

f_T	Fraction of cells in tissue, Chapter 10
F	Applied force (N)
F	Faraday's constant, Chapter 9
F_x	Force required to move particle through fluid (g-cm/s^2)
g	Gravitational acceleration (cm/s^2)
G	Shear modulus (N/cm^2), Chapter 5
G', G''	Storage and loss moduli, Chapter 5
h	Height of fluid channel (cm)
H	Hydrodynamic coefficient, Chapter 9
$H(t)$	Unit step function, Chapter 5
I	Moment of inertia (cm^2), Chapter 5
j_A	Mass flux of component A (mg/cm^2-s) in a binary mixture with respect to a coordinate system that is moving with the mass average velocity of the mixture
J	Radial moment of inertia, Chapter 5
J	Net cell flux (cell/cm^2-s), Chapter 7
k	First-order elimination rate constant (s^{-1})
$k(\ )$	Relaxation function, Chapter 5
k^+	Diffusion-limited reaction rate constant (s^{-1})
k_B	Boltzmann constant (1.3807 × 10^{-23} J/K)
k_f	Rate constant for forward (association) reaction in binding (s^{-1})
k_{off}	Intrinsic binding kinetic off rate constant (s^{-1})
k_{on}	Intrinsic binding kinetic on rate constant (s^{-1})
k_p	Rate constant for cell proliferation (s^{-1})
k_r	Rate constant for reverse (dissociation) reaction in binding (s^{-1})
K	Overall mass transfer coefficient (cm/s), Chapter 13
K	Equilibrium partition coefficient, Chapter 9
K_a	Equilibrium association constant (M^{-1})
K_b	Binding constant (M^{-1})
K_d	Equilibrium dissociation constant (M)
K_M	Michaelis–Menton coefficient (M)
L	Length of a hollow fiber (cm), Chapter 13
L_p	Hydraulic conductance, Chapter 9
L_{path}	Length of total path (cm), Chapter 7
m	Molecular mass (g/molecule)
M	Total body mass (mg)
M_w	Molecular weight (daltons)
n^-	Cell flux in − direction (cell/cm^2-s), Chapter 7
n^+	Cell flux in + direction (cell/cm^2-s), Chapter 7
n_A	Mass flux of component A (mg/cm^2-s) in a binary mixture with respect to a stationary coordinate system
n_i	Number density of particles i (1/cm^3), Chapter 8
N	Number of cells (#/cm^3)
N	Flux of solute across a membrane (mg/cm^2-s)
N	Number of hollow fibers in a dialysis unit, Chapter 13
N_{Av}	Avagadro constant (6.0220 × 10^{23} mol^{-1})

N_b	Number of bound cell surface receptors (molecules/cm^3-s), Chapter 7
N_{ij}	Rate of collision of particles i and j (1/cm^3-s), Chapter 8
N_T	Total solute flow across a membrane (mg/s)
N_T	Total number of receptors on cell surface (molecules/cm^3-s), Chapter 7
N_x	Local flux of solute across a membrane (mg/cm^2-s), Chapter 13
p^-	Probability of direction change for cells in $-$ direction (cells/s), Chapter 7
p^+	Probability of direction change for cells in $+$ direction (cells/s), Chapter 7
P	Cell persistence time (min)
P	Hydrostatic pressure (N/cm^2)
P	Cell persistence time (s), Chapter 7
P	Permeability (cm/s), Chapter 9
Pe	Peclet number, Chapter 9
Q_B	Flowrate of blood through an artificial organ (mL/min)
Q_D	Flowrate of dialysate through an artificial organ (mL/min)
Q_{in}	Flowrate at reactor inlet (mL/min), Chapter 13
Q_{out}	Flowrate at reactor outlet (mL/min), Chapter 13
r_N	Rate of cell production (cell/cm^3-s), Chapter 13
R	Ligand production rate (mg/cm^3-s), Chapter 4
R	Gas constant (8.314 J/mol K), Chapter 9
R	Radius (cm), Chapters 5 and 8
R_T	Total number of receptors (#/cell)
S	Secretion rate (mg/cm^2-s), Chapter 4
S	Cell motile speed (µm/min), Chapter 7
S	Total surface area of dialysis membrane (cm^2), Chapter 13
t	Time (s)
$t_{1/2}$	Time constant (s)
t_D	Doubling time (s)
T	Temperature (K)
T	Cortical tension (N/cm), Chapter 5
T	Torque (N-cm), Chapter 5
T	Time of treatment (dialysis, for example, s), Chapter 13
T_p	Modified persistence time (s), Chapter 7
U	Velocity (cm/s), Chapter 5
U_0	Strain energy (N/cm^2)
v_i	Velocity of fluid in i-direction (cm/s)
v_i	Volume of particles of size i (cm^3), Chapter 8
v_{rms}	Root-mean-square velocity (cm/s)
v_x	Velocity of particle movement (cm/s)
V	Molar volume (cm^3/mol)
V_B	Fluid volume in body (cm^3), Chapter 13
V_c	Chemotactic velocity, Chapter 7
V_{max}	Maximum rate of reaction (1/s), Chapter 9

w	Cross-sectional area per unit length for fiber bundle, Chapter 13
W	Hydrodynamic coefficient, Chapter 9
$W(x, y)$	Mean time to capture (s), Chapter 7
X	Mass of a region of interest (mg)
Y	Mass of a region of interest (mg)
$Y_{N/S}$	Yield coefficient (mg/cell), Chapters 4 and 13
z	Relative rate of blood to dialysate flow, Chapter 13
z_{ion}	Valence of ion, Chapter 9
ΔG_0	Free energy of the standard state (J), Chapter 6

Greek symbols

α, β	Parameters in model of stochastic process, Chapter 7
β	Collision frequency function, Chapter 8
γ	Relative rate of mass transfer to blood flow, Chapter 13
δ	Distance moved between changes in direction for a particle executing a random walk (cm), Appendix B
$\delta(t)$	Delta function
η	Fluid viscosity (g/cm-s)
λ	Ratio of solute to pore radius
μ	Random motility coefficient (cm^2-s), Chapter 7
μ	Spring constant (N/cm), Chapter 5
v_{xy}	Poisson's ratio
π	Osmotic pressure (N/cm^2), Chapter 9
ρ	Mass density (mg/cm^3)
ρ_A	Mass concentration of A (g/cm^3)
σ	Reflection coefficient, Chapter 9
σ	Applied stress (N/cm^2)
τ	Time interval between changes in direction for a particle executing a random walk (s)
τ	Time constant (sec), Chapter 4
τ	Stress response (N/cm^2), Chapter 5
τ_{xy}	Viscous shear stress in the x-direction exerted on a fluid surface of constant y (N/cm^2)
ϕ	Phase angle, Chapter 5; Orientation bias, Chapter 7
Φ	Equilibrium partition coefficient for particles in pores
χ	Chemotaxis coefficient (cm^5/mg-s), Chapter 7
ψ_A	Rate of generation of A per volume (g/cm^3-s)
ψ_A^m	Molar rate of generation of A per volume (mol/cm^3-s)
ω	Frequency (s^{-1})
ω_A	Mass fraction of A

D.2 Abbreviations

| CAM | Chorioallantonic membrane |
| CHO | Chinese hamster ovary |

DRG	Dorsal root ganglion
ECM	Extracellular matrix
EGF	Epidermal growth factor
EPO	Erythropoietin
EVAc	Poly(ethylene-*co*-vinyl acetate)
FGF	Fibroblast growth factor
FPR, FRAP	Fluorescent photobleaching recovery
G-CSF	Granulocyte colony-stimulating factor
GFP	Green fluorescent protein
GVHD	Graft versus host disease
HEMA	Methyl methacrylate
HEV	High endothelial venule
HIV	Human immunodeficiency virus
HSC	Hematopoietic stem cell
HUVEC	Human umbilical vein endothelial cells
IGF-I	Insulin-like growth factor I
IL-2	Interleukin-2
LAK	Lymphokine activated killer cells
MMA	2-hydroxyethyl methacrylate
MRI	Magnetic resonance imaging
MW	Molecular weight (daltons)
N-CAM	Neural cell adhesion molecule
NGF	Nerve growth factor
NK	Natural killer
PBS	Phosphate-buffered saline
PDGF	Platelet-derived growth factor
PEG	Poly(ethylene glycol)
PEO	Poly(ethylene oxide)
PET	Positron emission tomography
PET	Poly(ethylene terephthlate)
PGA	Poly(glycolic acid) or polyglycolide
PH	Pleckstrin homology
pHEMA	Poly(2-hydroxyethyl methacrylate)
PLA	Poly(lactic acid) or polylactide
PLGA	Lactide–glycolide copolymers, poly(lactide-*co*-glycolide)
PLLA	Poly(L-lactic acid)
pMMA	Poly(methyl methacrylate)
PNAd	Peripheral node addressin
PP	Polypropylene
PS	Polystyrene
PTFE	Polytetrafluoroethylene
r.m.s.	Root mean square
RBC	Red blood cell
SIV	Simian immunodeficiency virus
TCPS	Tissue culture polystyrene
TGF	Transforming growth factor

TGF-β1	Transforming growth factor-β1
TIL	Tumor-infiltrating lymphocytes
TNF	Tumor necrosis factor
VEGF	Vascular endothelial growth factor

D.3 Glossary

Note: A separate glossary on terms that are used in developmental biology is provided at the end of Chapter 3.

Allometric	The study of growth relative to a standard, or the growth of one region with respect to the whole organism.
Anisotropic etching	Etching processes that exploit the crystalline structure of certain materials, for example silicon, to etch at different rates in different directions.
Autocrine	Secretion of a substance that influences the cell that secreted it.
Bicoid protein	A transcription factor protein that is produced in Drosophila by a maternal effect gene; mRNA from the maternal gene is segregated to the anterior pole of the developing egg, resulting in spatially localized synthesis of Bicoid protein.
Chemokine	Cytokines that are chemotactic for leukocytes.
Chondrocytes	Cartilage cells.
Cytokine	Proteins secreted by inflammatory leukocytes that are not antibodies and that act as intercellular mediators.
Darcy's law	An empirical statement that the volumetric flow rate in a porous medium is linearly proportional to the applied pressure gradient.
Electrokinetic	Various phenomena involving the motion of fluids containing charged particles or ions in electric fields.
Electroosmosis	The motion of a liquid, relative to a stationary charged surface, that is induced by an applied electric field.
Endocrine	Pertaining to internal secretions and hormones.
Genotype	The genetic composition of an organism.
Gliadel®	Biodegradable wafers of polyanhydride loaded with a chemotherapy drug that can be implanted in the brain for local controlled release at a tumor resection site.
Growth factor	A substance that affects growth of a cell or organism.
Hepatic	Pertaining to the liver.
In situ	Latin, in the natural or normal place. Used to indicate procedures that are performed at the normal site of an organ or tissue.
In vitro	Latin, in glass. Used to indicate procedures that are performed outside of a living body, in a test tube or culture dish.
In vivo	Latin, in the living body. Used to indicate procedures that are applied within a living body.

Mitogen	An agent that stimulates cell division.
Morphogens	Biological agents, often proteins, that influence a change in cell behavior.
Neotissues	Assemblies of cellular, protein, and synthetic elements, in which the various components are physically arranged to encourage development into a functional replacement tissue.
Norplant®	Cylindrical silicone implants loaded with contraceptive steroids which provide constant steroid release for up to 5 years.
Ohmic heating	The generation of heat due to the passage of an electrical current through a medium with electrical resistance.
Paracrine	A kind of chemical signaling in which the target cell is close to the cell that is secreting the chemical, as in neurotransmission.
Peclet number	A dimensionless number whose numerical value estimates the relative importance of mass transfer by convection compared with mass transfer by diffusion.
Phenotype	The traits that are expressed by an organism.
Piezoelectric	A property of certain materials, for example quartz, that produces a physical deformation proportional to an applied potential difference.
Progenitor	An ancestor in a direct line of descendants.
Renal	Pertaining to the kidney.
Reynolds number	A dimensionless number whose numerical value estimates the relative importance of inertial forces compared with viscous forces in flowing fluids.

Index